METHODS FOR COMMUNITY-BASED PARTICIPATORY RESEARCH FOR HEALTH

METHODS FOR
COMMUNITY-BASED
PARTICIPATORY
RESEARCH FOR HEALTH

Second Edition

BARBARA A. ISRAEL

EUGENIA ENG

AMY J. SCHULZ

EDITH A. PARKER

EDITORS

Foreword by David Satcher

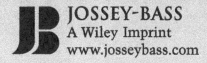

JOSSEY-BASS
A Wiley Imprint
www.josseybass.com

Published by Jossey-Bass
A Wiley Imprint
One Montgomery Street, Suite 1200, San Francisco, CA 94104-4594—www.josseybass.com

Jossey-Bass books and products are available through most bookstores. To contact Jossey-Bass directly call our Customer Care Department within the U.S. at 800-956-7739, outside the U.S. at 317-572-3986, or fax 317-572-4002.

Wiley publishes in a variety of print and electronic formats and by print-on-demand. Some material included with standard print versions of this book may not be included in e-books or in print-on-demand. If this book refers to media such as a CD or DVD that is not included in the version you purchased, you may download this material at **http://booksupport.wiley.com**. For more information about Wiley products, visit **www.wiley.com**.

Library of Congress Cataloging-in-Publication Data
Methods for community-based participatory research for health / Barbara A. Israel ... [et al.], editors ; foreword by David Satcher. – 2nd ed.
    p. ; cm.
  Rev. ed. of: Methods in community-based participatory research for health / Barbara A. Israel ... [et al.], editors. 1st ed. c2005.
  Includes bibliographical references.
  ISBN 978-1-118-02186-6 (pbk.); ISBN 978-1-118-28588-6 (ebk.); ISBN 978-1-118-28212-0 (ebk.); ISBN 978-1-118-28253-3 (ebk.)
  I. Israel, Barbara A. II. Methods in community-based participatory research for health.
  [DNLM: 1. Community-Based Participatory Research–methods. 2. Public Health–methods. 3. Consumer Participation–methods. 4. Healthcare Disparities. 5. Research Design. 6. World Health. W 84.3]
  362.1'072_dc23
2012022689

Printed in the United States of America
SECOND EDITION

PB Printing SKY10048051_051723

CONTENTS

FIGURES AND TABLES

FIGURES

TABLES

FOREWORD

As director of the Centers for Disease Control and Prevention (CDC) in the mid-1990s, I had the opportunity to initiate the Urban Research Centers Program. At that time, we were able to fund three inaugural programs representing partnerships between communities and academic institutions. The original programs were in Detroit, Michigan, Seattle, Washington, and New York, New York. Although we were not able to expand the programs as we had hoped, we learned valuable lessons from them. Many of these lessons were included in the first comprehensive federal programs geared toward the reduction and ultimate elimination of disparities in health: the CDC's Racial and Ethnic Approaches to Community Health (REACH). More than forty communities have been funded through REACH. These communities have been funded and empowered to contract with academic health centers to conduct community-based participatory research.

Community-based participatory research brings the best and latest technology for design and measurement together with the insights of community members regarding the major issues affecting community health. In communicating the goals, objectives, and strategies of Healthy People 2010, we settled on a design that showed the interaction among determinants of health. The major components included the individual and his or her behavior (downstream), the physical and social environment including health care (midstream), and the various policies that impact this interaction (upstream). We tried to show that the components do not exist in isolation; there is intense interaction among them.

From 2005 to 2008, I served as a member of the World Health Organization (WHO) Commission on Social Determinants of Health (CSDH). We examined the conditions in which people are born, grow, learn, work, and age and their impact on health outcomes. In the process, we visited several countries through-out the world and had one meeting in the United States. We recommended a major focus on these social determinants as a component of our commitment to achieve global health equity in a generation. The report was accepted by the WHO and the Director-General of the WHO launched the report in 2008 with strong support for this focus and goal. This focus has been affirmed and extended in Healthy People 2020, which incorporates a substantial emphasis on social determinants of health. It is increasingly clear that in order to reach the goals of improving quality as well as increasing years of healthy life and eliminating dis-parities in health among different racial, ethnic, and socioeconomic groups, we must target all of the determinants of health where disparities have their roots. We must close the gaps that exist in access to quality health care, practice of healthy lifestyles, quality of physical and social environments, and policies that impact these areas. For research aimed at understanding and closing these gaps, community-based participatory research is a viable approach.

As more and more programs in community-based participatory research are funded and initiated, it is important that the lessons learned and problems solved in this area over the last thirty or more years are captured and shared. This book, *Methods for Community-Based Participatory Research for Health*, provides a major contribution to this field. The editors are some of our most outstanding leaders in community-based participatory research. This second edition of the book incorporates experiences engaging the social determinants of health, including the very important "food environments" relative to overweight, obesity, diabetes, and cardiovascular disease. These chapters add tremendously to the value of this book, as well as its currency. The writing of this book represents an unusual partnership among diverse participants whose involvements with communities make them experts in their own right. They bring a broad range of perspectives to this research approach, grounded in extensive community involvement and experience. What brings them together in this book is their respect for the dignity of community and the tremendous challenges and opportunities found in communities for enhancing health. Because they have found each other, and have come together around this common theme from their diverse backgrounds of race, ethnicity, and perspective, we are the beneficiaries of this outstanding text.

Critical to each case example of community-based participatory research discussed in this book is the development of meaningful partnerships. These partnerships must exist in order that when the question "Who is the community?" is asked, the answer can reliably be, "We are the community," we who have engaged in meaningful partnerships, made the investments, developed the relationships, suffered the pains, and reaped the benefits of the community. These partnerships are entrenched in the community, they are as diverse as the community, and they are devoted to meaningful change and progress in the community. They share knowledge, resources, and control at every level of the community. They are trusted, not because of what they say, but because of who and where they are, and with whom they share information, methodology, and control of the research agenda. They are interested in bringing the best technology and methodology to bear on problems and opportunities within the community. Community-based participatory research deals with all the determinants of health and the dynamic nature of the interactions within the community. This research approach holds the promise of getting to the root cause of health disparities and of strategies for enhancing health as well as the involvement of persons at every level of community. In her book *Night Falls Fast*, which deals with teenage suicide, Kay Redfield Jamison says, "The gap between what we know and what we do is lethal." Community-based participatory research holds the promise of removing these tremendous gaps and adding significantly to what we know.

To move our field forward in accomplishing these aims, this volume provides an excellent compendium of chapters on the methods and processes of community-based participatory research.

David Satcher, MD, PhD
Director, Satcher Health Leadership Institute
at the Morehouse School of Medicine
16th U.S. Surgeon General

ACKNOWLEDGMENTS

This book would not have been possible without the insightful contributions from the numerous authors, who so graciously shared their time and experiences in writing these chapters. It was important to us that each chapter reflected the principles of community-based participatory research, involving community partners as well as academics and professionals as coauthors. We extend to each writing team, therefore, our deepest appreciation for the privilege of witnessing, and temporarily joining, their collaboration throughout the writing process.

And to those with whom we have collaborated through our CBPR partnerships over the years, we are tremendously indebted. We consider ourselves most fortunate to have worked with, learned from, and been inspired by many partners. To our community and health practitioner partners and staff, we are especially grateful for your wisdom and tireless efforts to effect meaningful change with your communities, and in us. We have also been most fortunate to count among our academic partners fellow faculty members, students, and postdoctoral fellows whose hard work and enthusiastic engagement continue to renew our energy and perspectives on the value of CBPR. Specifically, although too numerous to mention by name, we would like to acknowledge and thank the following community and academic partners, who have been involved with us through the following CBPR partnerships: Bi-Cultural Bi-Lingual Medicaid Managed Care Project, Broome Team in Flint, Carolina-Shaw Partnership to Eliminate Health Disparities, Chatham Communities in Action, Chatham Social Health Council, Community Action Against Asthma, Detroit Community-Academic Urban Research Center, Detroit-Genesee County Community-Based Public Health Consortium, East Side Village Health Worker Partnership, Greensboro Health Disparities Collaborative, Health Literacy Partnership, Healthy

Environments Partnership, Men As Navigators for Health, Neighborhoods Working in Partnership, North Carolina Community-Based Public Health Initiative, Partners for Improved Nutrition and Health, Project GRACE, Promoting Healthy Eating in Detroit, REACH Detroit Partnership, Save Our Sisters, Strengthening The Black Family, Inc., Stress and Wellness Project, The Partnership Project of Greensboro, and United Voices of Efland-Cheeks, Inc.

We are also indebted to friends and colleagues who were not involved with these partnerships but who have had important impacts on our thinking and commitment to CBPR. Current and former colleagues and mentors at the University of Michigan include Cleo Caldwell, Barry Checkoway, Mark Chesler, Noreen Clark, Jim Crowfoot, Libby Douvan, Lorraine Gutierrez, Cathy Heaney, Hy and Joyce Kornbluh. Similarly, at the University of North Carolina at Chapel Hill, we are indebted to Alice Ammerman, Marci Campbell, Tim Carey, Leonard Dawson, Paul Godley, John Hatch, Michel Ibrahim, Ethel Jean Jackson, Laura Linnan, Betsy Randall-David, Allan Steckler, Guy Steuart, Jim Thomas, Rosalind Thomas, and Steve Wing.

We also thank the many other academic and practitioner colleagues who have influenced and supported our CBPR endeavors, including Clive Aspin, Heather Danton, Nancy Epstein, Jean Forester, Mark Freedman, Jack Geiger, Myles Horton, Ron Labonté, Mubiana Macwangi, Kathleen Parker, Baba Phillip-Ouattara, Ted Parrish, Jesus Ramirez-Valles, Sarena Seifer, Jackie Smith, Meera Viswanathan, and Tony Whitehead. For Barbara, a special debt is owed to her colleagues in New Zealand at the Department of Public Health and the Eru Pōmare Center, University of Otago, Wellington, for hosting and supporting her during the two sabbatical years in which much of the work on both editions of the book occurred, including Peter Crampton, Richard Edwards, Philippa Howden-Chapman, Anna Matheson, Bridget Robson, Clare Salmond, Louise Signal, and Alistair Woodward.

We have been most fortunate and appreciative of the funding we have received from a number of federal and foundation sources, which has enabled us to engage in CBPR endeavors. We are especially indebted to the following institutions and individuals, who are presently or were formerly involved in these institutions, for the leadership they have provided in supporting CBPR for us and countless others. These include: the W.K. Kellogg Foundation and Tom Bruce, Barbara Sabol, Steven Uranga-McKane, and Terri Wright; the National Institute of Environmental Health Sciences and Linda Birnbaum, Gwen Coleman,

Allen Dearry, Liam O'Fallon, Kim Gray, Ken Olden, Shobha Srinivasan, and Fred Tyson; the Centers for Disease Control and Prevention and Lynda Anderson, Larry Green, Donna Higgins, Shawna Mercer, and David Satcher; the National Institute on Minority Health and Health Disparities and John Ruffin, Khu Rhee, Francisco Sy; the National Cancer Institute and Jon Kerner; and the Agency for Healthcare Research and Quality and Kaytura Felix-Allen.

An edited book such as this involves considerable organizational skills and attention to details. We owe a tremendous thanks to Sue Andersen, whose continuous assistance and ability to anticipate what needed to be done was invaluable for the completion of this volume. A special thanks is also due to Linnea Evans who played a critical role in several aspects of pulling this volume together, including the development of the downloadable supplements that accompany this second edition of the book.

We have been most fortunate to have worked with Andy Pasternak, senior editor at Jossey-Bass. His knowledge of the publishing process, flexibility and sense of humor were instrumental in guiding our efforts. We thank Seth Schwartz, associate editor at Jossey-Bass, for his attention to details and thorough and good-natured help with our questions, and production editor Kelsey McGee and copy editor Donna J. Weinson, for their assistance.

We recognize the importance of social justice as both a core value and guiding principle for this book, and hence, are grateful to have parents and grandparents who instilled this commitment in us and encouraged our work. We would like to specifically acknowledge our parents, Archie and Adelaide Israel, Wah and Alice Eng, Robert and Gail Stegmier, and Jim and Hallie Parker.

To our partners and children, Richard Pipan, Ilana Israel, Daniel Goetz, Mira Eng-Goetz, Gabriel Eng-Goetz, David Schulz, and David Cohen, whose support and love are always given so unconditionally, we could not have completed this book without you.

THE EDITORS

Barbara A. Israel, DrPH, MPH, is a professor of Health Behavior and Health Education at the School of Public Health, University of Michigan, where she joined the faculty in 1982. She received her Masters of Public Health and Doctorate of Public Health degrees from the University of North Carolina at Chapel Hill. She was deputy editor of *Health Education & Behavior* from 1989 to 2003. Dr. Israel has authored or coauthored more than one hundred and twenty-five journal articles and book chapters on community-based participatory research, social support and stress, social determinants of health and health inequities, and evaluation. She has over thirty years of experience conducting CBPR in collaboration with partners in diverse ethnic communities, and is presently involved in several CBPR partnerships in Detroit addressing: environmental triggers of childhood asthma; social and physical environmental factors and cardiovascular disease; approaches to policy advocacy, and education and health. She is the principal investigator of the Detroit Community-Academic Urban Research Center, funded initially through the Centers for Disease Control and Prevention, and presently funded through the National Institute on Minority Health and Health Disparities, and the University of Michigan; and principal investigator for Neighborhoods Taking Action, with funding from the Robert Wood Johnson Foundation, The Skillman Foundation, and the W. K. Kellogg Foundation.

Eugenia Eng, DrPH, MPH, is a professor of health behavior at the Gillings School of Global Public Health, University of North Carolina at Chapel Hill, where she joined the faculty in 1984. She received her Masters of Public Health and Doctorate of Public Health degrees from the University of North Carolina at Chapel Hill. She directed the MPH degree program from 1987 to 2006 and has directed the Kellogg Health Scholars Postdoctoral Program since 1998. Dr. Eng has authored or coauthored over one hundred fifteen journal articles, book chapters, and monographs on the lay health advisor intervention model, the concepts of community competence and natural helping, and the community assessment procedure, "Action-Oriented Community Diagnosis." She has over thirty years of CBPR experience including field studies conducted with rural communities of the U.S. South, Sub-Saharan Africa and Southeast Asia to address socially stigmatizing health problems such as pesticide poisoning, cancer, and STI/HIV. Dr. Eng's CBPR projects include the CDC-funded Men As Navigators for Health, the NCI-funded Cancer Care and Racial Equity Study, the NHLBI-funded CVD and the Black Church: Are We Our Brother's Keeper?, and the NCI-funded CBPR Training Core for the Carolina Community Network Center to Reduce Cancer Health Disparities.

Edith A. Parker, DrPH, MPH, is professor and chair of the Department of Community and Behavioral Health at the University of Iowa College of Public Health. Before joining the University of Iowa in 2010, she was on the faculty at the University of Michigan, School of Public Health for fifteen years. She received her Masters of Public Health and Doctorate of Public Health degrees from the University of North Carolina at Chapel Hill. Dr. Parker has authored or coauthored more than sixty journal articles and book chapters on community-based participatory research, community capacity, childhood asthma and related areas. Dr. Parker has over twenty years of research experience focusing on the development, implementation, and evaluation of community-based participatory interventions to improve health status. Currently, she serves as the principal investigator (PI) of the Centers for Disease Control and Prevention–funded University of Iowa Prevention Research Center for Rural Health, and as director of the Community Engagement Key Function for the University of Iowa Clinical and Translational Science Award. Previously, she served as PI of the Community Action Against Asthma (CAAA) CBPR household intervention research component of the NIEHS/EPA-funded Michigan Center for the Environment and Children's Health, the NIEHS-funded CAAA "Community Organizing Network for Environmental Health" and "Community Based Participatory Research (CBPR) Intervention for Childhood Using Air Filters and Air Conditioners" research projects.

Amy J. Schulz, PhD, MPH, is professor, Department of Health Behavior and Health Education, University of Michigan School of Public Health, where she joined the faculty in 1997, and associate director for the Center for Research on Ethnicity, Culture and Health. She received her PhD degree in sociology and MPH in health behavior and health education from the University of Michigan. Her research focuses on social determinants of health in urban communities, with a particular focus on the role of racism, socioeconomic position, and social and physical environments in shaping health and health inequities, and in the design, implementation, and evaluation of interventions to promote health and contribute to the elimination of health inequities. She has over twenty years experience in the field and has authored or coauthored more than seventy journal articles and book chapters on the development, implementation, and evaluation of community-based participatory research partnerships, social determinants of health, and related topics. She serves as principal investigator for the Healthy Environments Partnership, a CBPR partnership that has been active since 2000 with funding from the National Institute for Environmental Health Sciences and the National Institute on Minority Health and Health Disparities. She also serves as a board member for the Detroit Community-Academic Urban Research Center, and served as an active member of the Detroit Eastside Village Health Worker Partnership and Promoting Healthy Eating in Detroit, two other CBPR efforts in Detroit.

Alex J. Allen III, MSA, is a non-profit consultant who specializes in organizational development, project management, grant writing, fundraising, and evaluation. Prior to consulting, Allen was a program officer with the Skillman Foundation, a private grant making organization with three chief aims: to help develop good schools, good neighborhoods, and support good opportunities that accomplish significant results for children. Allen was vice president of the Community Planning and Research division at Isles, Inc., a nonprofit organization in Trenton, NJ, that is committed to fostering self-reliant families in healthy, sustainable communities. He has been involved in various aspects of community development work for the past 25 years. He has collaborated and addressed a broad range of community issues, including his work with the Detroit Community-Academic Urban Research Center and other organizations. He has expertise in CBPR and participatory neighborhood planning.

Carol Allen is a community health education consultant at Public Health Seattle-King County and is skilled in working with diverse populations of low to moderate income. Previously she worked as project coordinator for the Seattle King County Healthy Homes (SKCHH) Project, providing supervision and overall guidance to outreach workers, conducting asthma trainings, monitoring progress, and overseeing quality control of intervention activities, ensuring the proper application of established protocols. She served as a community board member of the Seattle Partners for Healthy Community (SPHC). She is a master home environmentalist (MHE) through the American Lung Association and a certified asthma trainer by the Asthma and Allergies Foundation of America.

Robert Aronson, DrPH, MPH, is an associate professor of the Department of Public Health Education at the University of North Carolina Greensboro. He is a founding member of the Greensboro Health Disparities Collaborative, and is currently serving as cochair. His research has focused on health disparities affecting African American and Latino communities and the development and evaluation of community-based programs. For the past ten years much of his work has been with African American male college students, using CBPR to understand the influence of masculinity ideology on sexuality, and developing culturally and contextually congruent approaches to HIV prevention in this population. He received his MPH in health behavior and health education at UNC-Chapel Hill and his DrPH in international health from Johns Hopkins Bloomberg School of Public Health.

Magdalena Avila, DrPH, is an assistant professor of Health Education, Health Exercise and Sports Science, College of Education at the University of New Mexico. She has been working and partnering with communities of color for over twenty-five years to address environmental health disparities and inequalities. She has been using activism scholarship to develop grassroots and culturally appropriate public health education interventions. For the past ten years she has been involved in two NIEHS-funded research grants in Albuquerque's South Valley, both of which have incorporated CBPR into the research process with New Mexican Communities. Recently her involvement has included participatory research with New Mexican/Chicano/Immigrant communities to examine the role of CBPR in informing community residents to engage in the land use zoning and planning policy process, health impact assessments, and environmental health literacy.

Elizabeth A. Baker, PhD, MPH, is a professor and chair of the Department of Behavioral Science and Health Education at Saint Louis University School of Public Health. Her research areas include social networks and social support, control, and other social determinants of health (such as race and income) and the ways in which they influence community and individual capacity to create desired changes. She has extensive experience in CBPR in both urban and rural communities. She received her MPH and PhD degrees from the University of Michigan School of Public Health.

Ellen Barnidge, PhD, MPH, is an assistant professor at Saint Louis University School of Public Health and serves as an administrative manager and research coordinator for the Prevention Research Center in St. Louis. She has experience managing the research activities of community-based participatory research projects in urban and rural communities. She has trained community partners to engage in the design, implementation, and evaluation of interventions that address both chronic disease and social determinants of health. Her research interests include CBPR, social determinants of health, and qualitative methodology. She received her MPH and PhD degrees from Saint Louis University School of Public Health.

Stuart Batterman, PhD, MS, is a professor in the Department of Environmental Health Sciences at the University of Michigan, School of Public Health. He is the director of the University of Michigan Education and Research Center funded by the National Institute for Occupational Safety and Health. He is an environmental health scientist and engineer working mostly in human and ecological exposure research with application to risk and epidemiological studies in occupational, indoor, and environmental settings. In the past six years, he has worked with the Community Action Against Asthma, a CBPR partnership in Detroit, as an investigator on four research projects that address the health effects of both indoor and outdoor air pollutants.

Adam B. Becker, PhD, MPH, is executive director of the Consortium to Lower Obesity in Chicago Children (CLOCC), a nationally recognized broadbased network of over 1,300 organizations working to promote healthy eating and physical activity through individual, community, and policy change. He has used CBPR approaches to examine and address the impact of stressful community conditions on the health of women raising children, youth violence, and the impact of the social and physical environment on physical activity. Before becoming the executive director for CLOCC, he was the director of evaluation and research at the Louisiana Public Health Institute and a faculty member at Tulane University's School of Public Health and Tropical Medicine where he taught courses in community change and CBPR.

Lorenda Belone, PhD, MPH, is an assistant professor in the Health Education Program, Department of Health, Exercise, and Sports Science, University of New

Mexico College of Education. She is a member of the Navajo Nation and a Robert Wood Johnson Center for Health Policy Postdoctoral Fellow and has worked on several National Institutes of Health and Centers for Disease Control and Prevention funded research projects with American Indian communities in the Southwest. Currently, Dr. Belone is principal investigator of an intergenerational family prevention program and a coinvestigator to a national study to better understand CBPR projects in American Indian and Alaska Native and other communities facing health disparities.

Marlene J. Berg, MUP, was associate director for training and cofounder of the Institute for Community Research (ICR), Hartford, CT. She was an anthropologist and participatory action research (PAR) methodologist whose work promotes social justice through social science research. She served as project director on federal and state funded action research-based programs and studies involving adults, children, and youth. Since 2002 she managed ICR's PAR efforts, training youth, youth workers, teachers, community residents, and university students and faculty to conduct PAR to address issues stemming from structural inequities including teen hustling and structural determinants of racism. Throughout her career, she mentored and inspired high school, college, and graduate students and faculty to use PAR for personal, group, and social change. Marlene Berg passed away on May 29, 2012. She was the recipient of the 2012 Hartford Woman of the Year award, awarded posthumously, and ICR's twenty-fifth anniversary celebration on October 19, 2011 was dedicated to her.

Nicole S. Berry, PhD, was trained as a medical anthropologist and is an assistant professor in the Faculty of Health Sciences at Simon Fraser University, British Columbia. Her research focuses on the study of social change through an examination of reproductive health in a globalizing world. As a post-doctoral Kellogg Health Scholars Fellow, she worked collaboratively with members of the Durham Hispanic Community and El Centro Hispano (ECH) in North Carolina on a CBPR project that developed a curriculum for immigrant parents who had teens or preteens in their household. She is the author of *Unsafe Motherhood: Mayan Maternal Mortality and Subjectivity in Post-War Guatemala,* and currently holds funding from the Social Science and Humanities Research Council (SSHRC) of Canada for the study "Development from the North: Correspondence Between Concepts of Modernity and Development Practice."

Wilma Brakefield-Caldwell received her BS in nursing from Wayne State University and worked for twenty-eight years with the Detroit Health Department (DHD). During her time with the DHD, she worked as a public health nurse and supervisor, a project coordinator, a public health nursing administrator, and most recently, as health care administrator. In that capacity, Ms. Brakefield-Caldwell served as the DHD representative to the Detroit Community-Academic Urban Research Center. Ms. Brakefield-Caldwell retired in 1998 but continues to serve as a community representative on the Community Action Against Asthma Steering Committee. She is a frequent speaker and consultant on CBPR, has coauthored several articles on CBPR, and is a member of the External Advisory Committee for the National Children's Study.

Linda Burhansstipanov, DrPH, MSPH, is a member of the Cherokee Nation of Oklahoma and has worked in public health since 1971, primarily with Native American issues. She taught full-time at California State University Long Beach for eighteen years and part-time for the University of California Los Angeles for five years. She developed and implemented the Native American Cancer Research Program at the National Cancer Institute from 1989 to 1993. She worked with the AMC Cancer Research Center in Denver for five years before founding Native American Cancer Initiatives, Incorporated (1998) a for-profit business, and Native American Cancer Research Corporation (1999), an American Indian–operated nonprofit. She serves on multiple federal advisory boards for NIH and CDC. She currently is the principal investigator and subcontractor for more than five NIH grants. She has over a hundred peer-reviewed publications, most of which address Native American cancer, public health, and data issues.

Milyoung Cho, MPH, MS, was the project coordinator of the New York City Health Equity Project (HEP). In that role, she collaborated on the development of the HEP curriculum, worked closely with young people to conduct research on health disparities and food environments in New York City, and facilitated youth-led policy and action projects stemming from that research. She has an MPH from Hunter College's School of Urban Public Health and a Masters of Science in Chinese Medicine. She was formerly a community organizer and acupuncturist.

Suzanne Christopher, PhD, is a professor in the Department of Health and Human Development at Montana State University. She received her doctorate in the Department of Health Behavior and Health Education from the University of North Carolina at Chapel Hill, School of Public Health. She is on the Coordinating Committee for the Spirit of 1848 Caucus of the American Public Health Association (the Caucus is devoted to issues of social justice in health). She worked as a health education consultant with the Montana Breast and Cervical Health Program from 1995 to 1997. During this time she began working with Alma Knows His Gun-McCormick and members of the Apsáalooke Nation to develop and implement a community-based cervical health program, Messengers for Health. She does this work because she believes in health equality and that equality will happen with everyone walking and working side by side.

Nettie Coad was a community organizer, advocate, leader, and founding member of the Partnership Project and Greensboro Health Disparities Collaborative. She worked for twenty-two years in various management capacities for the Sears Catalog Distribution Center. She was an experienced trainer for the People's Institute for Survival and Beyond (PISAB), a nationally recognized antiracist training and consulting organization. She served on a broad array of active community organizational boards, including the Community Foundation of Greater Greensboro and the City of Greensboro Re-Development Commission. Nettie was a trustee for the Wesley Long-Moses Cone Community Health Foundation and steadfast organizer in her Greensboro neighborhood for over twenty-eight years, serving eight terms as president of the board for her neighborhood association. In that capacity, she successfully organized her neighborhood to prevent the widening of Martin Luther King Jr. Boulevard and assumed management of a multifamily housing unit, which was named the Nettie Coad Apartments in her honor. Nettie Coad died on April 10, 2012. Yet, her unwavering commitment to change, beautiful spirit, and sweet memory will continue to inspire each person she touched.

Jason Corburn, PhD, MCP, is an associate professor jointly appointed in the Department of City and Regional Planning and the School of Public Health at the University of California, Berkeley. He has published two award-winning books: *Street Science: Community Knowledge and Environmental Health Justice* (MIT Press, 2005) and, *Toward the Healthy City: People, Places and the Politics of Urban Planning* (MIT Press, 2009). His work is focused on engaged scholarship aimed at addressing urban health inequities. He received both a Masters in City

Planning (1996) and a PhD in Urban Environmental Planning (2002) from MIT.

Bonnie Duran, DrPH, is an associate professor in the Department of Health Services, University of Washington School of Public Health, and director of the Center for Indigenous Health Research, Indigenous Wellness Research Institute (http://www.iwri.org). She is the principal investigator of two NIH-funded research projects in "Indian Country." Working with the National Congress of American Indians Policy Research Center, and the University of New Mexico, she is studying the promoters, barriers, and mechanisms of change in CBPR (http://narch.ncaiprc.org/). With the Northwest Indian College and the American Indian Higher Education Consortium, she is conducting a needs and capacity study of behavioral health at 34 tribal colleges (http://iwri.org/tcu-dapss/research-resources/). The overall aims of her research are to work with communities to design public health treatment and prevention efforts that are empowering, culture-centered, sustainable, and that have maximum public health impact.

Katherine K. Edgren, MSW, has held leadership positions in a variety of settings for over thirty years. Most recently, she served as director of the Health Promotion and Community Relations (HPCR) Department at University Health Service at the University of Michigan. She was project manager of Community Action Against Asthma, a CBPR partnership in Detroit, and was based at the University of Michigan School of Public Health. She also served as executive director of two nonprofit organizations working with adults with serious mental illnesses, and as a city council member in Ann Arbor, Michigan. Her interests include CBPR, citizen participation in the political process, college health and wellness, strategic planning, and psychosocial rehabilitation.

Kevin Foley, PhD, has been in the Native American mental health field for almost thirty years. He is the clinical director at the Na'Nizhoozhi Center, Inc. (NCI) in Gallup, New Mexico, the largest treatment program in the country. He oversees the Hinaah Biits'os Society, a Navajo-based traditional Native American residential treatment program. He was the principal investigator of HRSA's five-year American Indian/Alaskan Native Special Projects of National Significance "Four Corners American Indian Circle of Services Collaborative" grant. He was the co-investigator of NIDA's Clinical Trials Network Job Seekers Workshop,

Navajo version, at NCI and the co-investigator of the Methamphetamine Use and Treatment in Native American Communities in the Southwest. He writes about cultural competency and clinical issues related to American Indian psychological treatment.

Nicholas Freudenberg, DrPH, is the Distinguished Professor of Public Health at the City University of New York School of Public Health at Hunter College, where he directs its Doctor of Public Health Program. He has been working with and for community organizations, advocacy organizations, and public agencies in New York City for more than thirty years designing, implementing, and evaluating community-based activities to change health damaging policies and programs. He has written on urban health, health advocacy, and health policy. His recent interests have been on food policy and strategies to modify harmful business practices. He is founder and director of Corporations and Health Watch (http://www.corporationsandhealth.org), a network for researchers, health professionals, and activists concerned about the health consequences of business practices.

Derek M. Griffith, PhD, is an associate professor of medicine, health and society and general internal medicine and public health at Vanderbilt University. He has an MA and PhD in clinical-community psychology from DePaul University. He completed a two-year fellowship as a W.K. Kellogg Foundation–funded Community Health Scholar at the University of North Carolina at Chapel Hill School of Public Health, and he served as an academic mentor for the Community-Track of the Kellogg Health Scholars Program when he was a faculty member at the University of Michigan School of Public Health site. He is currently an associate editor of *Progress in Community Health Partnerships: Research, Education, and Action* and he conducts CBPR primarily on African American men's cancer prevention and control and men's health disparities.

Jeanette Gustat, PhD, MPH, is a clinical associate professor of epidemiology and the principal investigator of the core research project for the Prevention Research Center (PRC) at the Tulane University School of Public Health and Tropical Medicine in New Orleans, Louisiana. The Tulane PRC studies the impact of the social and physical environment on obesity and collaborates with community partners through policy, education, and communication strategies to build healthier communities in New Orleans using a CBPR approach. As part of this work, she is a member of the Physical Activity and Policy Research Network funded by the Centers for Disease Control and Prevention. Additionally, she teaches research methods courses in the Department of Epidemiology.

J. Ricardo Guzmán, MSW, MPH, is the chief executive officer of Community Health and Social Services Center, Inc. (CHASS). CHASS is a Section 330–funded Federally Qualified Health Center (FQHC) with two locations in the city of Detroit. He is a long-standing community leader and activist in southwest Detroit. He has played a strong role in increasing access to culturally appropriate, high-quality, affordable, patient-centered services to community members who historically have not had access to such services. He is also a member of the National Association of Community Health Centers Executive Committee and in 2010 was named Social Worker of the Year by the National Association of Social Workers, Michigan Chapter. He is a founding member of the Detroit Community-Academic Urban Research Center and directs the REACH Detroit Partnership, two long-standing CBPR partnerships.

Nehanda Imara is an Oakland, California resident, activist, and educator. She is the East Oakland organizer for Communities for a Better Environment (CBE). She is also an adjunct lecturer in African American and Environmental Studies at Merritt College. She created the first environmental racism/justice course at the Peralta Community College District. She is on the steering committee for Sustainable Peralta, and the board of directors of Leadership Excellence, a non-profit African American youth organization in Oakland. She organized the first Environmental Justice Hip Hop event at Laney College to bring awareness to Environmental Racism in Oakland.

Betty T. Izumi, PhD, MPH, RD, is an assistant professor in the School of Community Health at Portland State University where her research and teaching focus on issues of sustainability, health, and equity. Before joining the faculty at Portland State University, she was a postdoctoral research fellow with the W.K. Kellogg Health Scholars Program at the University of Michigan, School of Public Health where she gained skills in CBPR. As a fellow, she worked with the Healthy Environments Partnership on multilevel interventions to reduce health disparities among Detroit residents. She continues to work with the Healthy Environments Partnership and is also involved in CBPR partnerships in Oregon and Alaska.

Srimathi Kannan, PhD, is an assistant professor of nutrition at the University of Massachusetts (UMASS), Amherst School of Public Health and Health Sciences and is director for the UMASS Community Nutrition Biomarkers Laboratory. She served as co-principal investigator for the National Institute of Environmental Health Sciences funded Healthy Environments Partnership CBPR project (2000–2005). Her research interests are the assessment of biological risk and protective (micro) nutrient markers in the context of acute and chronic exposure to air pollution in culturally diverse populations. In collaboration with Columbia and Harvard Universities, she is assessing cardio-pulmonary nutritional health of multiethnic populations of mother-child dyads in New York and Massachusetts. Funded by USDA, she has developed and implemented multisensory nutrition interventions promoting fruits and vegetables in early childhood settings (Head Start).

Edith (Edie) C. Kieffer, PhD, MPH, is associate professor, University of Michigan School of Social Work. Her research addresses ethnic and geographic disparities in maternal and child health, obesity, and diabetes. Using CBPR approaches, she and her community partners have identified weight, diabetes, eating, and exercise-related beliefs and practices of Latino and African American Detroit community residents, including pregnant and postpartum women, and have conducted multilevel interventions supported by NIH, CDC, and HRSA/ MCHB. She is a REACH Detroit Partnership team leader and co-investigator of Community Health Worker Diabetes RCT for Latinos. She is analyzing data from Healthy Mothers on the Move (NIH/NIDDK) and other completed studies. She teaches courses in health care services and policies, health ethics, and CBPR.

Alma Knows His Gun McCormick is a member of the Apsáalooke (Crow) Nation of Montana and fluently speaks her language. From 1996 to 2000 she was the outreach coordinator for the Centers for Disease Control and Prevention–funded Montana Breast and Cervical Health Program. She first conducted outreach education with Apsáalooke Indian women, feeling a breakthrough about the awareness of the importance of the Pap test and mammograms. Later, she provided culturally sensitive education to all Indian women on the seven reservations and in urban Indian clinics in Montana. Her compassion for working with cancer stems from her personal experience of losing her daughter to cancer. Her focus has been on cervical health education with the dream of continuing her work with women on the Crow reservation. She has fulfilled that dream by being the project coordinator for the Messengers for Health Program. She is a single mother with two sons, one daughter, and two grandchildren.

James (Jim) Krieger, MD, MPH, is chief of the Chronic Disease and Injury Prevention Section at Public Health—Seattle and King County, clinical professor of Medicine and Health Services at the University of Washington and attending physician at Harborview Medical Center. He has led multiple asthma CBPR studies, including examining the effectiveness of in-home community health worker asthma education programs, how integrated systems of asthma control and asthma coalitions can improve outcomes, and the impact of improving housing conditions on asthma. He has contributed to improving asthma control serving the NIH Asthma Guidelines Implementation Panel and taking care of patients with asthma. He has received numerous awards for his work, including the U.S. Secretary of Health and Human Services' Innovation in Prevention Award, the U.S. Environmental Protection Agency's Children's Environmental Health Excellence Award, and U.S. Department of Housing and Urban Development Healthy Homes Innovator Award.

Paula M. Lantz, PhD, MS, is a professor and chair of the Department of Health Policy of the George Washington University School of Public Health and Health Services. As a social demographer/social epidemiologist, her research is focused on policies, programs, and interventions that improve population health and reduce health inequities. She has particular expertise in the areas of cancer prevention and control, social determinants of health, and the role of public health in health care reform.

Toby Lewis, MD, MPH, is an associate professor in the Department of Pediatrics at the University of Michigan, School of Medicine. She is a pediatric pulmonologist with expertise in environmental epidemiology. Her research focuses on environmental factors involved in the development and persistence of childhood asthma, particularly characteristics which increase vulnerability to environmental exposures, and interventions that can reduce the health impact of environmental hazards among vulnerable populations. She has served as a co-investigator on the initial Community Action Against Asthma (CAAA) Household Intervention and Epidemiology projects and the current NEXUS and Diesel Exposure Studies, and is the principal investigator on the CAAA Air Filter Intervention Study and the AIRWAYS studies, all CBPR projects in Detroit.

Richard Lichtenstein, PhD, MPH, is an associate professor of Health Management and Policy at the University of Michigan, School of Public Health. He received his MPH and PhD in Medical Care Organization from the University of Michigan, and a BS in Industrial and Labor Relations from Cornell University. He has taught graduate courses on the U.S. health care system for over thirty-five years. He was the principal investigator for the Detroit Community-Academic Urban Research Center's (Detroit URC) Eastside Access Partnership—an effort to enroll uninsured children in Detroit in Medicaid, and he is the codirector of the Detroit Community-Academic Urban Research Center. He is on the board of directors of Neighborhood Service Organization in Detroit and the Corner Health Center in Ypsilanti, Michigan, and is the trustee for two retiree health plans.

Murlisa Lockett, MA, previously assistant community health coordinator, Detroit Department of Health and Wellness Promotion, and a member of the Healthy Environments Partnership Steering Committee, a CBPR partnership in Detroit. She coordinated the Eastside Village Health Worker Partnership (1996–2004), an innovative lay health adviser program that worked on Detroit's eastside community, and oversaw the development of minimarkets that brought healthy produce into areas of Detroit with few retail outlets providing healthy foods. She also served as project manager for the Healthy Connections Advocate Program (2004–2008) and supervisor for Kin Keeper, a community health worker cancer prevention project (2006–2011). She continues to be active in the community health worker field.

Ellen D. S. López, PhD, is an assistant professor at the University of Alaska at Fairbanks where she holds a joint appointment with the Department of Psychology and the Center for Alaska Native Health Research. She is developing partnerships with tribal and community-based organizations with the goal of forming a collaborative cancer research program focused on cancer prevention and survivorship for Alaska Native people and their communities. Her research program is devoted to integrating CBPR principles with innovative research methods (such as photovoice and photo-mapping) to gain perspectives on cancer prevention, control, and survivorship among rural and underserved communities.

Martha Matsuoka, PhD, MCP, is an assistant professor in the Urban and Environmental Policy Department at Occidental College where she teaches courses on environmental justice, community development, organizing, and regional economic development. Her research focuses on community-based regionalism and regional equity, the environmental justice movement, and the role of community and labor in ports and goods movement policy and planning. She is currently involved in assessment projects focused on environmental justice policy in Los Angeles and regional work and health collaboratives. She is coauthor with Manuel Pastor and Chris Benner of *This Could Be the Start of Something Big: How Social Movements for Regional Equity Are Reshaping Metropolitan America* (Cornell University Press, 2009).

Robert J. McGranaghan, MPH, is the Aurora Community Liaison for the Community Engagement Core of the Colorado Clinical Translation Science Institute at the University of Colorado School of Medicine. He was the project manager for the Detroit Community-Academic Urban Research Center (Detroit URC) from its inception in 1995 to 2012, and was based at the University of Michigan School of Public Health. His current interests include working to disseminate lessons learned and recommendations for conducting CBPR, helping new and emerging community-institutional partnerships to understand and use the CBPR model, and advocating for community-based interests in public health.

Chris McQuiston, PhD, RN, was an associate professor of nursing at the University of North Carolina at Chapel Hill School of Nursing. Her research, teaching, and service focused on improving access to care for minority groups, in general, and on developing interventions that address the unique heath care needs of immigrant Latino populations, in particular. She was a member of El Centro Hispano, a Latino community-based organization located in Durham, North Carolina, Café de Mujeres, the UNC-Chapel Hill Coalition for AIDS Research, the Chancellor's Advisory Committee on AIDS, the National Coalition of Hispanic Health and Human Services, and the National Center for Minority Health. Working collaboratively with these community partners, Dr. McQuiston secured external funding to develop and deliver culture-specific HIV interventions, such as "Protegiendo Nuestra Comunidad," a lay health adviser program that empowers community members to teach HIV prevention to fellow Latinos, and identified measurement concerns with data collected from recently arrived Mexicans. She received the Research in Minority Health Award from the Southern Nursing Research Society for her extensive research on HIV and STD prevention with Latino populations to develop culturally sensitive prevention models that reflect the values, culture, and sexual practices of this population. She is retired.

Elvira M. Mebane is president and founding member of United Voices of Efland-Cheeks, Inc. Retired after thirty-two years of service with the Orange County Health Department as the Deputy Registrar of Vital Records, she continues to serve her community as a member of the Orange County Healthy Carolinians Board, the Northern Orange NAACP, and the Orange County Educational Taskforce. Additionally, she is a volunteer driver for the Orange County Meals on Wheels program sponsored by Orange Congregations and Missions and an apheresis donor for the Red Cross. As a member of McCoy's Temple United Holy Church, she serves on the administrative board for the pastor.

Meredith Minkler, DrPH, is professor and director of Health and Social Behavior, School of Public Health, University of California, Berkeley, where she was founding director of the UC Center on Aging. She has over thirty-five years' experience teaching, conducting research, and working with underserved communities on community-identified issues through community building, community organizing, and CBPR. Her current research and service includes documenting the impacts of CBPR on healthy public policy, an ecological CBPR study of immigrant worker health and safety in Chinatown restaurants, and a community building and organizing project for and with older activists in California. She is coauthor or editor of eight books and over one hundred thirty peer-reviewed articles and book chapters including the edited books *Community Organizing and Community Building for Health* (3rd edition, 2012), and *Community Based Participatory Research for Health* (with Wallerstein) (2nd edition, 2008).

Rachel Morello-Frosch, PhD, MPH, is an associate professor in the Department of Environmental Science, Policy, and Management and the School of Public Health at the University of California, Berkeley. Her research integrates environmental health science with social epidemiologic methods to assess potential synergistic effects of social and environmental factors in environmental health disparities. In collaboration with scientific and community colleagues, she has developed scientifically valid and transparent tools for assessing the cumulative impacts of chemical and nonchemical stressors to inform regulatory decision making to advance environmental justice goals. She is assessing the application of these methods for implementation of climate change policies in California. Her most recent book is *Contested Illnesses: Citizens, Science and Health Social Movements* (2011, coauthored with Phil Brown and Steve Zavestovski). Her research is supported by the National Institute of Environmental Health Sciences, National Science Foundation, U.S. EPA, Cal-EPA, and private foundations.

Freda L. Motton, BS, MPH is a community/academic liaison currently working on a R24 grant with the National Institute on Minority Health and Health Disparities (Men on the Move: Growing Communities), and with the Prevention Research Center in St. Louis in the Bootheel and Ozark Regions of Missouri. She is a past chair of the Centers for Disease Control and Prevention, Prevention Research Centers National Community Committee (NCC), where she played a critical role in identifying Special Interest Project 13: Increasing Physical Activity Among Adults in Racially/Ethnically Diverse Communities in the United States, one of the first of its kind. She also served NCC in a partnership with the Center of Public Health and Community Genomics at the University of Michigan–Ann Arbor to facilitate the 2007 Midwest Genomics Forums. She served on the Planning Committee for GenoCommunity Think Tank: First National Meeting collaboration between the NCC and the Center for Public Health and Community Genomics, University of Michigan School of Public Health. In addition, she has contributed to peer-reviewed publications. She received her MPH from Saint Louis University School of Public Health.

Saritha Nair, PhD, Scientist C, is an applied social scientist researcher at the National Institute for Research in Reproductive Health (Indian Council of Medical Research), Mumbai, India. She has received a number of distinguished awards including Government of India fellowship for pursuing PhD program

(1999–2002) and Population Council, India, Fellowship for Health and Population Innovation for 2004–2006. For her work on community-based research promoting gender equity, she has received funding from both the government of India and the U.S. NIH for projects to enhance participation of men in reproductive health, develop positive partnerships to improve maternal health, address the role of violence on health outcomes of new mothers seeking care in a Mumbai slum, and reduce the use of smokeless tobacco among women of reproductive age in a low-income community of Mumbai. She has authored more than ten articles in peer-reviewed journals.

Angela M. Odoms-Young, PhD, MS, is an assistant professor in Kinesiology and Nutrition, College of Applied Health Sciences, University of Illinois at Chicago. Her research focuses on understanding social, cultural, and environmental determinants of dietary behaviors and diet-related diseases (cancer, diabetes, and cardiovascular disease) in low-income and minority populations. Her current studies include evaluating the impact of the new WIC food package on dietary intake, weight status, and chronic disease risk in two- to three-year-old low-income children; examining relationships between neighborhood food availability, eating behaviors, and weight status in Latino families; and understanding the influence of marketing on food consumption in African American families. She previously completed Family Research Consortium and Kellogg Community Health Scholars postdoctoral fellowships at the Universities of Pennsylvania and Michigan, respectively.

Julio César Olmos-Muñiz is a computer system technician from Tamaulipas, Mexico, who came to the United States over a decade ago with his wife, Aide Arredondo. They have two children, Julio Jr. and Naomi. Olmos-Muñiz worked as a volunteer for the National AIDS Prevention Program (CONASIDA) in Monterrey, N.L. Mexico. On his arrival in the United States, he worked as a lay health adviser for HIV/STD prevention and as an outreach worker for the Syphilis Elimination Project at the local Health Department. He has been a guest lecturer at workshops on CBPR and teenage pregnancy prevention as well as an outreach coordinator for Project LIFE, an HIV/STD education and prevention program. In his current job as director of community organizing at El Centro Hispano (ECH) in Durham, North Carolina, he is working on building leadership capacity in the Hispanic community.

Ashley O'Toole, MPH, MSW is the manager of the Detroit Community-Academic Urban Research Center and is based at the University of Michigan School of Public Health. She is the former project manager of Community Action Against Asthma, a CBPR partnership in Detroit, a position she held for over three years. She has several years of experience as a health educator in both the private and public sectors.

Gloria Palmisano, MA, BS, is the project manager of the REACH Detroit Partnership, which addresses diabetes disparities among African Americans and Latinos. She is employed by Community Health and Social Services Center, a federally qualified health center in Detroit. She has over thirty years' experience in program implementation, staff development, and managing federal, local, and grant-funded public health, education, and employment training programs. She developed and coordinated a comprehensive training program for REACH Detroit Community Health Workers (CHWs). She has a national reputation as a steadfast advocate for recognition and adequate CHW compensation, speaks and consults on CHW models and community-based participatory approaches for eliminating health disparities, and has increased the linkages and collaborative efforts that further the work of the REACH Detroit Partnership.

Emilio Parrado, PhD, is an associate professor of sociology at the University of Pennsylvania. His research focuses on issues of health, migration dynamics, and adaptation among Latinos. Recently, he has concentrated on Latino migration to new areas of destination in the Southwestern United States, including issues of occupational representation, social demands, and HIV risks. In addition, he has worked collaboratively with the Durham, North Carolina, Latino community to better understand the social and cultural forces shaping migrants' lives. He is currently principal investigator of a binational NIH–funded study investigating the health consequences of the economic recession on immigrant sending communities in Mexico and receiving areas in the United States.

Manuel Pastor, PhD, MA, is a professor of American Studies and Ethnicity at the University of Southern California and director of USC's Program for Environmental and Regional Equity. His most recent books include *Just Growth: Inclusion and Prosperity in America's Metropolitan Regions* (2012, coauthored with Chris Benner) and *Uncommon Common Ground: Race and America's Future* (2010, coauthored with Angela Glover Blackwell and Stewart Kwoh). Along with Morello-Frosch and Sadd, he works on issues of environmental disparities with support from foundations and agencies, including the California Air Resources Board and the National Science Foundation, and in collaboration with a range of environmental justice advocates and organizers.

Regina Y. Petteway, MSPH, BSPH, is the division director for administration with Wake County Human Services in North Carolina. She holds BSPH and MSPH degrees from the University of North Carolina at Chapel Hill and has been an adjunct professor in the Department of Health Behavior and Health Education since 2001. For the past eighteen years she has worked with Wake County Government serving as the director for the Office of Community Affairs, and currently as the division director for administration. She was one of the representatives for Wake County with the Project DIRECT partnership (diabetes initiative) and was vital in facilitating the Project DIRECT partnership becoming institutionalized with Strengthening the Black Family, Inc. in Raleigh, North Carolina. She has received numerous awards, including an award from the Triangle Lost Generation Task Force. She is involved in group facilitation and organizational capacity-building projects.

Michele Prichard, MA, is the director of Common Agenda at the Liberty Hill Foundation where she coordinates policy initiatives on environmental health and social justice. As Liberty Hill's executive director from 1989 to 1997, she helped create new grant programs addressing poverty, race relations, and environmental health. She has served on the boards of many nonprofit and philanthropic organizations, including the Southern California Association for Philanthropy, the L.A. Urban Funders, the Funding Exchange, the L.A. County Federation of Labor's Community Service Program, the Venice Community Housing Corporation, and the Advisory Board of the Los Angeles Coalition to End Hunger and Homelessness. She is currently vice president of the Harbor Community Benefit Foundation, a newly established foundation to address the health and environmental impacts from the Port of Los Angeles on local neighborhoods. She was a Senior Fellow in the UCLA School of Public Affairs during 2007–2008. She received her MA from the UCLA School of Urban Planning in 1989.

Angela G. Reyes, MPH, is the founder and executive director of the Detroit Hispanic Development Corporation (DHDC). Founded in 1997, DHDC is a nonprofit community-based organization that has developed integrated services for youth and families including gang prevention and intervention, youth development, prisoner reentry, HIV prevention, adult education, parenting education, and community organizing for social justice. She has over thirty years of experience as a community activist, working with at-risk and gang-involved youth. She is the recipient of several awards for her community work, including the 1992 Michiganian of the Year and Detroit Public Schools Community Service Award. *Corp! Magazine* named her one of Michigan's Most Influential Hispanic Leaders. She is a founding board member of the Detroit Community-Academic Urban Research Center.

Scott D. Rhodes, MPH, PhD, is a professor in the Division of Public Health Sciences, Wake Forest School of Medicine. He has an MPH from the University of South Carolina and a PhD from the University of Alabama at Birmingham. He completed a two-year postdoctoral fellowship with the W.K. Kellogg Foundation-funded Community Health Scholars Program at the University of North Carolina at Chapel Hill, gaining valuable skills in establishing a CBPR partnership with Latino communities. He is currently principal investigator for several federally-funded CBPR studies designed to reduce the risk of HIV and sexually transmitted disease infection and understand the role of partnerships in health disparity reduction in infection rates.

Thomas G. Robins, MD, MPH, is a professor in the Department of Environmental Health Sciences at the University of Michigan School of Public Health. He is the director of the University of Michigan Southern Africa Program in Environmental and Occupational Health funded by the NIH. He is an occupational and environmental physician and epidemiologist. He has served as the principal investigator on a number of large-scale epidemiologic studies of environmental exposures and health outcomes, both in United States and internationally. He was the principal investigator for the initial Community Action Against Asthma (CAAA) Epidemiology Research project and is principal investigator for CAAA's Diesel Exposure Study, both CBPR projects in Detroit.

Naomi Robinson, MA, BA, earned her bachelor's degree in Business Administration from North Carolina Central University and her Masters of Arts degree in Teaching from Trinity College. Now retired, she spent her career in service to her community. For five years she served as a social worker for the Department of Social Services in Washington, North Carolina, and as a case manager for

Comprehensive Interventions Incorporated. As a community research adviser (CRA) on the Surviving Angels—Inspirational Images Project, and then through her work with the Eastern North Carolina Witness for Life Program, she helped to guide and sustain efforts to improve quality of life for African American breast cancer survivors.

Frank Rose III has worked with a number of community organizations in Pemiscot County, Missouri. His main interests are in the social support of men and youth (for example, jobs, education, family). Rose is the farm manager of the Men on the Move Program: Growing Communities, a community-campus partnership between Community Partners in Pemiscot County and Saint Louis University. He also serves on the Pemiscot Initiative Network Board of Directors, and is vice chair of Word Outreach, Inc.

Zachary Rowe, BBA, is executive director of Friends of Parkside, a grassroots community-based organization on Detroit's eastside, which provides programs for youth, a computer learning center, health and safety projects, and linkages for residents to employment opportunities. He has been involved with various CBPR projects for more than fifteen years and is a founding member of the Detroit Community-Academic Urban Research Center Board.

James Sadd, PhD, MS, is a professor of Environmental Science, and chair of the Geology Department at Occidental College in Los Angeles, California. A founding board member of the Harbor Community Benefit Foundation, his research includes spatial analysis using geographic information systems and remote sensing tools particularly to evaluate environmental justice questions. He also has active research programs in the historical reconstruction of sedimentation and pollution histories in coastal and marine environments. His current research is supported by grants from the U.S. Army Corps of Engineers, U.S. Navy Office of Naval Research, U.S. Environmental Protection Agency, California Sea Grant, and the California Endowment.

Yamir Salabarría-Peña, DrPH, MPHE, is lead epidemiologist at the Centers for Disease Control and Prevention (CDC), Division of Global AIDS/HIV, Epidemiology and Strategic Information Branch. She provides expert capacity-building consultation on design and use of empowerment evaluation, participatory evaluation, utilization-focused evaluation, implementation/process evaluation, qualitative methodology and mixed methods to colleagues in HIV/STI/TB control and prevention, and maternal and child mortality in the United States, Latin America, Asia, and Africa. She was a W.K. Kellogg post-doctoral scholar at the University of Michigan, School of Public Health where she was a co-investigator of multiple CBPR and evaluation projects of chronic-disease prevention interventions utilizing ecological frameworks.

Sharon Sand, MPP, has been involved with the Healthy Environments Partnership (HEP), since 2002 in both evaluation and project management capacities, and is based at the University of Michigan, School of Public Health. She is currently managing HEP's Walk Your Heart to Health program, a program designed to engage Detroit community members and organizations in developing and sustaining walking groups to enable community members to exercise together to improve their heart health. Her interests include social determinants of health and community-based participatory research. She received her MPP degree from the University of Michigan.

Jennifer C. Schaal, MD, completed her residency in Obstetrics and Gynecology at the University of Minnesota and practiced gynecology in a small private practice until she retired in 2006. During her practice she was a clinical investigator for the Heart and Estrogen-Progestin Replacement and Estrogen Replacement and Atherosclerosis studies and was on the Community Advisory Board of the Women's Health Initiative. A founding member of the Greensboro Health Disparities Collaborative, she has served as cochair of the Collaborative for two years and currently serves as secretary. She participated as an interviewer and critical incident technique analyst for the Collaborative's Cancer Care and Racial Equity Study. She has been an active participant in the development and implementation of the Collaborative's Health Equity Training.

Jean J. Schensul, PhD, an anthropologist, is founding director (1987–2004) and full time senior scientist (2005-ongoing) of the Institute for Community Research, an independent community-based research organization committed to reducing inequities in health, education, and cultural representation, with collaborative projects in the United States, China, and India. She continues to create infrastructure for many forms of collaborative research, intervention, dissemination, and participatory action research (PAR). She is the recipient of many NIH,

SAMHSA, and other federal and foundation grants for health-related projects built on principles of collaborative research and PAR, which she has implemented globally. She is past president of the Council on Anthropology and Education and the Society for Applied Anthropology and a member of the executive board of the American Anthropological Association. Lead editor and coauthor of the *Ethnographer's Toolkit* (1999, 2nd edition, 2010–11), she has published extensively on public health topics including substance use, democratization of science, collaboration research methods, and PAR.

Kate Shirah, MPH, BSPH, is the program director for the John Rex Endowment, a private foundation focused on improving the health and well-being of children and youth in Wake County, North Carolina. She works to concentrate the John Rex Endowment's resources on the best strategies for making change, directs the proposal development process, and conducts evaluation activities for the foundation. Before joining the John Rex Endowment, she worked as an instructor and the field training coordinator in the Department of Health Behavior and Health Education at the University of North Carolina at Chapel Hill Gillings School of Global Public Health. Her BSPH degree in Health Policy and Administration and MPH degree in Health Behavior and Health Education are from the University of North Carolina.

Carmen Stokes, MSN, BSN, is an assistant professor at the University of Detroit-Mercy McAuley School of Nursing. She teaches courses in fundamentals of nursing, community health nursing, and a family crises nursing course. A resident of northwest Detroit, she has been a member of the Healthy Environments Partnership Steering Committee, a CBPR partnership in Detroit, since 2001. She has served as a member of the HEP Survey Committee, assisted in conducting focus groups with community residents, and represented HEP in a variety of venues, including the American Public Health Association meetings. She received her MSN degree from the University of Detroit-Mercy, her BSN from Wayne State University, is a certified family nurse practitioner (FNP), and is currently working on her doctorate in Educational Studies.

Karen Strazza, MPH, BA, is a public health analyst with Research Triangle Institute International in the Community Health Promotion Research Program. She has worked at both the state and local level in developing, implementing, and evaluating collaborative community health interventions, and providing technical assistance and training programs for chronic disease, injury and violence prevention, and maternal and child health. Most recently she served as assistant director of education and outreach for the University of North Carolina Injury Prevention Research Center. Prior positions include clinical instructor, Department of Health Behavior and Health Education, University of North Carolina at Chapel Hill; lead health educator, North Carolina Breast and Cervical Cancer Control Program; and project director, North Carolina Community-Based Public Health Initiative. In Southeast Asia, she was involved in refugee assistance and community development with UNICEF, CARE, and Save the Children.

Samara Swanston, JD, an environmental lawyer and an educator, has worked for and volunteered with many community-based organizations in New York City including ten years as the executive director of the Watchperson Project as well as many years as a volunteer with the New York City Environmental Justice Alliance and WEACT. Currently, she is counsel to the Environmental Protection Committee of the New York City Council, and a visiting professor at both the Pratt Institute Graduate School for Urban Planning and the Environment and the Hunter College Graduate Program for Urban Affairs and Planning. Her interests are air quality, protection of public health, renewable energy, and sustainability.

Tim K. Takaro, MD, MPH, MS, is a physician-scientist and associate professor in the Faculty of Health Sciences at Simon Fraser University, Vancouver, BC. His research examines linkages between occupational or environmental exposures and disease and tests public health-based preventive solutions for such risks. One area of focus has been environmental exposures in childhood asthma. In addition to directing intervention trials, he is a lead investigator for the environmental assessment component of the Canadian Health Infant Longitudinal Development birth cohort examining the mechanisms of asthma development through study of gene and environment interactions. A new area of research is in human health effects and adaptive capacity to climate change.

Emma Tsui, PhD, MPH, is an assistant professor in the Masters of Public Health Program at Lehman College, City University of New York. As a postdoctoral fellow at the City University of New York School of Public Health at Hunter

College, she participated in several policy and research projects focused on the role of community mobilization and social movements in reshaping food systems to help achieve public health goals. Her research interests include food access and food policy; urban spaces and health, labor, and social movements; and the relationships between workforce development, economic development, employment, and health. She has worked primarily in Baltimore and New York City on a range of qualitative, ethnographic, policy-oriented, and participatory research projects.

Nina Wallerstein, DrPH, professor in the Public Health Program, and director of the Center for Participatory Research, School of Medicine, University of New Mexico, has been developing participatory research methodologies and empowerment intervention research for thirty years, with her latest coedited volume covering these fields, *Community-Based Participatory Research for Health* (with Meredith Minkler, 2008). She has worked in North American and Latin American contexts, in participatory evaluation of healthy city initiatives, in adolescent and women's health, and in translational research, developing strengths-based assessments and culturally centered interventions with tribal communities. Since 2006, she has been involved in NIH research to advance the science of CBPR, by identifying best partnering practices and processes that contribute to CBPR capacity-building and systems changes leading to reduced health disparities.

Vanessa Watts Simonds, ScD, member of the Crow Nation of Montana, is an assistant professor in the Department of Community and Behavioral Health at the University of Iowa's College of Public Health. Her current research interests include using participatory approaches to address health issues, and incorporating indigenous knowledge into intervention development.

Lucille Webb, MA, is a long-time resident of Wake County, North Carolina. She is a former teacher and founding president of the board of directors at Strengthening the Black Family, Inc. For lasting contributions made to the city of Raleigh, North Carolina, she and her husband, Harold Webb, were inducted in 2011 into the Raleigh Hall of Fame. She has served as an exemplary community mentor for numerous postdoctoral fellows through the W.K. Kellogg Foundation's Community Health Scholars Program.

Donele Wilkins has demonstrated leadership in her hometown, Detroit, for nearly twenty years. Her work on the front lines of the local movement for environmental justice has inspired many, particularly young people, to join the cause. Her achievements include participation in the development and adoption of an environmental justice policy in Michigan. As the founding director for Detroiters Working for Environmental Justice, she conceived and launched the first Green Jobs training program in Detroit. She is an advocate for citizen involvement in Brownfield Redevelopment and other environmental issues, placing environmental stewardship on the agenda of many community leaders and decision makers. As the founder of the Green Door Initiative, she is involved in taking Detroit to the next level of environmental stewardship.

Sharla K. Willis, DrPH, MPH, has worked in Los Angeles, Chicago, Detroit, and Columbus conducting research that has focused on the use of qualitative research methods in collaboration with Latino and African American women to identify community-based health needs and strategies to address those needs. She has an MPH degree in international and population and family health, an MA degree in Latin American studies from the University of California-Los Angeles, and a DrPH degree from the University of Illinois at Chicago. The research in which she was involved that is discussed in this book was conducted during a W.K. Kellogg Foundation–funded Community Health Scholars postdoctoral program at the University of Michigan School of Public Health. She currently runs a small business with her family.

Michael Yonas, DrPH, MPH, is an assistant professor in the Department of Family Medicine at the University of Pittsburgh. His MPH and DrPH degrees were both awarded by the Johns Hopkins University, Bloomberg School of Public Health in Baltimore, Maryland. Concentrating on the health, wellness, and chronic disease prevention for children and adolescents, his research employs a participatory, creative, and ecological perspective for understanding and promoting health of individuals and communities. He is committed to exploring and preventing disparities in child and adolescent health, specifically in conducting research examining the impact of community social and contextual influences such as violence and stress upon asthma. He has specialized training and experience in the application and teaching of principles of CBPR. He is a founding member of the Greensboro Health Disparities Collaborative.

Anna Yun Lee was a staff researcher and scientist at Communities for a Better Environment (CBE) in Oakland, California, at the time of writing this chapter. She is now on the staff of the Alameda County Department of Public Health.

Shannon N. Zenk, PhD, MPH, MSN, RN, is an assistant professor of Health Systems Science at the University of Illinois at Chicago College of Nursing. She is a leading scholar in the area of social and built environmental contributions to racial and socioeconomic disparities in health, with a particular interest in the identification of environmental and policy interventions to reduce disparities in obesity. She has been, and continues to be, actively involved in a number of CBPR efforts including the Healthy Environments Partnership and the East Side Village Health Worker Partnership in Detroit, as well as the Englewood Neighborhood Health Center in Chicago.

METHODS FOR COMMUNITY-BASED PARTICIPATORY RESEARCH FOR HEALTH

PART ONE

INTRODUCTION TO METHODS FOR COMMUNITY-BASED PARTICIPATORY RESEARCH FOR HEALTH

Chapter 1

INTRODUCTION TO METHODS
FOR CBPR FOR HEALTH

BARBARA A. ISRAEL

EUGENIA ENG

AMY J. SCHULZ

EDITH A. PARKER

Public health problems are complex, and their solutions involve not only political and social but also biomedical dimensions. Researchers, practitioners, community members, and funders continue to recognize the importance of comprehensive and participatory approaches to research and intervention, and opportunities for such partnership approaches continue to emerge. As they do, so does the demand for concrete skills and knowledge about how to conduct community-based or other participatory approaches to research. Both new and established partnerships continue to search for information about strategies, skills, methods, and approaches that support the equitable participation and influence of diverse partners in developing a clearer understanding of public health problems and in working collectively to address them. Like the first edition, this book is a resource for students, practitioners, researchers, and community members seeking to use community-based participatory research (CBPR) approaches to improve the health and well-being of communities in general and to eliminate health inequities in particular. In the introduction to this volume, we discuss the background to and support for CBPR, principles of CBPR, core components/phases of CBPR, and the broad cultural, socioeconomic, and environmental context in which CBPR is conducted. Finally, we describe the purposes and goals of this book, and present the organization and brief descriptions of the chapters.

BACKGROUND

Over the past decade, there has continued to be increasing recognition that more comprehensive and participatory approaches to research and interventions are needed in order to address the complex set of social and environmental determinants associated with population health and those factors associated more specifically with racial and ethnic inequities in health (Commission for the Social Determinants of Health, 2008; Commission to Build a Healthier America, 2009; Israel, Schulz, Parker, & Becker, 1998; Mercer & Green, 2008; Minkler & Wallerstein, 2008; Schulz, Williams, Israel, & Lempert, 2002). Concomitantly, funding opportunities that support partnership approaches to research addressing these problems continue to grow (Catalani & Minkler, 2009; Chen, Diaz, Lucas, & Rosenthal, 2010; Cook, 2008). These include, for example, the National Institute on Minority Health and Health Disparities' Community-Based Participatory Research Initiative (NIMHD, 2011); the Centers for Disease Control and Prevention's Prevention Research Centers program (CDC, 2011); the National Cancer Institute's Center to Reduce Cancer Health Disparities Community Networks Program (NCI, 2012); the National Institutes of Health's Clinical and Translational Science Awards Program, Community Engagement Core (NIH, 2011); and the Office of Behavioral and Social Sciences Research's opportunities for community participation in research (OBSSR, 2012).

Partnership approaches to research exist in many different academic disciplines and fields. In the field of public health, partnership approaches to research have been called, variously, "community-based participatory," "community-involved," "collaborative," and "community-centered-research" (see Israel et al., 1998, for a review of this literature). In addition, a large social science literature has examined research approaches in which participants are actively involved in the process. Examples include discussions of "participatory research" (deKoning & Martin, 1996; Green et al., 1995; Hall, 1992; Kemmis & McTaggart, 2000; Park, 1993; Tandon, 1996), "participatory action research" (Whyte, 1991), "action research" (Peters & Robinson, 1984; Reason & Bradbury, 2006, 2008; Stringer, 2007), "participatory feminist research" (Maguire, 1987, 1996; Joyappa & Miartin 1996), "action science/inquiry" (Argyris, Putnam, & Smith, 1985; Torbert & Taylor, 2008), "cooperative inquiry" (Heron & Reason, 2001; Reason, 1994), "critical action research" (Kemmis & McTaggart, 2000), "participatory community research" (Jason, Keys, Suarez-Balcazar, Taylor, & Davis, 2004), "tribally driven participatory research" (Mariella, Brown, Carter, & Verri, 2009), "community engagement" (Clinical and Translational Science Awards Community Engagement Key Function Committee Task Force, 2011), and "community-based collaborative action research" (Pavlish & Pharris, 2012). Although there are differences among these approaches, they all involve a commitment to conducting research that to some degree shares power with and engages community partners in the research process and that benefits the communities involved, either through direct intervention or by translating research findings into interventions and policy change.

In public health, nursing, social work, and related fields, the term *community-based participatory research* (CBPR) has been increasingly used to represent such collaborative approaches (Israel et al., 2001; Minkler & Wallerstein, 2008; Viswanathan et al., 2004), while recognizing that there are other approaches with different labels that share similar values and methods. CBPR in public health is a partnership approach to research that equitably involves, for example, community members, organizational representatives, and researchers in all aspects of the research process and in which all partners contribute expertise and share decision making and ownership (Israel et al., 1998, 2008). The aim of CBPR is to increase knowledge and understanding of a given phenomenon and integrate the knowledge gained with interventions and policy and social change to improve the health and quality of life of community members (Israel et al., 1998, 2008).

Associated with the developments described above, the Institute of Medicine Report, *Who Will Keep the Public Healthy? Educating the Public Health Professionals for the 21st Century* (Gebbie, Rosenstock, & Hernandez, 2003), identifies CBPR as one of the eight areas in which all public health professionals need to be trained. As stated in the report, "the committee believes that public health professionals will be better prepared to address the major health problems and challenges facing society if they achieve competency in the following eight content areas," and then lists and discusses CBPR as one of "these eight areas of critical importance to public health education in the 21st century" (p. 62).

Further recognition of the relevance of CBPR for professionals can be found in the increasing number of participatory research courses being taught in schools and departments of public health, nursing, sociology, social work, and psychology, among others. In addition, the number of CBPR workshops and conference sessions offered in local communities as well as at regional, national and international meetings has expanded over the past decade as participants strive to enhance their knowledge and skills related to partnership approaches to research. A number of excellent books examine the theoretical underpinnings of participatory approaches and provide case studies that illustrate implementation issues (see, for example, deKoning & Martin, 1996; Jason et al., 2004; Minkler & Wallerstein, 2008; Reason & Bradbury, 2006, 2008; Stringer, 2007). In 2004, the Agency for Healthcare Research and Quality commissioned a systematic, evidence-based review examining definitions of, and the evidence base regarding implementation and outcomes of CBPR approaches in population health interventions (Viswanathan et al., 2004). Over the past decade, several journals, such as the *Journal of General Internal Medicine* ("Community-Based Participatory Research," 2003) and *Health Education & Behavior* ("Community-Based Participatory Research—Addressing Social Determinants of Health: Lessons from the Urban Research Center," 2002), published entire issues devoted to CBPR, and special sections on CBPR appeared in such journals as the *American Journal of Public Health* ("Community-Based Participatory Research," 2001) and *Environmental Health Perspectives* ("Community-Based Participatory Research," 2005). In 2007, a new journal was launched dedicated entirely to CBPR, *Progress in Community Health Partnerships: Research, Education and Action*. Indicative of these activities may be the increase in the use of the term, "Community-Based Participatory Research," in the title or abstract of PubMed cited articles from 25 in 2001 to 226 in 2011. There have also been a number of training manuals and downloadable courses developed on CBPR (Israel, Coombe, & McGranaghan, 2010; Zimmerman, Tilly, Cohen, & Love, 2009).

As opportunities for conducting and learning about CBPR expand, so does the demand for knowledge and skills in this area. Practitioners and scholars ask for information about specific participation structures and procedures needed to establish and maintain equitable partnerships among individuals and groups from diverse cultures. They ask how specific data collection methods, such as survey questionnaires, in-depth interviews, focus groups, ethnography, and mapping can be designed and implemented to follow participatory principles, and how to engage all CBPR partners in disseminating research findings and translating results into action and policy change. This book is designed as a resource for students, practitioners, community members, and researchers in public health and related disciplines to expand their repertoire of skills and methods for supporting partnership approaches to research intended to improve the health and well-being of communities in general and to eliminate health inequities in particular.

PRINCIPLES OF CBPR

Based on an extensive review of the literature, the following discussion briefly presents nine guiding principles of CBPR (see Israel et al., 1998 and 2008, for a more detailed examination). These principles are offered with the caution that no one set of principles is applicable to all partnerships. Rather, the members of each research partnership need to jointly decide on the core values and guiding principles that reflect their collective vision and basis for decision making. However, as partnerships go about the process of making these decisions, they may be informed by the considerable experience and lessons learned over the past several decades of participatory forms of research as well as by the literature on partnerships and group functioning. Developing or existing partnerships may choose to draw on the principles presented here, as appropriate, as well as to develop additional or alternative principles that facilitate equitable participation and influence in each partnership's particular context. We suggest that partnerships consider the principles they adopt as ideals or goals to strive toward, and evaluate the extent to which they are able to adhere to those principles as one aspect of partnership capacity building (Cornwall, 1996; Green et al., 1995; Israel et al., 2008). We clearly do not think that there is one "best" set of principles, and believe that such principles can also be considered on a continuum, for example, by differing levels of community involvement. At the same time, we argue that as CBPR continues to grow in recognition and stature, care should be taken that its more widespread adoption not result in CBPR being "selectively invoked to accomplish predetermined aims or goals not collaboratively developed or locally defined" (Trickett, 2011, p. 1353). As will be evident throughout this volume, the principles described here and similar principles have been applied in numerous ways by the authors of these chapters, reflecting multiple approaches to CBPR, while at the same time having an overarching commitment to equity and power sharing in the process of research and action.

1. *CBPR acknowledges community as a unit of identity.* Units of identity refer to entities in which people have membership, for example, a family, social

network, or geographical neighborhood; they are socially created dimensions of identity, created and re-created through social interactions (Hatch, Moss, Saran, Presley-Cantrell, & Mallory, 1993; Steuart, 1993). Community as a unit of identity is defined by a sense of identification with and emotional connection to others through common symbol systems, values, and norms; shared interests; and commitments to meeting mutual needs. Communities of identity may be geographically bounded (people in a particular physical neighborhood may form such a community, for example) or geographically dispersed but sharing a common identity or sense of common interests (as members of an ethnic group or gay men may do, for example). A city, town, or geographical area may represent a community of identity, or may be an aggregate of individuals who do not have a common identity, or it may comprise multiple overlapping communities of identity (Gaffikin & Morrissey, 2011). CBPR partnerships seek to identify and work with existing communities of identity, extending beyond them as necessary, to improve public health (Israel et al., 1998, 2008).

2. *CBPR builds on strengths and resources within the community.* CBPR recognizes and builds on the strengths, resources, and assets that exist within communities of identity, such as individual skills, social networks, and organizations, in order to address identified concerns (Balcazar et al., 2004; Israel et al., 1998, 2008; McKnight, 1994; Steuart, 1993).

3. *CBPR facilitates a collaborative, equitable partnership in all phases of research, involving an empowering and power-sharing process that attends to social inequalities.* To the extent possible, all partners participate in and share decision making and control over all stages of the research process, such as defining the problem, collecting and interpreting data, disseminating findings, and applying the results to address community issues (Balcazar et al., 2004; deKoning & Martin, 1996; Green et al., 1995; Israel et al., 1998, 2008; Park, Brydon-Miller, Hall, & Jackson, 1993; Stringer, 2007). Researchers involved in CBPR recognize the inequalities that exist between themselves and community partners and attempt to address these inequalities by developing relationships based on trust and mutual respect and by creating an empowering process that involves open communication and sharing information, decision-making power, and resources (Blankenship & Schulz, 1996; Israel et al., 1998, 2008; Labonté, 1994; Suarez-Balcazar et al., 2004).

4. *CBPR fosters colearning and capacity building among all partners.* CBPR is a colearning process that fosters the reciprocal exchange of skills, knowledge, and capacity among all partners involved, recognizing that all parties bring diverse skills and expertise and different perspectives and experiences to the partnership process (deKoning & Martin, 1996; Freire, 1973; Israel et al., 1998, 2008; Stringer, 2007; Suarez-Balcazar et al., 2004).

5. *CBPR integrates and achieves a balance between knowledge generation and intervention for the mutual benefit of all partners.* CBPR aims to contribute to science while also integrating and balancing the knowledge gained with interventions and policies that address the concerns of the communities involved (Green et al., 1995; Park et al., 1993; Israel et al., 1998, 2008). Although a given CBPR project may not include a direct intervention component, it will have a commitment to the translation of research findings into action strategies that will benefit the community (deKoning & Martin, 1996; Green et al., 1995; Israel et al., 2008; Schulz, Israel, Selig, Bayer, & Griffin, 1998).

6. *CBPR focuses on the local relevance of public health problems and on ecological perspectives that attend to the multiple determinants of health.* CBPR addresses public health concerns that are of local relevance to the communities involved, and emphasizes an ecological approach to health that pays attention to individuals, their immediate context (for example, the family or social network), and the larger contexts in which these families and networks exist (for example, the community and society) (Bronfenbrenner, 1990; Israel et al., 1998, 2008; Stokols, 1996). Thus CBPR efforts consider the multiple determinants of health and disease, including biomedical, social, economic, cultural, and physical environmental factors, and necessitate an interdisciplinary team of researchers and community partners (Freudenberg, Klitzman, & Saegert, 2009; Israel et al., 1998, 2008; Suarez-Balcazar et al., 2004).

7. *CBPR involves systems development using a cyclical and iterative process.* CBPR addresses systems development, in which a system, such as a partnership, draws on the competencies of each partner to engage in a cyclical, iterative process that includes all the stages of the research process including, as appropriate, community assessment, problem definition, research design, data collection and analysis, data interpretation, dissemination, determina-

tion of intervention and policy strategies, and action taking (Altman, 1995; Israel et al., 1998, 2008; Stringer, 2007).

8. *CBPR disseminates results to all partners and involves them in the wider dissemination of results.* CBPR emphasizes the dissemination of research findings to all partners and communities involved in ways that are understandable, respectful, and useful (Israel et al., 1998, 2008; Schulz, et al., 1998). This dissemination principle also emphasizes that all partners engage in the broader dissemination of results, for example as coauthors of publications and copresenters at meetings and conferences (Israel et al., 2008).

9. *CBPR involves a long-term process and commitment to sustainability.* In order to establish and maintain the trust necessary to successfully carry out CBPR endeavors, and to achieve the aims of addressing multiple determinants of health, CBPR involves a long-term process and commitment to sustainability (Hatch et al., 1993; Israel et al., 2008; Mittelmark, Hunt, Heath, & Schmid, 1993). This long-term commitment frequently extends beyond a single research project or funding period. Although partners may reach a point at which they decide to discontinue the partnership, they retain a commitment to the relationships that exist and that can be called on in the future (Israel et al., 2006, 2008).

Core Components/Phases in Conducting CBPR

As depicted in Figure 1.1, there are seven broad core components in conducting CBPR (Israel, Coombe, & McGranaghan, 2010).[1] These components may be considered as phases or stages, and though there is some sequential order to conducting CBPR, the process is more circular than linear, and some elements may continue throughout an entire CBPR effort. For example, as indicated by the large circle in the center of the figure, maintaining and sustaining a partnership occurs throughout the different phases of the process, as partners work on an ongoing basis to strengthen trust, resolve conflicts, develop and share knowledge and skills, and as they work together to carry out the tasks involved in conducting the research. Similarly, evaluation of the partnership's effectiveness needs to start at the beginning and continue throughout a CBPR project. This

1. This section is adapted from Israel, Coombe, & McGranaghan, 2010.

FIGURE 1.1 Core Components/Phases in Conducting CBPR

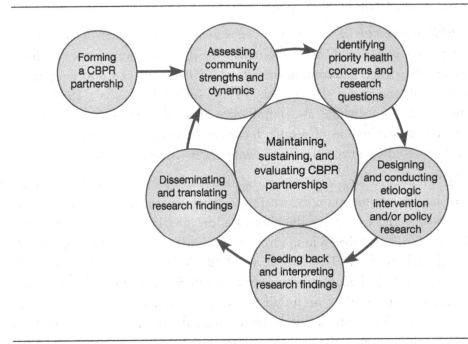

Source: Israel, B. A., Coombe, C., & McGranaghan, R., 2010.

model provides the basis for the organization of the book, as described below, and each of these components is briefly presented here. Throughout the book, aspects of these different phases will be discussed in more depth.

The first core component is *forming a CBPR partnership.* This involves such processes as identifying potential partners and communities to be involved, building trust and relationships, establishing operating norms and CBPR principles to ensure equity and power sharing, and creating an infrastructure for carrying out the research process.

The second component entails *assessing community strengths and dynamics.* This involves asking questions, such as: What are the strengths and resources in the community? What are key cultural and historical dimensions? Which are the influential organizations? Where's the power in the community? Who needs to be involved to ensure community voice?

The third component is *identifying priority local health concerns and research questions.* Key questions here include: What are the major health problems that have an impact on the community that a partnership might address? How are these problems identified and prioritized? What are the factors (for example, social, economic) that contribute to these health concerns? What are the key research questions that this study is intended to answer?

The fourth component involves *designing and conducting etiologic, intervention, and/or policy research.* This involves, for example, deciding which research design and data collection methods to use, and, as appropriate, what the most appropriate intervention strategy is, as well as determining how to implement the design and the strategies selected.

The fifth component is *feeding back and interpreting the findings* within the partnership. This involves sharing the findings from the research, such as the results of the analysis of survey or in-depth interview data, and engaging all partners in making sense of what was found.

The sixth component is *disseminating and translating research findings.* Critical questions here include: What is most important from the findings to share with the community? What are the most appropriate ways to disseminate results to the community? What is the role of community partners in publishing the results? How can the results be translated and disseminated into more broadscale interventions and policy change?

The last core component is *maintaining, sustaining, and evaluating the partnership*—which, as depicted in Figure 1.1, is an ongoing process that is at the center of all these phases and occurring throughout them. Relevant questions to address include: How well is the partnership working? How can the partnership process be improved? What aspects of the partnership need to be considered regarding sustainability, for example, enhanced relationships and capacity?

As we hope is apparent from this discussion and will be elaborated below, CBPR is an approach to research and not a specific method. Indeed, similar phases apply to the application of any approach to research. What is unique to CBPR is its emphasis on the diverse partners involved, and on striving for equal participation and ownership, reciprocity, colearning, and change.

CBPR AND HEALTH INEQUITIES: CULTURAL, SOCIAL, ECONOMIC, AND ENVIRONMENTAL CONTEXT

Although CBPR is appropriate for addressing many health problems in different community contexts, in the United States such partnership efforts have been carried out primarily in predominantly low-income communities, often communities of color (Minkler, 2004). African American, Latino, Native American, and other ethnic communities have historically been economically and politically marginalized and have compelling reasons to distrust research and researchers (Gamble, 1997; Minkler, 2004; Ribisl & Humphreys, 1998; Sloane et al., 2003). Furthermore, communities of color and low-income communities disproportionately experience the burden of higher rates of morbidity and mortality (Braveman, Cubbin, Egerter, Williams, & Pamuk, 2010; Commission for the Social Determinants of Health, 2008; Commission to Build a Healthier America, 2009; House & Williams, 2000; Schulz et al., 2002). These health inequities are associated with numerous socio-structural and physical environmental determinants of health status, such as poverty, inadequate housing, racism, lack of access to community services and employment opportunities, air pollution, and exposure to toxic substances (Braveman et al., 2010; Commission for the Social Determinants of Health, 2008; Commission to Build a Healthier America, 2009; Marmot, 2007; Schulz et al., 2002; Schulz & Northridge, 2004; Wilkinson & Pickett, 2009). Thus, it is critical that CBPR efforts strive to understand the historical and contemporary social, economic, and environmental contexts that have a significant impact on the communities involved, and work to improve the conditions that foster these health inequities. In addition, as elaborated here, it is essential that the cultural context of communities be understood and respected, explicitly informing partnership approaches to research.

CBPR is intended to bring together researchers and communities to establish trust, share power, foster colearning, enhance strengths and resources, build capacity, and examine and address community-identified needs and health problems. Given that academically-based researchers involved in CBPR are often from "outside" the community in which the research is taking place and are often different from community partners in terms of, for example, class, ethnicity, and culture, a number of power issues and tensions may arise and need to be addressed (Chávez, Duran, Baker, Avila, & Wallerstein, 2008; Minkler, 2004; Nyden & Wiewel, 1992; Ross, 2010). These differences require researchers to gain the self-awareness, knowledge, and skills to work in multicultural contexts.

Two concepts are particularly germane to our focus on CBPR and to efforts to work effectively in cultures different from the researcher's own. First, the concept of *cultural safety* originated in nursing education and has been applied to medical education in New Zealand (Crampton, Dowell, Parkin, & Thompson, 2003; Ramsden, 1997). Second, the concept of *cultural humility* has its roots in medical education in the United States (Chávez et al., 2008; Juarez et al., 2006; Ross, 2010; Tervalon & Murray-García, 1998). We provide brief descriptions of the ways in which each concept provides a framework for considering the many methods and issues addressed in this volume.

Cultural safety was first defined in New Zealand during the processes of (1) examining how relationships and power imbalances affect, and are affected by, racism, and (2) investigating the health inequities that exist between Maori (the colonized indigenous peoples of New Zealand) and non-Maori (Crampton et al., 2003; Ramsden, 1997). A policy of cultural safety gives the power to community members to say whether or not they feel safe, and professionals need to enable the community members to express the extent to which they feel risk or safety, resulting in changes in the behaviors of health professionals as appropriate. The concept of cultural safety purports that cultural factors, such as differences in worldview and language, have a major influence on current relationships between professionals and communities. Hence professionals need to acknowledge and understand that these cultural factors, as well as the social, economic, political, and historical determinants of health inequities, can contribute to communities' distrust of, and feeling unsafe about, collaboration (Ramsden, 1997). To achieve cultural safety within a CBPR partnership, it is essential to: establish deliberation and decision-making structures and procedures whereby all partners are required to express and critically examine their own realities and the attitudes they bring to the issue at hand; be open-minded toward others whose views are different from their own; consider the influences of social and historical processes on their present situation; and work toward becoming members of a partnership that anticipates differences and conflict by addressing them through processes that have been defined by all partners; and particularly by community partners, as culturally safe (Crampton et al., 2003; Ramsden, 1997).

As articulated by Tervalon and Murray-García (1998), cultural humility, rather than *cultural competence*, is the *goal* for professionals to strive to achieve, because achieving a "static notion of competence" (p. 120) is not possible. That is, professionals cannot fully master another's culture. Tervalon and Murray-García recommend a process that requires humility and commitment to ongoing self-reflection and self-critique, including identifying and examining one's own patterns of unintentional and intentional racism and classism, addressing existing power imbalances, and establishing and maintaining "mutually beneficial and non-paternalistic partnerships with communities" (p. 123). Cultural humility has three areas of focus that researchers and practitioners need to address: (1) knowledge—such as understanding the social determinants of health and health inequities (Ross, 2010; Smith, et al. 2007); (2) attitudes—which includes conscious and subconscious stereotyping and bias, and the recognition of power and privilege (Ross, 2010; Tervalon & Murray-García, 1998); and (3) skills—such as, nonhierarchical communication, and the ability to identify power imbalances and share decision making and power (Ross, 2010; Smith et al., 2007; Tervalon & Murray-García, 1998). Achieving cultural humility is reflected in the principles of CBPR, given its emphasis on colearning, which requires relinquishing one's role as the "expert" in order to recognize the role of community members as full partners in the learning process. The concepts of cultural humility and cultural safety are integral to the purpose and goals of this book.

PURPOSE AND GOALS OF THIS BOOK

As in the first edition, the overall purpose of this book is to provide students, practitioners, researchers, and community members with the knowledge and skills necessary to conduct research that is guided by community-based participatory research (CBPR) principles. CBPR is *not* a particular research design or method. Rather, it is a collaborative *approach* to research that may draw on the full range of research designs (from case study, etiological, and other nonexperimental designs to randomized control trial, longitudinal, and other experimental or quasi-experimental designs). CBPR data collection and analysis methods may involve both quantitative (for example, psychometric scaling and exposure assessment instruments) and qualitative (for example, in-depth interview and participant observation), as well as mixed-methods approaches. What distinguishes CBPR from other approaches to research is the integral link between the researcher and the researched whereby the concepts of cultural humility and cultural safety are combined with process methods and procedures to establish and maintain the research partnership.

The chapters in this volume provide a wide range of concrete examples of CBPR study designs, specific data collection and analysis methods, and innovative partnership structures and process methods. There are six new chapters in this second edition and all remaining chapters have been revised and updated. Each chapter addresses one or more methods for data collection and analysis and presents a detailed case example of CBPR from the authors' experience to examine challenges, lessons learned, and implications that can be applied to other contexts. The purpose is to describe and provide examples of how to conduct research across a variety of methods in ways that involve all partners and that attend to issues of equity, power sharing, cultural differences, dissemination, and mutual benefits to all partners. Thus, our goal is not to provide detailed explanations of how to administer data collection methods per se, for example, survey questionnaires and in-depth interviews; numerous excellent books provide such guidance (for example, Denzin & Lincoln, 2011; Fowler, 2009; Nardi, 2006; Patton, 2002), and they are referred to throughout this volume. Rather, the chapters discuss different processes for engaging community partners in research, providing numerous examples from the authors' experiences in multiple settings. In keeping with the principles of CBPR, all chapters have community partners as coauthors, ensuring that community partners' voices are reflected in the descriptions and recommendations provided.

Our work has been greatly enhanced by Minkler and Wallerstein's 2008 excellent second edition of their volume *Community-Based Participatory Research for Health*, which provides an in-depth discussion of: what CBPR is, its history, and its theoretical roots (Wallerstein & Duran, 2008); issues related to power and trust (Chávez et al., 2008); and case examples of CBPR efforts that examine topics such as ethical considerations (Farquhar & Wing, 2008) and conducting CBPR with and by diverse populations (Cheatham-Rojas & Shen, 2008). *Community-Based Participatory Research for Health* is an outstanding companion volume for this one.

We also acknowledge the international body of work in participatory research that has laid the foundation for CBPR (for examples of work in Australia and Canada and in Asia, Latin America, and Africa, see deKoning & Martin, 1996; Fals-Borda & Rahman, 1991; Park et al., 1993; Reason & Bradbury, 2006, 2008; Smith, 1999; Stringer & Genat, 2004). While recognizing and drawing upon this important work, we have chosen to focus this CBPR methods book on case examples from the United States, given the importance of attending to the context within which CBPR is conducted (Minkler & Wallerstein, 2008). Our intent is that readers will embrace the lessons learned by the authors of the chapters in this book and gain the skills needed to apply them throughout the United

States and to adapt them as appropriate to the particular context of other countries as well.

ORGANIZATION OF THIS BOOK

The chapters in this book are organized into six parts. The first introductory part provides an overview of CBPR and the entire book. The remaining five parts combine to correspond with the core components or phases in conducting CBPR presented in Figure 1.1, collapsing those seven components into the five parts of the book. The parts of the book are listed below.

1. An introduction to methods in CBPR and to the seven specific phases of the CBPR approach that are discussed in the subsequent parts.

2. Partnership formation and maintenance (phases 1 and 7 described above in Figure 1.1).

3. Community assessment and diagnosis (phase 2).

4. Definition of the issue, design and conduct of the research (phases 3 and 4).

5. Documentation and evaluation of the partnership process (phase 7, occurs throughout the process).

6. Feedback, interpretation, dissemination, and application/translation of results (phases 5 and 6).

Although these phases are presented in the book as distinct entities, as depicted in Figure 1.1, CBPR is an iterative process in which a partnership will cycle through different phases at various points in time.

Each chapter examines one or more methods organized around a case study and includes: an overview of each method; background on the CBPR partnership and project to be discussed; a description of how the method was designed and implemented within a particular phase of CBPR; an analysis of the challenges and limitations of the method within the context of CBPR; an examination of the lessons learned, implications, and recommendations for using the data collection method in CBPR projects more broadly; and a list of discussion questions to stimulate the readers' reflection and understanding of the topics covered.

When a method examined in relation to a particular phase of CBPR is also applicable to another phase, readers are referred to relevant chapters elsewhere in the book. In addition, a few methods are covered in more than one part of the book given that their application differs depending on the phase of CBPR in which they are used.

Part Two (Chapters Two, Three, and Four) focuses on one of the most critical aspects of CBPR, partnership formation and maintenance. In any CBPR project, regardless of the specific focus of the project and the data collection methods used, a number of important questions need to be addressed regarding the creation of a partnership. Such questions include the following: How is the community defined? Who will be involved, and who decides on that involvement? Are community members involved as individuals or representatives of organizations? To what extent do members of the partnership represent the community in terms of class (income and education level), gender, race, or ethnicity, and language(s) spoken? How will partners be involved? How will trust and open communication be established and maintained? How will issues of power and conflict be addressed? How will equitable participation and influence be achieved across all partners? To address these and more questions and the issue of developing and maintaining effective partnerships, Chapters Two, Three, and Four examine *process methods* that can be used. Although this phase is presented as the start of a CBPR effort, as presented in Figure 1.1, it is essential to recognize that while the initial formation of a partnership happens only once (at the beginning), continued attention needs to be paid to these partnership process methods throughout all phases of a CBPR endeavor in order to maintain the partnership.

In Chapter Two, Duran, Wallerstein, Avila, Belone, Minkler, and Foley share their experiences in building and maintaining university-community research partnerships working with tribes and rural and urban community-based organizations in New Mexico and California. They describe the "how-to" methods and challenges of partnership development and maintenance, framed specifically for academic and other outside research partners. However, all readers, including community partners and those new to CBPR, will benefit from the self-reflection and dialogue methods provided. They examine different starting points and strategies for establishing partnerships, process methods for creating and incorporating collaborative principles to foster effective partnerships, the dilemmas and challenges of collaboration between outside researchers and communities that are built into the various contexts represented and strategies for addressing these challenges (such as ways to achieve cultural humility), and process methods for maintaining partnerships over the long haul.

In Chapter Three, Becker, Israel, Gustat, Reyes, and Allen describe group process methods and facilitation strategies to establish and maintain effective partnerships. Based on concepts and findings from the field of group dynamics, they present specific techniques and activities for facilitating CBPR groups, drawing from a number of CBPR efforts in which they have been involved in Michigan and Louisiana, as well as several other locations. This chapter is organized around 12 elements of group dynamics (including equitable participation and open communication, developing trust, addressing power and influence, conflict resolution, and working in culturally diverse groups) relevant to CBPR partnerships. For each element the authors provide useful strategies and techniques for improving the partnership process with the aim of achieving the ultimate outcomes of a given CBPR effort.

In Chapter Four, one of the new chapters in the second edition, Yonas, Aronson, Coad, Eng, Petteway, Schaal, and Webb discuss structures and mechanisms that can be used by CBPR partnerships to create an infrastructure for equitable participation in decision making that anticipates and manages conflict, and is transparent and accountable to all partners. The six structures and mechanisms examined are: (1) *Undoing Racism Training* for developing a common language and framework on health equity to address power differences and historical challenges; (2) *Full Value Contract* for identifying the specific set of values, affirmed by each member of the partnership; (3) *Research Ethics Training and Certification* for community partners; (4) *Partnership Bylaws* for explicitly stating long-term principles and procedures for the partnership; (5) *CBPR Conflict Management Procedures*; and (6) *Publications and Dissemination Guidelines* for ensuring co-ownership and control of dissemination. The authors draw on the experiences of the North Carolina Community-Based Public Health Initiative Consortium and the Greensboro Health Disparities Collaborative to highlight the impetus, process, and application of these six structures and mechanisms.

Part Three (Chapters Five and Six) examines the important phase of community assessment and diagnosis. Unlike a needs assessment that focuses on identifying health needs and problems often out of context, this phase focuses on gaining a better understanding of what it is like to live in a given community.

Such understanding includes, for example, the strengths and resources that exist within the community; the history and involvement of its members and organizations; community values, culture, language, communication, and helping patterns; and community needs and concerns (Eng & Blanchard,1991); Kretzmann & McKnight, 1993; Minkler & Hancock, 2008; Steuart, 1993).

In Chapter Five, Eng, Strazza, Rhodes, Griffith, Shirah, and Mebane refer to this phase as *Action-Oriented Community Diagnosis* (AOCD). As in the phase of partnership formation, although it is necessary for AOCD to occur early in a CBPR partnership, gaining entry to a community and establishing relationships is a long-term, ongoing process for outsiders. Eng and colleagues examine several different methods for collecting and interpreting data (participant observation, key informant in-depth interviews, key informant focus group interviews, and community forums) as part of this systematic and in-depth community assessment process. They provide a case example of their experience with conducting an AOCD in Efland-Cheeks, North Carolina, describing in detail the CBPR approach they have used to engage community members and outsider researchers throughout the process, including formulating the AOCD case study research design, selecting and using multiple data collection methods, analyzing data using the technique of constant comparison to identify differences and similarities, and interpreting the findings and determining next action steps to address them. They highlight the challenges, lessons learned and implications of using this multi-method community assessment approach within the context of CBPR.

In Chapter Six, a new chapter in the second edition, Schensul, Berg, and Nair describe ways in which ethnography can be used to assess communities in the context of CBPR in health and other sectors. Ethnographic methods provide accessible ways for academically trained researchers and community researchers to partner to gather information about community life, processes, organizational structures, cultural factors, beliefs, and norms that can be used to help in planning interventions. In this chapter, the authors define ethnography, describe why it is a useful participatory community assessment approach, and how it can be used to conduct a community assessment. They present an overview of ethnographic methods including mapping, surveys, photography, GIS, semi-structured and in-depth interviews with community residents, and consensus modeling. The chapter illustrates with an example from the Institute for Community Research in Hartford, Connecticut, involving their youth action research work in which a group of youth identified hustling as a major issue. The ethnographic participatory assessment process they describe provides an in-depth and rigorous analysis of the multiple factors that contribute to underlying health inequities and the resources available to solve them.

As discussed in Part Four (Chapters Seven through Twelve), whether a CBPR project is examining a basic research question, an intervention evaluation question, or both, two major phases that go hand in hand are defining the issue or health problem that will be the focus of the project, and the design and conduct of the research. As in all phases of CBPR, a key aspect is obtaining the active involvement of all partners in the process, ideally from the very beginning. These chapters examine various data collection methods, including quantitative (for example, survey questionnaires, systematic observations) and qualitative (for example, focus group interviews, ethnography) used to identify the issues that a research partnership will investigate and address, and provide examples of different research designs and implementation processes. Although the methods examined in each chapter are quite different, there are some similar lessons learned with regard to their application as part of a CBPR effort. For example, lessons are offered on the role of community partners in developing measurement instruments, in tailoring language and data collection procedures to the local culture of the community, and in training and involving community members as data collectors.

In Chapter Seven, Schulz, Zenk, Kannan, Israel, and Stokes draw on their experience with the Healthy Environments Partnership in Detroit, Michigan. Their case example illustrates collaboration among community and academic partners in jointly developing and implementing a population-based survey administered to a stratified random sample of community residents. The survey was conducted to provide the communities involved with data that documented community concerns as well as strengths. This information helped to establish connections between those phenomena and the health of community residents, and provided information to inform specific community level interventions and policy change efforts. The authors give particular attention to processes through which representatives from diverse groups were actively engaged and the contributions of these various forms of engagement to such aspects of the survey as conceptualization, identification of specific topics and items, selection of language and wording, and administration. The authors' discussion of challenges, recommendations, and lessons learned for addressing these challenges, and implications for CBPR partnerships seeking to jointly develop and implement community surveys is particularly valuable.

In Chapter Eight, Christopher, Burhansstipanov, Knows His Gun McCormick, and Watts-Simonds discuss the CBPR process they used to modify interviewer training protocols developed originally for use with non-Native groups, in order to increase the cultural acceptability and accuracy of the survey data gathered by and from women on the Apsáalooke Reservation in Montana. They describe a history of inequality, manifest in the community's past disrespectful interactions with researchers and the community's inability to access, influence, or make use of information generated through research to improve the health of community members. The authors discuss how this history has shaped the community's current perspectives and responses to research, and the implications for training survey interviewers. Some of the training implications they address relate to issues of recruitment and enrollment of interviewees, the manner of interviewers, beginning the interview, language use, and dissemination of findings. The authors provide a summary of the lessons learned and the implications for research and interventions. Their description of the CBPR process used offers a model for partnerships seeking to improve the cultural acceptability of interview protocols, as well as the reliability of survey data gathered.

In Chapter Nine, Guzman, Kieffer, Odoms-Young, Palmisano, Salabarria-Peña, and Willis describe a multistage process that engaged community residents and policymakers in focus groups to define and develop concrete strategies to address challenges faced by women as they sought to maintain healthy diets and physical activity levels during and following pregnancy. They draw upon their experiences with several CBPR projects in Detroit, emphasizing the role and contributions of community partners throughout the focus group interview process. The process includes developing focus group guides, recruiting and training focus group moderators and note takers, recruiting participants, collecting and analyzing data, reporting the findings to the community, and engaging community members in the interpretation of results. The authors discuss challenges and limitations, lessons learned, and the implications for using a participatory approach in conducting focus group interviews. This is an important chapter offering concrete strategies for identifying community factors that contribute to health problems while engaging community women, local organizations, and state decision makers in a problem-solving discussion of future potential action strategies.

In Chapter Ten, another new chapter in this second edition, Zenk, Schulz, Izumi, Sand, Lockett, and Odoms-Young describe a series of participatory approaches used in the design and implementation of systematic observational instruments for documenting food availability, quality and costs, store characteristics, and linking the information gathered through these observational data collection instruments to dietary-related health outcomes in Detroit. The authors describe how partners based in community-based organizations, health service providers, and academic institutions worked together to design the Healthy Environments Partnership's food store audit instrument, Food Environment Audit for Diverse Neighborhoods. The authors provide direct and concrete examples of specific contributions made by community and academic partners through this participatory process to the development of this observational tool. They offer a cogent discussion of challenges faced as well as lessons learned in the process of applying a CBPR approach to the design of this food environment observational tool. This is an insightful and instructive chapter for CBPR efforts seeking to apply systematic observation to establish links between community contexts and health outcomes.

In Chapter Eleven, Berry, McQuiston, Parrado, and Olmos describe a CBPR approach to gathering ethnographic data, with the aim of understanding the social context of health and illness in a population of recent immigrants. Community-based ethnographic participatory research (CBEPR) focuses on culture and cultural interpretation and uses a participatory process. The authors discuss a case example from their experiences in Durham, North Carolina, involving Latinos who have recently immigrated to the area. They examine the roles of community and academic partner organizations and community members in proposal development, ethnographic survey development and administration, training community members as ethnographers and participant observers, and analysis and interpretation of findings. The process of cultural interpretation that they describe provides a model for conducting collaborative research that is critical and self-reflective. The authors also reflect on the capacity building of the partners involved and provide a cogent discussion of challenges and limitations, lessons learned, and implications for practice.

In Chapter Twelve, Krieger, Allen, and Takaro describe their efforts using a community-based participatory process to apply exposure assessments within two community-level interventions developed and implemented as part of the Seattle-King County Asthma Program aimed at reducing household asthma triggers in

Seattle, Washington. Their discussion of the application of different methods (for example, GIS mapping, home environmental checklists, surveys, dust samplings) using a CBPR approach to collect information on exposure to indoor environmental asthma triggers is an important one in illuminating both challenges and contributions made by joining together epidemiologists, toxicologists, community residents and community health workers. The collaborative efforts of the partners as they worked together to address challenges illustrate the emergence of trust and trustworthiness on the part of both the academic and community partners as they learned to understand and value the contributions that each made to the success of the project. The discussion of lessons learned offers insights for researchers as well as community members who are seeking to adapt complex and sophisticated technologies to address public health concerns.

As discussed in Part Five (Chapter Thirteen), it is essential that CBPR partnerships continually document and evaluate their progress toward achieving an effective collaborative process (Brooks, 2010; Butterfoss, 2009; Cheadle, Hsu, Schwartz, Pearson, Greenwald, Beery, et al., 2008; Israel et al., 2008; Lasker, Weiss, & Miller, 2001; Schulz, Israel, & Lantz, 2003; Sofaer, 2000; Tolma, Cheney, Troup, & Hann, 2009; Wallerstein et al., 2008). Such an evaluation involves focusing on the partnership's adherence to its CBPR principles, such as those described earlier (determining, for example, whether the partnership fosters colearning and capacity building; involves equitable participation, influence, and power sharing; and achieves balance between knowledge generation and action). A determination of whether and how effectively a partnership is collaborative and participatory (for example, in its project implementation process), and whether and how effectively it achieves its intermediate or impact objectives (for example, those considered essential to attaining ultimate health outcomes), can occur long before it is possible to assess the partnership's impact on health (Butterfoss, 2009; Cheadle et al., 2008; King et al., 2009; Rossi, Lipsey, & Freeman 2004; Schulz, Israel, & Lantz, 2003; Wallerstein et al., 2008). Such documentation and evaluation of the partnership process can be used by the partnership to improve its actions and in turn the achievement of its ultimate goals (Butterfoss, 2009; Brooks, 2010; Lantz, Viruell-Fuentes, Israel, Softley, & Guzman, 2001; Schulz, Israel, & Lantz, 2003; Wallerstein et al., 2008).

In Chapter Thirteen, Israel, Lantz, McGranaghan, Guzman, Lichtenstein, and Rowe describe the use of two data collection methods, in-depth, semi-structured interviews and closed-ended survey questionnaires, for assessing the process and impact of the collaborative dimensions of CBPR partnerships (for example, participatory decision making, two-way open communication, and constructive conflict resolution). They also present a conceptual framework for assessing CBPR partnerships and how it has been used to guide the Detroit Community-Academic Urban Research Center's application of these two data collection methods. The authors emphasize the role of academic and community partners in the participatory process used in designing, conducting, feeding back, and interpreting the results of these two data collection methods for evaluating this CBPR partnership. Their discussion of the strengths and weaknesses of using multiple methods is particularly informative. They provide a thorough examination of the challenges and limitations, lessons learned, and implications for the use of these methods in other CBPR contexts.

Part Six (Chapters Fourteen through Nineteen) focuses on the CBPR phases of ensuring active engagement of all partners in the feedback, interpretation, dissemination, and application/translation of results. Feedback and interpretation of findings involves all partners in reviewing results from data analysis for the purpose of sharing reactions and interpretations of what the findings mean in the context of their community. Of equal importance to the CBPR process is dissemination of findings to all partners and community members more broadly through multiple venues and in ways that are understandable, respectful and useful. Lastly, the translation and application of research findings for broadscale intervention development and policy formation is a critical link to CBPR's commitment to action and social change. The chapters in Part Six show how various data collection methods used (for example, photovoice, economic assessment, secondary data analysis) within the context of CBPR relate to these four elements of data feedback, interpretation, dissemination, and application/translation of research findings.

In Chapter Fourteen, Parker, Robins, Israel, Brakefield-Caldwell, Edgren, O'Toole, Wilkins, Batterman, and Lewis describe how they established and implemented dissemination guidelines in a CBPR partnership in order to ensure widespread dissemination of results and participation of all partners in the process. The case example draws on their experience with Community Action Against Asthma, a CBPR effort affiliated with the Detroit Community-Academic Urban Research Center. The authors examine the role of community and academic partners in deciding how to address issues in the dissemination guidelines. These issues included developing a process for selecting members to participate in presentations, establishing ground rules for collaborative authorship, drafting a list of proposed core articles and presentations, and providing feedback of results to participants and the wider community. The authors discuss the challenges and the lessons learned in creating and applying dissemination guidelines, and provide a thoughtful discussion of implications for practice.

In Chapter Fifteen, a new chapter in this edition, Baker, Motton, Barnidge, and Rose argue for the use of multiple data collection methods to provide different types of data and answers to different types of questions, which together enhance understanding of the complex set of factors that contribute to health disparities, and are essential for the development of viable and effective interventions. The authors describe the use of multiple methods in their *Men on the Move* CBPR project to assess individual, environmental, and social determinants of cardiovascular disease in a rural community in Southeast Missouri. The methods presented include community forums, economic assessment, and photo-elicitation focus groups. The authors also discuss the impact of collaboration on the development of tools, data collection, and interpretation. They provide a cogent and compelling description of how the use of multiple methods and the active engagement of community and academic partners enabled them to identify mechanisms through which individual, environmental, and social determinants influence health outcomes, and to develop interventions that address these multiple determinants.

In Chapter Sixteen, another new chapter in this volume, Corburn, Lee, Imara, and Swanston describe how map making is an essential aspect of CBPR and offer two case studies—one from East Oakland, California, and a second from Brooklyn, New York—to show how community groups use map making to highlight health equity issues in their neighborhoods. In this chapter, the authors emphasize that there are multiple approaches and technologies that can be used for the purposes of mapping, for example, hand-drawn maps, Geographic Information Systems, web-based mapping tools, and Global Positioning Systems. The two case examples of collaborative mapping processes provide compelling examples of the challenges and opportunities for community members, scientists and decision makers interested in generating visual representations of community and professional knowledge, and how that knowledge can be used to inform action.

In Chapter Seventeen, López, Robinson, and Eng discuss the use of photo-voice in the context of a CBPR approach. Photovoice is a participatory method in which community members use cameras to take pictures that represent their experiences and communicate those experiences to others (Wang & Burris, 1994). Following a brief review of the origins, diverse applications, and theoretical underpinnings of photovoice, the authors present a case example of the Inspirational Images Project that was conducted in three counties in rural, eastern North Carolina using photovoice as the primary data collection method. They provide a thorough examination of the role of academic and community partner organizations and individual breast cancer survivors, who were coinvestigators in this effort, in deciding on the design of the study and research protocol, the selection and recruitment of participants, photovoice training, data collection and theoretical sampling, data management and grounded theory analysis, data feedback and interpretation, and the engagement of local policymakers in discussing the findings. The authors share lessons learned, and draw from feedback provided by photovoice participants in providing thoughtful implications of the method for CBPR efforts more broadly.

In Chapter Eighteen, also a new chapter in this edition, Tsui, Cho, and Freudenberg define community-based participatory policy work (CBPPW), an approach to policy activism that combines CBPR and community-based policy advocacy. The authors focus on the methods that CBPPW practitioners use to collect, interpret, and apply the data that guide their activities. To illustrate the methods used in CBPPW, they draw from the experiences of three collaborative efforts to change food-related policies in New York City. The methods described in the chapter (for example, literature reviews, surveys, elicitation dialogues, participatory mapping) can help CBPPW practitioners interested in food policy work to explore multiple topics, including eliciting data on experiences of current policies, collecting and/or analyzing data on food environments, policy scanning and analysis, and eliciting views on policy opportunities. Based on the case examples, the authors note several limitations and challenges, followed by several lessons learned about conducting research to support CBPPW.

In Chapter Nineteen, Morello-Frosch, Pastor, Sadd, Prichard, and Matsuoka discuss how the Los Angeles Collaborative for Environmental Health and Justice has applied a CBPR approach to conduct research using secondary data sources. They discuss the rationale for the use of secondary data analysis and focus on how the collaborative has collectively developed research projects, interpreted data, disseminated study findings, and leveraged the results of secondary data to promote policy change and bolster organizing. The authors explore how their research approach has sought to transform traditional scientific approaches to studying community environmental health. They conclude with a discussion of some of the challenges they have faced and the lessons learned from their work. The authors provide a compelling argument that the work of the Collaborative shows that CBPR projects that emphasize secondary data analysis can be powerful agents for policy change without compromising scientific rigor.

This book ends with 13 appendixes that give the readers examples of the process methods tools, procedural documents, and data collection instruments discussed by some of the chapter authors. The intent of these appendixes is to provide further detail on methods for CBPR and the instruments developed as a result of the process. Among the process methods and procedural documents included are an informed consent form, guidelines for establishing research priorities, and dissemination guidelines. The data collection instruments include a key informant in-depth interview protocol, open-ended and closed-ended questionnaires for evaluating partnership functioning, and focus group interview guidelines. The appendixes are intended to further assist researchers, practitioners, and community partners in developing and implementing strategies and methods that strengthen the use of community-based participatory research. To expand upon these resources, a new aspect of the second edition of the book is the inclusion of downloadable supplements for each chapter which are available on the publisher's Web site. These supplements are organized to include the following categories of materials, as appropriate for each chapter: toolkits, measurement instruments, experiential learning activities/small group exercises, guideline/procedures, and PowerPoint presentations. Every item listed includes a reference, brief description of the item, and a link to a Web site, where appropriate. The inclusion of these downloadable supplements greatly expands the resources available to the reader for enhancing the use of community-based participatory research.

SUMMARY

As is evident throughout this volume, there is no one approach to community-based participatory research, and there are no process methods or data collection methods that are applicable to all CBPR efforts. Rather, community-based participatory research is a fluid, iterative approach to research, interventions, and policy change that draws from a wide range of research designs and methods and pays particular attention to issues of trust, power, cultural diversity, and equity. Furthermore, CBPR is one of many different approaches to research and action. The case examples provided throughout this book illustrate methods used by various CBPR partnerships whose goal has been to move the public health field forward by generating new knowledge (such as better information on the ways social and physical environmental factors influence health), identifying the factors associated with intervention success, and determining actions (based on partnership findings and colearning) that will effect social and behavioral change in order to eliminate health inequities.

REFERENCES

Altman, D. G. (1995). Sustaining interventions in community systems: On the relationship between researchers and communities. *Health Psychology, 14*(6), 526–536.

Argyris, C., Putnam, R., & Smith, D. M. (1985). *Action science: Concepts, methods and skills for research and intervention.* San Francisco: Jossey-Bass.

Balcazar, F. E., Taylor, R. R., Keilhofner, G. W., Tamley, K., Benziger, T., Carlin, N., et al. (2004). Participatory action research: General principles and a study with a chronic health condition. In L. A. Jason, C. B. Keys, Y. Suarez-Balcazar, R. R. Taylor, & M. I. Davis (Eds.), *Participatory community research: Theories and methods in action* (pp. 17–36). Washington, DC: American Psychological Association.

Blankenship, K. M., & Schulz, A. J. (1996, August 17). *Approaches and dilemmas in community-based research and action.* Paper presented at the Society for the Study of Social Problems, Annual Meeting, New York.

Braveman, P. A., Cubbin, C., Egerter, S., Williams, D. R., & Pamuk, E. (2010). Socioeconomic disparities in health in the United States: What the patterns tell us. *American Journal of Public Health, 100*(Suppl 1), S186–S196.

Brooks, P. E. (2010). Ethnographic evaluation of a research partnership between two African American communities and a university. *Ethnicity & Disease, 20*(Suppl 2), S2–21–29.

Bronfenbrenner, U. (1990). *The ecology of human development: Experiments by nature and design.* Cambridge, MA: Harvard University Press.

Butterfoss, F. D. (2009). Evaluating partnerships to prevent and manage chronic disease. *Preventing Chronic Disease, 6*(2), A64.

Catalani, C., & Minkler, M. (2009). Photovoice: A review of the literature in health and public health. *Health Education & Behavior, 37*(3), 424–445.

Centers for Disease Control and Prevention. (2011). Prevention Research Centers Program. Retrieved from http://www.cdc.gov/prc/

Chávez, V., Duran, B. M., Baker, Q. E., Avila, M. M., & Wallerstein, N. (2008). The dance of race and privilege in CBPR. In M. Minkler & N. Wallerstein (Eds.), *Community-based participatory research for health: From process to outcomes* (2nd ed., pp. 91–106). San Francisco: Jossey-Bass.

Cheadle, A., Hsu, C., Schwartz, P. M., Pearson, D., Greenwald, H. P., Beery, W. L., et al. (2008). Involving local health departments in community health partnerships: Evaluation results from the partnership for the public's health initiative. *Journal of Urban Health*, *85*(2), 162–177.

Cheatham-Rojas, A., & Shen, E. (2008). CBPR with Cambodian girls in Long Beach, California: A case study. In M. Minkler & N. Wallerstein (Eds.), *Community-based participatory research for health: From process to outcomes* (2nd ed., pp. 121–135). San Francisco: Jossey-Bass.

Chen, P. G., Diaz, N., Lucas, G., & Rosenthal, M. (2010). Dissemination of results in community-based participatory research. *American Journal of Preventive Medicine*, *39*, 372–378.

Clinical and Translational Science Awards Community Engagement Key Function Committee Task Force. (2011). *Principles of community engagement* (2nd ed.). Washington, DC: NIH Publication No. 11–7782.

Commission for the Social Determinants of Health. (2008). *Closing the gap in a generation: Health equity through action on the social determinants of health.* Retrieved from http://www.who .int/social_determinants.en

Commission to Build a Healthier America. (2009). *Beyond health care: New directions to a healthier America.* Retrieved from http://www.commissiononhealth.org/Report.aspx ?Publication=64498

Community-based participatory research. (2001). Special section of *American Journal of Public Health*, *91*(12), 1926–1943.

Community-based participatory research. (2005). Special section of *Environmental Health Perspectives.*

Community-based participatory research—Addressing social determinants of health: Lessons from the Urban Research Center (2002). Special section of *Health Education & Behavior*, *29*(3).

Community-based participatory research. (2003). Special section of *Journal of General Internal Medicine*, *18*(7).

Cook, W. K. (2008). Integrating research and action: A systematic review of community-based participatory research to address health disparities in environmental and occupational health in the USA. *Journal of Epidemiology & Community Health*, *62*, 668–676.

Cornwall, A. (1996). Towards participatory practice: Participatory rural appraisal (PRA) and the participatory process. In K. deKoning & M. Martin (Eds.), *Participatory research in health: issues and experiences* (pp. 94–107). London: Zed Books.

Crampton, P., Dowell, A., Parkin, C., & Thompson, C. (2003). Combating effects of racism through a cultural immersion medical education program. *Academic Medicine, 78,* 595–598.

deKoning, K., & Martin, M. (Eds.). (1996). *Participatory research in health: Issues and experiences.* London: Zed Books.

Denzin, N. K., & Lincoln, Y. S. (Eds.). (2011). *The Sage handbook of qualitative research* (4th ed.). Thousand Oaks, CA: Sage.

Eng, E., & Blanchard, L. (1991). Action-oriented community diagnosis: A health education tool. *International Quarterly of Community Health Education, 11,* 93–110.

Fals-Borda, O., & Rahman, M. A. (1991). *Action and knowledge: Breaking the monopoly with participatory action research.* New York: Intermediate Technology Publications/Apex.

Farquhar, S., & Wing, S. (2008). Methodological and ethical considerations in community-driven environmental justice research: Two case studies from rural North Carolina. In M. Minkler & N. Wallerstein (Eds.), *Community-based participatory research for health: From process to outcomes* (2nd ed., pp. 263–284). San Francisco: Jossey-Bass.

Fowler, F. J., Jr. (2009). *Survey research methods* (4th ed.). Thousand Oaks, CA: Sage.

Freire, P. (1973). *Education for critical consciousness.* New York: Seabury Press.

Freudenberg, N., Klitzman, S., & Saegert, S. (2009). *Urban health and society: Interdisciplinary approaches to research and practice.* San Francisco: Jossey-Bass.

Gaffikin, F., & Morrissey, M. (2011). *Planning in divided cities: Collaborative shaping of contested space.* Oxford: Wiley-Blackwell.

Gamble, V. N. (1997). The Tuskegee Syphilis Study and women's health. *Journal of the American Medical Women's Association, 52*(4), 195–196.

Gebbie, K. M., Rosenstock, L., & Hernandez, L. M. (Eds.). (2003). *Who will keep the public healthy? Educating public health professionals for the 21st century.* Washington, DC: National Academies Press.

Green, L. W., George, M. A., Daniel, M., Frankish, C. J., Herbert, C. J., Bowie, W. R., et al. (1995). *Study of participatory research in health promotion.* Vancouver, BC: University of British Columbia, Royal Society of Canada.

Hall, B. (1992). From margins to center? The development and purpose of participatory research. *American Sociologist 23,* 15–28.

Hatch, J., Moss, N., Saran, A., Presley-Cantrell, L., & Mallory, C. (1993). Community research: Partnership in black communities. *American Journal of Preventive Medicine, 9*(6, suppl.), 27–31.

Heron, J., & Reason, P. (2001). The practice of cooperative inquiry: Research "with" rather than "on" people. In P. Reason & H. Bradbury (Eds.), *Handbook of action research: participative inquiry and practice* (pp. 179–188). Thousand Oaks, CA: Sage.

House, J. S., & Williams, D. R. (2000). Understanding and reducing socioeconomic and racial/ethnic disparities in health. In B. D. Smedley & S. L. Syme (Eds.), *Promoting health: inter-*

vention strategies from social and behavioral research (pp. 81–124). Washington DC: National Academy Press.

Israel, B. A., Coombe, C., & McGranaghan, R. (2010). *Community-based participatory research: a partnership approach for public health* [CD-ROM]. Available from http://sitemaker.umich.edu/cbpr/home

Israel, B. A., Schulz, A. J., Parker, E. A., & Becker, A. B. (1998). Review of community-based research: Assessing partnership approaches to improve public health. *Annual Review of Public Health, 19*, 173–202.

Israel, B. A., Lichtenstein, R., Lantz, P., McGranaghan, R., Allen, A., Guzman, J. R., et al. (2001). The Detroit Community-Academic Urban Research Center: Development, implementation and evaluation. *Journal of Public Health Management and Practice, 7*(5), 1–19.

Israel, B. A., Krieger, J. W., Vlahov, D., Ciske, S. J., Foley, M., Fortin, P., et al. (2006). Challenges and facilitating factors in sustaining community-based participatory research partnerships: Lessons learned from the Detroit, New York City, and Seattle Urban Research Centers. *Journal of Urban Health, 83*(6), 1022–1040.

Israel, B. A., Schulz, A. J., Parker, E. A., Becker, A. B., Allen, A., & Guzman, J. R. (2008). Critical issues in developing and following CBPR principles. In M. Minkler & N. Wallerstein (Eds.), *Community-based participatory research for health: From process to outcomes* (2nd ed., pp. 47–66). San Francisco: Jossey-Bass.

Jason, L. A., Keys, C. B., Suarez-Balcazar, Y., Taylor, R. R., & Davis, M. I. (Eds.). (2004). *Participatory community research: Theories and methods in action.* Washington, DC: American Psychological Association.

Joyappa, V., & Miartin, D. (1996). Exploring alternative research methodologies for adult education: Participatory research, feminist research and feminist participatory research, *Adult Education Quarterly, 47*, 1–14.

Juarez, J. A., Marvel, K., Brezinski, K. L., Glazner, C., Towbin, M. M., & Lawton, S. (2006). Bridging the gap: A curriculum to teach residents cultural humility. *Family Medicine, 38*(2), 97–102.

Kemmis, S., & McTaggart, R. (2000). Participatory action research. In N. K. Denzin & Y. S. Lincoln (Eds.), *Handbook of qualitative research* (pp. 567–605). Thousand Oaks, CA: Sage.

King, G., Servais, M., Kertoy, M., Specht, J., Currie, M., Rosenbaum, P., et al. (2009). A measure of community members' perceptions of the impacts of research partnerships in health and social services. *Evaluation and Program Planning, 32*(3), 289–299.

Kretzmann, J. P., & McKnight, J. L. (1993). *Building communities from the inside out: A Path toward finding and mobilizing a community's assets.* Chicago: ACTA Publications.

Labonté, R. (1994). Health promotion and empowerment: Reflections on professional practice. *Health Education Quarterly, 21*, 253–268.

Lantz, P., Viruell-Fuentes, E., Israel, B. A., Softley, D., & Guzman, J. R. (2001). Can communities and academia work together on public health research? Evaluation results from a community-based participatory research partnership in Detroit. *Journal of Urban Health*, *78*(3), 495–507.

Lasker, R. D., Weiss, E. S., & Miller, R. (2001). Partnership synergy: A practical framework for studying and strengthening the collaborative advantage. *The Milbank Quarterly*, *79*(2), 179–205.

Maguire, P. (1987). *Doing participatory research: A feminist approach*. Amherst: University of Massachusetts School of Education.

Maguire, P. (1996). Considering more feminist participatory research: What's congruency got to do with it? *Qualitative Inquiry*, *12*(1), 106–118.

Mariella, P., Brown, E., Carter, M., & Verri, V. (2009). Tribally-driven participatory research: State of the practice and potential strategies for the future. *Journal of Health Disparities Research and Practice*, *3*, 41–58.

Marmot, M. (2007). Achieving health equity: From root causes to fair outcomes. *Lancet*, *370*(9593), 1153–1163.

McKnight, J. L. (1994). Politicizing health care. In P. Conrad & R. Kern (Eds.), *The sociology of health and illness: Critical perspectives* (4th ed., pp. 437–441). New York: St. Martin's Press.

Mercer, S. L., & Green, L. W. (2008). Federal funding and support for participatory research in public health and health care. In M. Minkler & N. Wallerstein (Eds.), *Community-based participatory research for health: From process to outcomes* (2nd ed., pp. 399–406). San Francisco: Jossey-Bass.

Minkler, M. (2004). Ethical challenges for the "outside" researcher in community-based participatory research. *Health Education & Behavior*, *31*, 684–697.

Minkler, M. & Hancock, T. (2008). Community-driven asset identification and issue selection. In M. Minkler & N. Wallerstein (Eds.), *Community-based participatory research for health: From process to outcomes* (2nd ed., pp. 153–169). San Francisco: Jossey-Bass.

Minkler, M., & Wallerstein, N. (Eds.). (2008). *Community-based participatory research for health: From process to outcomes* (2nd ed.). San Francisco: Jossey-Bass.

Mittelmark, M. B., Hunt, M. K., Heath, G. W., & Schmid, T. L. (1993). Realistic outcomes: Lessons from community-based research and demonstration programs for the prevention of cardiovascular diseases. *Journal of Public Health Policy*, *14*(4), 437–462.

Nardi, P. M. (2006). *Doing survey research: A guide to quantitative research methods* (2nd ed.). Boston: Allyn & Bacon.

National Cancer Institute. (2012). Center to Reduce Cancer Health Disparities Community Networks Program. Retrieved from http://crchd.cancer.gov/cnp/overview.html

National Institutes of Health. (2011). Clinical and Translational Science Awards Program. Retrieved from http://www.ncrr.nih.gov/clinical_research_resources/clinical_and_translational_science_awards/

National Institute on Minority Health and Health Disparities. (2011). Community-Based Participatory Research Initiative. Retrieved from http://www.nimhd.nih.gov/our_programs/communityParticipationResearch.asp

Nyden, P. W., & Wiewel, W. (1992). Collaborative research: Harnessing the tensions between researcher and practitioner. *American Sociologist, 24*(4), 43–55.

Office of Behavioral and Social Sciences Research. (2012). *Community participation in research.* Retrieved from: http://obssr.od.nih.gov/scientific_areas/methodology/community_based _participatory_research/index.aspx

Park, P. (1993). What is participatory research? A theoretical and methodological perspective. In P. Park, M. Brydon-Miller, B. Hall & T. Jackson (Eds.), *Voices of change: Participatory research in the United States and Canada* (pp. 1–19). Westport, CT: Bergin & Garvey.

Park, P., Brydon-Miller, M., Hall, B., & Jackson, T. (Eds.). (1993). *Voices of change: Participatory research in the United States and Canada.* Westport, CT: Bergin & Garvey.

Patton, M. Q. (2002). *Qualitative research and evaluation methods* (3rd ed.). Thousand Oaks, CA: Sage.

Pavlish, C. P., & Pharris, M. D. (2012). *Community-based collaborative action research: A nursing approach.* Sudbury, MA: Jones & Bartlett Learning.

Peters, M., & Robinson, V. (1984). The origins and status of action research. *Journal of Applied Behavioral Science, 29*(2), 113–124.

Ramsden, I. (1997). Cultural safety: Implementing the concept. The social force of nursing and midwifery. In P. T. Whaiti, M. McCarthy, & A. Durie (Eds.), *Mai I Rangiatea* (pp. 113–125). Auckland: Auckland University Press, Bridget Williams Books.

Reason, P. (1994). Three approaches to participative inquiry. In N. K. Denzin & Y. S. Lincoln (Eds.), *Handbook of qualitative research* (pp. 324–339), Thousand Oaks, CA: Sage.

Reason, P., & Bradbury, H. (Eds.). (2006). *Handbook of action research* (Concise Paperback ed.). London: Sage.

Reason, P., & Bradbury, H. (Eds.). (2008). *The SAGE handbook of action research: Participative inquiry and practice* (2nd ed.). London: Sage.

Ribisl, K. M., & Humphreys, K. (1998). Collaboration between professionals and mediating structures in the community: Towards a third way in health promotion. In S. A. Shumaker, J. Ockene, E. Schron, & W. McBee (Eds.), *The handbook of health behavior change* (2nd ed., pp. 535–554). New York: Springer.

Ross, L. (2010). Notes from the field: Learning cultural humility through critical incidents and central challenges in community-based participatory research. *Journal of Community Practice, 18*, 315–335.

Rossi, P. H., Lipsey, M. W., & Freeman, H. E. (2004). *Evaluation: A systematic approach* (7th ed.). Thousand Oaks, CA: Sage.

Schulz, A. J., Israel, B. A., Selig, S. M., Bayer, I. S., & Griffin, C. B. (1998). Development and implementation of principles for community-based research in public health. In R. H. MacNair (Ed.), *Research strategies for community practice* (pp. 83–110). New York: Haworth Press.

Schulz, A. J., Williams, D. R., Israel, B. A., & Lempert, L. B. (2002). Racial and spatial relations as fundamental determinants of health in Detroit. *Milbank Quarterly, 80*, 677–707.

Schulz, A. J., Israel, B. A., & Lantz, P. (2003). Instrument for evaluating dimensions of group dynamics within community-based participatory research partnerships. *Evaluation and Program Planning, 26,* 249–262.

Schulz, A. J., & Northridge, M. E. (2004). Social determinants of health and environmental health promotion. *Health Education & Behavior, 31,* 455–471.

Sloane, D. C., Diamant, A. L., Lewis, L. B., Yancey, A. K., Flynn, G., Nascimento, L. M., et al. (2003). Improving the nutritional resource environment for healthy living through community-based participatory research. *Journal of General Internal Medicine, 18,* 568–575.

Smith, L. T. (1999). *Decolonizing methodologies: Research and indigenous peoples.* London: Zed Books Ltd. and Dunedin, New Zealand: University of Otago Press.

Smith, W. R., Betancourt, J. R., Wynia, M. K., Bussey-Jones, J., Stone, V. E., Phillips, C.O., et al. (2007). Recommendations for teaching about racial and ethnic disparities in health and health care. *Annals of Internal Medicine, 147*(9), 654–665.

Sofaer, S. (2000). *Working together, moving ahead: A manual to support effective community health coalitions.* New York: Baruch College School of Public Affairs.

Steuart, G. W. (1993). Social and cultural perspectives: Community intervention and mental health. *Health Education Quarterly, 20*(suppl 1), 99–111.

Stokols, D. (1996). Translating social ecological theory into guidelines for community health promotion. *American Journal of Health Promotion, 10,* 282–298.

Stringer, E. T. (2007). *Action research: A handbook for practitioners* (3rd ed.). Thousand Oaks, CA: Sage.

Stringer, E. T., & Genat, W. (2004). *Action research in health practice.* Upper Saddle River, NJ: Prentice Hall.

Suarez-Balcazar, Y., Davis, M. I., Ferrari, J., Nyden, P., Olson, B., Alvarez, J., et al. (2004). University-community partnerships: A framework and an exemplar. In L. A. Jason, C. B. Keys, Y. Suarez-Balcazar, R. R. Taylor, & M. I. Davis (Eds.), *Participatory community research: Theories and methods in action* (pp. 105–120). Washington, DC: American Psychological Association.

Tandon, R. (1996). The historical roots and contemporary tendencies in participatory research: Implications for health care. In P. Reason & H. Bradbury (Eds.), *Participatory research in health: Issues and experiences* (2nd ed., pp. 19–26). London: Zed Books.

Tervalon, M., & Murray-García, J. (1998). Cultural humility vs. cultural competence: A critical distinction in defining physician training outcomes in medical education. *Journal of Health Care for the Poor and Underserved, 9*(2), 117–125.

Tolma, E. L., Cheney, M. K., Troup, P., & Hann, N. (2009). Designing the process evaluation for the collaborative planning of a local turning point partnership. *Health Promotion Practice, 10*(4), 537–548.

Torbert, W. R., & Taylor, S. S. (2008). Action inquiry: Interweaving multiple qualities of attention for timely action. In P. Reason & H. Bradbury (Eds.), *Handbook of action research: Participative inquiry and practice* (pp. 239–251). Thousand Oaks, CA: Sage.

Trickett, E. J. (2011). Community-based participatory research as worldview or instrumental strategy: Is it lost in translation(al) research? *American Journal of Public Health*, *101*(8), 1353–1355.

Viswanathan, M., Ammerman, A., Eng, E., Gartlehner, G., Lohr, K., Griffith, D., et al. (2004). *Community-Based Participatory Research*. RTI International-University of North Carolina Evidence-Based Practice Center, Contract No. 290–02–0016, Agency for Healthcare Research and Quality. Retrieved from: http://www.ahrq.gov/clinic/epcsums/cbprsum.htm

Wallerstein, N., & Duran, B. M. (2008). The theoretical, historical, and practice roots of CBPR. In M. Minkler & N. Wallerstein (Eds.), *Community-based participatory research for health: From process to outcomes* (2nd ed., pp. 25–46). San Francisco: Jossey-Bass.

Wallerstein, N., Oetzel, J., Duran, B., Tafoya, G., Belone, L., & Rae, R. (2008). What predicts outcomes in CBPR? In M. Minkler & N. Wallerstein (Eds.), *Community-based participatory research for health: From process to outcomes* (2nd ed., pp. 371–394). San Francisco: Jossey-Bass.

Wang, C., & Burris, M. A. (1994). Empowerment through photo novella: Portraits of participation. *Health Education Quarterly*, *21*, 171–186.

Whyte, W. F. (1991). *Participatory action research*. Newbury Park, CA: Sage.

Wilkinson, R., & Pickett, K. (2009). *The spirit level: Why more equal societies almost always do better*. London: Allen Lane.

Zimmerman, S., Tilly, J., Cohen, L., & Love, K. (2009). *A manual for community-based participatory research: Using research to improve practice and inform policy in assisted living*. Retrieved from http://www.shepscenter.unc.edu/research_programs/aging/publications/CEAL-UNC%20Manual%20for%20Community-Based%20Participatory%20Research-1.pdf

PART TWO

PARTNERSHIP FORMATION AND MAINTENANCE

Partnership formation and maintenance are fundamental components of all community-based participatory research efforts. Many of the guiding principles for conducting CBPR focus on the roles of partners and partnerships in the process. As described in the Introduction to this volume and elsewhere (Israel, Schulz, Parker, & Becker, 1998; Israel et al., 2008), these principles include an emphasis on developing collaborative, equitable partnerships; promoting capacity building and colearning among all partners; disseminating results to all partners and involving all partners in the dissemination process; and involving a long-term process and commitment. At the same time, community-researcher partnerships are complex and multidimensional and can range from driven and initiated by the community on one end of a continuum to initiated and controlled by university or other outside researchers on the other end (Minkler & Wallerstein, 2008). Although numerous benefits have been identified from partners working together successfully across diverse backgrounds, values, priorities, and expertise (Israel et al., 1998, 2008; Northridge et al., 2000; Schulz et al., 2003), developing and maintaining successful partnerships is considered one of the most challenging aspects of CBPR efforts (Green et al., 1995; Israel et al., 2001; Sullivan et al., 2003).

In Part Two, we focus on methods for forming and maintaining research partnerships regardless of the specific focus of the project and data collection methods used. A range of "process methods" that can be used to establish and maintain research partnerships are examined in Chapters Two, Three, and Four.

As discussed in these chapters, and Chapter One (see Figure 1.1 of the core phases of CBPR) although it is essential to pay attention to partnership-related issues during the initial phases of a CBPR endeavor, continual attention to maintaining the partnership over time is equally essential. Together these chapters illustrate numerous formal and informal strategies, techniques, structures, and mechanisms that can be used by CBPR partnerships to ensure ongoing attention to and success in maintaining authentic, equitable partnerships.

In Chapter Two, *Developing and Maintaining Partnerships with Communities*, Duran, Wallerstein, Avila, Belone, Minkler, and Foley draw upon their experiences working directly with American Indian tribes and urban and rural community-based organizations in New Mexico and California. They describe the "how-to" methods and challenges of partnership development and maintenance. They examine different starting points and strategies for establishing partnerships, process methods for creating and incorporating collaborative principles to foster effective partnerships, the dilemmas and challenges of collaboration between outside researchers and communities that are built into the various contexts represented and strategies for addressing these challenges, and process methods for maintaining partnerships over the long haul.

The authors' case examples reflect the diversity of conceptualizations of community partners, which in turn highlights the relevance of their recommended strategies to the diversity of the settings in which we work. Throughout the chapter, the authors stress the need for critical self-reflection and ongoing attention to deeply rooted issues, such as historic legacies and current identities and contexts, as these influence the development and maintenance of CBPR partnerships.

In Chapter Three, *Strategies and Techniques for Effective Group Process in Community-Based Participatory Research Partnerships*, Becker, Israel, Gustat, Reyes, and Allen draw upon the literature on the evaluation of CBPR partnerships and group dynamics to argue for the necessity of CBPR partnerships to attend to group processes in order to achieve the goals and objectives of the research and action projects involved. The chapter is organized around twelve elements of group dynamics that are relevant to CBPR partnerships (for example, equitable participation and open communication, establishing norms for working together, developing goals and objectives, addressing power and influence, resolving conflicts, working in culturally diverse groups). For each of these elements, the authors provide concrete examples of numerous strategies, techniques, and specific exercises that they have used for developing and maintaining effective CBPR partnerships in their work in Michigan, Louisiana, and several other locations. The strategies and techniques described in this chapter are useful in multiple contexts for strengthening CBPR partnerships through appropriate attention to group dynamics.

In Chapter Four, *Infrastructure for Equitable Decision Making in Research*, Yonas, Eng, Aronson, Coad, Petteway, Schaal, and Webb discuss structures and mechanisms that can be used by CBPR partnerships to create an infrastructure for equitable participation in decision-making. This framework emphasizes decision-making processes that anticipate and effectively addresses conflict, is transparent and that is accountable to all partners. The six structures and mechanisms examined are: (1) *Undoing Racism Training* for developing a common language and framework on health equity to address power differences and historical challenges; (2) *Full Value Contract* for identifying the specific set of values, affirmed by each member of the partnership; (3) *Research Ethics Training and Certification* for community partners; (4) *Partnership Bylaws* for explicitly stating long-term principles and procedures for the partnership; (5) *Managing and Addressing Conflict* strategies; and (6) *Publications and Dissemination Guidelines* for ensuring coownership and control of dissemination. The authors draw on the experiences of the North Carolina Community-Based Public Health Initiative Consortium and the Greensboro Health Disparities Consortium to highlight the impetus, process, and application of these six structures and mechanisms.

REFERENCES

Green, L. W., George, M. A., Daniel, M., Frankish, C. J., Herbert, C. J., Bowie, W. R., et al. (1995). *Study of participatory research in health promotion.* Vancouver, BC: University of British Columbia, Royal Society of Canada.

Israel, B. A., Schulz, A. J., Parker, E. A., & Becker, A. B. (1998). Review of community-based research: Assessing partnership approaches to improve public health. *Annual Review of Public Health, 19*, 173–202.

Israel, B. A., Lichtenstein, R., Lantz, P., McGranaghan, R., Allen, A., Guzman, J. R., et al. (2001). The Detroit Community-Academic Urban Research Center: Development, implementation and evaluation. *Journal of Public Health Management and Practice, 7*(5), 1–19.

Israel, B. A., Schulz, A. J., Parker, E. A., Becker, A. B., Allen, A., & Guzman, J. R. (2008). Critical issues in developing and following community-based participatory research principles.

In M. Minkler & N. Wallerstein (Eds.), *Community-based participatory research for health: From process to outcomes* (2nd ed., pp. 47–66). San Francisco: Jossey-Bass.

Minkler, M., & Wallerstein, N. (Eds.). (2008). *Community-based participatory research for health: From process to outcomes* (2nd ed.). San Francisco: Jossey-Bass.

Northridge, M. E., Vallone, D., Merzel, C., Greene, D., Shepard, P. M., Cohall, A. T., et al. (2000). The adolescent years: An academic-community partnership in Harlem comes of age. *Journal of Public Health Management & Practice, 6*(1), 53–60.

Schulz, A. J., Israel, B. A., Parker, E. A., Locket, M., Hill, Y., & Wills, R. (2003). Engaging women in community-based participatory research for health: The East Side Village Health Worker Partnership. In M. Minkler & N. Wallerstein (Eds.), *Community-based participatory research for health* (pp. 293–315). San Francisco: Jossey-Bass.

Sullivan, M., Chao, S., Allen, C. A., Koné, A., Pierre-Louis, M., & Krieger, J. (2003). Community-research partnerships: Perspectives from the field. In M. Minkler & N. Wallerstein (Eds.), *Community-based participatory research for health* (pp. 113–130). San Francisco: Jossey-Bass.

Chapter 2

DEVELOPING AND
MAINTAINING PARTNERSHIPS
WITH COMMUNITIES

BONNIE DURAN

NINA WALLERSTEIN

MAGDALENA M. AVILA

LORENDA BELONE

MEREDITH MINKLER

KEVIN FOLEY

Most of the guiding principles for conducting community-based participatory research are directed at partners and partnerships. CBPR is described as supporting "collaborative, equitable partnerships in all phases of the research," which will "promote co-learning and capacity building among partners," "disseminate findings and knowledge gained to all partners and involve all partners in the dissemination process" (Israel et al., 2008).

CBPR *is* dependent on partnerships, yet the skills and methods we need to develop and maintain collaborative research partnerships often are not taught or explored in academic settings. In addition, academic research partners, based in universities, health and social service agencies, and other institutions, may read about the importance of partnerships, yet neglect to engage in ongoing **self-reflection** about the inevitable challenges of initiating, nurturing and maintaining partnerships. Finally, community research partners may not sufficiently be aware of the imperatives of university and other institutional settings which may challenge the development of mutually beneficial partnerships.

Community-academic research partnerships are multi-dimensional and range across a continuum with partnerships initiated and driven by the community at one end and initiated and controlled by university or other "outside expert" collaborations at the other (Minkler & Wallerstein, 2008). Traditionally, universities or health and social service agencies have identified funding sources and approached communities for their involvement in a research effort. Increasingly, however, ongoing partnerships are being developed to which multiple groups of stakeholders bring their concerns and skills to create a partnership or community-initiated research pursuits. Most often, in the course of a CBPR project, relationships evolve with projects, which may have been initiated by one partner, becoming more collaborative and equitable in their decision making over time.

It is still rare, however, for community partners to serve as the sole principal investigator to lead a CBPR project, as the protocols and governing structures of research most often reside in academic institutions, which have the benefit of methodological expertise, resources to execute grant proposals, regulatory bodies to protect human subjects, and the explicit scholarly mission of the academy. Although some important exceptions exist (for example, the research structures being instituted in some tribal nations [Becenti-Pigman, et al., 2008] and community-based organizations, such as West Harlem Environmental Action and the Hartford Hispanic Council), the current concentration of research resources in the academy requires careful attention to redressing power imbalances with community partners for mutually beneficial collaborations.

Those of us who are professionally trained researchers may be fortunate to build on existing relationships for **Community Partnerships,** either through groundwork laid by our academic and community colleagues or our own more personal connections with the community. Some of us may share common identities with the community; or may be "insider-outsiders" with bonds to the community based on ethnic identity, gender, sexual orientation, or disability, for example, yet we are outsiders based on other factors, such as our educational attainment or a change in class status, and the privileges that they convey. We may have to start de novo and therefore face challenges in being accepted. Many times we have to leave our communities to pursue opportunities, and the context of our rootedness to our communities' changes. We may face failure and have to leave a community. If our partnership relationships are less than optimal during a certain period, we may be tempted to blame our institutions or our community partners, yet it is essential that we reflect on our own roles. In all cases, we need to ask ourselves questions, such as: "Why do we want to work with a particular community? What are the benefits to us? To the community? What is the mutual benefit?"

Those of us who have engaged in CBPR to bring about change will recognize that the process is fluid, dynamic, at times fast-paced and at times slow, and always requires long-term commitment. The old axiom "plan and then implement the plan" is too simplistic. To succeed, CBPR processes, like other forms of research, must be open to permutations and reformulations. Unexpected obstacles can surface, such as staff turnover or changes in leadership, or even just a better idea. For example, when community partners in Tar Creek, Oklahoma, objected to the idea of using white children as controls, given that only Native Americans would receive the potential benefits of an intervention to reduce lead exposures, the academic research partners agreed to the change. The community partners' objection involved the fact that as Native Americans, they had often been excluded from benefits that were available to members of the dominant culture, and they did not want to be part of a study in which exclusion—in this case, of white children—was involved, especially as all children in the area were experiencing the same problematic exposures. Although including white children in the intervention group and, thereby eliminating the control group, somewhat weakened the research design, the processes and outcomes of this change proved positive (since showing the benefits to white children as well improved the study's political value) and further helped in building initial trust and collaboration (Petersen et al., 2007). Partnership means spending the time to develop trust and, most important, spending time to develop the structures that support trust, so that unexpected new directions or setbacks can be seen as part of a long-term process that will continue.

The purpose of this chapter is to describe the "how-to" methods and challenges of partnership development and maintenance, primarily for academic and other outside research partners. We expect, however, that all readers, including community partners and those new to CBPR, will benefit from the self-reflection and dialogue presented. In this chapter we discuss strategies and different starting points for developing partnerships, methods for incorporating and developing collaborative principles to support effective partnerships, and skills for maintaining partnerships over the long haul.

In this chapter, we draw on our own research experience and that of colleagues, working directly with tribes and community-based organizations (CBOs). Although we often use the shorthand "university" (when referring to researchers) and "community" partners, the reader is reminded that researchers may be housed in many institutions, such as health and human service departments, government and private nonprofit agencies, and integrated care systems. Community members and partners may be the staff and membership of CBOs, including professionals with research expertise, or the term may refer to residents of shared neighborhoods, grassroots organizations, or communities of identity, such as gay or bisexual men who are HIV-positive. In the sections that follow, we have purposely chosen diverse case examples that utilize different conceptualizations of community partners as we illustrate questions for critical reflection by researchers.

HOW DO WE START?

There is no one starting place, no single technique, no magic bullet for the development of relationships and partnerships with communities. For the purposes of this chapter, we define community as a group of people having a shared identity, whether it is based on geography; political affiliation; culture or race/ethnicity; faith; sovereign tribal nationhood; institutional connection, such as schools or workplaces; or shared group identification (Minkler, 2012; Minkler & Wallerstein, 2008; Rothman, 2008). Sometimes, when outside researchers partner with geographic communities, there is a tendency to accept outside-defined boundaries, such as census or zip code tracts used for data collection. It is critical, however, that we recognize that residents within a geographic area may have their own designations, for example, the neighborhood across the tracks, or the location of important history. It is this shared identity that facilitates partnerships, and outside researchers must begin by getting to know how community members define their own communities (see Chapter One for a discussion of community as a unit of identity).

Getting to know the "community" in all its complexity and in ways that are consistent with the principles of CBPR also means looking at communities through new lenses. For several decades, Kretzmann and McKnight (1993; McKnight & Kretzmann, 2012), have admonished health and social service professionals to look for community assets, rather than simply community needs, an approach espoused by the more recently articulated community-building strategies (Walter & Hyde, 2012). These strengths may reside within individuals, and within those community-based organizations that give the community voice, such as parent-teacher organizations, safety watch groups, or environmental justice coalitions. In an example of a CBPR project with Tribal Colleges and Universities (TCU) across the rural United States, tribal college expertise in accommodating multitribal student bodies was essential for developing common measures to assess capacities for drug and alcohol identification and interventions. In addition, high-capacity TCUs (College, 2011) with long-standing mechanisms for tribal review shared their materials and provided training to other colleges just initiating these protections.

When we develop academic-community research partnerships that do not come directly from the community, it is important that they not be window dressing, put together at the last minute because of a grant mandate. We need to consider how to make our partnerships reflect the culture of the community, respecting the community's expert knowledge concerning its assets as well as its needs, and not simply replicate "professional cultures" to forge egalitarian CBPR partnerships. (See Chapter Five for a discussion of the use of in-depth interviews and focus groups to assess community strengths as well as challenges.)

Starting a research relationship for a specific project is always easier if we have a previous positive connection with the community. Students as research assistants have often facilitated trust and rapport if they come from similar ethnic/ racial or other social identities shared with the communities. University reputations and previous institutional histories have not always been positive however. Many times communities feel "mined" by research partnerships, with consequences of mistrust. Most often, we face a constellation of these facilitators and challenges.

Without any previous connections, we need to rely on hard work and time to build the relationships. Public health professor and CBPR partner Mary Northridge's admonitions (2003) to university faculty who desire to engage in CBPR are apropos: listen, show up, be yourself, believe in social justice, and demonstrate respect through willingness to meet on the community's turf, rather than expecting residents to come to the university. Just showing up, however, may make the situation worse if outside researchers are inflexible about their research agenda, or if they underestimate the knowledge of community partners. Respect is an earned quality, which includes being responsive to the diverse needs of different constituents and partners. For example, former health department employees Galen Ellis and Sheryl Walton in West Contra Costa County, California, write about how it was important not merely to show up but also to help cook for a community memorial service after a drive-by shooting as part of gaining credibility (Ellis & Walton, 2012). The Healthy Neighborhood Project they helped create went on to become an effective community-health department collaboration for research and action (Ellis & Walton, 2012). This partnership may never have achieved success had not the health department staff literally and figuratively shown up for multiple events important to local residents.

Five strategies are helpful for university or other institutional-based researchers as we seek to begin and sustain a community partnership:

1. Self-reflecting on our own and our institutional base's capacities, resources, and potential liabilities as health professionals/academics interested in engaging with the community, including identifying historical and current relationships between the university and community;

2. Identifying potential partners and partnerships through appropriate networks, associations, and leaders;

3. Negotiating a research agenda based on a common framework on mechanisms for change;

4. Using up, down, and peer mentoring and apprenticeship across the CBPR partnership; and

5. Creating and nurturing structures to sustain partnerships, through constituency building and organizational development.

These strategies are not sequential and steps 3–5 may take place simultaneously, yet all require continual attention; earlier strategies also need to be revisited, especially when new partners join a long-standing relationship.

Strategy 1: Reflect on Own Capacities and Those of Our Institutions to Engage in Research Partnerships

To assess our capacities and resources as researchers working with communities, it is important to think about: our own strengths as individuals and as the institutions we represent; our weaknesses as individuals and institutions; the benefits we might gain; and the dangers or concerns we might face. These issues include being self-reflective about our own positions of power in relation to the communities with whom we partner, which includes the historical and current relationship of our institution to these same communities (Tuhiwai-Smith, 2005; Israel et al., 2008; Wallerstein, 1999).

One of the most important skills in this assessment of our own capacities is the ability to listen to ourselves, as well as to, and with, our community partners. Such active and introspective listening requires concrete and measureable skills that include patience, silence, and an attitude of openness, humility, discovery, and nondefensiveness (Chávez, Duran, Baker, Avila, & Wallerstein, 2008).

For CBPR researchers in academic settings, part of listening to our history involves reflecting on and learning from the activist scholar traditions that reemerged in the 1960s, when many researchers moved out of the academy to participate in social movements to improve economic conditions (MacDonnel, 1986). For activist scholars, these historical roles included shining a spotlight on resistance among marginalized communities; the role of culture in everyday practices; and the reality of community agencies to define their agendas and identities as decision makers (Ong, 1987).

In the 1970s and 1980s, a key innovation of poststructuralist analysis and the *new social movements* was the shift from a predominantly Marxist analysis, to a deeper understanding of the way dominant society served to exclude and disadvantage cultures or groups due to race, gender, sexuality, and class, or an intersection of these (Laclau & Mouffe, 1985). Academics engaged in participatory research began to see themselves as moving beyond the legacy of ventriloquism (or speaking *for* community partners) to making room for the voice of people's lived experiences, with the belief that "only those directly concerned can speak in a practical way on their own behalf" (MacDonnel, 1986, pg. 16). Yet, beyond giving voice, the role of the academic can shift toward "weaken[ing] the existing links between power and knowledge" to prevent local knowledge from being devalued and undermined (MacDonnel, 1986, pg. 16). We can help create multiple spaces (for example, meetings and publications) in which the lived experience, core values, and diverse epistemologies of our partners can be heard and validated (Quijano, 2007; Spivak, 1990).

One example of this space was at a recent "facilitated CBPR discussion" at the national Native Research Network (NRN) meeting (http://nativeresearchnetwork .org/National%20Conference.htm). The NRN is comprised of academic and community indigenous scholars, and includes non-Native allies. The planners rightly assumed everyone would be CBPR practitioners, and organized the event around lessons learned, problem solving, and considerations of the unique position of Indigenous CBPR researchers. After a rich joint discussion, indigenous and ally participants separated and a palpable energy shift occurred. The diverse but all-indigenous group identified a "third space" of knowledge development, defined as neither Western nor exclusively indigenous, and spoken about in shorthand terms as a "felt sense," not captured adequately by research concepts. Due to the exclusively indigenous space, community scholars with traditional knowledge credentials felt at ease to express their truths about the partnered research process and their ideas about **culture-centered interventions.** The group identified gaps in the current knowledge base and began to identify "alter/native" research agendas. Dependent upon an exclusively indigenous space for discussion, it was the highest rated event of the conference and this "Third Space" of Indigenous Knowledge Development became the theme of the next annual conference. Although the non-Native research allies meeting separately may not have fully understood the need for an exclusively indigenous space, allies promote voice and theory development when they offer opportunities for and support community-group caucusing.

The second process of listening involves making explicit historical abuses (for example, the academic invention of "primitive societies" in part as a justification for colonization [Said, 1978]). Stories of alleged abuse (as in the Havasupai tribe's multimillion-dollar lawsuit against Arizona State University for nonconsenting use of blood samples) add potency in the face of historical realities (Potkonjak, 2004). One strategy to reduce mistrust involves what Foucault has termed, "effective history"—a retelling of the past that refutes the dominant perspective (Dean, 1994), that is, creating space for community partners to construct the histories of previous relationships with universities that contribute to mistrust and misunderstanding. CBPR researchers can then articulate a new approach that is not an inevitable outcome of the past.

The third process of listening is to uncover the role of power dynamics in our own collaborative processes; "expert" or "scientific knowledge," for example, may inadvertently prevent community knowledge from being viewed as equally legitimate. Many white or middle-class academics working in communities of color may fail to recognize the ways in which "unearned privilege" may foster or may maintain internalized oppression of community members who assume they themselves have less to offer. In addition, as institution-based researchers, we often have the power of resources. For example, our capacity to develop subcontracts with community partners may be potentially problematic if community members become more interested in resources, rather than in the research questions per se. Increasingly, however, savvy community partners are expecting a shared distribution of resources to build their own research capacities. Finally, as part of self-reflection, we encourage each of us who has privilege to consider how best to be an ally to our research colleagues of color and to the communities with which we work. All of us have intersecting contexts, being in the dominant group in terms of power in some domains (for example, race/ethnicity, class, sexual orientation, ability/disability) but not others (Graham, Brown-Jeffy, Aronson, & Stephens 2011). For example, junior minority faculty may lead research projects, but not have the power to influence their institutions' priorities for hiring, promotion, or student recruitment toward diversity (Stanley, 2006).

Although we may face formidable obstacles to changing power imbalances (for example, funding mandates and norms that support the superior validity of "expert knowledge"), as Foucault (1980) reminds us, power is inherently unstable and therefore able to be challenged. Seifer and colleagues noted the importance of centers in the academy which support community-engaged scholarship; interdisciplinary values; and community coinvestigators (Calleson, Siefer, & Maurana 2002; Seifer, 2008).

Although some academics share identities with communities, it is important to live with the contradictions of finding how our lived experiences of oppression intersect with those of our partners, yet not take advantage and claim the same level of marginalization. By recognizing our privilege, our power bases, we can have the integrity to create authentic partnerships (Labonté, 2012), which honor the strengths and knowledge each partner brings.

Strategy 2: Identify Potential Partners and Partnerships Through Appropriate Networks, Associations, and Leaders

An important CBPR task is to identify potential community partners, and consider the practical, political, and personal implications of partnership choices. Ideally in CBPR, the research topic comes from the community, and a concerned CBO may approach the university, health department, or other research entity about partnering. Frequently, however, the university wishes to initiate a partnership, and these steps may therefore be useful.

First, outside researchers should plan to spend considerable time getting to know the community before they approach individuals, groups or organizations about partnering. This process is important for credibility (Hancock & Minkler, 2012; Lewis & Ford, 1990) and for learning who may be most appropriate partners.

One of the authors of this chapter (Minkler) and her primary research partner (a graduate student with a disability) had each been involved with the local disability community for many years before they discussed the possibility of conducting a CBPR project with that community. Because the topic was a controversial one (that is, broadening the dialogue within the disability community about attitudes toward "death with dignity" legislation), assessing key community stakeholders' interest in advance was imperative; they agreed that they would not proceed without community buy-in. Their status, as an able-bodied ally and a member of the community, helped them know which stakeholders to approach for guidance, which organizations to approach about potential partnering, and, once an agreement was achieved, how to form a diverse advisory committee whose membership reflected differences of opinion about this topic in the larger disability community (Fadem et al., 2003).

For researchers who are not as familiar with the community with which they hope to partner, a variety of tools may be useful. Action-oriented community assessment and methods for identifying "movers and shakers" can help find community partners and learn about community-perceived assets and concerns (Eng & Blanchard, 1990–1991; Hancock & Minkler, 2012; Chapter Five in this volume). Such techniques, however, are best used with community partners, who can help determine which methods will most appropriately capture the unique context of their community.

In a project in which chapter authors Duran and Foley were involved, a farsighted division of the tribal health department received a large federal grant, aimed at developing and integrating HIV services with a large tribe in the Southwest. The tribal council Health Committee, however, as the "lead" agency responsible for research oversight, had factions that were opposed to this work; some members thought people with HIV should be quarantined. After the stigma was uncovered, Duran and Foley deliberately chose to work with a nongovernmental agency (NGO) and those supporters within the tribal health department to steer clear of more contentious tribal council elements. (See Exhibit 2.1 for a more detailed discussion of this example from the perspective of the community-based organization.)

Exhibit 2.1: The CBO Perspective

From a community-based organization (CBO) perspective, universities, health departments or other research institutions need to understand a range of concerns, that is, the potential for draining resources, talent or money from the community; the potential competition among different agencies and their regulations; the distinct relations that agencies and community members have with the university; and the potential that university guidelines might not reflect collaborative relationships. All of these issues were epitomized in one community-initiated research project in the Southwest.

In 2001, the clinical director of a Native American alcohol treatment CBO (Foley, one of the authors of this chapter) contemplated the possibility of applying for an integration of services research project, and called another community-based agency serving Native clients that provided HIV case management services. The executive director of the case management agency was interested, so a meeting was called with medical and social services providers and university researchers (led by Duran, one of the authors of this chapter) to discuss forming a collaborative to apply for the grant. From the outset, there was an agreement to start from culturally centered interventions and to make traditional healers central.

Partnership concerns remained, however. The HIV case management agency, with the Indian Health Service and the tribal government, had worked for five years on the first round of funding with Dr. Duran and wanted her as evaluator on the next five-year submission. Dr. Foley expressed his concern that his board might not buy into contracting for evaluation services. The CBO board had a policy of not hiring outside contractors because in the past outside contractors were not invested in the organization; the board's preference was to hire local evaluators to develop local capacity. Drs. Foley and Duran had known each other for several years, however, and trust had already been established. Hence Dr. Foley convinced his board to participate and to contract with the university. As part of the buy-in to working with the university, Dr. Duran assisted in arranging for training all CBO staff on motivational interviewing at no cost. University guidelines however made it difficult to view Dr. Foley as an equal partner. Although he was Principal Investigator for the federal funding, the university institutional review board (IRB) refused to allow his name to be placed on the participant consent form. The research collaborative was forced to accept the IRB's conditions, although they dishonored the community partner. Because of the long-standing relationship between Drs. Duran and Foley and the evolving relationship with other partners, the partnership has continued and been able to openly reflect on and negotiate the issues as they emerge.

Recognizing the multiple voices of a "single" community acknowledges the challenges of community participation. It is often easier to attract service professionals and policymakers to board meetings than it is to expect community members (such as parents, low-wage workers, and the elderly) to come out on a regular basis, although service providers may also be community members, especially staff of local CBOs. Selection criteria for new partners might include:

people (and organizations) who are well respected, knowledgeable about the community, with a long-standing history of working on community issues, and with prior positive history of working in partnerships. For policy-oriented CBPR, it is increasingly recognized that strong community partners with their own history of organizing are essential for advocacy work required in translating science into policy change (Minkler et al., 2011; Wing, Avery Horton, Muhammad et al., 2008). In a recent NIEHS-funded project on health and safety issues for restaurant workers in San Francisco's Chinatown, having the long-standing and well-respected Chinese Progressive Association as the community partner was instrumental in furthering media advocacy and development and signing into law the first wage theft ordinance in the nation (Chang, Salvatore, Tau Lee, Liu, & Minkler, 2012). With effective implementation, the ordinance, which attempts to end such practices as paying below minimum wage, withholding back wages, sometimes for months, and having the boss take tip money, could make a substantial contribution to the health and well-being of low-wage workers and their families living in poverty. Community partners may consider their own criteria for academic partners, such as people who have demonstrated commitment to the community independent of specific funding.

Some of the most obvious barriers to attendance for community members at partnership meetings can be overcome by providing food, transportation, and child care; and holding meetings at the community partner organizations, though job and family demands can take priority. In the Healthy Neighborhoods Project, the health department began granting flex time to employees whose ability to work from noon to 9 p.m. and on weekends enabled them to be more available for times that worked best for community residents. As the partnership matured, this show of respect was reciprocated, as community members began arranging their schedules to be able to attend daytime events at the health department (Ellis & Walton, 2012).

Encouraging active participation in CBPR activities also requires methods to reduce the intimidation community members may feel in groups characterized by status differences, including nominal group processes (Delbecq, Van de Ven, & Gustafson, 1975); collaborative mapping of community risks and assets (Hancock & Minkler, 2012); establishing partnership norms (Israel et al., 2008); and support for bringing community voices to the table. (See Chapters Three and Four in this volume for a discussion of different methods that can be used to foster equitable relationships.)

Although the importance of constantly working to deepen the participation of community partners cannot be overstated, outside researchers also need to be aware of the impacts of racism on both the context and process of the work. Camara Jones's analysis of institutional, interpersonal, and internalized racism is helpful for understanding their impact on partnering (Jones, 2000). Community members may have differential access to knowledge and representation in institutions to enable them to connect as community partners. They may feel uncomfortable with the potential for stereotyping and believe they do not have opinions to offer. Or they may want to protect the community's hidden voices from perceived threats (Scott, 1990). To avoid such situations, and to confront them more honestly when they do arise, the concept of **cultural humility** (Chávez et al., 2008; Tervalon & Murray-García, 1998) has proven useful. Cultural humility is more realistic and useful, we believe, than the more popular term *cultural competence*—an end point that we can never truly achieve, because we cannot truly be "competent" in another's culture. As a term promoting life-long self-evaluation and self-critique to redress power differences, *cultural humility* practices might include willingness to acknowledge institutional racism, including through university-sponsored anti-racism or crosscultural trainings (Ellis & Walton, 2012; see Chapter Four for an example of the use of undoing racism training).

Strategy 3: Negotiate a Research Agenda Based on a Common Framework on Mechanisms for Change

Ideally, all CBPR research projects become a negotiated process between community and outside research partners. With a newly formed partnership, or an existing partnership where there is flexibility in choosing the research agenda, one of the first strategies would be to gather information on community needs, concerns, resources, and strengths. Out of a data gathering and prioritization strategy, research questions would emerge.

Beyond the typical participatory data collection and prioritization methods used to identify needs and strengths however (Duran & Duran, 2000; Hancock & Minkler, 2012; Wallerstein & Sheline, 1998; see also Part Four of this volume), a CBPR partnership would benefit from identifying the culturally defined etiologic theories and culturally specific mechanisms for change. No true prioritization can happen without the community's perspective being paramount.

Typically, universities have privileged empirically derived knowledge, or empirically supported interventions (ESIs); yet increasingly there is a recognition of another valuable source of research, that of culturally supported interventions (CSIs), the indigenous theories and practices from communities (Hall, 2001). Many widespread health practices within communities, that is, traditional healers or cultural revitalization practices, have never been formally studied or evaluated; neither have many community programs. As Larry Green (2008) suggests, "evidence-based practice" has not been accompanied by an equally important accent on "practice-based evidence," which deserve rigorous research as to their effectiveness for a specific population. Recognizing academic AND community streams of knowledge would be helpful for legitimizing the community perspective within a partnership. For example, the case study outlined in Exhibit 2.1 highlights the integration of culturally supported traditional medicine with motivational-interviewing treatments within the CBPR partnership.

Traditional healers integrate healing not only for diseases, but also for the psychological, physical, and emotional impact of "historical trauma," or the collective injuries over the life span and across generations, resulting from histories of genocide or other oppressions (Brave Heart, Chase, Elkis, & Altschul 2011; Duran, 1996; Duran & Walters, 2004). Recently, historical trauma, within Native communities as well as other communities of color, has emerged as an important theory of etiology for many social and health problems. Understanding and appreciating culturally embedded concepts like historical trauma may prove critical to outsiders' abilities to partner effectively.

Strategy 4: Use Up, Down, and Peer Mentoring and Apprenticeship, Across the CBPR Partnership

Mentorship is a vibrant component of CBPR partnerships, especially as the academy expands to greater numbers of students, staff, and faculty of color and community members who are connected to the communities where research is taking place. Inclusive mentorship models have been shown to be effective through fostering skill development and culturally supportive environments (Viets et al., 2009; Waitzkin et al., 2006; Yager et al., 2007), which promote indigenous knowledge and offer safe peer spaces to navigate career tensions related to latent prejudices and emotional legacies of discrimination (Tuhiwai-Smith, 2005; Walters & Simoni, 2009).

Within CBPR teams, authentic partnerships, among senior and junior researchers and community members, eschew the historic academic process of appropriating knowledge, but rather put in place an iterative process that is characterized by respect, dignity, mutual learning, and an opportunity for up, down, and peer mentoring. This comprehensive approach recognizes epistemological diversity, and the value of listening deeply and integrating the perspectives and values from each partner, including community science, the inherited knowledge that stems from community-based legacies. Mentorship becomes a multidimensional and nonhierarchical process that builds on mentee identities, rather than deconstructing them in order to build them up into "socialized" academics under a singular scientific paradigm. The totem pole, as a storyboard detailing the achievements and history of communities, can be seen as an anchor metaphor of CBPR. In this artistic yet symbolic creation of community history, there is no such thing as "low man on the totem pole," an expression Hollywoodized as a pop culture expression. Totem poles, on the contrary, have no rank based on where their story carvings are situated; rather, the seeds of knowledge and legacy start at the base, reflecting collective history and community rootedness. An indigenous person does not view the totem pole as a status symbol of top to bottom, but rather a holistic representation of the entire tribe, clan, or community. Herein is where CBPR makes a strategic link as a research venue. As a research orientation and as a mentoring model, inherent in CBPR are the values, principles, and respect for multiple sources of knowledge. There is no hierarchy in who is driving the quest for knowledge but rather a sense of equity and collectiveness to move all CBPR partners forward in a collaborative and comentoring way.

In up, down, and peer mentoring, community partners learn about academic research processes and increase their capacity building in research skills. In reciprocity, academic partners learn how to work with communities using parameters that are contextually defined and not merely theoretically or academically driven. The academic senior faculty also learns how to more effectively mentor up-and-coming scholars of color by adopting this same reciprocal model. Oftentimes, it is the junior faculty member of color, university staff person of color, or key community member who bridges the community and academic settings, and who provides essential brokering knowledge to sustain effective partnerships, at the same time that they are mentoring each other. Ultimately, the methodologies that shape our mentoring approach are important, as they also shape the approach of those who will be replacing us. Reflexive dialogue among all partners builds on auto-ethnographic, narrative, performative, and collaborative methodologies (Fine et al., 2003; Tuhiwai-Smith, 2005); and enables us to create the critical, ethical, and respectful legacy of CBPR. As Belone (2010) found in her dissertation examining challenges faced by Native researchers in the academy, through bringing the reflexivity and mutuality back into the academy CBPR can empower minority scholars to better navigate career challenges. Utilizing CBPR principles "allows for a full circle of reciprocity throughout the research process" (Belone, 2010, p. 171), from the lead researcher to graduate students, staff, and community members; and then back up to the lead researcher, creating beneficial and supportive co-learning and mentoring among all partners.

Strategy 5. Create and Nurture Structures to Sustain Partnerships, Through Constituency Building and Organizational Development

The success of a CBPR partnership is heavily dependent on our ability to develop strong personal relationships with communities in part through showing up, demonstrating cultural humility, and demonstrating our willingness to share power and resources. In addition, however, **sustaining lasting partnerships** requires (1) careful attention to the development of joint institutional structures, (2) collaboratively agreed-upon agreements and principles, and (3) having communities codefine research deliverables. Although Israel and her colleagues have articulated a common set of principles that are widely used in the field, they advise each new and ongoing partnership to develop their own principles to ensure local appropriateness and ownership (Israel et al., 2008). The Oakland Community Health Academy provides one example of collaborative development of principles (Brown & Vega, 1996). Located in the heart of an economically depressed but culturally vibrant urban area, the Academy is comprised of local residents and representatives of the health department and the University of California, Berkeley's School of Public Health. Together, they crafted a research protocol designed to initiate wider dialogue on the relevance of academic research to the health needs of the community. Protocol questions include: "How will research processes and outcomes serve the community?" and "Are the research methods sufficiently rigorous yet true to community-based principles that incorporate perspectives and beliefs of community residents?" (Brown & Vega, 2008, p. 396).

Such questions and principles become even more codified when working with tribes, as tribal codes expand the general principles of respect to emphasize government-to-government relationships in research, such as who controls the data (see, for example, Turning Point, 2003). The Navajo Nation, which has its own Institutional Review Board, articulates a research process for research with Navajo people on or near the reservation, involving tribal resolutions from local "chapters" (or governing bodies), tribal ownership of data, IRB approval of dissemination, and strategies for community benefit (Becenti-Pigman et al., 2008).

In addition to collaboratively developing principles and guidelines as a basis for CBPR, sustaining partnerships means continuing to work with organizational bureaucracies in examining and revising policies and practices that mitigate against authentic partnerships. A new conceptual model of CBPR incorporates this idea of revising university policies as an appropriate target for CBPR partnerships (Wallerstein, et al., 2008). As an example, some Southwest tribes and one of the authors (Wallerstein) successfully challenged the university IRB to reduce the "boilerplate" survey consent form from four pages to a single page. By mobilizing letters of support from tribal leaders, Wallerstein was able to convince her institution's IRB to adopt a more community-accessible product.

In addition to starting from principles, and viewing our own institutional systems as potential change targets, several organizational strategies are helpful for developing early success. These include: providing an immediately recognizable service to community partners; developing mission statements; and creating memoranda of agreement on such things as decision making, ownership of data, publication authorship, and other research deliverables (see Chapter Four in this volume for examples of the use of some of these mechanisms).

In working with communities, it is crucial to establish the benefit of working with the university, and to establish mechanisms for feedback to the community in short action-research cycles. This is especially important because traditional epidemiologic or intervention research can take multiple years. Potential shorter-term benefits for communities might include researchers providing trainings, help with grants, or technical assistance, which may not be directly related to the research. In a collaboration between West Harlem Environmental Action (WE ACT) and their research partners at Columbia University Children's Environmental Health Center, a faculty member has offered sessions for WE ACT's ambitious community leadership training program in environmental health issues. At the same time, WE ACT staff continue to be invaluable research partners with the Center (personal communications from Peggy Shepard and Patrick L. Kinney, March, 2004).

A key structural issue is recognizing each partner's imperatives and needs, which may overlap but be different from each other. The dimension of time, for example, is a key difference between academic and community partners. Academic calendars are driven by grant deadlines, student research assistant availability during semesters, or faculty needs for tenure and promotion products. Community calendars are driven by a desire for research results that can be disseminated quickly in support of action objectives.

Potential structural university challenges become more acute for junior faculty, who need to develop a productive research career in a timely manner. The time-intensive relationship building in CBPR and coauthorship with community partners, including community review processes that honor community involvement (and in tribes, which may require formal approvals for publication), can lengthen considerably the time before publication, and in some cases may inhibit release of data. Many universities are considering community-engaged scholarship criteria now for tenure and promotion (see www.ccph.info/), as well as urging junior faculty to join existing CBPR teams as a way to jump-start their careers (Seifer, 2008).

Building in structures to deal with conflict is an important organizational development strategy. Although conflicts are inevitable, resolution of conflict may strengthen the commitment to the partnership. As Gutierrez and Lewis (2012) suggest, particularly when researchers and community members are of different racial/ethnic or other groups, recognizing and embracing conflicts within cross-cultural work can be a critical step in the development of respectful collaborative work. (See Chapters Three and Four in this volume for strategies for addressing conflict within CBPR partnerships.)

Reliability-tested guidelines exist to help academic researchers clarify their involvement with community partners (Mercer et al., 2008). The questions ask about community involvement in different aspects of research, for example, setting the research agenda, collecting and analyzing data, and whether there is community capacity building in research. Many partnerships have developed their own qualitative and quantitative process and outcome measures (see Chapter Thirteen in this volume; Pearson et al., 2011; Sandoval et al., 2011). Parker and colleagues have developed a tool to evaluate the capacity of health departments for engaging community partners (Parker, Margolis, Eng, & Renriquez-Roldan,

2003). These instruments can be applied over time as partnerships change throughout the process.

Although such tools are helpful, they do not fully capture some of the core issues within partnerships, for example, the role of self-reflection about our personal and institutional relationships, the ability to create new interdependent partnering structures and policies, and the ability to create internal change within each participating member's institution. A CBPR conceptual model (Wallerstein et al., 2008) has proven useful as a collective reflection tool for partnerships to assess their current partnering practices and goals for the future (http://hsc.unm.edu/SOM/fcm/cpr/cbprmodel.shtml).

SUMMARY

We have provided principles and methods for developing and maintaining collaborative partnerships with communities for the purpose of more effective research and improved health outcomes. This work demands interdependence, with all partners being open to change. Our challenge is to uncover and address our historic legacies and current identities and contexts as they affect our ability to successfully engage in CBPR. Some excellent guidelines, protocols, and other tools now exist for assessing and supporting collaboration between the community and outside researchers. As we have suggested, however, without the necessary self-reflection and continued attention to many deep-rooted issues, such partnerships may have a difficult time thriving and achieving their goals. In the final analysis, as Maurana and colleagues (2000) suggest, two of the most important questions for assessing CBPR may well be: "Would the community work with the scholar again?" and "Would the scholar work with the community again?" Through continued reflection and culturally centered approaches, laying the groundwork in the critical early stages of developing the partnership may strengthen our ability to answer these questions in the affirmative.

KEY TERMS

Community partnerships

Cultural humility

Culture-centered interventions

Self-reflection

Sustaining lasting partnerships

DISCUSSION QUESTIONS

1. What are the challenges for partnering identified in this chapter?

2. Describe the facilitating factors for overcoming the challenges to partnership development identified in this chapter.

3. What strategies or skills may be useful for creating a sustainable partnership?

REFERENCES

Becenti-Pigman, B., White, K., Bowman, B., Palmanteer-Holder, L., & Duran, B. (2008). Research policies, processes and protocol: The Navajo Nation human research review board, in Minkler, M., and Wallerstein, N. (Eds.), *Community-based participatory research for health: From process to outcomes* (2nd ed., pp. 441–446). San Francisco: Jossey Bass.

Belone, L. (2010). An examination of communicative dialectical tensions and paradoxes encountered by Native American researchers in the field and in the academy. Unpublished dissertation, University of New Mexico. http://www.WorldCat.org (2010–09–09T21:55:10Z 2010–09–09T21:55: 10Z 2010–09–09 July 2010).

Brave Heart, M. Y. H., Chase, J., Elkis, J., & Altschul, D. (2011). Historical trauma among indigenous peoples of the Americas: Concepts, research, and clinical considerations. *Journal of Psychoactive Drugs 43*, 282–290.

Brown, L., & Vega, W. A. (1996). A protocol for community-based research. *American Journal of Preventive Medicine, 12*(4), 4–5.

Brown, L., & Vega, W. (2008). A protocol for community based research. In M. Minkler and N. Wallerstein (Eds.), *Community-based participatory research in health: From process to outcomes* (2nd ed., pp. 395–398). San Francisco: Jossey Bass.

Calleson, D., Siefer, S. D., & Maurana, C. (2002). Forces affecting community involvement of academic health centers: Perspectives of institutional and faculty leaders. *Academic Medicine, 77*(1), 72–81.

Chang, C., Salvatore, A., Tau Lee, P., Liu, S. S., & Minkler, M. (2012). Popular education, Participatory research and community organizing with immigrant restaurant workers in San Francisco's Chinatown: A case study. In M. Minkler (Ed.) *Community organizing and community building for health and welfare* (3rd ed.). New Brunswick, NJ: Rutgers University Press.

Chávez, V., Duran, B., Baker, Q., Avila, M., & Wallerstein, N. (2008). The dance of race and privilege in community based participatory research. In M. Minkler and N. Wallerstein (Eds.), *Community-based participatory research in health: From process to outcomes* (2nd ed., pp. 91–106). San Francisco: Jossey Bass.

College, S. K. (2011). *Salish Kootenai college institutional review board policy.* Retrieved October 23, 2011.

Dean, M. (1994). *Critical and effective histories: Foucault's methods and historical sociology.* London, New York: Routledge.

Delbecq, A., Van de Ven, A. H., & Gustafson, D. H. (1975). *Group techniques for program planning: A guide to nominal group and delphi processes.* Glenview, IL: Scott, Foresman.

Duran, B. (1996). Indigenous versus colonial discourse: Alcohol and American Indian identity. In E. Bird (Ed.), *Dressing in feathers: The construction of the Indian in American popular culture* (pp. 111–128). Boulder: Westview Press.

Duran, B., & Duran, E. (2000). Applied postcolonial research and clinical Strategies. In M. Battiste (Ed.), *Reclaiming indigenous voice and vision* (pp. 86–100). Vancouver, Toronto: UBC Press.

Duran, B., & Walters, K. (2004). HIV/AIDS prevention in "Indian Country": Current practice, indigenous etiology models and postcolonial approaches to change. *AIDS Education and Prevention, 16,* 187–201.

Ellis, G., & Walton, S. (2012). Local government and resident collaboration to improve health: A case study in capacity building and cultural humility. In M. Minkler (Ed.), *Community organizing and community building for health*, 3rd ed. New Brunswick, NJ: Rutgers.

Eng, E., & Blanchard, L. (1990–1991). Action oriented community diagnosis: A health education tool. *International Quarterly of Community Health Education, 11*(2), 96–97.

Fadem, P., Minkler, M., Perry, M., Blum, K., Moore, L., & Rogers, J. (2003). Ethical challenges in community based participatory research: A case study from the San Francisco Bay Area disability community. In M. Minkler & N. Wallerstein (Eds.), *Community-based participatory research in health* (pp. 242–262). San Francisco: Jossey-Bass.

Fine, M., & Demakis, J. (1993). The Veterans Health Administration's promotion of health equity for racial and ethnic minorities. *American Journal of Public Health, 93*(10), 1622–1624.

Foucault, M. (1980). Two lectures. In M. Foucault (Ed.), *Power/knowledge: Selected interviews and other writings, 1972–1977* (pp. 78–108). New York: Pantheon Books.

Graham, L., Brown-Jeffy, S., Aronson, R., & Stephens, C. (2011). Critical race theory as theoretical framework and analysis tool for population health research. *Critical Public Health, 21,* 81–93.

Green, L. W. (2008). Making research relevant: If it is an evidence-based practice, where's the practice-based evidence? *Family Practice, 25*: i20–i24.

Gutierrez, L. M., & Lewis, E. (2012). Education, participation, and capacity building in community organizing with women of color. In M. Minkler (Ed.), *Community organizing and community building for health* (3rd ed.). New Brunswick, NJ: Rutgers University Press.

Hall, G. C. (2001). Psychotherapy research with ethnic minorities: Empirical, ethical, and conceptual issues. *Journal of Consulting & Clinical Psychology, 69*(3), 502–510.

Hancock, T., & Minkler, M. (2012). Community health assessment or healthy community assessment: Whose community? Whose assessment? In M. Minkler (Ed.), *Community organizing and community building for health* (3rd ed.). New Brunswick, NJ: Rutgers University Press.

Israel, B. A., Schulz, A., Parker, E., Becker, A., Allen, A., & Guzman, J. R. (2008). Critical issues in developing and following community based participatory research principles. In M. Minkler and N. Wallerstein (Eds.), *Community-based participatory research in health: From process to outcomes* (2nd ed., pp. 47–66). San Francisco: Jossey Bass.

Jones, C., (2000). Levels of racism: A theoretic framework and a gardener's tale. *American Journal of Public Health*, 8, 1212–1215.

Kretzmann, J. P., & McKnight, J. L. (1993). *Building communities from the inside out: A path toward finding and mobilizing a community's assets*. Chicago: ACTA Publications.

Labonté, R. (2012). Community, community development, and the forming of authentic partnerships: Some critical reflections. In M. Minkler (Ed.), *Community organizing and community building for health* (3rd ed.). New Brunswick, NJ: Rutgers University Press.

Laclau, E., & Mouffe, C. (1985). *Hegemony and socialist strategy: Towards a radical democratic politics*. London and New York: Verso.

Lewis, E., & Ford, B. (1990). The network utilization project: Incorporating traditional strengths of African Americans into group work practice. *Social work with groups*, 13(3), 7–22.

MacDonnel, D. (1986). *Theories of discourse: An introduction*. Oxford and Cambridge: Basil Blackwell.

Maurana, C., Wolff, M., Beck, B. J., & Simpson, D. E. (2000). *Working with our communities: Moving from service to scholarship in the health professions*. San Francisco: Community-Campus Partnerships for Health.

McKnight, J. L., & Kretzmann, J. P. (2012). Mapping Community capacity. In M. Minkler (Ed.) *Community organizing and community building for health and welfare* (3rd ed.). New Brunswick, NJ: Rutgers University Press.

Mercer, S., Green, L. W., Cargo, M., Potter, M. A., Daniel, M., Olds, R. S., et al. (2008). Reliability tested guidelines for participatory research in health promotion. In M. Minkler and N. Wallerstein (Eds.), *Community-based participatory research in health: from process to outcomes* (2nd ed., pp. 407–418). San Francisco: Jossey Bass.

Minkler, M. (Ed.). (2012). *Community organizing and community building for health and welfare*, 3rd ed. New Brunswick, NJ: Rutgers University Press.

Minkler, M., & Wallerstein, N. (Eds.). (2008). *Community-based participatory research in health: From process to outcomes* (2nd ed.). San Francisco: Jossey Bass.

Minkler, M., Breckwich-Vasquez, V., Chang, C., Miller, J., Rubin, V., Blackwell, A. G., et al. (2011). *Promoting healthy public policy through community-based participatory research: Ten case studies*. Oakland, California: PolicyLink. Retrieved from http://www.policylink.org/atf/cf/%7B97C6D565-BB43–406D-A6D5-ECA3BBF35AF0%7D/CBPR_Promoting-HealthyPublicPolicy_final.pdf

Northridge, M. E. (2003). Partnering to advance public health: Making a difference through government, community, business, and academic vocations. *American Journal of Public Health*, *93*(8), 1205–1206.

Ong, A. (1987). *Spirits of resistance and capitalist discipline: Factory women in Malaysia*. Albany: State University of New York Press.

Parker, E., Margolis, L. H., Eng, E., & Renriquez-Roldan, C. (2003). Assessing the capacity of health departments to engage in community-based participatory public health. *American Journal of Public Health*, *93*(3), 472–476.

Pearson, C. R., Duran, B., Martin, D., Lucero, J., Sandoval, J., Oetzel, J., Tafoya, G., Belone, L., Avila, M., Wallerstein, N., & Hicks, S. (2011). CBPR variable matrix: Research for improved health in academic/community partnerships. *CES4HEALTH* Dec. http://hsc .unm.edu/SOM/fcm/cpr/cbprmodel.shtml

Petersen, D., Minkler, M., Brechwich, V. A., Kegler, M. C., Malcoe, L. H., Whitecrow, S. (2007). Using community-based participatory research to shape policy and prevent lead exposure among Native children. *Progress in Community Health Partnerships*, *1*, 249–256.

Potkonjak, M. (2004, March 17). Havasupai tribe files $50 M lawsuit against Arizona State University. *East Valley Tribune*.

Quijano, A. (2007). Coloniality and modernity/rationality. *Cultural Studies*, *21*, 168–178.

Rothman, J. (2008). Multi modes of community intervention. In J. Rothman, J. L. Erlich, & J. E. Tropman (Eds.), *Strategies of community intervention* (7th ed., pp. 141–170). Peosta, IA: Eddie Bowers.

Sandoval, J. A., Lucero, J., Oetzel, J., Avila, M., Belone, L., Mau, M. B., et al. (2011). Process and outcome constructs for evaluating community-based participatory research projects: A matrix of existing measures. *Health Education Research*, doi: 10.1093/her/cyr087

Scott, J. (1990). *Domination and the arts of resistance: Hidden transcripts*. New Haven, CT: Yale University Press.

Said, E. (1978). *Orientalism*. New York: Vintage Books.

Seifer, S. (2008). Making the best case for community engaged scholarship in promotion and tenure review. M. Minkler and N. Wallerstein (Eds.), *Community-based participatory research for health: From process to outcomes* (2nd ed., pp. 425–430). San Francisco: Jossey-Bass.

Shepard, P., & Kinney, P. L. (1994). Personal communication.

Spivak, G. (1990). Can the subaltern speak? In S. Haraasym (Ed.), *Post colonial critic: Interviews, strategies and analysis*. New York: Rutledge.

Stanley, C. A. (2006). *Faculty of color: Teaching in predominantly white colleges and universities*. Bolton, MA: Anker.

Tervalon, M., & Murray-García, J. (1998). Cultural humility vs. cultural competence: A critical distinction in defining physician training outcomes in medical education. *Journal of Health Care for the Poor and Underserved*, *9*(2), 117–125.

Tuhiwai-Smith, L. (2005). *Decolonizing methodologies: Research and Indigenous peoples.* London: Zed Books.

Turning Point. (2003). Thirteen policy principles for advancing collaborative activity among and between tribal communities and surrounding jurisdictions. In M. Minkler and N. Wallerstein (Eds.), *Community-based participatory research in health* (pp. 436–437). San Francisco: Jossey Bass.

Viets, V. L., Baca, C., Verney, S. P., Venner, K., Parker, T., & Wallerstein, N. (2009). Reducing health disparities through a culturally centered mentorship program for minority faculty: The Southwest Addictions Research Group (SARG) experience. *Academic Medicine, 84,* 1118–1126.

Waitzkin, H., Yager, J., Parker, T., & Duran, B. (2006). Mentoring partnerships for minority faculty and graduate students in mental health services research. *Academic Psychiatry, 30*(3), 205–217.

Wallerstein, N. (1999). Power between evaluator and community: Research relationships within New Mexico's healthier communities. *Social Science and Medicine, 49*(1): 39–53.

Wallerstein, N., & Sheline, B. (1998). Techniques for developing the community partnership in community-oriented primary care. In R. Rhyne, H. Bogue, G. Kukulka, & R. Fulmer (Eds.), *Health care for the 21st century* (pp. 88–116). Washington, DC: American Public Health Association Press.

Wallerstein, N., Oetzel, J., Duran, B., Tafoya, G., Belone, L., & Rae, R. (2008). What predicts outcomes in CBPR? In M. Minkler & N. Wallerstein (Eds.), *Community-based participatory research for health: From process to outcomes* (2nd ed., pp. 371–392). San Francisco: Jossey Bass.

Walter, C., & Hyde, C. (2012). Community building practice: An expanded conceptual framework. In M. Minkler (Ed.) *Community organizing and community building for health and welfare* (3rd ed.). New Brunswick, NJ: Rutgers University Press.

Walters, K. L., & Simoni, J. M. (2009). Decolonizing strategies for mentoring American Indians and Alaska Natives in HIV and mental health research. *American Journal of Public Health, 99*(Suppl. 1), S71–76.

Wing, S., Avery Horton, R., Muhammad, N., et al. (2008). Integrating epidemiology, education, and organizing for environmental justice: Community health effects of industrial hog operations. *American Journal of Public Health, 98,* 1390–1397.

Yager, J., Waitzkin, H., Parker, T., & Duran, B. (2007). Educating, training, and mentoring minority faculty and other trainees in mental health services research. *Academy of Psychology, 31,* 146–151.

Chapter 3

STRATEGIES AND TECHNIQUES FOR EFFECTIVE GROUP PROCESS IN CBPR PARTNERSHIPS

ADAM B. BECKER

BARBARA A. ISRAEL

JEANETTE GUSTAT

ANGELA G. REYES

ALEX J. ALLEN III

Researchers, practitioners, and community partners who have participated in CBPR projects note the benefits of successfully integrating partners' different expertise, values, and priorities (Israel, Schulz, Parker, & Becker, 1998; Schulz et al., 2003). Many have also noted, however, that the development and maintenance of successful partnerships can be challenging (Green et al., 1995; Israel et al., 2008; Sullivan et al., 2003). Israel and colleagues (1998) describe a number of challenges that are relevant to the development of successful partnerships. These include lack of trust and respect among partners; inequitable distribution of power and control; and conflicts associated with partner diversity. These partnership-related issues in CBPR are also elements of group dynamics that are relevant to the effectiveness of any collaborating group (Forsyth, 2009; Johnson & Johnson, 2008). CBPR process evaluation literature points to the importance of attending to group dynamics to increase partnership success (Israel et al., 2001; Plumb, Collins, Cordeiro, & Kavanaugh-Lynch, 2008). CBPR evaluation studies have noted that democratic leadership that attends to task goals, relationship maintenance, equitable participation, open communication, and a climate that supports group cohesion contribute to partnership effectiveness (Israel et al., 2001; Schulz, Israel, & Lantz, 2003).

These integral elements of effective CBPR partnerships have been well examined by group dynamics researchers (Forsyth, 2009; Johnson & Johnson, 2008). Johnson and Johnson (2008) list characteristics of effective groups identified through group dynamics research: clear and operational group goals that emphasize cooperation and reflect individual interests; open communication; equitably distributed participation and leadership; and influence and power derived from members' capacities. In addition, effective groups use decision-making procedures that match specific situations, create an environment that encourages the creative use of conflict, emphasize group members' skills, and endorse individuality while advancing cohesion through high levels of inclusion, support and trust (Johnson & Johnson, 2008). Processes and strategies for helping groups develop these characteristics are critical for effective CBPR partnerships.

In this chapter we describe group process methods and facilitation strategies for establishing and maintaining effective partnerships, based on findings from the field of group dynamics. We discuss specific techniques and activities that we have used in facilitating CBPR partnerships using examples from initiatives in which we have been involved (Israel et al., 2001; Parker, Schulz, Israel, & Hollis, 1998; Parker et al., 2003; Schulz et al., 2011; Israel et al., 2010; Israel, Schurman, & House, 1989; Schulz et al., 2003; Becker, Willis, Joe, Baker, & Shada, 2002; Becker, Randels, & Theodore, 2005; Gustat, Rice, Parker, Becker, & Farley, 2012).

ELEMENTS OF GROUP DYNAMICS RELEVANT TO CBPR PARTNERSHIPS

This chapter is organized around 12 elements of group dynamics pertinent to CBPR partnerships: group membership; equitable participation and open communication; establishing norms for working together; developing trust; selecting and prioritizing goals and objectives; identifying community strengths and concerns; leadership, power, and influence; addressing conflict; decision making; strategies for working across diversity; and partnership assessment. For each element, we review group dynamics literature and describe strategies we have used. We conclude with broad lessons learned through applying group dynamics techniques to CBPR partnership development and maintenance.

Group Membership

Most definitions of an effective group refer to mutual recognition among members and a sense of belonging to the group (Forsyth, 2009; Johnson & Johnson, 2008). Definitions also refer to shared norms and values, goal interdependence (setting goals that cannot be met by one individual alone), mutual influence, a sense of shared purpose, and the ability of members to unite for action. Fostering a sense of membership early in a CBPR partnership's development increases the likelihood of success (Schulz, Israel, & Lantz, 2003). A number of activities that can help partners identify common ground can be equally useful when new members join partnerships or when existing partners need to refresh relationships.

The recruitment process itself can be an important step toward fostering a sense of membership. Members may be self-selected, invited strategically by a small core group, or recruited through a combination of methods. Many of the partnerships referred to in this chapter relied on the "reputational method" of recruitment whereby early partners recommend others whose work and values they know (Jackson & Parks, 1997; Service, Salber, & Jackson, 1979). In the PACE project (Gustat et al., 2012), researchers invited individuals and organizations they knew and trusted to serve on the steering committee. Once geographic focus was determined and programmatic decisions were made, a second round of recruitment ensued. Original community partners recommended others with expertise in the focus community and intervention approaches of interest. This method of recruitment helped to build a foundation of trusting relationships that served the partnership well.

Initial partnership meetings present important opportunities for developing a sense of membership. In the early stages, meetings can include activities that help group members learn about each other and develop effective working relationships. For example, in a study involving four community-based research projects (Becker et al., 2002), a subcommittee charged with attending to group process asked members to bring to a meeting one object that reminded them of home. Each object was given a number corresponding to a number on another partner's name tag. Partners described their objects and their meaning to the group and then gave them to each other based on matching numbers. We have used brief interviews in which members at a meeting pair up, interview and then introduce each other to the group. In a *human bingo* activity we have used, members identify and obtain the signatures of others who have specific characteristics (for example, someone who speaks two languages), helping them to connect on a personal level. Other partnership-building activities can be found in *A Handbook of Structured Experiences for Human Relations Training, Vols. 1–10* (Pfeiffer, 1975–1985).

Equitable Participation and Open Communication

Equitable participation and open communication are at the crux of all other group processes (Schwarz, 2002). Groups are most effective when all members' knowledge and skills are used fully to accomplish tasks and maintain productive relationships (Forsyth, 2009; Johnson & Johnson 2008; Schwarz, 2002). For this to occur, all members must have opportunities to participate openly in group discussion and action. Appropriate patterns, or *networks*, of communication can help a group achieve this goal (Forsyth, 2009). A communication network may be centralized (one or a few members are responsible for receiving and sharing information with all others) or decentralized (all members freely share information) (Forsyth, 2009; Johnson & Johnson, 2008). Different types of networks may be needed, depending on the complexity of a task. A centralized network may be more effective for simple tasks (for example, informing partners of a meeting date). When a task requires multiple perspectives or broadbased support, decentralized networks may be more appropriate—particularly if all members are present when the information is transmitted and discussed (Forsyth, 2009). A number of techniques, described below, can help CBPR partnerships foster equitable participation and open communication.

Establish Appropriate Group Size

Group dynamics research suggests that smaller group size (eight to twelve) is best for effective communication (Johnson & Johnson, 2008; Watson & Johnson, 1972). Most research acknowledges, however, that decisions about group size should be based on the purpose of the group (Johnson & Johnson, 2008). There are several reasons to keep groups relatively small. Studies have shown that members of larger groups are less likely to see their participation as essential and thus less likely to actively engage in discussion and decision making, reducing group effectiveness (Johnson & Johnson, 2008; Kerr, 1989). The greater the complexity of the group's structure and the more effort it takes to coordinate, the less effective the group will be (Johnson & Johnson, 2008).

Keeping CBPR partnerships small, however, can be challenging. Inclusion is an important value of CBPR, and partners often want to engage many stakeholders. In order to reduce challenges to group process, large partnerships often establish structures that minimize the numbers of participants in any one task. For example, a steering committee may be responsible for overall project management and decision making, with specific duties assigned to subcommittees. When large numbers of people must be present at meetings, a number of strategies can be used to facilitate effective communication.

Use Individual and Small-Group Work

One technique for maximizing participation is to first allow individuals to organize and write down their thoughts before discussion begins. For example, during the initial formation of a partnership, a meeting facilitator might ask members individually to identify three community issues that they would like to address, giving them time to write each issue on a separate sticky note and then post the notes around the room. As a group, or in several small groups, members then organize the responses into categories and these become the starting point for further discussion and prioritization. Another strategy is to break the initial group into small groups that discuss an issue or generate ideas and then come back together for large-group discussion. Individual reflection time and small groups give more people the opportunity for input. Starting with time for individual reflection and writing can minimize inequities that may stem from some members needing more time than others to develop and articulate their ideas. Small-group work enables the participation of members who may be uncomfortable speaking in large groups or who are in "low-power" positions relative to others who are present (for example, a staff member in relation to a supervisor, or a community resident in relation to a government partner).

Employ the Nominal Group Technique

In the *nominal group technique* (NGT) (Delbecq, Van de Ven, & Gustafson, 1975), members form groups of five to fifteen persons. The facilitator poses a question and each individual writes out a list of responses. One at a time, group members share one of their responses with the rest of their group. A facilitator writes each idea verbatim where it is visible to all members (on sheets of newsprint, for example). Members are asked to raise their hand if they have written exactly the same idea. Through a show of hands, the facilitator tallies the number of members who have the exact same idea on their list. This process continues, without discussion, until all individuals' lists have been exhausted. Members then clarify ideas and collapse those that are very similar. The facilitator must be careful at this stage not to eliminate ideas in an attempt to reduce the number of responses posted, and all members must agree that integration does not result in the loss of anyone's ideas. If two or more small groups engage in this process simultaneously, they share their results and then collectively discuss and integrate their ideas. NGT is particularly useful for questions that might generate a large list of responses. For example, "What are the barriers to walking and biking in this neighborhood?" or "What three priorities should our partnership address this year?" Studies have shown that groups produce more ideas and members feel more satisfied when NGT is used (Forsyth, 2009).

Apply Facilitation Strategies

Facilitators can use a number of strategies to encourage participation. A facilitator may encourage quieter members to participate by asking if anyone else has a comment to make or by explicitly noting that not everyone has been heard from. Facilitators should be careful, however, not to pressure members to participate or put them on the spot by calling their names. After a meeting, the facilitators may ask the less vocal members if they are satisfied with their level of participation or invite suggestions for techniques that would help them participate more freely. The group may also use evaluation to elicit partners' feelings about group participation and communication (see section on partnership assessment later in this chapter).

Some groups use the process known as Robert's Rules of Order. In this process, members are formally recognized, one at a time, to discuss a formal motion. Following discussion, members cast a binding vote. Although many groups use this approach because the rules are concrete and provide a structure for getting through a meeting's agenda, we suggest that this process be used with caution as it may inhibit open communication. When this process is applied strictly, group members do not have the opportunity to ask questions freely, negotiate and jointly problem solve, or engage in open discussion. In addition, the "majority-rules" nature of voting may make it difficult for the minority to support the majority's decision. Finally, the formality of the process may be intimidating to partners who prefer less formal approaches, are not familiar with the procedures, or who are not comfortable speaking in front of the group. We encourage CBPR partnerships to use other approaches, such as the consensus approach described in the section on decision making. In considering the use of Robert's Rules of Order, groups should discuss the benefits and challenges or try the approach and move to alternative processes if members are not comfortable with the results.

Use Agendas and Take Minutes

Communication between meetings is as important as communication during meetings. Decisions about who sets the agenda, who takes minutes, and when minutes will be distributed can all affect group effectiveness. Although these activities are often seen as simple coordination tasks, they may actually transfer power to those who take them on. For example, those responsible for creating the agenda have more control than other members over what gets discussed at a meeting. Those in charge of minutes have control over the official record of the partnership. Rotating these responsibilities may distribute control more equitably. It is important to recognize, however, that these tasks require resources (for example, personnel to create and distribute agendas and minutes). In CBPR partnerships, academic partners may be responsible for these tasks due to greater access to administrative support or to their role as evaluators. We have used a number of procedures to ensure that these processes are carried out equitably and do not constitute undue control by the academic partners. These include: reserving time at the end of each meeting to brainstorm ideas for the next meeting's agenda; including "new business" or "other" as a permanent agenda item; and distributing a draft agenda ahead of meetings, which partners may revise.

Before the minutes of a particular meeting are distributed to all partners, draft minutes may be distributed for revisions to those who were present. Some groups review minutes at the beginning of meetings and make changes as appropriate. This may not be effective if the process is rushed or members have not seen the minutes beforehand. A group may develop minutes jointly during a meeting by having the facilitator summarize each discussion and the decisions made, list those who have agreed to carry out actions, and check with the group for accuracy before moving on. With this process, meeting participants can clarify and ensure shared understanding of the decisions made. This technique also gives the note taker guidance by identifying the aspects of the discussion that are most important to record in the minutes.

Establishing Norms for Working Together

One approach to effective communication is for the partnership to develop a set of operating norms. Different from the CBPR principles that guide the overall work (Israel et al., 1998, 2001, 2008), group norms guide day-to-day functioning of the partnership and often include guidelines for communication, decision making, and addressing conflict. For example, a group might "agree to disagree" or choose to make decisions by consensus. Group norms have been defined as "emergent consensual standards that regulate group members' behaviors" (Forsyth, 2009, p. 145). Once accepted and regulated by the group, norms help group members to behave consistently (Johnson & Johnson, 2008).

Norms can be written and formally adopted, or may emerge gradually as members work together (Johnson & Johnson, 2008). We recommend that CBPR partnerships, because they have explicit values pertaining to equity and openness, discuss norms jointly and decide on those to which they will adhere. The degree of formality of these norms will depend on the interests of the group. Whether formal or informal, norms are most effective when developed collaboratively. In developing CBPR partnerships we often use a "norming exercise" (Israel et al., 2001). In this exercise, the facilitator asks group members to take several minutes to independently complete the following task:

Think about groups in which you have been a member that have been positive experiences—groups in which you enjoyed participating . . . Considering these groups, write down the three to five factors that contributed to this being a positive experience . . . That is, what was it about the group that made it successful? If you have not had any such experiences working with groups, then think about groups in which you were a member that you did not think were effective and consider what are three to five factors that would have needed to change in order to have made it a more effective group. (Israel et al., 2001, p. 5)

Using NGT or some other process for sharing ideas, partners then present the factors that they think contribute to effective groups. The facilitator writes down all factors and the group discusses which ones they will adopt as their norms. Groups can distribute the norms to all members as they join, and agree to assess them periodically to ensure they are adequately followed or revise them as needed. These norms may also be used to help guide the evaluation of the partnership process.

Developing and Maintaining Trust

Trust among partners is another important element of successful group process. Trust is especially important in CBPR partnerships because of historical experiences that some members may have had with the institutions that others represent (for example, a university that has bought community land and displaced residents). Community-based organization representatives, for example, have described feeling an initial need to be "gatekeepers" in CBPR partnerships, to keep researchers from doing harm in the communities they serve (Israel et al., 2001). Academic researchers may mistrust community partners—fearing, for example, that community members will act to limit, rather than facilitate, the research process or that community influence will result in a decrease in scientific rigor. Developing trust among CBPR partners, though time-consuming, is among the most important aspects of creating effective partnerships. Partners in CBPR efforts must demonstrate trustworthiness throughout the life of the partnership. In keeping with the principle of addressing social inequalities, higher-power partners (for example, academic partners) in particular must demonstrate trustworthiness and not simply expect trust from others (Israel et al., 1998). There are a number of ways in which partners can display trustworthiness and gain each other's trust.

Show Respect

Partners can display trustworthiness by seriously considering the ideas and opinions of others. Feeling heard and respected can be as important as being agreed with (Becker, 1999), and members who feel they have been listened to during decision-making processes are more likely to support the final decisions, even if they did not go the way they had hoped (Johnson & Johnson, 2008). In our work, partners have set group norms that foster showing respect through listening, agreeing to allow members to finish their statements before interjecting, or to change the subject only when all partners agree to move on.

Follow Through

Trustworthiness can also be demonstrated by following through on commitments. Although lack of follow-through may not be intentional, it can lead to a lack of confidence among partners. Taking accurate minutes can help with follow-through, as partners can see in writing and be reminded of what they committed to do. When a partner agrees to take on a particular task, it can be entered in the minutes as an *action item*. Progress on the action item can be checked at subsequent meetings, with adjustments made as needed. Partners should be careful to follow through on anything to which they commit and not to commit to anything on which they cannot follow through.

Respect Confidentiality

Demonstrating respect for confidentiality is another dimension of trustworthiness. CBPR, by definition, involves partners from diverse institutions with power differentials. Partners may discuss the institutional challenges they face in their individual work environments. Knowing that such comments will be kept confidential helps partners trust each other. Numerous other issues may arise within a partnership for which respecting confidentiality is of utmost importance (for example, events going on in the community or challenges with funders). Again, the adoption of a group norm explicitly stating that partners will respect confidentiality helps to enhance trust and trustworthiness.

Attend to Each Other's Interests and Needs

Acting as allies can help CBPR partners establish trustworthiness. Partners may be asked to participate in activities that are not directly related to their shared work. In our experiences, academic and practice partners have written grant proposals and participated in community activities that are beyond the specific work of the CBPR partnership. Community and practice partners have interviewed candidates for university positions and worked with students on class projects not related to the specific CBPR effort. Partners have developed trust and friendship by attending significant events in each other's nonwork lives (such as birthday celebrations or other important family events). These activities help to solidify trusting relationships (Israel et al., 2001) that can help keep the partners together even without specific funding. Informal networking time at meetings, especially over a meal, helps partners establish relationships and can sustain people through long meetings.

Engage in Ongoing Relationship Building

Displaying trustworthiness and gaining trust is an ongoing component of building partnership relationships. Trust is not established once and for all; rather it must be continually earned and maintained. In addition to the strategies already discussed, ongoing relationship building can be accomplished by acknowledging the contributions of partners at monthly meetings, celebrating "successes" on an ongoing basis with food and informal gatherings, and carrying out team-building exercises on a regular basis. The Healthy Environments Partnership (Schulz et al., 2005), over the course of a year, started each of its monthly steering committee meetings with a 15- to 25-minute team-building exercise, designed and facilitated by a different partner at each meeting. Exercises were designed to enhance partners' knowledge of each other and to be fun. In one exercise, each member of the steering committee shared the name of one individual, alive or deceased, with whom they would like to have lunch, and explained why. In another, each person shared a memory involving someone either 5 years old or younger or 60 years old or older.

Selecting and Prioritizing Goals and Objectives

To be effective, groups must set goals to which all members can agree and commit and to which all partners are willing and able to contribute (Johnson & Johnson,

2008). When partners operate under different understandings of the partnership's goals, success can be diminished. Although it is appropriate for groups to have goals that differ from those of individual members, conflicts can arise when individuals' goals are not made explicit (that is, when people have hidden agendas) (Johnson & Johnson, 2008). Although members may only reveal their individual goals over time, as the group builds trust and develops effective communication, a number of activities can be used to facilitate cooperative goal-setting and the expression of individual interests and motivations for participating, perhaps increasing the likelihood that those interests will be incorporated into the overall group goals.

CBPR partnerships often start with brainstorming activities, using nominal group technique or small- and large-group discussion, to identify priority activities for the partnership. For example, a facilitator may ask each member to complete the phrase, "by the end of our first five years we will have accomplished . . . ," listing all of the goals they would like to see the partnership attain. These lists can then be narrowed down and prioritized according to established criteria (for example, resources available, skills and interests of partners, community health statistics) and established as the goals for the partnership. Specific theoretical frameworks (for example, a conceptual model of the stress process) may be used to structure brainstorming (see Israel et al., 2001; also Chapter Seven in this volume). The Partnership for an Active Community Environment (PACE; Gustat et al., 2012) used an interactive exercise, informed by an existing conceptual model (Glanz, Sallis, Saelens, & Frank, 2005), to generate a list of environmental barriers and promoters of physical activity in the intervention neighborhood, based on committee members' experiences. Facilitators posed the following questions: What kinds of physical activity do you see in this community? What features of the community environment make these kinds of physical activities easy to do? What features of the community environment make these or other kinds of physical activity hard to do? What actions could create additional environmental features that support physical activity or reduce or eliminate the features that make physical activity hard to do? Researchers then synthesized the responses to these questions and the emerging themes were used to develop survey questions. Theoretically guided brainstorming can help to ensure that CBPR projects and activities will contribute to the partnership's overall research and action agendas. The use of a Force Field Analysis, a group-process activity, can help partnerships to identify facilitating factors and barriers and their potential impact on achieving project goals (Johnson & Johnson, 2008; Lewin, 1944; also see Appendix A). Force Field Analysis can be particularly useful to partnerships setting policy and advocacy goals. Identifying forces for and against such goals can help partnerships prioritize goals and action steps according to their political viability.

Partnerships can also engage in goal setting and prioritizing exercises that help the group to think creatively. Partners may use *visioning* activities to describe, for example, the ideal community or specific environmental improvements they hope to make. Creative exercises that move away from verbal lists and toward visual images and products can give partners with diverse backgrounds and experiences a common set of tools to work with. In the East Side Village Health Worker Partnership training (Parker et al., 1998; Schulz et al., 2003), for example, trainees working in small groups used arts and crafts materials to "build" their ideal community—discussing its elements while representing them visually. Group discussions of feasibility is another method for setting priorities—and one in which multiple perspectives from academic, practice-based, and community-based partners can be most useful. The PACE project used a group-driven process to determine which environmental changes it would implement to promote physical activity in the project neighborhood. The steering committee used open brainstorming to list all the strategies they thought might be appealing to community residents and that would fit into the existing cultural and physical environment. The university and practice-based members of the team then conducted research on each option to assess feasibility and potential impact and presented the findings to the steering committee. Outside experts were brought in to supplement the information the team gathered. The steering committee reached final consensus-based decisions (see below) by weighing both the desirability and the feasibility of each option.

Identifying Community Strengths and Concerns

CBPR seeks to identify and mobilize the strengths and resources available in the community and among partners to address research questions and communal health concerns (Israel et al., 1998, 2008). All communities possess strengths, such as the knowledge and skills of individuals, the contributions of organizations, and desirable features of the physical environment (green space, for example). Identifying strengths can help community members feel valued and respected, as partners recognize the strengths in a community rather than empha-size its problems (Minkler & Hancock, 2008; Steuart, 1993). Community assets, once identified, can enhance CBPR partners' efforts. For example, one of the partners in the Detroit URC was a city-owned multipurpose center. This center was identified in the early stages of partnership development as an important community resource and its staff was invited to participate in proposal-writing. Once the project was funded, the center's director provided office and meeting space. This centrally located physical space in the community was a critical factor in the project's success.

A number of exercises can help CBPR partnerships identify and mobilize assets. For example, this chapter's first author and a community colleague adapted a skills inventory activity (Kretzmann & McKnight, 1993) for a lay health adviser training on the importance of personal strengths and community assets. Facilita-tors listed, on separate pieces of newsprint around the room, the skills and experiences that the trainees might have (for example, "can drive a van," "orga-nized a party of twenty guests or more") and asked them to sign their names under those that applied to them. The facilitated discussion then focused on the community-organizing and community-building activities that the trainees could accomplish given their skills and experiences. Other partnerships have used mapping to identify and categorize institutional resources available to the part-nership and the community (for example, schools and health care facilities) (Kretzmann & McKnight, 1993). (See Chapter Sixteen for further discussion of mapping). *Windshield tours*, in which partners familiar with the community educate other partners about its history, culture, and environment (Minkler & Hancock, 2008; Parker et al., 1998); in-depth interviews with key informants; and a review of historical documents can also help partnerships learn about com-munity strengths and resources (Warren & Warren, 1977; Eng & Blanchard, 1990–1991; also see Chapter Five in this volume).

Leadership

Shared leadership has been identified as an important element of CBPR approaches that seek to create equitable partnerships among diverse individuals (Schulz, Israel, & Lantz, 2003; Wallerstein et al., 2008). One particularly relevant theory of leadership is the distributed-actions theory, which posits that any group member can provide leadership by taking actions that help the group to achieve its goals and maintain effective working relationships. The theory suggests that groups are more successful when two kinds of leadership are present: leadership that helps the group to complete tasks (task leadership) and leadership that helps maintain interpersonal relationships (maintenance leadership) (Forsyth, 2009; Johnson & Johnson, 2008). Examples of task leadership actions include asking for or giving opinions or information and summarizing discussions. Examples of maintenance leadership actions include encouraging participation, relieving tension, and praising group members.

Task and maintenance leadership actions need to be distributed among CBPR partners in keeping with the principles of equity and shared ownership (Israel et al., 2001). We have used a number of strategies to assist CBPR partnerships to distribute task and maintenance leadership functions among members. Having partners rotate facilitation tasks emerged from one partnership assessment as a desired strategy. Not all partnerships are interested in rotating facilitation, however. For example, the Detroit URC Board stated its preference for an academic partner with substantial experience in group facilitation to serve as permanent facilitator (Israel et al., 2001). Regardless of who facilitates meetings, leadership actions should go beyond the facilitators. Strategies for distributing task and maintenance leadership functions include modeling by those who are comfortable with task and maintenance leadership actions so that others eventually take them on; specifically integrating task and maintenance actions into the group norms; and reflecting periodically on how group members are feeling after discussions or at the end of meetings until this type of maintenance leadership becomes routine (partnership assessment strategies are discussed later in this chapter).

Power and Influence

Balancing power and influence is important but challenging in CBPR partnerships (Chávez, Duran, Baker, et al., 2008; Israel et al., 2008), because members, by definition, represent multiple levels of social hierarchy (Israel et al., 1998). CBPR partnerships may include leaders of community-based organizations and community residents; leaders, staff, and clients of public health departments; and senior and junior university faculty. CBPR members represent different power levels *within* each system represented (community, practice agency, or university) and levels *across* systems in terms of status and control over resources.

Group process literature states that principles of equity, mutual influence, colearning, and maintaining a balance of power are critical for successful group efforts. Power and influence in a group can come from expertise, personal attraction, access to information, the ability to reward or punish, authority based on role, verbal skill, or even self-confidence (Johnson & Johnson, 2008; Mansbridge, 1973). Most group dynamics studies have found that a group's effectiveness is improved when power is balanced among members and based upon competence, expertise, and information (Johnson & Johnson, 2008) as opposed to personality or position. Mansbridge (1973) maintains that "in groups committed to the ideal that all members have an equal influence on decisions, continuing inequalities can be disastrous" (p. 361) and recommends beginning group initiatives and activities with "more than one task or with a task that depends on the skills of many members" (p. 362) to ensure a balance of power and influence.

Equitable participation is one component of balancing power and influence (see strategies and techniques described above) but it may not be sufficient on its own. Mansbridge (1973) makes several suggestions that may be helpful in addressing imbalances of influence and power. If influence is skills based, members can transfer skills through training. If verbal fluency is a source of influence, members can work together to develop verbal skills and confidence among all. If information results in power, all members can be given the same information as soon as possible. A number of other strategies can help to balance power among partners. Small-group work, described previously, may enable lower-power members to participate more freely than they might in large-group discussions. Partnerships might discuss up front issues of equity in power and influence, or pose and work to solve hypothetical situations in which power imbalances occur, developing a set of solutions that partners might actually use if imbalances begin to play out in the partnership.

Decentralized decision making is another strategy that we have used to balance power in CBPR partnerships. We have established subcommittees with representation from community, practice, and academic contexts to make proposals to the larger group on, for example, policies and procedures for writing manuscripts, content and methods of partnership evaluation, and hiring staff. Multiple subcommittees give a greater number of members the opportunity to shape decisions, thus balancing power and influence among partners. The role of community, practice, and academic partners in hiring staff (for example, project managers, interviewers) is particularly important. We have actively engaged partners in hiring processes in many of our partnerships. In each case, hiring subcommittees have written job descriptions, reviewed applications, interviewed candidates, and selected the candidate to be hired. The use of a hiring subcommittee comprising members from each partner context (community, practice organization, university) ensures shared power and influence throughout the hiring process.

Addressing Conflict

Conflict is often one of the most challenging issues for a group to address. Although some group members may believe that all conflict should be avoided, group dynamics literature suggests that conflict is a necessary part of group development (Forsyth, 2009; Johnson & Johnson, 2008). Many group dynamics experts suggest that when conflict is welcomed and addressed successfully, decisions are more creative and effective (Johnson & Johnson, 2008). Forsyth (2009) categorizes conflict according to its sources, including: personal (individuals' personalities conflict); substantive (members disagree over ideas); or procedural (members' preferred operating methods clash). Conflict may be caused by competition among individual members or be related to group-level experiences of oppression connected to social identity (for example, race, gender, sexual orientation). Some types of conflict influence group goals and effectiveness more than others. For example, when members disagree over substantive or procedural issues, systematic approaches to addressing the conflict can lead to stronger relationships among members and better decisions and outcomes for the entire group (Johnson & Johnson, 2008). When members have interpersonal conflicts, more targeted approaches with just those members involved may be more useful. All types of conflict, when not appropriately addressed, can be damaging to a group temporarily or permanently.

One group process we have used early on in partnership development to limit conflict avoidance is to establish norms for addressing conflict. Discussing conflict explicitly before it occurs is one way to encourage group members to see it as something that can lead to positive results if handled effectively. A common norm in our work is to "agree to disagree." This norm sets the tone that conflicts do not have to end with one position winning out over another. When supported by appropriate decision making, such as consensus as opposed to unanimous agreement (as discussed later), agreeing to disagree can help a group resolve a conflict and reach a decision that all members can support.

In Community Action Against Asthma (Parker et al., 2003), the partnership was faced with a conflict in trying to decide whether to take a stand on an environmental issue. Some of the partners were not in favor of supporting the issue for fear that funders would not approve, whereas others considered supporting the issue as essential for advancing the agenda of the partnership, regardless of how funders would respond. Using the norm of "agree to disagree" and the 70% rule for consensus decision making (described in the next section), the partners discussed the issue in depth over several steering committee meetings. Ultimately, the partnership decided to stop the consensus decision-making process and take a majority vote. The majority voted in favor of action, but agreed that those opposing could opt out without sacrificing their standing in the partnership.

Johnson and Johnson (2008) describe a constructive use of conflict and controversy. In this approach, group members who disagree over a substantive or procedural issue each first present their case, using all available supporting information. Each member agrees to keep an open mind and listen carefully to the others' cases. Members then work first to understand and then to challenge each other's cases. Members clarify the differences in their ideas and integrate where possible so that aspects of all ideas are included in the final decision. This approach helps to ensure that different points of view generate the best-informed and most appropriate solutions.

Other types of conflict may not be as systematically addressed. Personality conflict, for example, may need to be addressed outside the group setting, perhaps with a mediator. Conflict that stems from competition may be reduced by setting up a cooperative goal structure in which any success is a group success, all members have opportunities to contribute, and members are assigned tasks and roles according to their interests and capacities. Conflict that stems from histories of oppression may benefit from the sharing of experiences and efforts by all members to understand the others' experiences.

Decision Making

Groups that sufficiently address the dimensions of group process described thus far have the best chance of making effective decisions. Decision-making methods themselves can also influence effectiveness. Johnson and Johnson (2008) present several decision-making methods, including decision by authority, expert member decision making, majority or minority control, and consensus. We suggest that groups engage in discussion to develop processes for decision making—essentially "deciding how to decide." Too often groups enter into a decision-making process before determining how the decision will be made, and the process itself then leads to conflict. Partners may set one process for all decisions, or they may take time before each decision to discuss how it will be made. When all members know what the process will be, they can engage in the process with more appropriate contributions and clear expectations.

Decision making is facilitated when all members know ahead of time what will be discussed at a particular meeting. Alerting members to upcoming decisions by distributing the meeting agenda in advance, reviewing it at the beginning of the meeting, and following it throughout, can be helpful. Members will know in advance the issues to be discussed and can formulate opinions before coming to the meeting. Before a new topic is opened for discussion, the previous agenda item can be closed with a decision and agreement on action steps. This process helps to ensure that decisions are clearly articulated and enables members to fully focus on each agenda item in turn.

Certain topics may be especially important to include on the agenda for group decision making to ensure a balance of power and influence (as previously discussed above). For example, creating a transparent process for budget development and decisions about the allocation and monitoring of funds are essential to equity among partners. In the Detroit URC, staff prepares budgets with the involvement of community partners most directly involved in the project. Draft budgets are shared with the board prior to monthly meetings, at which time they are discussed and revised as needed. In addition, expenditure spreadsheets are periodically shared with the board to engage them in monitoring and revising as appropriate.

Group dynamics researchers agree that different types of decisions require different methods (Forsyth, 2009; Johnson & Johnson, 2008). Using a time-consuming consensus-building process to make a decision in which partners have a low emotional stake (for example, determining the color of a flyer) would be frustrating. Conversely, unilateral decision making on a high-stakes decision (how to cut a jointly developed budget, for example) is likely to have far-reaching negative implications. Decentralized decision making, with committees or work groups assigned to make certain decisions, is a common way to distribute decision-making responsibility. Well-thought-out committee membership that is agreed to by the group (rather than appointed by the leaders) may be an effective method for making decisions that do not require everyone's input. The important feature of decentralized decision making is that the deciding group is actually allowed to make a decision without needing to be reviewed or approved by the larger group or formal leadership.

For complex decisions, **consensus decision making** may be useful. Johnson and Johnson (2008) describe consensus as an opinion arrived at through collective discussion when group members work together under conditions in which communication is sufficiently open and all members feel they have had a chance to influence the decision. Consensus does not necessarily mean unanimity. The Detroit URC, for example, has agreed to use a "70% rule" as their form of consensus in which "everyone still has to support a decision but they do not have to be behind it 100 percent. Rather, if all members can buy into a decision with at least 70 percent of their support, then an overall consensus has been reached" (Israel et al., 2001, p. 5). In applying this rule, there have been numerous times at URC board meetings when, after an extensive discussion about a particular issue in which consensus does not appear to exist, one of the partners asks "can we all get behind this decision 70%?" If the answer is "no," the board continues to discuss the issue until everyone on the board agrees to a resolution with at least 70% of his/her support.

Specific Strategies for Working in Diverse Partnerships

CBPR partnerships are diverse by definition, including partners with different educational backgrounds and areas of expertise, diverse social backgrounds, and often different values and beliefs. In the early partnership development stages, a number of activities can help diverse partners identify and respect differences, similar to the gift exchange exercise described earlier. Another is Culture Box, developed by the University of Michigan's Program on Intergroup Relations (http://www.igr.umich.edu/). In this exercise, partners share items that they feel represent aspects of their identity (for example, cultural heritage, religious beliefs, or gender). Through discussion of these items and their significance, members can begin to understand and value the personal diversity among them.

To deal with diversity of affiliation (community, practice, or academia), one partnership developed an exercise that enabled partners to express hopes and concerns for working across their differences. The exercise is described below as a guide to facilitators, with instructions to participants embedded.

1. Divide the partners into the three groups (community, practice, academia). Ask each group to complete the task following the instructions below:

    a. List separately for each of the other two groups the things that you hope they will contribute to our work together, based on your understanding of their skills, knowledge, backgrounds, and resources.

    b. Next, list the things you believe will be challenges in working with each of the other two groups because of who they are and the contexts they represent.

2. Reconvene the large group and ask each group to present their lists to each other. Allow the groups to ask for clarification when necessary but ask that they hold off on discussing issues that emerged until the end of the activity.

3. Divide the groups again, as before, providing them with the lists the other groups created about them in the previous step. To complete this step, give the small groups these instructions:

    a. Review the contributions and challenges that the other two groups thought you would bring to our work.

    b. Discuss strategies that your group or the entire partnership can use to increase the likelihood that your group will be able to contribute the things listed and decrease the likelihood that your group will present the challenges listed.

4. Reconvene the large group for the last time. Ask each group to discuss the strategies each small group had developed, propose additional strategies, and the next steps the entire collaborative can take to support these new strategies.

This exercise helped the partners engage more effectively with their diversity of affiliation. Some of the strategies shared during the exercise were integrated as new group norms to ensure that the exercise had long-lasting benefits.

Importance of Partnership Assessment

Partnership effectiveness is influenced in part by the extent to which groups reflect on how well they are functioning (Johnson & Johnson, 2008) by providing individual and group feedback. CBPR partnerships can benefit from devoting time to evaluating their process and reviewing their progress (Plumb et al., 2008; Schulz et al., 2003; Wallerstein et al., 2008). Acting expediently on feedback can help a CBPR partnership improve functioning. Participation of all members in the assessment process should be encouraged so that all points of view are considered. Such evaluation can take a number of forms, and partnerships may engage in one or several over the course of their work together. We describe several techniques to evaluate the *process* through which partnerships work together, as distinct from the health-related or social outcomes they are trying to achieve.

Several approaches to evaluate and improve group process can be implemented at specific meetings. A brief questionnaire can ask participants to rank the group's performance using a scale from least to most effective on a number of the process dimensions reviewed earlier (for example, communication and trust). Responses to these anonymous questionnaires can be tallied, distributed, and discussed at a subsequent meeting, with group discussion about revisions of procedures as indicated by the findings. Another method asks those present to answer three open-ended questions in writing: "What was the most helpful aspect of this meeting?" "What was the least helpful aspect of this meeting?" and "What should we do differently next time?" Written responses can be summarized and distributed, or provided verbally and discussed at the next meeting. The key is that members have an opportunity to offer input based on their experience in one meeting in order to make improvements in subsequent meetings. In both of these approaches it is important for the group to review members' input and make appropriate changes as soon as possible.

More formal and in-depth approaches to evaluating group dynamics, employing both qualitative and quantitative methods, are also useful. Such approaches are described in Chapter Thirteen (also see Schulz et al., 2003) and will not be repeated here. All groups are different, and each evaluation method may be more or less appropriate for any CBPR partnership. For individuals as well as groups, however, reflection and subsequent feedback form a significant stage in an experiential learning cycle (Johnson & Johnson, 2008).

SUMMARY

We have briefly reviewed key principles and common challenges to the successful functioning of CBPR partnerships. We have drawn from evaluation literature on CBPR partnerships and from group dynamics literature to emphasize that CBPR partnerships need to attend to group process in addition to achieving goals and completing research and action projects. Johnson and Johnson's book (2008) on group process is particularly useful for understanding and addressing group dynamics and for describing activities that can foster effective group dynamics. We have described a number of strategies, techniques, and specific exercises used in CBPR partnerships to support effective partnership development and maintenance. Group dynamics are not always viewed as equally important by all partners; at various stages of our partnership work, partners have mentioned frustration with the time spent on group process, which is sometimes perceived as delaying action (Israel et al., 2001; Schulz, Israel, & Lantz, 2003). However, evaluation and assessment have indicated that in the long run, attention to group process is valued and seen as worthwhile in CBPR partnerships (Israel et al., 2001; Schulz, Israel, & Lantz, 2003; Wallerstein, et al., 2008). Partners often point to the up-front and ongoing group processes in which their partnership engages as contributing to the group's accomplishments and to the strong relationships the partners enjoy. For optimal goal attainment, attention to group process must be balanced with attention to tasks. We hope that the strategies provided in this chapter will help other CBPR partnerships develop mechanisms to strengthen their partnerships through careful attention to group dynamics.

DISCUSSION QUESTIONS

The premise of this chapter is that group process methods and facilitation strategies are particularly useful for establishing and maintaining effective partnerships in CBPR efforts.

1. What are the characteristics of CBPR partnerships that make group process methods so useful?

2. What are some key strategies for ensuring equitable participation and open communications in CBPR partnerships?

3. The authors present a number of approaches to addressing conflict. What are some potential sources of conflict in CBPR partnerships and what approaches seem best suited for addressing them?

KEY TERMS

Equitable participation   Conflict

Trust among partners   Consensus decision making

Shared leadership

REFERENCES

Becker, A. B. (1999). Perceived control as a partial measure of empowerment: Conceptualization, predictors, and health effects. Unpublished doctoral dissertation, University of Michigan, Ann Arbor.

Becker, A. B., Randels, J., & Theodore, D. (2005). Project BRAVE: Engaging youth as agents of change in a youth violence prevention project. *CYD Journal*, Special Peer Reviewed Issue, 39–52.

Becker, A. B., Willis, M., Joe, L., Baker, E. A., & Shada, R. E. (2002, November). A multi-site CBPR experience: Layers of collaboration and participation. Paper presented at the 130th annual meeting of the American Public Health Association, 130th Annual Meetings, Philadelphia, Pennsylvania.

Chávez, V., Duran, B., Baker Q. E., Avila, M. M., & Wallerstein, N. (2008). The dance of race and privilege in community based participatory research. In M. Minkler & N. Wallerstein (Eds.) *Community-based participatory research for health: From process to outcomes* (2nd ed., pp. 91–103). San Francisco: Jossey Bass.

Delbecq, A., Van de Ven, A., & Gustafson, D. (1975). *Group techniques for program planning.* Glenview, IL: Scott, Foresman.

Eng, E., & Blanchard, L. (1990–1991). Action-oriented community diagnosis: A health education tool. *International Journal of Community Health Education, 11*, 93–110.

Forsyth, D. R. (2009). *Group dynamics* (5th ed). Belmont, CA: Wadsworth, Cengage Learning.

Glanz, K., Sallis, J. F., Saelens, B. E., & Frank, L. D. (2005). Healthy nutrition environments: Concepts and measures. *American Journal of Health Promotion, 19*(5), 330–333.

Green, L. W., George, M. A., Daniel, M., Frankish, C. J., Herbert, C. P., Bowie, W. R., et al. (1995). *Study of participatory research in health promotion: Review and recommendations for the development of participatory research in health promotion in Canada.* Vancouver, British Columbia: Royal Society of Canada.

Gustat, J., Rice J., Parker, K., Becker, A. B., & Farley, T. A. (2012). Effect of changes to the neighborhood built environment on physical activity in a low-income African-American neighborhood. *Preventing Chronic Disease, 9*, 110–165.

Israel, B. A., Coombe, C. M., Cheezum, R. R., Schulz, A. J., McGranaghan, R. J., et al. (2010). Community-based participatory research: A capacity-building approach for policy advocacy aimed at eliminating health disparities. *American Journal of Public Health, 100*, 2094–2102.

Israel, B. A., Lichtenstein, R., Lantz, P., McGranaghan, R., Allen, A., Guzman, R., et al. (2001). The Detroit Community-Academic Urban Research Center: Lessons learned in the development, implementation, and evaluation of a community-based participatory research partnership. *Journal of Public Health Management and Practice, 7*(5), 1–19.

Israel, B. A., Schulz, A. J., Parker, E. A., & Becker, A. B. (1998). Review of community-based research: Assessing partnership approaches to improve public health. *Annual Review of Public Health, 19*, 173–202.

Israel, B. A., Schulz, A. J., Parker E. A., Becker, A. B., Allen, A. J., III, Guzman, J. R. (2008). Critical issues in developing and following community-based participatory research principles. In M. Minkler & N. Wallerstein (Eds.), *Community-based participatory research for health: From process to outcomes* (2nd ed., pp. 47–66). San Francisco: Jossey Bass.

Israel, B. A., Schurman, S. J., & House, J. S. (1989). Action research on occupational stress: Involving workers as researchers. *International Journal of Health Services, 19*(1), 135–155.

Jackson, E. A., & Parks, C. P. (1997). Recruitment and training issues from selected lay health advisory programs among African Americans: A 20-year perspective. *Health Education & Behavior, 24*(4), 418–431.

Johnson, D. W., & Johnson, F. P. (2008). *Joining together: Group theory and group skills*, 10th edition. Boston: Allyn & Bacon.

Kerr, N. (1989). Illusions of efficacy: The effects of group size on perceived efficacy in social dilemmas. *Journal of Experimental Social Psychology, 35*, 287–313.

Kretzmann, J. P., & McKnight, J. L. (1993). *Building communities from the inside out: A Path toward finding and mobilizing a community's assets.* Chicago: ACTA.

Lewin, K. (1944). Dynamics of group action. *Educational Leadership, 1*, 195–200.

Mansbridge, J. J. (1973). Time, emotion and inequality: Three problems of participatory groups. *Journal of Applied Behavioral Science, 9*(2/3), 351–368.

Minkler, M., & Hancock, T. (2008). Community-driven asset identification and issue selection. In M. Minkler & N. Wallerstein (Eds.), *Community-based participatory research for health: From process to outcomes* (2nd ed., pp. 153–169). San Francisco: Jossey-Bass.

Parker, E. A., Israel, B. A., Brakefield-Caldwell, W., Keeler, G., Lewis, T. C., Ramirez, E., Robins, T., Rowe, Z., & Williams, M. (2003). Community Action Against Asthma: Examining the partnership process of a community-based participatory research project. *Journal of General Internal Medicine, 18*, 558–567.

Parker, E. A., Schulz, A. J., Israel, B. A., & Hollis, R. M. (1998). Detroit's East Side Village Health Worker Partnership: Community-based lay health advisor intervention in an urban area. *Health Education & Behavior. 25*(1), 24–45.

Pfeiffer, J. W. (1975–1985). *A handbook of structured experiences for human relations training* (Vols. 1–10). San Francisco: Jossey-Bass/Pfeiffer.

Plumb, M., Collins, N., Cordeiro, J. N., & Kavanaugh-Lynch, M. (2008). Assessing process and outcomes: Evaluating community-based participatory research. *Progress in Community Health Partnerships, 2*(2), 85–97.

Schulz, A. J., Israel, B. A., Coombe, C., Gaines, C., Reyes, A., Rowe, Z., Sand, S., Strong, L., Weir, S. (2011). A community-based participatory planning process and multilevel intervention design: Toward eliminating cardiovascular health inequities. *Health Promotion Practice, 12*(6), 900–911.

Schulz, A. J., Israel, B. A., & Lantz, P. (2003). Instrument for evaluating dimensions of group dynamics within community-based participatory research partnerships. *Evaluation and Program Planning 26*, 249–262

Schulz, A. J., Israel, B. A., Parker, E. A., Lockett, M., Hill, Y. R., & Wills, R. (2003). Engaging women in community-based participatory research for health: The East Side Village Health Worker Partnership. In M. Minkler & N. Wallerstein (Eds.), *Community-based participatory research for health* (pp. 293–315). San Francisco: Jossey Bass.

Schulz, A. J., Kannan, S., Dvonch J. T., Israel, B. A., Allen, A., James, S. A., House, J. S., Lepkowski, J. (2005). Social and physical environments and disparities in risk for cardiovascular disease: The healthy environments partnership conceptual model. *Environmental Health Perspectives, 113*(12), 1817–1825.

Schwarz, R. M. (2002). *The skilled facilitator: New and revised.* San Francisco: Jossey-Bass.

Service, C., Salber, E. J., & Jackson, E. J. (1979). Identification and recruitment of facilitators. In C. Service & E. J. Salber (Eds.), *Community health education: The lay advisor approach* (pp. 26–32). Durham, NC: Health Care Systems.

Steuart, G. W. (1993). Social and cultural perspectives: Community intervention and mental health. *Health Education Quarterly, Suppl. 1*, S99–S111.

Sullivan, M., Chao, S. S., Allen, C., Kone, A., Pierre-Louis, M., & Krieger, J. (2003). Community-researcher partnerships: Perspectives from the field. In M. Minkler & N. Wallerstein (Eds.), *Community-based participatory research for health* (pp. 113–130) San Francisco: Jossey Bass.

Wallerstein, N., Oetzel, J., Duran, B., Tafoya, G., Belone, L., & Rae, R. (2008). What predicts outcomes in CBPR? In M. Minkler & N. Wallerstein (Eds.), *Community-based participatory research for health: From process to outcomes* (2nd ed., pp. 371–394). San Francisco: Jossey-Bass.

Warren, R. B., & Warren, D. I. (1977). *The neighborhood organizer's handbook.* Notre Dame, IN: University of Notre Dame Press.

Watson, G., & Johnson, D. W. (1972). *Social psychology: Issues and insights* (2nd ed.). Philadelphia: Lippincott.

Acknowledgments: The authors acknowledge the following groups (and the individuals involved with them) for their commitment to the development of effective CBPR partnerships and for contributing to the colearning environments from which the examples and lessons described here have emerged: Broome Team of the Detroit-Genesee County Community-Based Public Health Initiative; Building and Revitalizing an Anti-Violence Environment (Project BRAVE); Community Action Against Asthma; Detroit-Community Academic Urban Research Center; East Side Village Health Worker Partnership; Healthy Environments Partnership; Neighborhoods Working in Partnership; Partnership for an Active Community Environment (PACE); SIP23/24 Research Group; and Stress and Wellness Project. We thank the following organizations for supporting this work: U.S. Centers for Disease Control and Prevention (Prevention Research Centers Program; cooperative agreement #1-U48-DP-000047); National Institute on Alcohol Abuse and Alcoholism; United Auto Workers/General Motors National Joint Committee on Health and Safety; W.K. Kellogg Foundation; National Institute of Environmental Health Sciences; U.S. Environmental Protection Agency; National Institute on Minority Health and Health Disparities; Students at the Center in New Orleans; The Skillman Foundation; and the University of Michigan. We would especially like to acknowledge Rose M. Hollis for her ability to facilitate groups and help partnerships to work across difference and for her contributions to the development of some of the activities and strategies described in this chapter.

Chapter 4

INFRASTRUCTURE FOR
EQUITABLE DECISION
MAKING IN RESEARCH

MICHAEL YONAS

ROBERT ARONSON

NETTIE COAD

EUGENIA ENG

REGINA PETTEWAY

JENNIFER SCHAAL

LUCILLE WEBB

Calls from national governments, including the United States, for community participation to achieve health for all are not new. For example, the Alma Ata Declaration of 1978, which was ratified by 134 member nations of the World Health Organization (WHO), is considered a major public health milestone of the twentieth century (Rosato et al., 2008). A core principle of the declaration was that "people have a right and duty to participate individually and collectively in the planning and implementation of their health care" (WHO, retrieved 2011).

In the United States, the Economic Opportunity Act of 1964, which was the centerpiece for the nation's declared War on Poverty, mandated "maximum feasible participation" by the poor in planning programs, such as Community Health Centers and Head Start (Public Law 88–452). In reference to the mandated "maximum feasible participation," Sherry Arnstein (1969), chief adviser on Citizen Participation for the U.S. Department of Housing and Urban Development at the time, defined community participation as citizen power in decision making. In her eight-rung Ladder of Citizen Participation (Figure 4.1), Arnstein outlined the gradation of citizen power— from "manipulation" to "citizen control"—that she observed occurring in Community Action Agencies and the Model Cities Program.

More recently, a gradation for community participation in medical research has emerged in the second edition of *Principles of Community Engagement*, coauthored by the Clinical and Translational Science Award Consortium and the Community Engagement Key Function Task Force on the Principles of Community Engagement (United States Department of Health and Human Services, 2011). This *Continuum of Community Involve-*

FIGURE 4.1   Ladder of Citizen Participation

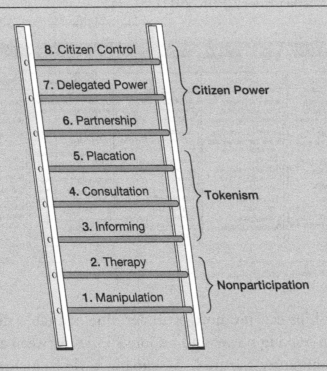

8. Citizen Control

7. Delegated Power

6. Partnership

Citizen Power

5. Placation

4. Consultation

Tokenism

3. Informing

2. Therapy

1. Manipulation

Nonparticipation

Source: The Ladder of Citizen Participation, Sherry R. Arnstein, *Journal of the American Planning Association,* 35(4), 216–224, 1969. Reprinted by permission of Taylor & Francis Ltd.

ment, Impact, Trust, and Communication Flow (Figure 4.2) describes five stages—from "outreach" to "shared leadership"—through which research collaborations involving researchers and communities are likely to move toward increasing community involvement. Different from Arnstein's Ladder, which is anchored in decision-making power, this continuum is anchored in several different dimensions, including level of community involvement, types of communication and information flow (that is, one-way versus bidirectional), and outcomes.

As heuristic tools, both the Ladder of Participation and Continuum of Community Involvement offer insights into the range and complexity of ways in which research

Increasing Level of Community Involvement, Impact, Trust, and Communication Flow →

Outreach	Consult	Involve	Collaborate	Shared Leadership
Some Community Involvement, which is described as follows:	*More Community Involvement, which is described as follows:*	*Better Community Involvement, which is described as follows:*	*Community Involvement, which is described as follows:*	*Strong Bidirectional Relationship, which is described as follows:*
Communication flow is from one to the other, to inform.	*Communication flows to the community and then back, answer seeking.*	*Communication flows both ways, participatory form of communication.*	*Communication flow is bidirectional.*	Final decision marking is at community level.
Provides community with information.	Gets information or feedback from the community.	Involves more participation with community on issues.	Forms partnerships with community on each aspect of project from development to solution.	Entities have formed strong partnership structures.
Entities co-exist.	Entities share information.	Entities are cooperating with each other.	Entities form bidirectional communication channels.	and outcomes: Broader health outcomes affecting broader community. Strong bidirectional trust built.
and outcomes: optimally, establishes communication channels and channels for research.	and outcomes: Develops connections.	and outcomes: visibility of partnership established with increased cooperation.	and outcomes: Partnership building, trust building.	

Source: http://www.atsdr.cdc.gov/communityengagement/images/figure1.1_lg.jpg

partnerships can promote or undermine equitable sharing of decision-making power and responsibilities between academic and community partners. Systematic reviews of articles on CBPR projects (Catalani & Minkler, 2009; Chen, Diaz, & Lucas et al., 2010; Cook, 2008; Viswanathan et al., 2004) as well as "conceptual" pieces on CBPR (Ahmed & Palermo, 2010; Cornwall & Jewkes, 1995; Hawe, Schiell, Riley & Gold, 2004; Rifkin, 1996; Trickett, 2011) have noted both the challenges and wide variation in activities to initiate, achieve, and sustain equitable participation between community and academic partners in the research enterprise. Community norms, institutional inertia, and internalized expectations all can enable more powerful partners, however well-intentioned, to determine what level of community participation is most valuable at which stage of research and for whom (Argyris et al.,

1985; Paez-Victor, 2002). Moreover, external policies and institutions that govern how research is organized, such as institutional review boards (IRBs), can dictate the level or form of community participation (Argyris et al., 1985; Downie & Cottrell, 2001; Flicker, Skinner, & Veinot, 2005; Israel, Schulz, Parker, & Becker, 1998; Schnarch, 2004).

In this chapter, we focus on explicit mechanisms and **structures for equitable decision making** for CBPR partnerships to create an infrastructure for integrating diverse expertise in decision making that anticipates and manages conflict, and is transparent and accountable to all research partners. These structures and mechanisms are:

Undoing Racism™ training for developing a common language and framework on health equity and social justice to address openly the power differences and historical challenges facing community-academic partnerships;

Full value contract for stating the specific set of values, affirmed by each member of the partnership, for investing time in, sharing experience with, giving and receiving open and honest feedback, and committing to the success of the partnership;

Research ethics training and certification for community partners, as an alternate to the conventional online Collaborative Institutional Training Initiative training modules;

Partnership bylaws for explicitly stating long-term principles and procedures to build the relationship among partners and governance of decision making;

Managing and addressing conflict that can be as formal as including a "conflict committee" in bylaws or as informal as a "pinch moment" group norm; and

> *Publications and dissemination guidelines* for ensuring co-ownership and control of how, when, and where findings and lessons learned are communicated.
>
> This chapter draws on the experiences of the North Carolina Community-Based Public Health Initiative Consortium and the Greensboro Health Disparities Collaborative to highlight the impetus, process, and application of these six structures and mechanisms.

BACKGROUND ON THE CBPR PARTNERSHIPS

The structures and mechanisms discussed here were developed by two CBPR partnerships in North Carolina (NC): The NC Community-Based Public Health Initiative Consortium (referred to as "the Consortium") and the Greensboro Health Disparities Collaborative (referred to as "the Collaborative"). the Consortium was established in 1992 by 11 partners in four contiguous counties with funding from the W.K. Kellogg Foundation, which included four local health departments, three African American community-based organizations (CBO), a county housing authority, a primary care center with satellite clinics in two counties, a university School of Public Health, and a regional Area Health Education Center (Margolis et al., 2000; Margolis, Parker, & Eng, 1999; Parker et al., 1998; Parker, Margolis, Eng, & Henriquez-Roldan, 2003). Since that time, one county's 400% growth in its Latino population caused the Consortium to add partners from this county that served Latino communities. The 11 current partners are concentrated in three of the four original counties and include two academic institutions, three CBOs, and six health agencies. CBPR projects include the CDC-funded *Men As Navigators for Health* and *Project DIRECT* (http://www.cdc.gov/diabetes/projects/direct.htm), and the Kate B. Reynolds Trust–funded *Project SELF* (Smoking, Exercise, Lifestyle and Fitness) Improvement (http://www.kbr.org/initiative-archive.cfm) (Engelgau et al., 1998; La Verne et al., 2003). The Consortium's mission is:

To improve the health of minority and/or high risk populations in selected communities by establishing collaborative structures and processes that respond to, empower, and facilitate communities in defining and solving their own problems. (WKKF, 1992, p. 1)

The "Collaborative" (http://www.greensborohealth.org) was established in 2004 through a planning grant from the Moses Cone-Wesley Long Health Foundation. The 35 members represent community, academic, and health professional organizations. The geographic focus of the Collaborative is Guilford County, North Carolina. The county seat of Greensboro has a population of nearly 270,000, and black or African American residents comprise more than 40% of the total population (U.S. Census, American Fact-Finder, 2011). CBPR projects include the NCI-funded *Cancer Care and Racial Equity Study*. The Collaborative's mission (Greensboro Health Disparities Collaborative, n.d.) is:

To establish structures and processes that respond to, empower and facilitate communities in defining and resolving issues related to racial disparities in health. Thus, the results of the work of the Collaborative will be used to reduce the racial disparities experienced by disadvantaged populations when interacting with health-care institutions.

The vision and leadership for the Collaborative to examine and address institutional racism and disparities in health was initiated by the Partnership Project, an anti-racism training organization in Greensboro, North Carolina, who approached the University of North Carolina (UNC) at Chapel Hill to identify a faculty research partner. After interviewing a number of faculty, the Partnership Project Board selected Dr. Eugenia Eng, which marked the beginning of this community-academic partnership. They were able to secure an 18-month planning grant from a local health care foundation to establish a health disparities task force of community leaders, academic and health professionals to explore the presence and nature of disparities in health and health care in Guilford County, North Carolina. Through support of the planning grant, the Collaborative was developed with a commitment to design and seek research funding to study how complexities in systems of health care, including historical and institutional racism, may help explain race-based differences in treatment and their potential association with racial disparities in health care treatment outcomes.

This chapter uses the experiences of the Consortium and the Collaborative to describe and analyze the application of the six structures and mechanisms (listed above) aimed at ensuring equity in decision making, power sharing, and transparency in community-academic partnerships.

INFRASTRUCTURE FOR CBPR PARTNERSHIP DEVELOPMENT

The following sections provide illustration and history associated with the utilization of participatory decision-making structures and tools for cultivating and sustaining CBPR partnerships.

Structure 1: Undoing Racism Training

To address the complex relationships of power differences and historical challenges among representatives of the academic, medical and wider communities, the Collaborative began its work with Undoing Racism training by the People's Institute for Survival and Beyond (PISAB, 2011), an anti-racism organization that has been recognized by the Aspen Institute (Fulbright-Anderson, 2004) as one of the top ten anti-racist training groups in the United States This 2.5-day training was identified by the Collaborative as an essential element in cultivating research to examine and address persistent and chronic racial disparities in health, as described in the Institute of Medicine report, *Unequal Treatment* (Smedley et al., 2003). To address such disparities, the Collaborative believed that it would be essential to come to an understanding of the history of the development of a race- and class-based health system that was a part of a social culture which is hundreds of years old. The primary purpose of having each member of the Collaborative complete the Undoing Racism training was to cultivate a common language and shared framework as a foundation for constructive dialogue associated with the dynamics of race, racism, and institutional culture in this country (Aronson et al., 2008a; Aronson et al., 2008b; Yonas et al., 2006).

PISAB's Undoing Racism training addresses controversial and emotional concepts such as racism, prejudice, privilege, institutional power, and internalized racism through a series of facilitated presentations, interactive dialogue, role playing and structured small-group activities. These are aimed at assessing, deconstructing, and generating a common awareness of power and privilege and their impact upon health disparities and health equity (Aronson et al., 2008a; Aronson et al., 2008b; Barnes-Josiah, 2004; Yonas et al., 2006). The five core objectives of the PISAB Undoing Racism training include (Aronson et al., 2008a):

- Defining racism and its different forms (individual, institutional, linguistic, and cultural);

- Recognizing the presence of institutional racism and its impact;

- Understanding why people are poor and the role of institutions in maintaining inequality;

- Understanding the historical and contemporary purpose and context for racial classifications within the United States; and

- Understanding how community organizing principles and strategies and multicultural coalition building are utilized as tools for Undoing Racism.

This formal and required training served as the foundation for the Collaborative's education about systems of power+race and how this dynamic affects all organizations at all levels. Members of the Collaborative came to understand collectively that the way people and organizations think about race and poor communities strongly influences the kinds of questions they ask and the solutions they seek. Although race is a biological myth, it is a political and institutional reality that continues to have consequences throughout our society, including in our health care system.

Using the Undoing Racism training as the central mechanism for the development of a common understanding of race and racism allowed for the development of a partnership to address health disparities with a unified focus. The training itself assisted in the production of the Full Value Contract (see Structure 2 below) based on the principles of mutual respect which are necessary for an in-depth discussion of race and racism. Though exceptionally challenging personally and collectively, participating together in the **Undoing Racism training** provided the unique and valuable opportunity to mutually explore our personal histories and develop a common language for learning how to address disparities. Throughout the life of the Collaborative, members have repeatedly referred back to the principles of Undoing Racism to facilitate understanding of the systems within which they are working.

Structure 2: Full Value Contract

The Full Value Contract (FVC) is a formal "living" document developed by a partnership, similar to a memorandum of understanding, to remind members of the guiding principles overseeing the CBPR project. For the Collaborative, the FVC was developed and signed by all members as an established set of beliefs and values which would guide the Collaborative's work together. Central to the FVC was the assumption that every member has equal worth (regardless of their diverse disciplines, expertise, and levels of power), and by the virtue of that worth, has a right and responsibility to give and receive open and honest feedback. In essence, the FVC helped to shape and codify a newly integrated identity for a group of individuals, each accountable to specific constituencies (for example, university, community organizations, and churches) and dedicated to understanding and addressing institutional racism in health and health care.

The Collaborative's one-page FVC (see Appendix B), developed through consensus and incorporating input from community and academic partners, affirmed the stated values of trust, mutual respect, accountability, confidentiality, active listening, integration of humor and patience, sharing of personal experience, and acknowledgment of everyone's strengths. To ensure that members would commit to maintaining trust, open communication, and shared power in decision making to achieve the goals of the Collaborative, each member agreed to sign the FVC as the foundation from which he or she would work. (For a description of other similar processes and tools for identifying operating norms and guidelines, see Chapter Three.)

Given the Collaborative's focus on understanding and addressing persistent inequities in health and health care through the systems-level framework of Undoing Racism, the FVC was used to inform the creation of collective decision-making expectations and structures and processes associated with research ethics training, partnership bylaws, and dissemination guidelines, as described in the following sections. In sum, the FVC has been essential throughout the Collaborative's history as a touchstone for why and how the partnership works collectively and with a common understanding grounding the purpose and process of research.

INFRASTRUCTURE FOR CONDUCTING RESEARCH

Structure 3: Research Ethics Training and Certification

The past two decades have witnessed an increasing number of major federal initiatives and funding opportunities for CBPR and community engagement in research (Catalani & Minkler, 2009; Chen et al., 2010; Cook, 2008; Viswanathan et al., 2004). With this growing support from the scientific sector for engaging communities in research, CBPR investigators and observers have noted that the values, guiding principles, and procedures of equitable participation can become entangled with the laws, regulations, and policies for protecting *human subjects* (Flicker et al., 2007).

Human subjects are people who participate in research, and whose rights and welfare are paramount. For universities, research involving human subjects is not a right, but a privilege. Any research proposed by faculty, staff, or students that involves human subjects must be reviewed and approved by an institutional review board (IRB) before studies may begin, and before related grants may be funded. Investigators and study personnel are required by their university to complete proper training in the ethical and regulatory aspects of research with human subjects. Processes and procedures differ from university to university as to how these training and regulatory aspects are handled in relationship to CBPR. In some instances, such as was the case with both the Consortium and the Collaborative, this requirement can be a "double-edged sword for CBPR studies." On the one hand, training in the ethical conduct of research to protect the rights and welfare of participants would be beneficial for community members who, for example, serve on CBPR steering committees; are hired by community and academic partners as project coordinators, recruiters, interviewers, or data managers; or fulfill a lay health adviser role in the intervention. On the other hand, because community members of the research team may not be affiliated with an institution that has an IRB, they may not be eligible to receive such training. Although human subjects training was an issue for both the Collaborative and Consortium as we describe in this section, we recognize that for other institutions, there may be other IRB-CBPR related issues that are problematic, or there may be no issues at all.

In the case of the Collaborative, we wanted all Collaborative members to be able to complete human subjects' research certification, regardless of whether or not they were listed as key personnel on the grant. If an IRB will not permit nonidentified personnel who are not affiliated with the institution to complete the training, in order to move forward with beginning the study, a CBPR partnership is forced to limit community partners' direct interaction with participants and access to identifiable data. In this section, we describe a mechanism established by the IRB of the University of North Carolina at Chapel Hill (UNC) for research ethics training and certification of community partners as *nontraditional investigators*. As an alternative to the more conventional online Collaborative Institutional Training Initiative (CITI) training modules (https://www.citiprogram.org/Default.asp), this mechanism not only can enable CBPR partnerships to fulfill the requirement for IRB approval, but also can build the capacity of community representatives to gain insights into the academic view on ethical conduct of research, the challenges of protecting the rights and welfare of participants, and their roles and responsibilities as community partners of the research team.

In the Collaborative, research ethics training for nontraditional investigators has been used to ensure their equitable participation into the research process at all phases, including data collection, data analysis, and to inform the ethical dynamics throughout the entire research process. Modeled after the traditional online CITI research ethics training, this 1.5- to 2.0-hour alternate training (see downloadable supplement for this chapter) is conducted in person and in a facilitated format using scenarios relevant to the specific research project. Comprising thirty PowerPoint slides with detailed inclusive notes pages, this interactive training uses historic photographs and a storyline to cover the same content found in the conventional CITI training:

- What it means to be a research participant;

- History of unethical research with examples of experiments conducted in Nazi Germany and the resulting Nuremberg trials and creation of the Nuremberg Code; a study of hepatitis A conducted at Willowbrook State School in New York; the establishment of the Declaration of Helsinki; the Tuskegee syphilis study and the resulting Belmont Report;

- Guiding principles of research ethics, which are respect for persons, protection from harm, and justice; and

- Rules guiding the ethical conduct of research, such as informed consent, training to protect participants in research, privacy protections, and requirement of IRB approval.

The trainer was required to be a senior university investigator from UNC. Questions and scenarios are built into the slides and notes pages for the trainer to trigger discussion about why participants may feel like "guinea pigs," and to critically examine ethical dilemmas that community and academic research partners may face while conducting their studies.

In short, by making this alternate research ethics training available for nontraditional investigators such as community partners, four issues that could undermine equitable participation and equitable decision making when using the CBPR approach are minimized: *accessibility, format, tailoring, and literacy. Accessibility* refers to the community-oriented presentation of the alternate research ethics training that is not dependent on access to the Internet and can be implemented in almost any community setting with an electrical power source for an LCD projector and laptop. If electricity is not available, paper copies of the PowerPoint slides can be substituted. The *format* in which the training is delivered is not one of sitting alone in front of a computer monitor and clicking response items on a test page. Rather, the format is a facilitated small-group discussion for exchanging interpretations, asking questions, and probing false assumptions with the trainer, project staff, and community partners. The alternate training also enables *tailoring* to the roles, interactions, and content that is specific to the study being conducted by the research partners receiving training. Finally, with regard to *literacy*, the alternate training is not dependent on either literacy levels or English language fluency of community partners. Guided by cues provided to the trainer in the PowerPoint slides and notes pages, oral comprehension is maximized and the slides can be translated into the language of participants. Upon completion of the alternate research ethics training, documentation of completion is certified by the senior university investigator, and then submitted to the IRB for entry into the database of nontraditional investigators who completed project-specific research ethics training. We describe below a case example of the effects from this alternate training on a CDC-funded study within the Consortium.

The Consortium was awarded funding from CDC to conduct a CBPR project, called Men as Navigators (MAN) for Health at three community sites (urban African American, rural African American, and rural Latino). An academic partner served as the fiscal agent, and three community partners each received a subcontract to hire a full-time project coordinator, form a community advisory group, and recruit and enroll "navigators" (male lay health advisers). The Consortium's steering committee served as the decision-making body for all aspects of the study, which included designing the intervention and evaluation instruments, and writing the application for funding. As a complex research intervention study, not only were skills in qualitative and quantitative research methods required, but also in the procedures and protocols for protecting the men who were participating in the research.

Given the newness of this training and certification in research ethics for nontraditional investigators, those who developed it also designed a brief evaluation form for all participants (that is, 4 project coordinators, 23 navigators, and 22 members of the MAN steering committee and 3 community advisory board members) to complete immediately after the training. MAN staff translated the form into Spanish for the Latino navigators. The training was conducted in community-chosen locations of convenience and facilitated primarily by the academic principal investigator.

With regard to who benefits from research, it is important to note that not one participant agreed with the statement, "Research will not help you, it will only help the researcher." About half agreed that research will help people outside their community. Whereas 70% of African American navigators and project coordinators agreed that research will help their own community, only 20% of the Latino counterparts did. Latino navigators and the project coordinators were still less sure than their African American counterparts, after training, about asking questions, or that the rules for people to follow will make research safe.

As an indicator of the relevance of this training to their role as coinvestigators with MAN, it is important to note that about three-quarters of both African American and Latino navigators and project coordinators felt better about the safety of research after undertaking the training. All but two of the African American and Latino investigators, respectively, felt that other lay health advisor studies should include this training.

To enable MAN's community partners, their community advisory board members, project coordinators, and navigators to be equitably involved as coinvestigators, they needed to understand, follow, and be certified in the principles of ethical research. University faculty, research staff, and graduate student research assistants were required to complete the online CITI course on the Protection of Human Research Subjects. For all coinvestigators, academic and community alike, training in research ethics was an essential component for the study to facilitate equitable decision making through a clear understanding of the history and ethics associated with research involvement.

Structure 4: Partnership Bylaws

Partnership bylaws have been found by some partnerships to serve as a useful tool in the governance of partnerships. The process of **bylaws development** and revision over time is as important as the content of the bylaws themselves. We describe two examples.

Development of Bylaws in Response to Funding Requirements

The Consortium was one of 15 selected from across the United States to participate in the W.K. Kellogg Foundation Leadership Model Program, a one-year preproposal period in 1991. During this year, the Consortium developed principles for collaboration, which included a commitment to move forward with implementing the proposed work *even if the application was not funded*. The full set of principles was stated in a written memorandum of understanding and signed by each partner organization's director, dean, or board president.

After funding was awarded in 1992, the Consortium established a steering committee that worked for more than nine months to complete the bylaws. During the time required for developing and receiving final adoption of the bylaws through consensus, the Consortium followed its initial principles of collaboration for equal partner participation, conflict management, and equitable distribution of resources to move forward with the tasks *as planned* and to address *unplanned* events that are inevitable during implementation.

The Important Role of Structure of the Consortium's Bylaws

The Consortium's bylaws mandated representation on the 24-member steering committee that would amplify the voice of community partners. The steering committee was comprised of 12 community representatives; 6 health agency representatives, including one from each of the four participating counties and two appointed by the Consortium chair; and 6 academic representatives. In addition, the bylaws designated specific roles and responsibilities for Consortium officers, the steering committee, county coalitions, university partners, and other partners. For example, the bylaws specified the responsibilities of the steering committee for handling administrative concerns and holding partners accountable for following the appropriate chain of communication, in all matters (see Appendix C for an example of bylaws).

The bylaws also specified a structure for shared leadership with the Consortium, for example, the president position rotated between a community partner and a health agency partner. University partners would hold the office of secretary-treasurer due to their responsibilities as the grant's fiscal agent. With regard to monitoring and revising protocols and procedures for making decisions and handling finances, the Consortium's bylaws established a resource panel. The resource panel was also charged with planning and recommending strategies to the steering committee in the areas of sustainability, policy development, and state expansion. Finally, the bylaws provided a specific mechanism for anticipating and managing conflict through the establishment of a conflict resolution committee (see Structure 5 below).

Development of Bylaws for Group Identity Development

Our second bylaws example was not driven by a funding agency requirement, but by a CBPR partnership's need to define and operationalize a unified sense of identity. In the case of the Collaborative, the development of the group as an entity (and later the development of the bylaws) was influenced by the shared principles, language, and framework for understanding racism gained through participating in the Undoing Racism training. The group developed through a process that evolved over two years during which time a grant proposal had been submitted and was funded by the National Cancer Institute (Yonas et al., 2006). When the process of securing the first research grant was complete and the Collaborative had begun to mature, it became clear that documents designed to sustain and maintain the Collaborative's mission through personnel and activity changes were needed. The organization had established group norms and expectations for membership, but these had not yet been codified in a formal document.

The Important Role of Process in the Development of the Collaborative's Bylaws

The first meeting at which the bylaws were proposed included a discussion emphasizing that the bylaws should not focus only on the currently funded study, but rather be broadly fashioned so as to apply to other funding mechanisms expected in the future. In addition, members emphasized that the bylaws should not hinder the leadership structure and that they should "incorporate humanistic approaches" toward accomplishing the work of the organization. Since the inception of the Collaborative, the "Full Value Contract," and the principles of Undoing Racism have been essential core values uniting all members. All activities of the Collaborative have maintained those principles, and the members, acting as a corporate body, have relied on each other to apply those principles to inform decision making, preparation of documents, planning of research, and interactions with the group. Recommendations were made from the group for the bylaws to contain specific descriptions of working committees, the frequency of meetings, and the number of allowed absences from meetings.

Subsequent Collaborative meetings focused on discussion of the balance of power between academic, community and health care members of the Collaborative which would be created by structural guidelines established in the bylaws. Throughout the development of the Collaborative, the balance of power between academic and community members was a primary concern. During the discussion of the bylaws, it was determined that the positions of chair and vice-chair should not be held by academics, in order to avoid the power imbalance which would result. Either members of the health care community or members of the general community were recommended to hold the positions of top leadership. Because the Collaborative had been developed in a fluid manner up to that point, and continued evolution was expected, the proposed bylaws were designed to easily incorporate changes over time to reflect the ongoing maintenance of the partnership.

Review of Membership in the Collaborative

After four years, the Collaborative recognized the need for a review of the membership status section of the bylaws. This identified need resulted in a review and revision of both the guidelines and other aspects of the bylaws, such as membership guidelines and leadership structures. Within the Collaborative, there was extensive discussion over the course of several meetings of the way to modify the bylaws to reflect members' active and inactive status. After extensive conversation, guided through consensus and incorporating input from both academic and community perspectives regarding the definition of membership, the bylaws committee was charged with modifying the membership to include two categories reflecting the levels of activity. The issue of membership was resolved when members agreed on the two categories of membership as: *Active* and *Inactive*. The Collaborative agreed that all members were required to have completed Undoing Racism training and to have signed the "Full Value Contract" as specified in the original bylaws, and to pay the annual dues. It was decided that Active members would be allowed to vote in all decisions made by the Collaborative; whereas Inactive members would serve as a valuable resource to further the mission and activities associated with the Collaborative, and could choose to continue their involvement as "Friends of the Collaborative."

As in the previous example of the Consortium, the development of the Collaborative bylaws required a great deal of time for discussion to eventually reach consensus. The development and the final adoption of the bylaws strengthened the unified identity of the Collaborative, stabilizing the group through common expectations and guidelines for ensuring equal partner participation, conflict resolution, and distribution of resources.

Structure 5: CBPR Conflict Management Procedures

In CBPR initiatives, it is common and expected that conflict will emerge during the honest and sincere integration of the perspectives, experiences and expectations of diverse partners. As with all relationships, those developed during partnered research are prone to growing pains and friction. As described in the following two examples, our CBPR partnerships have come to develop formal and informal **conflict negotiation** and management procedures (CMPs) in order to help facilitate the successful negotiation of these challenging and necessary experiences within CBPR. (Also see Chapter Three in this volume for a discussion of "Addressing Conflict" in the context of group process and CBPR partnerships.)

In the case of the Collaborative, an informal process for dealing with conflict emerged from the willingness of members to speak openly and honestly about issues, and from the culture of the group which includes a commitment to relationships and sensitivity to group dynamics. Because we believe that all members are important and have gifts and ideas to contribute, the Collaborative values equitable participation in discussion and decision making, which at times resulted in tension within the group. The recognition of tensions or potential conflicts led to the practice of discussing and examining what might be contributing to tensions as they arise, and this practice came to be called "pinch moments" by the group. An early example of a pinch moment occurred during the writing of the NIH proposal for the Cancer Care and Racial Equity Study (CCARES) project (http://www.greensborohealth.org), and related to the process of deciding on the project's budget. Failure to follow procedures, which included having the five community and one academic members of the budget subcommittee meet regularly to review and guide budget decisions for the proposal, led to resentments that threatened the level of trust within the group. By honestly discussing concerns and recommitting to equitable participation in the development of the budget, this pinch moment created a template for how conflict could be addressed in the future.

Later, there was a reemergence of distrust which could have been a threat to the partnership. After receiving a nonfundable score and reviewers' comments from the NIH Study Section, community partners were upset by their first experience with the academic research review process for funding. Community partners organized a series of meetings, which did not include university partners, to air opinions and feelings of distrust and frustration with the academic process. Meeting without university partners contributed to lack of transparency and inadequate understanding for the full Collaborative on the meaning and relevance of the reviewers' comments for revising and resubmitting the CCARES application. Resulting confrontations between community and university partners required multiple uses of the pinch moment mechanism to engage the full Collaborative in group processing. Reestablishing transparency and trust was required in order to move forward with equitable contributions to revising and resubmitting the proposal, which was ultimately funded. In sum, the culture of the Collaborative, which stresses the importance of relationships and includes the values codified in the Full Value Contract, allowed the partners to transform conflict situations into pinch moments, which strengthened the Collaborative and contributed to growth.

A second example involving the Consortium illustrates a more formal conflict resolution committee structure created initially to review and address issues associated with the distribution and access to financial resources for partnership activities and research. The conflict resolution committee comprised a chair who was a health agency member with degrees in both law and public health, and two additional members (one academic and one community) from the partnership, appointed by the Consortium president. The initial conflict incident leading to the establishment of the conflict resolution committee arose after subcontracts were issued by the university to community partners. Initially, invoices for sub-contracts were to be submitted by community agencies to the university grants management structure directly, as the federal fiscal agent. Per the grant proposal's established guidelines, the funding agency indicated that payments could be advanced to all subcontracted parties associated with the research. This was particularly important because the partnering community-based organizations and nonprofits lacked the available financial resources to pay for salaries and operational costs from internal resources, and relied on reimbursement from the university grants management system. Larger institutions and government agencies are more likely to possess such internal financial resources. Despite approval from the federal funding agency, it was not the policy of the university partner fiscal management office to advance subcontract funds.

The Consortium's steering committee agreed that with the necessary approvals from the funding agency, the community partners should be advanced the necessary payments needed to complete their responsibilities for the project. This issue was referred to the conflict resolution committee, which tasked the chair to negotiate the change in fiscal policy with the University Office of Sponsored Research. After six months, the university modified the fiscal policy to allow the advance release of funds—and it was apparent to the partnership that this change would not have occurred if not for the efforts and dedicated attention provided to the issue by the conflict resolution committee. Without a change in advance payment policy, it is likely that community partner organizations may not have been able to afford to remain active members of the Consortium and the valuable interdisciplinary partnerships developed may have been lost. Commitment of all partners, academic, health department, and community, was essential to the productive resolution which resulted. Keeping all partners informed and involved in the decision-making process was vital and, as illustrated in this example, "necessary conflict" that emerges can be resolved when a formal and transparent process is established.

INFRASTRUCTURE FOR DISSEMINATION PHASE

Structure 6: Publications and Dissemination Guidelines

When teams representing broad CBPR collaborations are engaged in preparing findings and reflections from the research process, shared learning occurs. Academics have traditionally monopolized the process of knowledge creation and dissemination, and in turn the process of learning (Hall, 1982). This has been apparent most notably in the conduct of research and the publication of findings in peer-reviewed scholarly journals. There is tremendous power in the act of knowledge creation, and when this process is monopolized, the power becomes concentrated in these same actors. In CBPR, opportunity for equitable participation in knowledge creation and dissemination is intentionally created (Farquhar & Wing, 2003; Parker et al., 2005). (For additional information on and examples of dissemination, see Chapter Fourteen in this volume.) With baseline data collection beginning in 1993 for the Consortium's four-county coalition's respective evaluations and the Kellogg Foundation's overall evaluation (1992), the Consortium's steering committee anticipated the need for a protocol that would ensure broad participation in identifying, articulating, and disseminating findings and other lessons learned. Furthermore, among the Consortium's academic members, four were junior faculty being reviewed the following year for tenure and one was a doctoral student intending to focus her dissertation on organizational capacity-building by the Consortium. Hence, the steering committee appointed an ad hoc committee to draft "Authorship Guidelines" for the Consortium (see downloadable supplement for this chapter). The preamble acknowledges formally that members have both an opportunity and responsibility to share their experiences with others. The intent was to make transparent that although several media are available, the most likely medium to be used is the written word, and it was recognized that faculty are likely to be most interested in writing for publication. However, faculty genuinely wanted to share credit and authorship with agency and community counterparts. Thus, the guidelines noted that contributions to publications could include: providing original ideas that were critical to the implementation of a project or development of a paper; making suggestions as to how to write about the Consortium's experience(s); or reviewing and commenting on a draft of a written paper. Moreover, the criteria for determining coauthorship were adapted from the International Committee of Medical Journal Editors' *Ethical Considerations in the Conduct and Reporting of Research: Authorship and Contributorship* (http://www.icmje.org/ethical_1author.html). In sum, the resulting Authorship Guidelines represented the Consortium's efforts to focus on a broader set of "contributors" to a written document, rather than the narrower definition of "writers" in defining authorship.

In the case of the Collaborative, these guidelines have been codified in the bylaws, which describe the organization, processes and policies of the Publications and Dissemination Committee, as well as guidelines for the development of manuscripts, presentations, brochures, and Web page content. The composition of this Committee includes at least two persons representing the three main constituencies of the collaborative: academics, health providers, and community members.

For the Collaborative, the process of disseminating research results can take many forms—presentations in informal and professional settings, communicating with the media, preparation of reports and manuscripts and information on our Web site. Members of the Collaborative felt that nonacademic as well as academic publications should be encouraged as an important form of knowledge dissemination. The content of the Collaborative's Publications and Disseminations Guidelines were developed by modeling those of the Consortium, described briefly above. For the purpose of the Collaborative dissemination document, the term "publication" refers to any and all forms of dissemination of information.

A standing Publications and Dissemination Committee of members of the Collaborative was formed to facilitate the review of proposed publications. The membership of the Collaborative decided that in order to maintain a balance of power and control, this committee would consist of seven representatives from the collaborative, including at least two members with university or college faculty affiliations, at least two members of the health care community, and at least two members of the wider community who do not have either of the previous affiliations. Any proposal for dissemination (for example, conference abstract, public presentation, manuscripts) submitted for review must include evaluation by a member from each Collaborative subgroup in order to be approved. Key example elements of the Collaborative's Guidelines include a clear description of the lead author's role, criteria for authorship, guidelines for authorship order, guidelines for publication review procedures, as well as guidelines for expedited or rapid review procedures.

Identification of a lead author, whether community or academic, was based on the individual member's interest and willingness to do the work and dedicate time necessary to complete and coordinate the Publications and Dissemination Guidelines procedures, including establishing and coordinating the publication working group, forwarding final draft to the Publications and Dissemination Committee for review, and presentation of oral publications to the Collaborative as a whole. Criteria for determining coauthorship reflected commonly accepted principles, such as including individuals whose original ideas were critical to the implementation of the related project, those who offered suggestions that contributed to the writing up and publication development of the related project experience, or both. All authors must have made substantial contributions to the following to be included as an author:

- Concept and design or analysis and interpretation,
- Drafting the document or article critically for important content,
- Reviewing the document or article critically for important content; and
- Approval of final version to be published.

Individuals who may have less experience writing for publication or presenting at formal conferences would qualify as coauthors if, either individually with the lead author or with the entire working group, they:

- Were involved with conceptual discussions about the work or interpretation of findings,
- Reviewed and made comments on at least one draft of the presentation or paper; and
- Reviewed the final version and gave approval.

A detailed example and guidelines established for structuring the dissemination of research partnership materials is available in the downloadable supplement for this chapter.

LESSONS LEARNED AND IMPLICATIONS FOR PRACTICE

It is essential that each of the structures described in this chapter *not* be adopted *as is* by other research partnerships. Rather, we recommend reviewing them to initiate conversations with all members of a partnership about making it transparent to all regarding how decisions are to be made and how accountability for equitable participation would be ensured, and adapting some of these structures, as appropriate. For example, should a partnership consider the Consortium's bylaws to be relevant and adaptable to their anticipated needs, then it would not likely require nine months to create and adopt as it did for the Consortium. It will require, nonetheless, dedicated time by the entire partnership or an ad hoc committee to tailor the bylaws and engage all partnership members in deliberating and adopting them.

It is also important to recognize that some of the structures and mechanisms discussed in this chapter may not be relevant for all participatory research partnerships. For example, investigators interested in working to understand and address the health of individuals living within native and tribal nations have a number of unique considerations. Indeed, the concept of tribal sovereignty is paramount to recognize in the research process with American Indian/Alaska Native partners (Brugge & Missaghian, 2006; National Congress of American Indians Policy Research Center, n.d.; and Schnarch, 2004). Based on the unique historical and treaty-based relationship between U.S. federal and tribal governments, a series of Executive Orders were issued between 1994 and 1998 to elevate the federal-tribal relationship to one of government-to-government. This recognition of tribal sovereignty has led to the emergence of structures that require equitable decision making with regard to investigators and the research process. Examples of such structures include institutional review boards governed by the Cherokee Nation and Navajo Nation and prenegotiated rates to cover Facilities and Administrative (F&A) costs of federally funded research (Becenti-Pigman et al., 2008; Indian Health Services Institutional Review Boards, 2012). These policies for equitable decision making in research are not in place, however, for community partners outside of federally recognized tribal nations. Nonetheless, recognition is growing that community research partners also warrant some degree of autonomy or sovereignty in decision making. To ensure equitable decision making, new structures may need to be established. Though these structures may take different forms than those found in tribal nations, an infrastructure at the community level can provide sustainability for equitable participation and community control that is necessary for the principles of CBPR to be put into practice. (For more information and key examples of participatory research being conducted with tribal communities, see Chapters Two and Eight in this volume.)

The deliberations and procedures for achieving consensus on developing an infrastructure for equitable decision making will likely reveal and confront difficult truths. For example, conversations about a community's history and current experiences with oppression or objectification of professors as being arrogant and out of touch will undoubtedly require courage from some and cause discomfort for all. Nonetheless, such conversations are necessary for research partnerships to foster a climate of diversity and inclusiveness, withstand transitions in leadership and membership, persevere through gaps in funding, and manage political and cultural conflicts. We have found, however, that although these conversations are necessary, they are not sufficient for maintaining the necessary partnership-guided principles needed for a research partnership to achieve its mission and goals. Based on our combined experience of 28 years as two CBPR partnerships in North Carolina, we conclude that an explicit infrastructure for equitable decision making must be in place to move up the rungs of Arnstein's Ladder of Citizen Participation or the levels of DHHS Continuum of Community Involvement.

Finally, as national recognition grows in the field of public health on the importance of research that is multidisciplinary, translational, and engages communities as partners, so have the inadequacies of current research policies and mechanisms for promoting research partnerships. Community-Campus Partnerships for Health, a nonprofit organization that promotes health through partnerships between communities and academic institutions, has adopted 10 Principles for Good Community-Campus Partnerships (http://depts.washington .edu/ccph/principles.html). The U.S. Department of Health and Human Services is proposing sweeping changes to the regulations that govern research involving human subjects. New infrastructures for equitable decision making are being created by tribal nations, for example through the National Congress of American Indians Policy Research Center to govern the ethical conduct of research with non-native investigators (www.ncaiprc.org). Hence, more work is needed to develop and examine the relevance and effectiveness of emerging innovations in structures for initiating and sustaining equitable decision making within research partnerships.

SUMMARY

Although the six structures described may serve to cultivate and sustain research partnerships, they are also central to and consistent with the CBPR principle of equitable participation by all partners. For all partnerships to thrive and endure, constant attention and hard work are required from each partner—regardless of the vows and good intentions expressed at the outset. And this is even more so for community-academic research partnerships, which are purposely formed to bring together worldviews and skill sets that are multidisciplinary and culturally diverse, on the one hand, with the challenges of managing contradictions and conflict while being inclusive, on the other. Hence, to anticipate these challenges, consideration should be given to the a priori creation of an infrastructure for equitable decision making that is transparent to all partners and accords accountability to the full partnership for each phase of the research enterprise. In this chapter, we offered examples of mechanisms and structures aimed at ensuring equitable decision making during the formative, implementation, and dissemination phases.

DISCUSSION QUESTIONS

1. Based on this chapter's discussion of creating and implementing an infrastructure for equitable participation in decision making, if you were a member of a newly formed CBPR partnership interested in applying for research grant funding, in what ways might you begin conversations among the partners regarding bylaws and ethical conduct of research?

2. Within a CBPR partnership that has been awarded research funding, what conflicts might you anticipate? If members of this partnership were uncomfortable with addressing conflict, how might you begin to structure conversations among all members to contribute differing insights and expertise on how to anticipate and manage "necessary conflict"?

3. Thinking back to the different dynamics of the Collaborative and Consortium illustrated within this chapter, what are the pros and cons associated with developing formal structures, such as written bylaws?

KEY TERMS

Bylaws development

Conflict negotiation

Structures for equitable decision making

Undoing Racism training

REFERENCES

Ahmed, S. M., & Palermo, A. S. (2010). Community engagement in research: Frameworks for education and peer review. *American Journal of Public Health, 100*, 1380–1387.

Argyris, C. et al. (1985). *Action science, concepts, methods, and skills for research and intervention.* San Francisco: Jossey-Bass.

Arnstein, S. R. (1969). The ladder of citizen participation. *AIP Journal,* 216–224.

Aronson, R. E., Yonas, M. A., Jones, N., Hardy, C., White, B., & Wiley, T. (2008a). Informing and developing research in the context of community-based participatory research and undoing racism. In B. Stanton, J. Galbraith & L. Kalijee (Eds.), *The unchartered path from clinic to community-based research.* New York: Nova Science.

Aronson, R. E., Yonas, M. A., Coad, N., Jones, N., Hardy, C., & Eng, E. (2008b). Undoing Racism training as a foundation for team building in CBPR (appendix). In M. Minkler & N. Wallerstein (Eds.), *Community-based participatory research for health: From process to outcomes* (2nd ed., pp. 447–451). San Francisco: Jossey-Bass.

Barnes-Josiah, D. L. (2004). Undoing racism in public health: A blueprint for action in urban MCH. Omaha: CityMatCH at the University of Nebraska Medical Center. Accessed January 5, 2012 at http://webmedia.unmc.edu/community/citymatch/CityMatCHUndoingRacism Report.pdf

Becenti-Pigman, B., White, K., Bowman, B., Palmanteer-Holder, L., & Duran, B. (2008). Research policies, processes and protocol: The Navajo Nation human research review board. In M. Minkler & N Wallerstein (Eds.), *Community-based participatory research for health: From process to outcomes* (2nd ed., pp. 441–446), San Francisco: Jossey Bass.

Brugge, D., & Missaghian, M. (2006). Protecting the Navajo people through tribal regulation of research. *Science and Engineering Ethics 12*(3).

Catalani, C., & Minkler, M. (2009). Photovoice: A review of the literature in health and public health, *Health Education & Behavior, 37*(3), 424–451.

Chen, P. G., Diaz, N., Lucas, G., et al. (2010). Dissemination of results in community-based participatory research. *American Journal of Preventive Medicine, 39*, 372–378.

Cook, W. K. (2008). Integrating research and action: A systematic review of community-based participatory research to address health disparities in environmental and occupational health in the USA. *Journal of Epidemiology and Community Health, 62*, 668–676.

Cornwall, A., & Jewkes, R. (1995). What is participatory research? *Social Science & Medicine, 41*, 1667–1676.

Downie, J., & Cottrell, B. (2001). Community-based research ethics review: Reflections on experience and recommendations for action. *Health Law Review, 10*, 8–17.

Engelgau, M. M., Narayan, K. M., Geiss, L. S., Thompson, T. J., Beckles, G. L., Lopez, L., Hartwell, T., Visscher, W., Liburd, L. (1998). A project to reduce the burden of diabetes in the African-American Community: Project DIRECT. *Journal of the National Medical Association, 90*, 605–613.

Farquhar, S., & Wing, S. (2003). Methodological and ethical considerations in community-driven environmental justice research. In M. Minkler & N. Wallerstein (Eds.), *Community-based participatory research for health* (pp. 221–241). San Francisco: Jossey-Bass.

Flicker, S., Skinner, H., Veinot, T., et al. (2005). Falling through the cracks of the big cities: Who is meeting the needs of young people with HIV? *Canadian Journal of Public Health, 96,* 308–312.

Flicker, S., Travers, R., Guta, A., Macdonald, S., & Meagher, A. (2007). Ethical dilemmas in community-based participatory research: Recommendations for institutional review boards. *Journal of Urban Health, 84*(4), 478–493.

Fulbright-Anderson, K., & Auspos, P. (Eds.) (2004). *Community change: Theories, practice, and evidence.* Washington, D.C.: The Aspen Institute.

Greensboro Health Disparities Collaborative. (n.d.). Accessed online March 20, 2012, at http://www.greensborohealth.org

Hall, B. L. (1982). *Creating knowledge: A monopoly?* Toronto and New Delhi: ICAE and PARI, p. 209.

Hawe, P., Shiell, A., Riley, T., & Gold, L. (2004). Methods for exploring implementation variation and local context within a cluster randomized community intervention trial. *Journal of Epidemiology and Community Health, 58,* 788–793.

Indian Health Services Institutional Review Boards, Department of Health and Human Services. (2012). Accessed January 8, 2012 at http://www.ihs.gov/Research/index.cfm?module=hrpp _irb

Israel, B. A., Schulz, A. J., Parker, E. A., & Becker, A. B. (1998). Review of community-based research: Assessing partnership approaches to improve public health. *Annual Review of Public Health, 19,* 173–202.

La Verne, R., Hatch, J., & Parrish, T. (2003). The role of a Historically Black University and the black church in community-based health initiatives: The Project DIRECT Experience. *Journal of Public Health Management & Practice, 9,* S70–S73.

Margolis, L., Stevens, R., Laraia, B., Ammerman, A., Harlan, C., Dodds, J., Eng., E., & Pollard, M. (2000). Educating students for community-based partnerships. *Journal of Community Practice, 7,* 21–34.

Margolis, L., Parker, E. A., Eng, E. (1999). Who speaks for health departments? *Journal of Public Health Management and Practice, 5,* 47–53.

National Congress of American Indians Policy Research Center (n.d.). Accessed March 20, 2012 at www.ncaiprc.org

Paez-Victor, M. (2002). Community-based participatory research: Community respondent feedback. Paper presented at 1st International Conference on Inner City Health, Toronto, Ontario.

Parker, E. A., Eng, E., Margolis, L. M., Laraia, B., Ammerman, A., & Dodds, J. (1998). Coalition building for prevention. *Journal of Public Health Management and Practice, 4*, 25–36. Reprinted in E. Baker (Ed.), *Topics in community-based prevention*, Gaithersburg, MD: Aspen, 1999.

Parker, E. A., Margolis, L. H., Eng, E., Henriquez-Roldan, C. (2003). Assessing the capacity of health departments to engage in participatory, community-based public health. *American Journal of Public Health 93*, 472–476.

Parker, E. A., Robins, T. G., Israel, B. A., Brakefield-Caldwell, W., Edgren, K. K., & Wilkins, D. J. (2005). Developing and implementing guidelines for dissemination: The experience of the Community Action Against Asthma Project. In B. Israel, E. Eng, A. Schulz, & E. Parker (Eds.), *Methods in community-based participatory research for health* (pp. 285–306). San Francisco: Jossey-Bass.

People's Institute for Survival and Beyond (PISAB). (2011). Accessed December 20, 2011. at http://www.pisab.org/

Rifkin, S. B. (1996). Paradigms lost: towards a new understanding of community participation in health programmes. *Acta Tropica, 61*, 79–92.

Rosato, M., Laverack, G., Grabman, L. H., Tripathy, P., Nair, N., Mwansambo, C., et al. (2008). Community participation: lessons for maternal, newborn, and child health. *The Lancet, 372*, 962–971.

Schnarch, B. (2004). Ownership, Control, Access, and Possession (OCAP) or self-determination applied to research. First Nations Centre, National Aboriginal Health Organization. *Journal of Aboriginal Health*, January: 80–95.

Smedley, B. D., Stith, A. Y., & Nelson, A. R. (2003). *Unequal treatment: Confronting racial and ethnic disparities in health care.* Washington, DC: National Academies Press.

Trickett, E. J. (2011). Community-based participatory research as worldview or instrumental strategy: Is it lost in translation(al) research? *American Journal of Public Health, 101*, 1353–1355.

U.S. Census, American Fact-Finder (2011). Accessed December 20, 2011 at URL http://factfinder.census.gov/home/saff/aff_transition.html

U.S. Department of Health and Human Services. (2011). Principles of community engagement (2nd ed.). Clinical and Translational Science Awards Consortium, Community Engagement Key Function Committee Task Force on the Principles of Community Engagement. Accessed December 12, 2011 at http://www.atsdr.cdc.gov/communityengagement/

Viswanathan, M., Eng, E., Ammerman, A., Gartlehner, G., Lohr, K. N., Griffith, D. et al. (2004). *Community-based participatory research: Assessing the evidence* (Evidence Report/Technology Assessment No. 99). Rockville, MD: Agency for Healthcare Research and Quality.

W.K. Kellogg Foundation. (1992). *Community-based public health initiative.* Battle Creek, MI: W.K. Kellogg.

World Health Organization. (2011). *WHO called to return to the Declaration of Alma-Ata.* Accessed online March 20, 2011, URL http://www.who.int/social_determinants/tools/ multimedia/alma_ata/en/index.html

Yonas, M. A., Jones, N., Eng, E., Vines, A., Aronson, R. E., Griffith, D. M., White, B., & DuBose, M. (2006). The art and science of integrating undoing racism with CBPR: Challenges of pursuing NIH funding to investigate cancer care and racial equity. *Journal of Urban Health, 83*(6), 1004–1012.

PART THREE

COMMUNITY ASSESSMENT AND DIAGNOSIS

In Part Three, we focus on *how to* acknowledge a community as a social and cultural unit of identity, which is a CBPR principle, and *how to* conduct a community assessment that is as much a process of community organizing and building relationships as it is a research process, which is a specific phase of CBPR. The objectives for this phase are to (1) gain entry to a community; (2) observe and record the collective dynamics and functions of relationships within a community; (3) observe and record the interactions between a community's Insiders and broader structures' Outsiders; and (4) promote the conditions and skills required for both Insiders and Outsiders to enlarge their roles and representation as research partners and program planners (Eng & Blanchard, 1991; Kretzmann & McKnight, 1993; McKnight & Kretzmann, 2012; Minkler & Hancock, 2008; Steuart, 1993).

For a community to function as a full partner in CBPR, it is essential to view a community as a social and cultural unit of identity; *not* as a setting (Israel, Schulz, Parker, & Becker, 1998; Israel, Schulz, Parker, Becker, Allen, & Guzman, 2008; Steuart, 1985). Within a community, people associate through multiple and overlapping networks, with diverse linkages based on different interests (Cornwall & Jewkes, 1995; Israel et al., 1998; O'Fallon & Dearry, 2002). Examples of community partners include members of a local community, such as citizens, residents of a neighborhood or hamlet, and members of community-based organizations (Green, Fullilove, Evans, & Shepard, 2002; Israel et al., 2008; Seeley, Kengeya-Kayonda, & Mulder, 1992; Wang, Burris, & Ping, 1996;

Wing, 2002). For these members, their community holds the strongest potential for collective power to negotiate the production and use of knowledge with the institutions and systems that govern the research enterprise (Boston, Jordan, MacNamara, Kozolanka, Bobbish-Rondeau, Iserhoff, 1997; Freudenberg, 2001; O'Fallon & Dearry, 2002). Institutions and systems may be represented, for example, by university faculty, elected officials, or professional staff at a workplace, such as managers, supervisors, medical practitioners, and other health and human service workers (Chesler, 1991; Ivanov & Flynn, 1999; Kovacs, 2000; McQuiston, 2000).

Enlarging the role and representation of communities as full research partners in taking action for social change and health status improvement is the particular emphasis of CBPR (Freudenberg, 2001; Israel et al., 1998, 2008; O'Fallon & Dearry, 2002). Two primary reasons that researchers need community partners are, first, to gain entry into the world of the people who experience the issue being studied and, second, to instill accountability and responsibility for what researchers learn to see, hear, and experience (Chesler, 1991; Kovacs, 2000; VanderPlaat, 1997; Williams, Bray, Shapiro-Mendoza, Reisz, & Peranteau, 2009). By examining multiple worldviews that community partners can provide, researchers can maximize reciprocity for study design, the construction and validation of instruments, planning the intervention, and interpretation and dissemination of findings (Badger, 2000; Ross et al., 2010; VanderPlaat, 1997).

Chapter Five by Eng, Strazza, Rhodes, Griffith, Shirah, and Mebane describes an approach for completing the community assessment phase of CBPR which meets the CBPR principle of acknowledging community as a social and cultural unit of identity. The purpose of the *Action-Oriented Community Diagnosis* (AOCD) is to understand the collective dynamics and functions of relationships within a community, as well as the interactions between Insiders and Outsiders, in order to promote the conditions and skills required to assist community members in taking action for social change and health status improvement (Eng & Blanchard, 1991). The authors trace the origins of AOCD to South Africa and the work of Guy Steuart, to whom this book is dedicated. They describe the details of AOCD's application of CBPR competencies, research assumptions, case study design, and use of multiple methods, that is, participant observation, use of secondary data, key informant one-on-one interview, key informant focus group interview, and a community forum to interpret findings and move toward action. The authors present a case example, which begins with a brief historical summary of United Voices of Efland-Cheeks, Inc. (UVE), a community-based organization, and its two-decade-long CBPR partnership with the University of North Carolina at Chapel Hill and local agencies. The structure of the partnership, its goals and objectives, and various funding streams are discussed to provide a vivid picture of the partnership context in which the AOCD occurred. The authors describe in detail the CBPR approach to engaging Insiders and Outsiders in: (1) formulating the AOCD case study research design; (2) selecting and using multiple data collection methods; (3) analyzing data; and (4) interpreting the findings and determining action steps to address them. Based on the Efland case example, they include an insightful examination of the challenges and lessons learned in conducting an AOCD.

Chapter Six is a new chapter in the second edition by Schensul, Berg, and Nair, who describe ways in which ethnographic methods can provide accessible ways for academic and community partners to assess communities (LeCompte & Schensul, 2010). The authors define ethnography, explain why it is a useful participatory approach for conducting community assessments, and describe how the methods used and findings generated can be relevant for health and other sectors. The ethnographic methods they present are mapping, surveys, photography, GIS, semi-structured and in-depth interviews with community residents, and consensus modeling. The information collected about a community's life, processes, organizational structures, cultural factors, beliefs, and norms can be used to help in planning interventions. The case example presented in this chapter comes from a CBPR partnership between the Institute for Community Research in Hartford, Connecticut and a group of youth, who had identified "hustling" as a major issue in their community. The participatory process and ethnographic procedures they used in conducting the community assessment provide an in-depth view and rigorous analysis of the multiple factors that contribute to underlying health inequities and the resources available to address them.

REFERENCES

Badger, T. G. (2000). Action research, change and methodological rigour. *Journal of Nursing Management, 8,* 201–207.

Boston, P., Jordan, S., MacNamara, E., Kozolanka, K., Bobbish-Rondeau, E., & Iserhoff, H. (1997). Using participatory action research to understand the meanings aboriginal Canadians attribute to the rising incidence of diabetes. *Chronic Disease in Canada, 18,* 5–12.

Chesler, M. A. (1991). Participatory action research with self-help groups: An alternative paradigm for inquiry and action. *American Journal of Community Psychology, 19,* 757–768.

Cornwall, A., & Jewkes, R. (1995). What is participatory research? *Social Science and Medicine, 41,* 1667–1676.

Eng, E., & Blanchard, L. (1991). Action-oriented community diagnosis: A health education tool. *International Journal of Community Health Education, 11,* 93–110.

Freudenberg, N. (2001). Case history of the Center for Urban Epidemiologic Studies in New York City. *Journal of Urban Health, 78,* 508–518.

Green, L., Fullilove, M., Evans, D., & Shepard, P. (2002). "Hey, mom, thanks!": Use of focus groups in the development of place-specific materials for a community environmental action campaign. *Environmental Health Perspectives, 110*(Suppl. 2), S265–S269.

Israel, B. A., Schulz, A. J., Parker, E. A., & Becker, A. B. (1998). Review of community-based research: Assessing partnership approaches to improve public health. *Annual Review of Public Health, 19,* 173–202.

Israel, B. A., Schulz, A. J., Parker, E. A., Becker, A. B., Allen, A., & Guzman, J. R. (2008). Critical issues in developing and following CBPR principles. In M. Minkler & N. Wallerstein (Eds.), *Community-based participatory research for health: From process to outcomes* (2nd ed., pp. 47–66). San Francisco: Jossey-Bass.

Ivanov, L. L., & Flynn, B. C. (1999). Utilization and satisfaction with prenatal care services. *Western Journal of Nursing Research, 21,* 372–386.

Kovacs, P. J. (2000). Participatory action research and hospice: A good fit. *Hospice Journal of Physical and Psychosocial Pastoral Care and Dying, 15,* 55–62.

Kretzmann, J. P., & McKnight, J. L. (1993). *Building communities from the inside out: A path toward finding and mobilizing a community's assets.* Chicago: ACTA Publications.

LeCompte, M. D., & Schensul, J. (2010). *Designing and conducting ethnographic research* (Vol. 1). Lanham, MD: AltaMira Press.

McKnight, J. L., & Kretzmann, J. P. (2012). Mapping community capacity. In M. Minkler (Ed.) *Community organizing and community building for health and welfare* (3rd ed.). New Brunswick, NJ: Rutgers University Press.

McQuiston, T. H. (2000). Empowerment evaluation of worker safety and health education programs. *American Journal of Industrial Medicine, 38,* 584–597.

Minkler, M., & Hancock, T. (2008). Community-driven asset identification and issue selection. In M. Minkler & N. Wallerstein (Eds.), *Community-based participatory research for health: From process to outcomes* (2nd ed. pp. 153–169). San Francisco: Jossey-Bass.

O'Fallon, L. R., & Dearry, A. (2002). Community-based participatory research as a tool to advance environmental health sciences. *Environmental Health Perspectives, 110*(Suppl. 2), S155–S159.

Ross, L. F., Loup, A., Nelson, R. M., Botkin, J. R., Kost, R., Smith, G. R., et al. (2010). The challenges of collaboration for academic and community partners in a research partnership: Points to consider. *Journal of Empirical Research on Human Research Ethics, 5*(1), 19–31.

Seeley, J. A., Kengeya-Kayondo, J. F., & Mulder, D. W. (1992). Community-based HIV/AIDS research—whither community participation? Unsolved problems in a research programme in rural Uganda. *Social Science and Medicine, 34,* 1089–1095.

Steuart, G. W. (1985). Social and behavioral change strategies. In H. T. Phillips & S. A. Gaylord (Eds.), *Aging and public health.* New York: Springer.

Steuart, G. W. (1993). Social and cultural perspectives: Community intervention and mental health. *Health Education Quarterly, 20*(suppl 1), 99–111.

VanderPlaat, M. (1997). *Emancipatory politics, critical evaluation and government policy.* Washington, DC: American Sociological Association.

Wang, C., Burris, M. A., & Ping, X. Y. (1996). Chinese village women as visual anthropologists: A participatory approach to reaching policymakers. *Social Science and Medicine, 42,* 1391–1400.

Williams, K. J., Bray, P. G., Shapiro-Mendoza, C. K., Reisz, I., & Peranteau, J. (2009). Modeling the principles of community-based participatory research in a community health assessment conducted by a health foundation. *Health Promotion Practice, 10,* 67–75.

Wing, S. (2002). Social responsibility and research ethics in community-driven studies of industrialized hog production. *Environmental Health Perspectives, 110,* 437–444.

Chapter 5

INSIDERS AND OUTSIDERS

ASSESS WHO IS

"THE COMMUNITY"

PARTICIPANT OBSERVATION, KEY INFORMANT INTERVIEW, FOCUS GROUP INTERVIEW, AND COMMUNITY FORUM

EUGENIA ENG

KAREN STRAZZA

SCOTT D. RHODES

DEREK GRIFFITH

KATE SHIRAH

ELVIRA MEBANE

"Professional strangers" is a term used by Merton (1970), a sociologist, for researchers who study groups or communities different from themselves. They differ in social status, frequently characterized by race and ethnicity, age, gender, social class, sexual orientation, or some combination thereof. Being different in social status from the communities they study can impede researchers from getting in, getting along with, and gaining an *emic* (Insider's) view on how people live (Cassel, 1976; Kauffman, 1994; Morris, Leung, Ames, & Lickel, 1999; Steuart, 1985; Young, 2005). An Insider's view is privileged knowledge that is: (1) borne through membership in a particular group, culture, and society; and (2) socialized by one's social position in that group, culture, and society (Merton, 1970; Steuart, 1985).

As "professional strangers," researchers do not have direct access to the Insider's view, and in some communities with prior negative experiences with and cultivated resentment of "professional strangers," researchers may be excluded from access to the Insider's view (Kauffman, 1994). At the same time, researchers can provide an *etic* (Outsider's) view of how people live, which is not complicated by membership in or socialization by the community being studied, and therefore, is relatively "objective." In addition, researchers can raise questions and seek new understanding about how people live— information that a community's insiders would be less likely to recognize without Outsider assistance (Kauffman, 1994; Merton 1970; Morris, Leung, Ames, & Lickel, 1999; Steuart 1985; Young, 2005).

Understanding how people live is fundamental to the mission of public health in the United States, which is to ensure the conditions in which people can be healthy (Institute of Medicine, 1988). As the Institute of Medicine (1988) concludes in *The Future of Public Health*, achieving this mission will require public health agencies to join forces with organizations of both Insiders and Outsiders to generate new learning for health status improvement. Through new learning about the conditions necessary for people to be in good health, each participating organization and community will be mutually changed. In addition, through such mutual change, participating organizations and communities will have developed new models for community-based education, research, and service. According to the Institute of Medicine,

> Its aim is to generate organized community effort to address the public interest in health by applying scientific and technical knowledge to prevent disease and promote health. The mission of public health is addressed by private organizations and individuals as well as by public agencies. But the governmental public health agency has a unique function: to see to it that vital elements are in place and that the mission is adequately addressed. (Institute of Medicine, 1988, p. 7)

This statement has four important implications for the field of public health in general and for Community-Based Participatory Research (CBPR) in particular. First, the conditions for people to be in good health are multidimensional—rooted in determinants that are not only biomedical and behavioral, but also social, political, economic, and cultural (Braveman, Cubbin, Egerter, Williams, & Pamuk, 2010; Cassel, 1976; Krieger, 2003; Taylor, 2002; Williams, 2003). Second, a **community assessment** is essential for service agencies, community-based organizations, and academic institutions to pool their resources to gain the **views of both Insiders and Outsiders** on the multiple dimensions of health *and* to organize collective action to improve them (Butterfoss, Goodman, & Wandersman, 1996;

Eng & Blanchard, 1991; Fetterman, 1989; Green, Krueter, & Krueter 1999; Hancock & Minkler, 2012; Parker et al., 1998; Steuart, 1985). Third, the procedures for conducting such a community assessment combine the principles and methods of scientific research with those of community organizing (Eng & Blanchard, 1991). Fourth, this blending of principles and methods is integral to the first three core components of CBPR: forming a CBPR partnership; assessing community strengths and priorities; and identifying priority local health concerns and research questions (see Chapter One in this volume).

In this chapter, we describe such a community assessment procedure, the *Action-Oriented Community Diagnosis* (AOCD). The purpose of AOCD is to understand the collective dynamics and functions of relationships within a community and the interactions between community members and broader structures that promote the conditions and skills required to assist community members in taking action for social change and health status improvement (Eng & Blanchard, 1991). The next section explains the origins of AOCD, describes its research assumptions and methods, and is followed by a case example. The case example begins with a brief historical summary of United Voices of Efland-Cheeks, Inc., a community-based organization, and its two-decade-long CBPR partnership with the University of North Carolina and local agencies. The structure of the partnership, its goals and objectives, and the various funding streams are described to provide a vivid picture of the partnership context in which the AOCD occurred. We then discuss in detail the CBPR approach to engaging Insiders and Outsiders in: (1) formulating the AOCD case study research design; (2) selecting and using multiple data collection methods to elicit the respective views of Insiders and Outsiders; (3)

analyzing data using the technique of constant comparison to identify differences and similarities; and (4) interpreting the findings and determining next action steps to address them. Based on the Efland AOCD case example, we highlight the challenges, lessons learned, and implications from triggering a dialogue between members of this rural, African American community and the agencies that serve them on the question of "Who is the Efland community?"

ORIGINS OF AOCD

The **origins** of AOCD can be traced to the pioneering work of a small group of South Africans at the Institute of Family and Community Health (Kark & Steuart, 1962). From 1945 to 1959, they trained their staff at seven primary health care centers in South Africa to conduct research in the communities they served on the connection between social relationships and health. The communities were of various incomes and ethnicities, urban and rural. The methodology and broad inclusion of social factors, such as poverty and discrimination, as determinants of health have been acknowledged as the fundamental work of the twentieth century in social epidemiology (Trostle, 1986).

The group's leader, Sidney Kark, credited Guy Steuart, the psychologist in the group, with calling their attention to the importance of social networks and primary groups, as community strengths and assets, on which to build their work in community health education (Israel, Dawson, Steckler, & Eng, 1993). Eng and Parker (2002) further noted:

> Steuart developed a unique procedure for recording the structure and functions of a community's natural helping system. His findings revealed sophisticated and complex skill sets and expertise on how to manage with life, deal with its frustrations, and strive to ensure the conditions for good health . . . even for communities whose life conditions, such as apartheid policy or rural poverty, would be expected to exert an undeniably harmful influence on health. (pp.128–129)

Steuart trained health center staff in conducting the procedure and using the findings to inform and incorporate new techniques into their daily practice at the health centers (Kark, 1951). They found that as a result of engaging social groupings of people in a 10-week mutual exchange of discussion-decision as a natural extension of their patient education activities, infant feeding practices changed in the desired direction (Steuart & Kark, 1962). Moreover, staff increased their own understanding of individuals within their family situation, families within their community situation, and what it was like to live in a community in relation to the social structure of South Africa (Kark, 1951).

This group of South African researchers, trained as epidemiologists and behavioral scientists, considered their experiment of gaining an Insider's view from communities and blending it with their own Outsider's view, to be among the Institute's most important work (Steuart & Kark 1962). Their experiment, however, came to an abrupt end in 1959, when the new South African government began to apply apartheid policy to the medical professions. The group dispersed to Israel, Kenya, and the United States.

From 1970 to 1984, Steuart chaired the Department of Health Education within the School of Public Health, University of North Carolina–Chapel Hill (UNC) where he refined his community assessment procedure and called it an "Action-Oriented Community Diagnosis." His rationale for using the term *diagnosis* was to indicate that when public health "professionals engage communities in assessing their own strengths and problems, they are ethically bound to take action to address the problems, as physicians are ethically bound to ensure medical treatment for patients they diagnose with an illness or disability" (Steckler, Dawson, Israel, & Eng, 1993, 45).

Steuart (1969) considered AOCD to be a critical first step in program planning and evaluation because it provides the foundation for a partnership approach:

- A collaborative relationship between professionals and communities, who can begin closing the gap between what we do not know and "what we ought to know";

- The selection of intervention methods and "units of practice" that are most authentic to a community's natural networks of communication and influence; and

- The establishment of baselines from which objectives, intended outcomes, and measures of change are to be derived (Steckler, Dawson, Israel, & Eng, 1993).

This foundation for a partnership approach to program planning is identical to the first three components of CBPR *prior to* designing and conducting etiologic, intervention, and/or policy research (Israel, Coombe, & McGranaghan, 2010, and see Figure 1.1 in Chapter One of this volume):

- Forming a CBPR partnership in which potential partners and communities are identified and involved in building relationships and principles for collaboration;

- Assessing community strengths and priorities so that both the CBPR partnership and research project will build on sources of power, influence, and communication within a community; and

- Identifying priority local health concerns and research questions.

Since 1971, the faculty of the Department of Health Behavior and Health Education at UNC has been training graduate students in conducting AOCD. Since 2002, postdoctoral fellows at the UNC training site for the Kellogg Community Health Scholars Program (Bowie, Eng, & Lichtenstein, 2009; Griffith, Citrin, Jerome, Bayer, Mebane, 2009) have been trained in how to guide student teams and collaborate with their community partners in integrating the principles of CBPR (Israel et al., 2008) with the theory and practice of AOCD. The following are the competencies necessary for conducting AOCD and the first three components of CBPR:

- Discovering and articulating a conceptual foundation for defining community, community participation, community capacity, and community competence;

- Adopting an ecological orientation to health promotion theories and interventions;

- Facilitating groups in consensus decision making and managing conflict;

- Gathering and interpreting secondary data sources;

- Interviewing, participant observation, and other forms of primary data collection and analyses in community settings; and

- Using empowerment education techniques for interpreting findings, determining priorities for next action steps, and conducting program planning.

General Description of AOCD Research Design and Methods

The following section focuses on the research design and methods of AOCD including data collection and analysis and dissemination of AOCD results.

Constructivist Research Paradigm

Research design and methods, such as those used in AOCD, reflect a specific research paradigm; defined as a set of basic beliefs about the nature of reality that can be studied and understood (Denzin & Lincoln, 2011; Lincoln & Guba, 2000; Tashakkori & Teddlie, 1998). These basic beliefs are accepted simply on faith, however well argued, and there is no way to establish their ultimate truth. The *positivist* and *postpositivist* research paradigms, for example, hold that a single reality on how things really are and really work exists to be studied and understood. The *positivist* research paradigm holds that this single reality can be fully captured; this paradigm is reflected in experimental research designs and methods, which are used most often in the basic sciences. Whereas the *postpositivist* research paradigm holds that this single reality can only be approximated and is reflected in quasi-experimental research designs and methods, used most often in the social and behavioral sciences. Both experimental and quasi-experimental methods require objective detachment between researchers and participants so that any influence in either direction (that is, threats to validity) on what is being studied can be eliminated or reduced.

For AOCD, the set of basic beliefs are those of a *constructivist* research paradigm, which holds that multiple realities exist to be studied and understood (Denzin & Lincoln, 2011; Lincoln & Guba, 2000; Tashakkori & Teddlie, 1998). Each reality is an intangible construction rooted in people's experiences with everyday life, how they remember them, and make sense of them. Individual constructions of reality are assumed to be more or less "informed" or "sophisticated," rather than more or less "true" and, consequently, are alterable. The aim is to generate a "consensus construction of reality" that is more informed and sophisticated than any of the predecessor constructions (including those of the researchers), and which moves both participants and researchers toward action and change. To achieve this aim, the methods used are those that require researchers and participants to be interactively linked so that the consensus construction of reality is literally created as the study proceeds. AOCD researchers are cast, therefore, in the roles of participant and facilitator. The research design they follow is the case study (Creswell, 2007).

Case Study Research Design

The case study research design, as defined by Creswell (2007, p.73), is "an exploration of a 'bounded system' or case (or multiple cases) over time through detailed, in-depth data collection involving multiple sources of information rich in context, [which] . . . include observations, interviews, audio-visual material, and documents and reports." The foundation of the case study design is purposeful sampling (Creswell, 2007), whereby the data to be collected are selected to represent what is considered to be the critical perspectives of the case. For AOCD, the case is a community and the critical perspectives to be represented in the data are those of Insiders and Outsiders. Insiders are those who are members of the community of interest. Outsiders, who may or may not be members of this community, are those who provide services or otherwise exert external influence on the community, such as elected officials and academic researchers (Eng & Blanchard, 1991). For AOCD, communities have typically been defined as geographic and locality-based, or as identity-based, in which members share a common culture or characteristics (Quinn, 1999).

AOCD is conducted by a team of researchers, who are typically Outsiders, guided by one or two community partners, who include an Insider (for example, local resident) and an Outsider (for example, staff of local agency serving this community), or just one individual who is both (for example, local agency staff who lives in this community). Being guided, accompanied, and introduced by community partners is critical to the team's entry into the community. In addition, community partners' roles in building relationships, trust, and respect for the team's commitment to the community are important foundations for the data collection process. Data collection and analysis cannot be separated from the interpersonal aspects of the overall AOCD process.

Data Collection and Analysis

With guidance from community partners, the AOCD team collects and analyzes data iteratively, using the process of constant comparison (Corbin & Strauss, 2008; Strauss & Corbin, 1998). AOCD data sources are the following: (1) demographic data to describe population characteristics of the community; (2) secondary data on social and health indicators that represent professionals' perspectives on the community; (3) secondary data on the community's history and geography including information on health and human service organizations serving the community; (4) field notes from each AOCD team member's participant observations of a community and agencies that serve its residents; (5) transcripts from interviews with key informants for Outsiders' views; and (6) transcripts from interviews with key informants for Insiders' views. As data are collected and de-identified, the AOCD team and their community partners immediately analyze them to inform the next lines of inquiry.

With regard to selecting and recruiting participants for key informant interviews with Insiders and Outsiders, community partners are essential for identifying the initial pool of potential participants and determining effective strategies for recruiting them. As community partners, they possess unique knowledge for identifying individuals with insights on the experiences and priorities among Insiders or Outsiders. In addition, community partners can help the AOCD team select effective modes for contacting and wording scripts for inviting key informants to be interviewed.

Incidents, actions, and events reported by Insiders are compared within and across data sources, using the qualitative research method of coding and retrieving. A code is a category of meaning or concept, such as *voice in government and politics*, which is identified by reading through text from interview transcripts and secondary data. To develop a list of codes, two team members independently read through the initial data, come to a consensus on the name and definition for each code, and present the list to the rest of the team and their preceptors for final refinement. Text lines representing the same concept are assigned the same code so that they can be retrieved and grouped to determine one or more patterns of meaning, or themes, such as: *Residents express a strong desire to be heard and understood by county officials, but because their town is unincorporated, there is no formal voice for residents.* The same is done with data sources that represent the perspectives of Outsiders (for example, interview transcripts and secondary data), and include those of individuals on the AOCD team (for example, field notes from participant observations). Convergent analysis of themes is conducted to examine similarities and differences between the perspectives of Insiders and Outsiders on the conditions for a community to be in good health.

Dissemination

As the findings emerge, the AOCD team and their community partners select Insiders and Outsiders who participated in key informant interviews to serve on an AOCD Forum Planning Committee. The committee reviews, interprets, and prioritizes the themes that emerge from Insiders' and Outsiders' views on a community's assets, challenges, and needs for change. This committee then determines the forum's content, format, and logistics for engaging community residents and local service providers in interpreting the results, constructing a "consensus construction" from the findings on the conditions necessary for a community to be in good health, and committing to next action steps (Eng & Blanchard, 1991; Quinn, 1999; Shirah, Eng, Moore, Rhodes, & Royster, 2002).

Duration

In short, AOCD is as much a process of relationship building and community organizing as it is a research process (Eng & Blanchard, 1991). Given the necessity of building relationships, it is important to anticipate the time required to complete an AOCD. Although the duration will vary according to the skills among individuals on the team, the readiness of a community, travel distance, and other variables, it is realistic to estimate a *minimum* of six to nine months. This time period is needed to build relationships, establish mutual commitment and norms for a partnership approach, and determine priorities and research questions from the assessment data *before* moving to the next stage of designing a study or program. Even when researchers are invited by a community to conduct AOCD, such as for the case example below, an optimal time period would be about 18 months (Yonas et al., 2006).

Application of AOCD Methods with United Voices of Efland-Cheeks, Inc.

This example describes the application of AOCD in a small rural community in North Carolina including the process by which students gained entrée into the community, collected secondary data and conducted participant observations and interviews with key informants. The section concludes with a description of how AOCD findings in this community were disseminated.

Partnership Background

United Voices of Efland-Cheeks, Inc. (UVE), is a community-based organization operating with its own governing structure and bylaws. Located in Orange County, North Carolina (NC), the communities served by UVE are rural and largely African American—separated historically and geographically from the health, business, education, and financial resources of Chapel Hill despite being in the same county. UVE's mission is to improve the quality of life for children, youth, adults, and seniors in Efland-Cheeks, North Carolina, by providing a variety of educational, literary, scientific, and charitable activities. Since 1992, UVE has sustained a partnership with the UNC Gillings School of Global Public Health through the North Carolina Community-Based Public Health Consortium's governing structures and processes aimed specifically at engaging all partners in Community-Based Participatory Research (CBPR). UVE board members include concerned community members and representatives from the Orange County Public Health Department, other local health agencies, and the UNC Gillings School of Global Public Health. Through these collaborations, UVE activities include serving as a CBPR training site for four postdoctoral fellows of the W.K. Kellogg Foundation's Community Health Scholars Program; providing *Community Voices Leadership Training* for local residents; designing, conducting, and evaluating a *Teens in Power Program* to prevent illicit drug use among local adolescents; serving as a community research partner for two federally funded intervention studies—*Men as Navigators for Health Project* to increase informed decision making about prostate cancer screening among rural African American men, and *The Black Church and CVD: Are We Our Brother's Keeper?*—to increase adherence to Cardiovascular Disease (CVD) care among rural African American men (Ayala et al., 2009; Griffith et al., 2007; Ornelas et al., 2009).

Of particular relevance to this chapter is the AOCD conducted in Efland from October 2002 to April 2003 by a team of six graduate students enrolled in a two-semester AOCD course sequence required for the MPH degree in the UNC Department of Health Behavior and Health Education. The Efland AOCD team members were all women with a college education, two were from North Carolina; five were white and one was African American. In the classroom, they learned the concepts and practiced the skills for conducting AOCD from a teaching team (two instructors, two teaching assistants, and two postdoctoral fellows). In Efland, the community partners simultaneously guided the students to apply their newly learned skills. The community partners were both African Americans born and raised in Efland. One community partner was the UVE president, a retired man, and the other community partner was a woman employed as deputy registrar of Vital Records at the Orange County Public Health Department who also was a founding member of UVE. With one being an Insider (male resident) and the other being both an Insider (female resident) and Outsider (agency staff), the AOCD team was given a wide range of access and perspectives on Efland as a community. For the purposes of this case example, which was conducted as a graduate course requirement, the two community partners are referred to as "preceptors."

The previous community assessment of Efland was conducted in 1990, as an important part of a planning year award to the UNC School of Public Health for the *Community-Based Public Health Initiative*, funded by the W.K. Kellogg Foundation. This Initiative led to the formation of UVE in 1992. Ten years later, UVE and two longtime UNC partners who teach the required AOCD course agreed that another community assessment was needed, and that the process of action and new knowledge to be generated through an AOCD would be mutually beneficial. UVE would be able to revitalize its agenda and membership based on a new understanding of changes in the conditions within and surrounding Efland. New public health professionals being trained at UNC would be guided by a community's Insiders in gaining skills through on-the-ground experience in community-based practice and participatory research. The full report, with complete appendixes of the Efland AOCD (Aulino et al., 2003) described in this chapter, can be downloaded from the UNC Health Sciences Library at http://www.hsl.unc.edu/phpapers/Efland2003.pdf.

Gathering Secondary Data

Gathering secondary data provided the AOCD team with an initial broad brushstroke on how a community is portrayed by Outsiders in the health and human service professions, political arena, and others. The Efland team used secondary data as background information to: (1) chart their entry into the community; (2) identify gaps in existing data; and (3) inform their interview guides. Secondary sources of statistics and qualitative data they collected were U.S. and N.C. census data; Web sites of government agencies for N.C. and Orange County (for example, the health department, planning department, school board, department on aging, chamber of commerce, transportation department, and the Environmental Protection Agency); an AOCD Report of the Efland-Mebane Corridor (Roodhouse, Siegfried, & Viruell, 1990); an evaluation report of UVE's Teens in Power program (Bruning, Eastwood, Gerhard, & Reid, 1993); and a master's thesis on a photovoice study conducted with Efland youth (Tucker, 2002). In addition, during interviews, the team solicited brochures, newspaper articles, annual reports, and grant applications.

Efland is a geographically defined community. Nonetheless, statistical data were either rarely collected at the community level or not extracted easily, efficiently, or cost-effectively from available sources. Because it is an unincorporated area of Orange County, its geographic boundaries are approximate—on Highway 70 between Hillsborough and Mebane. Its population size is also just an estimate at 500–600 families, of whom about one-fourth are African American. "For some, Efland is a state of mind" (Aulino et al., 2003, p. 14). Consequently, the team was forced to extrapolate from county-level statistics and make interpretations, while avoiding generalizations about Efland, to inform their application for IRB approval and prepare for entering the community.

Participant Observation and Gaining Entry

Participant observation is a primary data-gathering device used as part of an in-depth case study approach, which places researchers in direct involvement in people's lives, to "generate practical and theoretical truths about human life grounded in the realities of daily existence" (Jorgensen, 1989, p. 14). In preparing for entry to Efland, as a group of "professional strangers," the team and their preceptors needed a succinct way of introducing who they were and explaining why they were there. As recommended by Bogdewic (1992, p. 51), "An honest, jargon-free, down-to-earth explanation will suffice. Among other things, such an explanation is much easier for someone to pass on to the other members . . . [and] I was better off giving a much broader description of my purpose." The AOCD team's introduction was: *We are a group of six UNC students collaborating with community members in Efland to learn about the strengths and concerns of the Efland community.*

The AOCD team's first participant observation was a *windshield tour* (Minkler & Hancock, 2008), guided by their preceptors, of Efland and the surrounding area. They used the opportunity of UVE's annual Oktoberfest fundraiser to make initial contacts and volunteered in UVE's after-school program to begin developing collaborative relationships with residents and service providers. These relationships were essential for **gaining entrée to a community** through access to key people in the community and local agencies, and being entrusted with information that is pertinent and dependable (Bogdewic, 1992). Other observations suggested and facilitated by their preceptors included: the Efland Seniors Group's morning activities; board meetings of the county commissioners, school board, planning board, and transportation board; the PTA; and UVE monthly meetings.

Further, it was important for the team to record *field notes* systematically on their reactions, thoughts, and feelings about what they saw and heard. A participant observer consciously recording the details can construct patterns and meanings from analyzing field notes. Moreover, it is the team's views that will have an impact on their data collection, interpretation, and next steps. Recording field notes and debriefing with other members of the team on their respective perceptions, thoughts, and feelings are critical sources of data. Field notes were, therefore, entered into a database for analysis by the team. (For more details on the mechanics of recording and analyzing field notes, see Chapter Eleven in this volume.)

Key Informant Interviewing

In addition to collecting secondary data and primary data through participant observation to represent the views of Insiders and Outsiders, it is important to interview knowledgeable community members and representatives from local agencies and institutions. Given the constraints of time and resources, however, AOCD researchers cannot cultivate relationships with every knowledgeable Insider and Outsider. Instead, AOCD researchers conduct in-depth interviews with *key informants* (Goetz & LeCompte, 1984; LeCompte & Schensul, 2010; Spradley, 1979) who have been in the community or institution for sufficient time periods to accumulate special knowledge, relationships with people, and access to observations that are denied to researchers. Key informants who are thoughtful observers and informal historians are valuable to AOCD researchers (Bernard, 1988). Not only can they articulate important issues, but they can explain why they see those particular issues as important. (See Chapter Six in this volume for a complementary discussion of conducting in-depth interviews with community experts.)

Key informants' views on the history and culture of the community, social groupings and their relationships with institutions, perceived barriers to and facilitators for past and current health promotion efforts provide an indispensable foundation for interventions to promote good health. Their perspectives and expertise, however, often are eclipsed by secondary data to identify the problem areas and what a community needs to ameliorate the problems. By connecting with key informants through AOCD, their investment and expertise can increase the willingness of community members and local institutions to embrace, participate in, and sustain the process initiated by the team.

In Efland, the team identified key informants through referrals from their preceptors, public domain listings of leaders in institutions and agencies, and by asking other key informants at the end of each interview:

- Are there people or organizations with whom you think we should speak that you would be willing to gain permission for our team to contact?
- How would you describe the specific person or organization?
- Why would you think their opinion and views would be helpful for us to hear?

They recruited a total of 42 key informants (28 community members and 14 service providers). Of these, they conducted in-depth interviews with 10 community members and 14 service providers, and three focus group interviews with 12 youth and 6 adult community members of Efland.

Key Informant In-Depth Interview

The one-on-one interviews with adult key informants in Efland used an in-depth interview guide developed and pretested by the team with their preceptors (see Appendix D). Each interview began with introductions and a brief explanation of the interviewing process that was guided by a Fact Sheet. The Community Key Informant interview guide contained 22 open-ended questions that explored the following seven areas:

- General information about the Efland community

- Assets and needs of the community

- Problem-solving and decision-making patterns

- Services and businesses

- Recommended individuals to interview

- Recommendations for the community forum

- Any additional information

The Service Provider Key Informant interview guide contained the same areas and asked similar questions. The exception was the section on Services and Businesses, which asked the following seven questions:

- How long have you worked in this community? Why did you choose to work in Efland?

- What is your agency's role in the community? What is your source of funding?

- What services do you provide to residents of Efland?

- What services go underutilized?

- Who in the community is in the most need of your agency's services?

- What are your biggest barriers or challenges at work?

- Which community needs are not met by your agency or other organizations in Efland?

Each interview ranged from 45 to 90 minutes and was conducted and tape-recorded by two members of the AOCD team. A note taker accompanied the interviewer to record written verbal statements and nonverbal cues. After completing the interview, they met to debrief the interview and record written field notes on points made by the key informant that they considered important, as well as their personal reflections on the experience.

Key Informant Focus Group Interview

Youth were considered such an important part of UVE's mission that the preceptors needed their views represented through AOCD. The procedures and time required by IRB made it not feasible, however, to recruit and solicit signed informed assent from minors and signed informed consent from their guardians to participate in in-depth interviews with minors.

Instead, the team received IRB approval for youth to participate anonymously in focus group interviews. The preceptors assisted the team in distributing Focus Group Fact Sheets to youth and guardians. The focus group guide explored four topics: (1) their satisfaction with Efland and what they would change about it; (2) what they do for fun and to make money; (3) interactions at school and what they would change about the school; and (4) their recommendations for the community forum.

The focus group interviews ranged from 45 to 90 minutes. The procedures followed were identical to those for the key informant in-depth interview described above. (For further discussion of focus group interview procedures see Chapter Nine in this volume.)

Community Forum

The outcome from an AOCD is not only to produce a report but also to begin a process of action informed by and grounded in the primary and secondary data gathered on Insiders' and Outsiders' perspectives as part of the AOCD. (For further discussion of dissemination procedures and guidelines see Chapter Fourteen.) Although a report that includes data and its interpretation is valuable for both Insiders and Outsiders to document the needs and resources in a community (for example, Efland) for planning future interventions, it is equally important to document relationships and articulate the different perspectives regarding a community's priorities in order to create sustainable efforts that build on existing community structures and decision-making processes. One of the most valuable means for generating this outcome is for the process to culminate in a community forum that enables diverse groups in the community and those who serve them to gather, listen to, and discuss the results of the data collection process.

Facilitation of the community forum is critical, as the articulation of Insider and Outsider perspectives is done in an equitable fashion, whereby both Insiders and Outsiders are able to discuss the health, needs, and resources of their community, and prioritize the next steps in an action plan. There are three goals of the forum: (1) arrive at a consensus on priority needs and motivations for change; (2) examine possible causes and consequences of a priority problem; and (3) establish a partnership between communities and local agencies to develop a plan of action (Eng & Moore, 2003). The session should not be spent merely identifying what is "wrong" within the community; time should be dedicated to articulating strengths and resources available within the community. At the forum's culmination, persons will have self-identified and committed to accepting responsibility for following through with specific elements of the action plan, and segments of the group at the forum will plan a next meeting. Of equal importance, the forum should signal two important transitions: (a) from the assessment phase to program planning; and (b) for community/agency partners to take on more proactive responsibilities for program planning.

The Efland Community Forum Planning Committee was composed of 15 residents and service providers who began meeting weekly with the AOCD team and their preceptors in mid-March. Their goal was to organize a gathering that would help create new opportunities for citizens of Efland, and entitled it "Showcase for the Future: Spotlight on Efland." They developed the following strategies to promote the forum, which was held at the end of April in the local elementary school cafeteria.

- Fliers were posted in prominent places throughout the community, such as the post office, barbershops, the car wash, a local convenience store, and the Efland Community Center. In addition, each child at the elementary school received a flier to take home on the Wednesday before the forum. The school also posted a banner announcement outside the school the week before the forum.

- Personal invitations were delivered to church leaders and church announcements.

- Inserts about the forum were mailed with water bills by the Orange-Alamance Water System.

- Door prizes for forum participants were solicited from local businesses, such as passes to sport events, restaurant gift certificates, and movie tickets.

- Performances by the local youth step team and gospel singing group, and bakers for the "cake walk" were arranged.

Over 100 people, including 30 youth, participated in the forum. Planning committee members welcomed attendees, explained the goals of the forum, recognized the work of the AOCD team, and foreshadowed plans for follow-up. AOCD team members then briefly described the purpose of AOCD and the methods used, presented the major themes that had emerged, and invited participants to choose a small group of one of the four themes selected by the planning committee. Themes discussed were lack of recreation opportunities for youth, poor water and sewer infrastructure, lack of transportation, and the need for local services. For a more detailed discussion about each theme, see www.hsl.unc.edu/phpapers/Efland2003. pdf. Team members, trained in empowerment education techniques, used force field analysis (Lewin, 1997; see Appendix A) and SHOWED (Shaffer, 1983; Wallerstein, 1994) to facilitate the small-group discussions. Small-group participants discussed the causes and consequences of the particular theme and then reflected on how it affected them personally and the community as a whole. They then formulated action steps that were summarized and presented back to the large group by a community representative from each of the small groups. Action steps presented at the forum were incorporated into the AOCD final report (Aulino et al., 2003).

The planning committee also included entertainment at various times in the forum agenda in order to facilitate community cohesion, help alleviate some of the strong feelings that could arise from the group discussions, and to make the overall experience enjoyable. Entertainment included a "cake walk" and performances by the local 4-H Kinds of Unity Club and a gospel singing group. The date and location for a follow-up meeting, to be organized by the preceptors, was announced at the conclusion of the forum. The AOCD team expressed their appreciation, and before leaving, participants were asked to complete an interest form to indicate the issues they would like to pursue (Aulino et al., 2003).

CHALLENGES, LESSONS LEARNED, AND IMPLICATIONS FOR CONDUCTING AOCD

Although conducting a social diagnosis, such as AOCD, is considered an essential initial phase of program planning, it is too often skipped due to a variety of challenges (Green, Kreuter, & Kreuter 1999), of which four are highlighted here. These challenges are: the requirements for transitioning from assessment to action; the need for a team with skills from multiple disciplines; the need for professionals to be colearners; and time requirements.

As mentioned earlier, AOCD requires substantial investment in time—a minimum of six months—for gaining entrée to a community; building relationships; collecting, analyzing, and interpreting data; and planning and conducting the forum. Frequently, professionals engage in AOCD as part of their job responsibilities and students do so as part of their academic program. Their involvement in AOCD is "on a clock" that is paced and imposed by their institutions. The progress of the Efland AOCD, for example, was challenged by academia's inflexibility with IRB's meeting schedule, semester breaks, and deadlines for submitting grades. Similarly, community members' ongoing obligations to jobs and families competed with the time required to collaborate with the AOCD team, for example, as a preceptor, key informant, or forum planning committee member. To anticipate unexpected but inevitable challenges of time, the team itself met weekly, met biweekly with their preceptors, and designated a liaison to communicate more frequently with the preceptors by e-mail or phone. In addition, the teaching team held a lunch meeting every other month with the preceptors for Efland and seven other AOCD teams, and designated an instructor as the liaison to communicate with the preceptors.

One possibility for reducing the time period is to constrain AOCD to people served by one established local organization, such as UVE or a health department (Shirah et al., 2002). The advantage of working with a local organization for the AOCD team is quick access to those segments of the community closely associated with this particular organization and its affiliates. The disadvantage of this "short-cut" is the inadvertent reluctance of persons to express their views because they either do not feel represented by the organization or have a negative history with this organization. As a result, the AOCD may have missed opportunities for relationship building among diverse groups within a community. To reduce this disadvantage, the Efland AOCD team and their preceptors made a conscious effort *not* to function or be viewed as "sponsored by UVE." To cast a wide net, the team maintained a record of referrals to information sources and key informants to chart the diversity of views represented. In addition, although referrals included those made by the preceptors, they did not have access to the data until the team had removed all identifiers, and the team maintained confidentiality of the identities of those actually interviewed.

Another challenge is that AOCD requires colearning to be achieved by reconciling new knowledge generated with current understanding and experiences of a community (Perry, 1968). AOCD requires professionals to function as colearners with a community's Insiders and Outsiders. AOCD also requires one or two Insiders/Outsiders, who are willing to serve as points of entry for the AOCD team, to recognize that they have something new to learn about their community. Colearning, however, can sometimes frustrate Insiders and Outsiders. On a personal level, professionals engaged in AOCD often encounter and collaborate with people who differ in social status (Merton, 1970; Shirah et al., 2002). To make these differences explicit in the consciousness of students, the AOCD course organized the following three required workshops: institutionalized racism, invisibility of persons with disabilities, and homophobia. Members of the Efland AOCD team wrote extensively in their field notes about being conscious of their internalized privilege as being white or UNC graduate students, or both. They speculated on how being different from rural, low-income African Americans could limit their capacity to graft the cultural, historical, and experiential roots of Efland onto AOCD methods and findings. Being explicit about these differences was critical for establishing a research partnership with their preceptors and other Insiders.

A third challenge is that AOCD requires a range of concepts and skills from the fields of anthropology, epidemiology, health education, political science, community psychology, and community organizing. Learning and applying them adeptly would be impossible for a single person to achieve (Shirah et al., 2002). Hence, using a team approach that builds synergistically on each member's experience and skill set can maximize the quality of each method and task for completing the AOCD procedure. To ensure a range of skills among students assigned to each AOCD team, for example, the teaching team used the information from a 25-item "profile questionnaire" completed by each student on the assets he or she brings to AOCD. These included training in cultural competency or small-group facilitation; experience conducting surveys, qualitative interviews, or focus group interviews; proficiency with computer software programs; exposure to populations and cultures different from their own; languages; driver's license and access to a car.

Another challenge of AOCD is to sustain movement from data collection, analysis, and interpretation to the action steps generated during the community forum. For an AOCD team of students, such as in Efland, the natural inclination was to transfer responsibility to their preceptors and the community forum planning committee for the next phases. Preparing for the process for exiting a community needed to be as sensitive as the process for gaining entry.

For a nonstudent AOCD partnership, however, in keeping with the core phases of CBPR, the community and academic partners would engage the community forum planning committee and other forum participants in deciding which research design and data collection methods would be most appropriate for understanding and addressing the priority need. The research design could be etiologic, experimental with an intervention to be tested, or policy research—to be followed by several more phases, that is, feeding back and interpreting the findings, disseminating and translating research findings, and maintaining, sustaining, and evaluating the partnership (Israel, Coombe, & McGranaghan, 2010).

With regard to lessons learned from the Efland case example, defining community as relational, a geographic locality, or having the potential for political power (Heller, 1989) can have an important impact on the AOCD process. When an AOCD team uses geographic boundaries to define a community, they may overlook the assets and needs of subcommunities whose membership is based on common interests, history, or other relational characteristics that are not geographically based. When defining a community as relational, the potential risk is to neglect the impact of the physical environment on a community's identity. For communities whose geographic boundaries are not clear and common relationships are not clearly visible, designing a community-based intervention can be problematic to implement and evaluate (Shirah et al., 2002). It is essential, therefore, that in each encounter public health professionals develop a clear understanding of a community which has been mutually agreed upon with the community. To do this, AOCD is a viable option.

In an ideal world, AOCD would be conducted by public health organizations that respect and recognize a community's shared ownership of research procedures, findings, and dissemination. Organizations, however, do not always recognize when their own priorities are in conflict with those of a community.

Agencies have administrative and policy mandates that are likely to differ with a community's precedence of historical traditions and cultural norms. Funding organizations have expectations, which in most cases do not allow for flexibility in changing the focus of a study, even when the change requested is by the community being studied. Furthermore, organizations can place their professionals in the awkward position of negotiating on behalf of a community or, in some cases, speaking for a community. For these professionals, the pressures of competing interests are counterbalanced by the privilege of gaining entrée to and developing trust with a community.

In this less than ideal world, AOCD offers public health organizations and communities a process for beginning a new relationship—one that engenders a constant of open negotiation, colearning, and reciprocity. Entering into such a relationship can be a difficult transition for well-intentioned professionals who have been trained to be in control and to perceive themselves as having a larger skill set than that of their community partners. Yet, engaging in AOCD carries the long-term rewards of a CBPR partnership committed to understanding and addressing the conditions for a community to be in good health.

SUMMARY

The purpose of AOCD is to understand the collective dynamics and functions of relationships within a community and the interactions between community members and broader structures that can promote the conditions and skills required to assist community members in taking action for social change and health status improvement (Eng & Blanchard, 1991). Drawing upon the disciplines of anthropology, epidemiology, and community psychology, AOCD follows the assumptions of a constructivist research paradigm and combines both quantitative and qualitative methods to elicit and juxtapose the Insiders view with the Outsiders view.

Key to AOCD is its partnership approach that includes lay community members, community-based organization (CBO) representatives, health department and other agency staff, and university personnel, including students and faculty researchers. They share control over all phases of the research process, including community assessment, issue definition, development of research methodology, data collection and analysis, interpretation of data, dissemination of findings, and application of the results to address community concerns (action). This approach recognizes that lay community members are the experts in understanding and interpreting their own lives.

AOCD is an assets-oriented approach to understanding a community. Although identifying community needs and gaps is important in the quest to improve health outcomes, identifying assets to build on or further develop is equally important (McKnight & Kretzmann, 2012). Building on social structures and existing networks, decision-making processes, and local resources and strengths can yield intervention strategies that are rooted in the community, develop local critical-thinking and problem-solving skills, and ensure sustained efforts.

Finally, given that AOCD is one approach to assessing community strengths and dynamics, which is an early phase within the CBPR process, it is committed to movement toward action. This action may be loosely defined, including community organizing and mobilization; the development of new and authentic community member and agency partnerships with concrete tasks; and measurable plans for action with assigned responsibilities and defined time lines. The actions may be focused on immediate changes to improve health-related conditions, such as changes in public health department policies that increase access to services, or improved lighting on an outdoor neighborhood running/walking track. Furthermore, the actions may be focused on long-term changes in social determinants of health, such as improved racial equality in political representation through community mobilization and organization.

KEY TERMS

Community assessment

Insider and Outsider views

Gaining entrée to a community

DISCUSSION QUESTIONS

1. What are the pros and cons of conducting AOCD as the initial phase of designing a study or planning a program?

2. What are the roles and responsibilities of community partners, both while conducting AOCD and after its completion?

3. What is the value of pointing out the differences between the views and priorities of Insiders from those of Outsiders?

REFERENCES

Aulino, F., Farnsworth, J., Hunter, J., Jackson, T., Philpott, J., & Spurlock, D. (2003). *Efland, Orange County, An action-oriented community diagnosis: Findings and next steps of action.* Retrieved August 18, 2004, from http://www.hsl.unc.edu/phpapers/Efland2003.pdf

Ayala, G., Ornelas, I., Rhodes, S. R., Amell, J. W., Armstrong-Brown, J., Horton, E., et al. (2009). Correlates of dietary intake among men involved in the MAN for Health study, *American Journal of Men's Health, 3*, 214–223.

Bernard, H. R. (1988). *Research methods in cultural anthropology.* Newbury Park, CA: Sage.

Bogdewic, S. P. (1992). Participant observation. In B. F. Crabtree & W. L. Miller (Eds.), *Doing Qualitative Research.* Newbury Park, CA: Sage.

Bowie, J., Eng, E., & Lichtenstein R. (2009). A decade of postdoctoral training in CBPR and dedication to Thomas A. Bruce. *Progress in Community Health Partnerships: Research, Education, and Action, 3*(4), 267–270.

Braveman, P. A., Cubbin, C., Egerter, S., Williams, D. R., & Pamuk, E. (2010). Socioeconomic disparities in health in the United States: What the patterns tell us. *American Journal of Public Health, 100* Suppl 1, S186–S196.

Bruning, A., Eastwood, K., Gerhard, L., & Reid, A. (1993). *Teens in Power: A program for the prevention of illicit drug use by adolescents in the Efland-Cheeks community.* A report prepared for PUBH246: Public Health Program Planning and Evaluation: University of North Carolina at Chapel Hill.

Butterfoss, F. D., Goodman, R. M., & Wandersman, A. (1996). Community coalitions for prevention and health promotion: Factors predicting satisfaction, participation, and planning. *Health Education Quarterly, 23*, 65–79.

Cassel, J. C. (1976). The contribution of the social environment to host resistance: The Fourth Wade Hampton Frost Lecture. *American Journal of Epidemiology, 104*, 107–123.

Corbin, J., & Strauss, A. (2008). *Basics of qualitative research* (3rd ed.). Thousand Oaks, CA: Sage.

Creswell, J. W. (2007). *Qualitative inquiry and research design: Choosing among five traditions* (2nd ed.). Thousand Oaks, CA: Sage.

Denzin, N. K., & Lincoln, Y. S. (Eds.). (2011). *The Sage handbook of qualitative research* (4th ed.). Thousand Oaks, CA: Sage.

Eng, E., & Blanchard, L. (1991). Action-oriented community diagnosis: A health education tool. *International Journal of Community Health Education, 11*, 93–110.

Eng, E., & Moore, K. S. (2003) *The community forum*. Lecture in HBHE 241, Action-Oriented Community Diagnosis, University of North Carolina, School of Public Health.

Eng, E., & Parker, E. A. (2002). Natural helper models. In R. DiClemente, R. Crosby, & M. Kegler (Eds.), *Emerging theories and models in health promotion research & practice*. San Francisco: Jossey-Bass.

Fetterman, D. M. (1989). *Ethnography: Step by step*. Newbury Park, CA: Sage.

Goetz, J. P., & LeCompte, M. D. (1984). *Ethnography and qualitative design in educational research*. Orlando, FL: Academic Press.

Green, L. W., Kreuter, M., & Kreuter, M. W. (1999). *Health promotion planning: An educational and environmental approach* (3rd ed.). Mountain View, CA: Mayfield.

Griffith, D. M., Mason, M. A., Rodela, M., Matthews, D. D., Tran, A., Royster, M., et al. (2007). A structural approach to examining prostate cancer risk for rural southern African American men. *Journal of Healthcare for the Poor and Underserved*, *18*, 73–101.

Griffith, D. M., Citrin, T., Jerome, N. W., Bayer, I. S., & Mebane, E. (2009). The origins and overview of the W.K. Kellogg Community Health Scholars Program. *Progress in Community Health Partnerships: Research, Education, and Action*, *3*, 335–348.

Hancock, T., & Minkler, M. (2012). Community health assessment or healthy community assessment: Whose community? Whose assessment? In M. Minkler (Ed.), *Community organizing and community building for health*, (3rd ed.). New Brunswick, NJ: Rutgers University Press.

Heller, K. (1989). The return to community. *Journal of Community Psychology*, *17*, 1–15.

Institute of Medicine. (1988). *The future of public health*. Washington, DC: National Academy Press.

Israel, B. A., Coombe, C., & McGranaghan, R. (2010). Community-based participatory research: A partnership approach for public health [CD-ROM]. Available from http://sitemaker.umich.edu/cbpr/home.

Israel, B. A., Dawson, L., Steckler, A. B., & Eng, E. (1993). Guy W. Steuart: The person and his works. *Health Education Quarterly*, *Suppl*(1), S137–S150.

Israel, B. A., Schulz, A. J., Parker, E. A., Becker, A. B., Allen, A., & Guzman, J. R. (2008). Critical issues in developing and following CBPR principles. In M. Minkler & N. Wallerstein (Eds.), *Community-based participatory research for health: From process to outcomes* (2nd ed., pp. 47–66). San Francisco: Jossey-Bass.

Jorgensen, D. L. (1989). *Participant observation: A methodology of human studies*. Newbury Park, CA: Sage.

Kark, S. L. (1951). Health center service. In E. H. Cluver (Ed.), *Social medicine*. Johannesburg, South Africa: Central News Agency.

Kark, S. L., & Steuart, G. W. (1962). *A practice of social medicine, a South African team's experiences in different African communities*. Edinburgh: E. & S. Livingstone.

Kauffman, K. S. (1994). The Insider/Outsider dilemma: Field experience of a white researcher "getting in" a poor black community. *Nursing Research, 43,* 179–183.

Krieger, N. (2003). Does racism harm health? Did child abuse exist before 1962? On explicit questions, critical science, and current controversies: An ecosocial perspective. *American Journal of Public Health, 93,* 194–199.

LeCompte, M. D., & Schensul, J. (2010). *Designing and conducting ethnographic research* (Vol. 1). Lanham, MD: AltaMira Press.

Lewin, K. (1997/1948). *Resolving social conflicts and field theory in social science.* Washington, DC: American Psychological Association. (Original work published 1948.)

Lincoln, Y. S., & Guba, E. G. (2000). Paradigmatic controversies, contradictions, and emerging confluences. In N. K. Denzin & Y. S. Lincoln (Eds.), *The handbook of qualitative research* (2nd ed., pp. 163–188). Thousand Oaks, CA: Sage.

McKnight, J. L., & Kretzmann, J. P. (2012). Mapping community capacity. In M. Minkler (Ed.) *Community organizing and community building for health and welfare* (3rd ed.). New Brunswick, NJ: Rutgers University Press.

Merton, R. K. (1970). Insiders and Outsiders: A chapter in the sociology of knowledge. *American Journal of Sociology, 7,* 9–45.

Minkler, M., & Hancock, T. (2008). Community-driven asset identification and issue selection. In M. Minkler & N. Wallerstein (Eds.), *Community-based participatory research for health: From process to outcomes* (2nd ed., pp. 153–169). San Francisco: Jossey-Bass.

Morris, M. W., Leung, K., Ames, D., & Lickel, B. (1999). Views from inside and outside: Integrating emic and etic insights about culture and justice judgment. *The Academy of Management Review, 24,* 781–796.

Ornelas, I., Amell, J. W., Tran, A., Royster, M., Armstrong-Brown, J., & Eng, E. (2009). Understanding African American men's perceptions of racism, male gender socialization, and social capital through photovoice. *Qualitative Health Research, 19,* 552–565.

Parker, E. A., Eng, E., Laraia, B., Ammerman, A., Dodds, J., Margolis, L., & Cross, A. (1998). Coalition building for prevention: Lessons learned from the North Carolina Community-Based Public Health Initiative. *Journal of Public Health Management & Practice, 4,* 25–36.

Perry, W. G. (1968). *Forms of intellectual and ethical development in the college years: A scheme.* New York: Holt, Rinehart, & Winston.

Quinn, S. (1999). Teaching community diagnosis: Integrating community experience with meeting graduate standards for health educators. *Health Education Research, 14,* 685–696.

Roodhouse, K., Siegfried, J., & Viruell, E. (1990). *Orange County community diagnosis–1990: Needs assessment of Efland Mebane Corridor.* Report prepared for the Department of Health Behavior and Health Education: University of North Carolina at Chapel Hill.

Shaffer, R. (1983). *Beyond the dispensary.* Nairobi, Kenya: Amref.

Shirah, K., Eng, E., Moore, K., Rhodes, S. D., & Royster, M. O. (2002). *Insider's view and Outsider's view: Duality of cultural understanding and planned social change.* Paper presented at the American Public Health Association Annual Meeting, Philadelphia.

Spradley, J. P. (1979). *The ethnographic interview*. New York: Holt, Rinehart, & Winston.

Steckler, A. B., Dawson, L., Israel, B. A., & Eng, E. (1993). Community health development: An overview of the works of Guy W. Steuart. *Health Education Quarterly, Suppl, 1*, S3–S20.

Steuart, G. W. (1985). Social and behavioral change strategies. In H. T. Phillips & S. A. Gaylord (Eds.), *Aging and public health*. New York: Springer.

Steuart, G. W., & Kark, S. L. (1962). Community health education. In S. L. Kark & G. W. Steuart (Eds.), *A practice of social medicine: A South African team's experiences in different African communities*. Edinburgh and London: E. & S. Livingstone.

Steuart, G. W. (Ed.). (1969). Scientist and professional; the relations between research and action *Health Education Monographs, no. 29*. New York: Society of Public Health Educators.

Strauss, A., & Corbin, J. (1998). *Basics of qualitative research* (2nd ed.). Thousand Oaks, CA: Sage.

Tashakkori, A., & Teddlie, C. (1998). Introduction to mixed method and mixed model studies in the social and behavioral sciences. In *Mixed methodology: Combining qualitative and quantitative approaches* (pp. 1–2). Thousand Oaks, CA: Sage.

Taylor, R. B. (2002). Fear of crime, social ties, and collective efficacy: Maybe masquerading measurement, maybe déjà vu all over again. *Justice Quarterly, 19*(4), 773–792.

Trostle, J. (1986). Anthropology and epidemiology in the twentieth century: A selective history of the collaborative projects and theoretical affinities, 1920–1970. In C. R. James, R. Stall, & S. M. Gifford (Eds.), *Anthropology and epidemiology: Interdisciplinary approaches to the study of health and diseases (culture, illness, and healing)* (pp. 59–96). Norwell, MA: Kluwer.

Tucker, C. (2002). *The Efland Youth Photovoice Project: A participatory social assessment*. University of North Carolina, Chapel Hill.

Wallerstein, N. (1994). Empowerment education applied to youth. In A. C. Matiella (Ed.) *Multicultural challenge in health education* (pp. 153–176). Santa Cruz, CA: ETR Associates.

Williams, D. R. (2003). The health of men: structured inequalities and opportunities. *American Journal of Public Health, 93*, 724–731.

Yonas, M. A., Jones, N., Eng, E., Vines, A., Aronson, R. E., Griffith, D. M., et al. (2006). The art and science of integrating undoing racism with CBPR: Challenges of pursuing NIH funding to investigate cancer care and racial equity. *Journal of Urban Health, 83*, 1004–1012.

Young, J. (2005). On insiders (emic) and outsiders (etic): Views of self, and othering. *Systemic Practice and Action Research, 18*, 151–162.

Acknowledgments: The authors deeply appreciate the considerable support, commitment, and contributions of the following individuals and groups with whom we serve as coinvestigators and colearners. We thank the graduate students in Health Behavior and Health Education at the University of North Carolina School of Public Health, who set a high standard for following CBPR principles, including the Efland Action Oriented Community Diagnosis (AOCD) Team of Felicity Aulino, Jennifer Farnsworth, Jaimie Hunter, Julia Martin, Theresa Jackson, and Danielle Spurlock, and the AOCD teaching assistants, Molly Loomis and Lauren Shirey. We express our sincere gratitude to our CBPR partners of 18 years—the Orange County Public Health Department, The United Voices of Efland-Cheeks, Inc., and the Efland community—from whom we continue to learn the lessons about what is a community. To the W.K. Kellogg Foundation, we express our gratitude and recognize our good fortune in receiving continued support for preparing public health professionals with competencies in taking a CBPR approach to help address the major health problems and challenges facing society.

Chapter 6

USING ETHNOGRAPHY

IN PARTICIPATORY

COMMUNITY ASSESSMENT

JEAN J. SCHENSUL

MARLENE J. BERG

SARITHA NAIR

This chapter describes how **participatory** approaches to ethnography can be used to conduct **community assessment** in health and other sectors. Ethnographic data collection methods offer interactive, flexible, and readily accessible ways in which academically trained researchers and community members can conduct research together to better understand community settings; processes; organizational and cultural assets; and diversity of cultural resources, beliefs, and norms to suggest directions for their actions to remedy health inequities and reduce health disparities.

In this chapter, we define ethnography, describe why it is a useful participatory community assessment approach, and how it can be used to conduct a community assessment. We illustrate with a case example drawn from an ongoing program of participatory community assessment conducted by the Institute for Community Research with youth partners in the Hartford, Connecticut (CT) area. For more in-depth methodological knowledge and expertise we refer readers to texts and other relevant literature (Berg & Schensul, 2004; LeCompte & Schensul, 2010; Sydlo et al., 2000).

COMMUNITY-BASED PARTICIPATORY RESEARCH AND COMMUNITY ASSESSMENT

Community-based participatory research (CBPR) is an approach to community health research and activism that involves the people affected by a problem in the conduct of research to help them solve it, usually in conjunction with academically trained researchers (Berg & Schensul, 2004; Israel, Eng, Schulz, & Parker, 2005; Minkler & Wallerstein, 2008; Schensul,

1999). CBPR aims to make sure that the research responds to community needs, is improved through community involvement and voice, and leads to health improvement (Williams, Bray, Shapiro-Mendoza, Reisz, & Peranteau, 2009). CBPR calls for researchers to maintain their involvement in the partner community and for the use of the data to promote improvements in community health and well-being (Viswanathan et al., 2004; Wallerstein & Duran, 2006).

Introducing Participatory Community Assessment (PCA)

Participatory community assessment (PCA) is a collective approach to assessing: how a community is defined and organized; who are the key people with whom to discuss a joint effort; what issues and needs exist from a community perspective and what structural and other factors explain them; what resources and **assets** are available that residents could mobilize to resolve a community problem; and what changes might take place that could address existing disparities in new and transformative ways (Aronson, Wallis, O'Campo, Whitehead, & Schafer, 2007; Clark et al., 2003). These questions are important for researchers whose roots lie within the study community as well as for those from communities and institutions located elsewhere, both of whom may be engaged in a participatory community assessment process. Participatory ethnography offers a means of improving the quality of participatory community assessment, by seeking a broad and systematically accumulated informational base on which to make decisions.

Defining the Characteristics of Ethnography That Are Compatible with Participatory Community Assessment

Ethnography emphasizes the direct involvement of researchers with communities and residents over time (LeCompte & Schensul, 2010). Further, ethnographic approaches use an ecological framework to emphasize the interaction of local communities with broader political, social, and economic factors. A hallmark of ethnography is the requirement that the researcher learn to think, act, and view the world through the eyes of community members (Pelto & Pelto, 1978). In the process ethnographers discover many characteristics of local **culture** and community organization and problem solving that constitute cultural "assets" or resources that can be applied to the solution of health problems (Kretzmann & McKnight, 1993).

Through participation in community life, ethnographers often uncover significant community problems and struggles, and many become involved in organized problem-solving and advocacy efforts. Thus in the applied social sciences, including ethnography, there is a long history of critical participatory research and action for social change (Berg & Schensul, 2004; Brydon-Miller, Greenwood, & Maguire, 2003; Fals Borda & Rahman, 1991; Fine & Torre, 2006; Greenwood & Levin, 1998; Maguire, 2006). Ethnographic research approaches allow for flexibility and innovation, offering interactive methods and tools for participatory community assessment with adults and youth (Reason & Bradbury, 2006; Schensul, Berg, & Williamson, 2008).

Defining Participatory Community Assessment

PCA identifies a community's issues and priorities, assets and liabilities, from a historical, cultural, and systemic perspective (Kretzmann & McKnight, 1993; Van Willigen, 2005). By "politically and historically" we mean learning about or revisiting characteristics of the community's history, demographic changes, and shifts in power and political organization. The term "culturally" refers to the diversity of cultural beliefs, norms, and rituals that bind community residents together. "Systemically" refers to the ways in which community institutions, populations, and resources interact and intersect with regional, national, and global policies, a perspective that is central to holistic analysis that takes into consideration power dynamics and differentials.

The primary stakeholders in PCA are those experiencing the problem or injustice and who have the most at stake in its resolution—community residents. To ameliorate the multiple ways in which marginalized or affected communities bear the brunt of power differentials, including lack of voice, it is critical that they be involved in PCA through their own research and assessment. Henceforth, we will refer to them as nonacademically trained community researchers (CRs). The assessments carried out by CRs are strengthened through the collaboration of academically trained researchers who act as facilitators and collaborators in a participatory community assessment process. Part Two of this book discusses the variety of ways that such partnerships may be formed. Academically trained researchers may be from the study community, or may have background and experience similar to that of residents of the study community (both of these groups are sometimes referred to as "Insider researchers"), or they may be "Outsider researchers"—not from the study community but knowledgeable about it and committed to its well-being (Bartunek & Louis, 1996; Merriam et al., 2001). A good PCA involves a partnership between community researchers and academically trained researchers to accomplish a shared practical goal—the collection of information leading to community improvement and transformation. In the process, academically trained researchers learn that residents can teach them about their own communities and perspectives, and community researchers gain inquiry skills, self- and group-efficacy, methodology for more effective assessment of their own communities, and voice that enables more effective advocacy. A participatory community assessment should reinforce community solidarity through identifying the structural, historical, social, and cultural factors contributing to a problem, and the resources available at the institutional, cultural, and individual levels to solve it.

Defining Community

"Community" may be conceptualized as membership in a group defined by illness or ability; membership in a specific ethnic, racial, or national group; shared gender identity; or networked connections on the Internet. Linking personal identity with community is an important dimension of all these definitions (Israel, Schulz, Parker, & Becker, 1998). (For more information on communities of identity see Chapter One, in this volume.) Public health researchers as well as community residents often define community as a geosocial space (Schensul, 2009). Such spaces have included neighborhoods, towns or municipalities, and cities with governance structures that relate to local populations, generate and monitor policies and respond to higher-level political decision makers, policies, and regulations. Situating public health work in geosocial space is important because very often the results of a CBPR effort promote changes in governance, health, and other policies and related practices. Further, health disparities addressed in PCAs are often linked to broader structural inequalities that are expressed in features of the local spatial, political, and service-provider environments (LaVeist, Gaskin, & Trujillo, 2011).

Local spatial communities are often diverse in terms of national and racial/ethnic backgrounds, cultural experiences and histories, languages, and ways of solving problems. Residents may form ethnic enclaves or communities of identity or may be spread throughout a larger geographic space. A participatory community assessment must consider whether the focus is a community characterized by common identity, or a geographic space in which multiple groups with different identities want to or need to work together to solve a health problem that affects everyone (for example, asthma or environmental hazards).

ETHNOGRAPHIC METHODS IN PARTICIPATORY COMMUNITY ASSESSMENT

The goals of community assessment are to: (1) gain clarity on the problem and study it in greater detail; (2) identify the structural, social, cultural, and other resources that can be brought to bear on it; and (3) identify a direction for action and expand allies and stakeholders who can help address the problem. We describe how ethnographic methods can address these goals of participatory community assessment and further illustrate with a case example of community assessment work with a diverse group of urban youth.

Forming the Assessment Group

A participatory community assessment group generally consists of one or more academically trained researchers, often from a local university or research center, working together with community research partners (CRs). The PCA team (PCAT) may form in a variety of ways either because academically trained researchers learn about a problem and try to interest community residents in it, because CRs want to address a significant health problem in their community, or both. With many easily available sources of public epidemiologic data that highlight community health issues, more established coalitions, and more researchers who want to do CBPR work, it is easier now than before to form and build informed PCATs.

Ideally all PCA partners regardless of formal training should have a commitment to working on the selected health issue. It's best if there is an existing relationship among resident CRs and academically trained researchers that is built on prior work, because trust plus experience can make joint decision making easier and, if necessary, facilitate conflict resolution. But often new partners or new combinations of partners join forces in a venture. In the example below, academically trained researchers working in a community-based research institute sought out a new group of youth who could partner with them in a PCA and the youth, with their help, chose to assess a significant community health problem.

Introduction to Youth PAR at ICR

The Youth Action Research Institute (YARI) of the Institute for Community Research, Hartford, Connecticut, trains youth as CRs to conduct a PCA with guidance from academically trained researchers and youth development staff using interactive ethnographic methods, and to use the results to bring about some form of transformative social change (Berg, 2004; Berg, Coman, & Schensul, 2009; Berg & Schensul, 2004; Schensul, Berg, Schensul, & Sydlo, 2004; Sydlo et al., 2000). During the YARI summer program youth conduct a PCA using a process that enables them to gain consensus on a problem of importance to them, their peers, and their community, and the factors that contribute to it, and collect various forms of data which they triangulate to gain a clear understanding of the problem, and an action direction. Youth are recruited for summer work through the city's summer youth employment program which pays them as CRs. In the example we describe, youth applied, were interviewed and were hired in the 2005 Summer Institute. They were between the ages of 14 and 16, split approximately evenly by gender, and ethnically and racially diverse (38% African American, 17% West Indian, 43% Puerto Rican, 2% Bosnian, and 2% Irish American). The staff consisted of a team of African American and Latina youth workers in their 20s, living in Hartford and trained in adolescent development and participatory ethnographic methods for community assessment, and skilled graduate students of similar ethnic background. The team was led by Marlene Berg, an experienced anthropologist committed to democratizing science and enhancing urban youth voice. Together with youth, they formed the YARI 2005 PCAT. The 2005 YARI Summer Institute began with two day-long group exercises, first to develop a sense of group identity, and second, to enable youth to arrive at consensus on their public health problem of choice. Using photo essays, ranking and debating pros and cons of topics resulted in the selection of "teen hustling" as the 2005 PCA topic.

The main methodological components of ethnographic participatory community assessment are: (a) identifying the issue; (b) constructing assessment models; (c) deciding upon and conducting "cultural" or group level data collection;

(d) deciding upon and conducting individual level data collection; (e) developing data management systems; and (f) participating in joint data analysis and triangulation of data. This program of PCA activities ends with decisions about action steps as described in other chapters in this volume; see, for example, Chapters Fifteen, Sixteen, and Eighteen. Through the enactment of these components, PCA partners identify resources available to address the problem and engage allies and stakeholders important in finding solutions. These components of an ethnographically driven PCA can be sequenced or conducted simultaneously. They reflect standard approaches for rapid ethnographic assessment in a community (LeCompte & Schensul, 2010; Scrimshaw, 1992; Springgate et al., 2009), with the added elements of participatory research, and cultivation of resources and partners/stakeholders to address the problem.

Issue Identification

Issue identification builds group solidarity through dialogue, empathy, and consensus as important elements in the social construction of knowledge and action at the individual, group, and community levels. Issue identification can be facilitated by group listing of issues, issue ranking, and group discussion and negotiation. Participatory observation and photography in the community can also serve as the basis for discussion and prioritization. Creating, grouping, and analyzing photo essays involves individual views and group discussion about issues of social relevance (Catalani & Minkler, 2010; Hergenrather, Rhodes, Cowan, Bardhoshi, & Pula, 2009; Wilson et al., 2007) and provides the basis for debate and consensus. (See Chapter Three in this volume for a discussion of different strategies and techniques for effective group process within CBPR partnerships.)

Constructing Assessment Models

"**Assessment Modeling**" is a process that helps a PCAT to disaggregate the study problem and to identify the factors at multiple levels that contribute to the problem. The basic components of an assessment model consist of the problem, factors believed responsible for the problem, activities to reduce or eliminate the problem; and resources available to assist in problem solving. The result is a local explanatory theory guiding the community assessment, and a potential blueprint for the "intervention" or action to follow. Assessment modeling combines what members of the assessment team know with what they discover along the way, and how they plan to use it: it is an iterative process (Schensul et al., 2004; Sydlo, et al., 2000).

Several approaches to modeling can be used or combined. Kretzmann and McKnight (1993) invite collaboration to identify community assets (individuals, associations and institutions) for local problem solving (Kretzmann & Mc-Knight, 1993). Yosso (2005) refers to identifying cultural and other forms of capital including aspirational, navigational, social, linguistic, familial, and resistant capital (see also Soo Ah, 2008). Cultural and heritage arts resources, political capital, historical resources, religious rituals and beliefs, rituals that maintain cultural identity, and indigenous economic resources are all critical assets or resources that can be added to the Kretzmann and McKnight framework (Meinert, 2004; Schensul, 2005).

Ecological modeling (Bronfenbrenner, 1989; Latkin, Weeks, Glasman, Galletly, & Albarracin, 2010; Schensul, 2009; Trickett, 1997) uses a critical lens to provide a framework for enabling people to see problems as a result of the interaction of the individual with contextual/structural factors that influence their health. Linear modeling (LeCompte & Schensul, 2010; Schensul, Schensul, & LeCompte, 1999) or problem tree diagrams (Anyaegbunam, Mefalopulos, & Moetsabi, 2004; Chevalier & Buckles, 2008; DIFD, 2003; Thunhurst & Barker, 1999) help CRs to use their experiential knowledge to identify root causes, issues that develop from them, and their individual and community consequences. Once the PCAT has arrived at consensus on the problem, root causes, and consequences, it identifies the assets and resources that can be addressed to reverse the "causes," thus ameliorating the problem.

When "causal" domains are identified, the group discusses the hypotheses that connect them to the problem and then deconstructs each of the domains. Through this process the group learns where there is member concordance or disagreement and what information is missing. These questions, differences, and knowledge gaps drive the community assessment process. The following example describes how youth in the Teen Hustling project defined their topic and developed their model.

Teen Hustling Project Model Building

Youth defined teen hustling as "selling drugs, music CDs, clothing, DVDs, sex or other items illegally to make money for their survival." They identified concentric circles of influence on hustling, from proximate to distal and indirect influences. First they defined the important elements of teen hustling (for example, when, how, where, attitudes toward, consequences of). Next they identified which spheres of influence were more likely to be related to teen hustling. At the individual level, they specified the financial situation of the teen; at the family level, they specified family economic and other circumstances; and at the peer level, peer influences on behavior. Deconstructing further, under *financial situation* they identified specific reasons for needing money (for example, wanting material items, trying to keep up, getting back on their feet), and employment problems which included lack of opportunities for youth and adults including jobs in their neighborhoods; under *family problems* they identified such things as a baby on the way, stress, helping family survive, family hustlers. Under *peer influence* they identified having things required for achieving and sustaining popularity because their friends have those things, and that they are influenced by others to get those things. They linked each of the suggestions to hustling through "if-then" statements (for example, if people in your family hustle, then you are more likely to hustle) (See Figure 6.1: Model for Teen Hustling).

FIGURE 6.1   Model for Teen Hustling

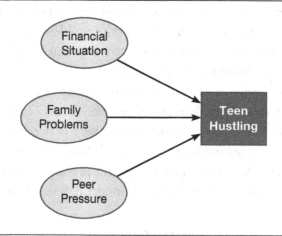

This form of participatory diagramming provides a blueprint for the collection of cultural/structural and individual level data.

Cultural (Community) Level Data Collection

Cultural/Structural level data are community assets, resources, problems, and policies that community spokespersons describe, including factors beyond the community that impact on community life. Typical methods used to collect cultural/community level data include: (a) social and physical mapping, (b) community expert in-depth interviewing, and (c) elicitation through pile sorts. We describe and then illustrate each of these data collection methods with examples from the Youth Hustling assessment.

Social and Physical Mapping

Participatory geosocial mapping has many useful learning and organizing functions. These include gaining a sense of the spatial arrangement and allocation of resources as well as learning about problems in the community, getting to know people and becoming familiar faces in the community, explaining the project that is under way and soliciting support, and identifying issues (if one has not yet been identified), allies, and locations where important activities happen. The most common forms of participatory ethnographic mapping are: (a) working together to locate landmarks and sites of activity or importance on a prepared map; (b) drawing a group map of the community and locating on it important ethnographic or structural details; and (c) asking community members to draw a map of important dimensions of their own community in response to PCAT questions (social mapping). These are activities that the assessment group participates in together. (See Chapter Sixteen in this volume for an examination of mapping to highlight health equity issues within CBPR efforts.) Most mapping activities benefit first from direct community contact through informal interviewing with storekeepers, people on the street, CBO staff, or others who work and live in the community about important aspects of the study community. In most cases it is not important to draw the map to scale but rather to use it as a means of collecting and organizing other detailed information about important activities, community history, the location and residence of specific groups, and of community, cultural, and other assets. Sometimes, as in our case example, the location of different types of activities is identified through brief surveys with groups of people in the community. The results of these surveys are mapped to illustrate where specific activities occur. Precise location using spatial coordinates and GIS software becomes significant when the assessment calls for showing relationships between population characteristics and health or environmental events or problems either across space or space/time such as distribution of toxic waste materials (Cromley & McLafferty, 2002; Skinner, 2005) and can be done in a participatory way. Though costly and time-consuming, GIS mapping can be very effective in community advocacy.

Mapping in the Youth Hustling Project

Mapping in this example focused on the "dependent domain," hustling. The mapping group identified what youth were likely to hustle (bootleg CDs, electronics, sneakers, clothes, drugs, tickets, and sex) and the kinds of places where they were most likely to be hustled (streets, bus stops, corner stores, schools, parks, and abandoned buildings). They combined a short survey with the mapping exercise by asking a sample of 50 youth in summer programs to identify three hustling locations they knew themselves, and what was hustled there. The data from these youth were entered into an Excel spreadsheet and geocoded. The youth assessment team then identified areas of concentration and looked at hustling activity in relation to gender and median household income of the surrounding neighborhood.

The data were imported into ArcInfo with the help of a graduate student intern, which resulted in clusters that illustrated the density of hustling in different places and the range of items in each cluster. These point-level data were layered on a household income map. Youth found that items were hustled in clusters, along central avenues in the center-south and northern lower-income areas of the city especially near downtown and on a major avenue, but not in the south, southwest, or western areas of the city. These clusters bore some relationship to neighborhood variations in household income levels.

In-Depth Community Expert Interviews (CEs)

At the cultural level, in-depth interviews with community experts (CEs) are an effective way to learn about community history, cultural events, social activities, local resources, and gaps in services (Schensul, Schensul, & LeCompte, 1999). The PCAT can identify CEs by listing everyone team members know who might be a community expert or who might know one. Other ways include (1) reviewing recent local newspaper issues to find community voices, listing organizations, and agencies that might house community experts and (2) using a chain referral strategy by asking everyone interviewed who else they know who might have useful information. In the first stages of an ethnographic community assessment, from 10 to 15 interviews with a diverse group of experts are sufficient to provide a good overview of issues and assets. Often these CEs become allies and can be revisited for additional insights.

In-depth interviews with CEs are tailored to the unique knowledge and contributions of the individual. Members of a PCAT may be new to individualized in-depth interviewing. The team should prepare as a group for an interview by deciding on its purpose, reviewing the conceptual model to remind themselves of the scope of the assessment, and generating open-ended questions together prior to the interview. In-depth interviews involve asking additional questions or probes to explore and expand the interviewee's responses. Because doing this well takes practice, it's helpful to gain experience by conducting "mock" interviews in pairs before the actual interviews where one CR takes notes and the other conducts the interview. Team interviewing ensures that important questions are included and allows the interviewers to discuss the interview after it is over. The interview can be digitally recorded and transcribed or recorded in writing and transcribed immediately afterward.

Confidentiality and respect for differences of opinion are important in CE interviewing. Some members of the PCAT may not agree with the CE's opinion and might even misrepresent or criticize the CE's position later on. CEs could inadvertently reveal private information about themselves or others. PCATs that choose CE interviews will need training in research ethics to understand why they should disassociate CE's names from their opinions and quotations and should ask permission beforehand to quote them directly and by name in the community. Signed consent forms may also be used with CEs, especially if the interview is recorded.

In-Depth Open-Ended Exploratory Interviews in Youth Hustling Project

Expanding the study model requires in-depth interviewing with local experts. Experts included an individual who works with gangs and street youth in Hartford, a policeman who works on juvenile crime, and an individual who had been engaged in hustling as a teen and was well connected within this community. With community experts the youth used an open-ended format to explore key areas including: what they viewed as teen hustling; how much they felt it occurred; why they felt it occurred; who they felt was involved in hustling; whether youth operated alone, in groups, or as part of larger networks; what were the major factors that they thought contributed to teens hustling (exploring issues of finances, role models, structural conditions in the neighborhoods, peer involvement and pressure); what they felt could be done to minimize hustling; and what types of programs, policies, or strategies they felt were (or might be) most effective in minimizing teen hustling.

Elicitation Through Pile Sorting: Cultural Consensus Modeling

Conducting sorting exercises to reveal cultural consensus is a simple way of learning about how people in a community organize their thinking about specific cultural domains (Weller, 2007; Weller & Romney, 1988). The standard sorting exercise calls for asking community residents to list items within cultural domains (for example, community problems, cultural assets, risk behaviors). The items selected most frequently are placed on cards and respondents are asked to sort them into groups or clusters by similarity. Because the "cultural level" or "aggregate" portrayal is designed to reflect the main way that community members organize items within the domain, the sample size for this exercise can be small—from 15 to 20 people. If there is known diversity in the community (for example by ethnicity, gender, or sexual preference), different groups can be recruited based on diversity criteria, and their consensus maps compared.

To conduct a sorting exercise, the assessment group first decides what cognitive cultural domain is important. In the next step the PCA group asks a small number of people in the identity community (up to 12) to answer the "listing question," for example, "What are the reasons that men drink in this community?" The most frequently mentioned items (no more than 30) are selected and placed on cards each with the item written on one side and a number (for example, from 1 to 30) on the back. A master list that pairs items and numbers is prepared. The assessment group then asks another set of respondents (approximately 15–30) to sort these items into piles according to similarity/difference. The data are entered into a matrix and analyzed using ANTHROPAC (Borgatti & Natick, 1998), a DOS-based program with a Windows interface that organizes all the items for the entire sample into a proximity matrix that produces a visual map of the sample's clustering of the items into groupings. The groupings are then named, and interpreted.

Sorting and Consensus Modeling in Youth Hustling Project

During the Summer Institute the youth used pile sorting to explore why teens hustle, family situations that influence teen hustling, and things that teens hustle, all domains in their model. They first asked their peers in the Summer Institute to list everything they could think of related to these three questions (a free list). Next they used ANTHROPAC to identify frequencies of these items in the family domain and in reasons for teen hustling. They then asked 50 additional youth and 20 adults to sort the items in each domain into groups according to similarity. The data were then analyzed using multidimensional scaling and cluster analysis features of ANTHROPAC (Borgatti & Halgin, 2012). For youth, an analysis of the family domain produced clusters that were named "money" (for example, no food, pressure to provide for family, inability to get a job), teen (for example, teen thrown out of household, teen has no family); home (for example, no father figure, head of household incarcerated); and environment (for example, area where family lives, immigration status, house burned down).

The clusters were read as falling along a continuum from those things teens perceived they had the most control over (money) to those things over which they had least control (environment and home situation). This analysis not only helped to explain the issue but was also important in influencing the selected action strategies, which focused on increasing opportunities for youth employment. There were also differences between adults and youth, and males and females in clustering (not shown here). These differences were useful in fine-tuning the employment approach by gender, and in knowing better how to approach adult allies with different views.

Individual-Level Data Collection

Individual-level data come from reports of respondents about themselves and usually include *semi-structured* open-ended interviews and *surveys* that ask individuals questions about their own experience and views. Below we describe each method, followed by an illustration from the Youth Hustling project.

Semi-Structured Open-Ended Interviews

Semi-structured interviews are important in obtaining detailed information about the same topics from a larger group of individuals. The intent is to identify areas of commonality and variation in the beliefs, opinions, and reported behaviors of a sample of residents from the assessment community about a topic (Schensul, Schensul, & LeCompte, 1999). These interviews are central to the assessment process because they reveal detailed descriptions of patterns in the ways that individuals experience the health problem that is the subject of the PCA. In addition, they offer the assessment group opportunities to meet others in the community and hear their stories. The PCA group reviews the in-depth CE interviews and sorting and mapping results, reviews and adjusts the assessment model, and creates a semi-structured interview schedule. The group negotiates and decides upon questions to be covered with each respondent that reflect their new knowledge and domains in their model. The process is similar to that used to prepare for CE interviews, but in the case of semi-structured interviews, the goal is to ask the *same* questions (with probes or subquestions) to every person interviewed.

Conducting semi-structured interviews is challenging for community assessment groups because the open-ended format sometimes takes interviewees away from the questions that need to be answered. To cover all topics, the interviewers must learn how to guide the respondents back to the interview questions while not disrupting the flow of the conversation. At the same time, inexperienced interviewers often rush through the questions and may not allow enough time for the person to think and expand on a question. To find the right balance and to gain these skills, community researchers must practice together.

Interviews in the Youth Hustling Project

Youth researchers interviewed parents and youth/adults who were known as knowledgeable about hustling as a result of their own experience. Through the interviews, they confirmed that the domains in their model were appropriate. Semi-structured interview questions included:

- What influenced you to hustle?
- Define hustling in your own words.
- Who or what kinds of people do you know who hustle?
- Do you or did you hustle with others? (explain)
- What places do you prefer to hustle? Why?

- Would you hustle in your area?

- How much do you make a day when you hustle?

- Have you ever thought about quitting?

One interview offered a good case example of a former hustler whose story illustrated well the meaning of each of the domains in the model. He agreed in a signed consent form prepared by the PCAT that his personal narrative and photographs could be used in a PowerPoint presentation to illustrate through his own experiences, how the domains in the model led to hustling, his own hustling activities, and the effects that hustling had on him, his peers, and his family. The PCAT took time to become confident that his disclosures about past hustling activities could not harm him in the present. The youth then combined his words with photographs they had taken to produce a multimedia case study (his words, photographs, story line). The case study acted as a powerful illustration and corroboration of other findings obtained through key informant interviews and surveys.

Locally Specific Survey Methodology

Many community assessments use survey methodology (Fowler, 2009; Manderson & Aaby, 1992; Smith, 1989). Surveys are important in identifying the range of variation in a population and avoiding biases and incorrect assumptions about the ways in which residents are affected by a problem. Ideally, the assessment group constructs the survey instrument with the assistance of experienced survey researchers (Schensul, Berg, & Williamson, 2008). To construct locally specific surveys, the PCA group creates "taxonomies" based on independent and dependent variable domains from the research model (Schensul, Schensul, & LeCompte, 1999). Questions and item responses are based on these taxonomies. The item responses should be derived from the semi-structured interviews which identify variations in responses in the study's main domains.

Local Survey Construction and Administration in Youth Hustling Project

In our example, with the help of adult researchers, youth members of the PCAT developed and administered a survey that included questions or items obtained from further deconstructing each of the conceptual domains in the model. Exhibit 6.1 presents an example of closed-ended questions on what items are hustled and where they are hustled.

Exhibit 6.1:   Sample Survey Questions

1. What kind of things do teens that you know hustle? (Check *all* that apply)
    ___ Electronics (such as TVs, DVD players, CD players)
    ___ Weed/marijuana
    ___ Ecstasy
    ___ Prescription drugs
    ___ Alcohol
    ___ Other hard drugs (such as cocaine, heroin, crack, etc.)
    ___ Bootleg CDs and DVDs
    ___ Clothes
    ___ Tricking (sexual favors for material things or favors)
    ___ Prostitution (sexual favors for money)
    ___ Food (such as junk food, candy)
2. Rank from 1 to 5 what kinds of locations teens hustle at, with **1 being the most common place and 5 being the least common place**?
    ___ In their house
    ___ At the corner store
    ___ At abandoned buildings
    ___ At school
    ___ On the street

CR members of the PCAT administered the paper survey to 120 city youth in other summer youth employment programs. They learned to use SPSS software to construct a database and entered their data. As a group they examined frequencies for all questions, considered gender differences in reasons for hustling and items hustled, among other things, and linked questions back to the PCA model.

Participatory Analysis and Triangulation of Data for Results

Triangulation is the process of comparing, contrasting, and synthesizing data gathered through different methods and from different researchers to tell a story (Duffy, 1987). For participatory ethnographic community assessment, this is a critical stage. It requires that all members of the assessment group participate in discussions and debates regarding the analysis process and the results of the analysis. It also involves them in debate about whether or not their predictors are correct, and whether they are verified by all or most sources of data collected. If the data all point to the same conclusions, the assessment group can have confidence in the findings. If either the hypotheses are contradicted or the data show disagreements across types of data collected, the assessment group will need to resolve them. Resolving differences based on data can be a challenge, especially for those with strong personal convictions and biases. For this reason, the idea of the "hypothesis," or educated guess, should be introduced early on and returned to repeatedly.

Triangulating Contradictory Findings in Youth Hustling Project

The PCAT research model hypothesized that the absence of a father-figure would result in higher levels of teen hustling. This perspective was upheld in interviews and in the pile sorting exercise, but the survey showed that father's absence had no effect on involvement in hustling. After discussion, the PCAT concluded that interview and pile sort data reflected the internalized "master narrative" (cultural beliefs and norms) regarding the negative effect of father's absence on teen behavior. In contrast, the hustling of other family members was an important influence on hustling. Family members were role models that endorsed and established the knowledge base and contacts that enabled teens to enter the world of hustling. The case examples and in-depth interviews also illustrated pathways to hustling and how hustling took place. Mapping showed where it took place and what was hustled. These data allowed the group to assess multiple influences on hustling and where it occurred, and to see it as a general economic enterprise in the informal economy. Policymakers, educators, and employed youth in other programs who were interviewed as part of the community assessment process endorsed the development of a youth employment program that could inform youth of occupational opportunities, and help to replace hustled income with wages derived from jobs.

IMPLEMENTATION CHALLENGES

The process of participatory community assessment using ethnographic methods is challenging. Here we detail a number of challenges we have encountered in doing this work, before moving to a discussion of lessons we have learned in the process.

1. *Inflexibility:* Academically trained researchers are not always flexible about adapting research methodology by integrating ideas from community researcher partners.

2. *Knowledge arrogance:* Academically trained researchers may not know enough about the community or the issue; community researchers may believe they know everything about their own community.

3. *Lack of belief in research results:* Universities or other research centers may not believe in the results of research conducted by or in partnership with community residents or CBOs, especially youth.

4. *Time limitations:* Good participatory ethnographic assessments take time because they require building group identity, addressing internal conflicts and resolving differences, establishing and carrying out methodology, and analyzing results.

5. *Conflicts:* Conflicts can arise at any point in the assessment process that need immediate resolution, which requires sensitivity to multiple perspectives and good facilitation skills that may be missing.

6. *Need for research technology that may be costly and require experience in use:* Research technology is required for some types of data collection (sorting exercises, GIS mapping, qualitative and survey data analysis). Some software (for example, ANTHROPAC for elicitation data) is free, but other software is not, and skills are needed to utilize the software.

7. *Limited literacy levels:* Math and reading levels of community researchers may be low, creating obstacles to data recording and analysis.

8. *Inexperience:* Working with young, inexperienced researchers requires adult researchers with experience in youth development as well as research and advocacy skills.

9. *Disrespect:* Community voices are not always heard by academically trained researchers and their opinions are not always incorporated into research designs, methods, and interpretations of outcomes.

LESSONS LEARNED

The lessons learned from conducting ethnographic participatory community assessment with youth are to some degree generalizable to working with adults. These lessons are as follows:

1. In tackling a complex community health problem, it is important to involve an interdisciplinary team of academically trained researchers in order to introduce to the PCA group different types of research expertise, personalities, and identities.

2. Members of the PCAT may reflect diverse populations within the community by age, culture, language, and ethnicity. The development of a strong sense of group identity comes from team members' commitment to a shared health problem as well as a recognition of members' history, cultural experience, and other dimensions of diversity that shape opinions and communication. Group facilitators should be knowledgeable about these topics, and should highlight both differences and similarities across participants, while recognizing their own positionality within the group.

3. Group facilitation is best shared by a community researcher (CR) and an academically trained researcher who work together to model the relationship, ensure technology transfer and knowledge exchange for community benefit, and help to address important local concerns.

4. PCA extends the reach of academically trained researchers and community researchers into sectors of the community with which they are less familiar. In this case the process taught all members of the PCAT about the hidden world of youth hustling.

5. PCA can dispel myths and misunderstandings about marginalized communities. In this case, it dispelled the stereotype that most urban youth hustle drugs, showing that many teens would prefer to work rather than to hustle, and that they hustle many other things before selling drugs.

6. Assessment group members should see themselves as learning and experimenting with data collection methods together. Academically trained researchers may be methodologically specialized and may not know how to apply research methods in a community setting. Community researchers may know the community but may be quite unfamiliar with research methodology.

7. All assessment team members should receive an introduction to all methods to ensure the option of choosing which methods will be most useful. Conducting focus groups alone is not sufficient for a participatory assessment

group; a good PCA uses multiple data collection methods and triangulates them for more rigorous analysis and improved understanding of the problem.

8. Using multiple methods of data collection is a means of engaging all members of the assessment team, by accommodating different learning and social styles.

9. Research software and technology including computers should be made available in advance, and the capacity to use specific software should be readily available in the team, or through technical assistance.

10. Community researchers, like academically based researchers, have time constraints. Thus care should be taken to respect schedules, which should be constructed and agreed upon together.

11. In-depth interviewing can be an emotional experience for all members of the assessment team, especially if they encounter illness, abuse, or violence, or structural inequities that have very negative effects on those being interviewed. The assessment group should be a safe place where group members can decompress and debrief and be supported in their concerns.

12. The ethnographic mandate of ongoing engagement in the community should remind all partners that knowledge development does not stop with the social construction of knowledge within the group, or through one-time data collection. It continues in interaction with the community in assessment, action, and reflection. PCA should deepen desire to continue learning and assessing community conditions over time.

IMPLICATIONS FOR PRACTICE

The approach that we have outlined has many advantages and implications for practice. Participatory ethnographic community assessment brings academically trained researchers and community residents together in a process that enables them to assess more effectively a health problem that they would like to tackle together. It offers a systematic approach to thinking through deeply the structural and social factors that contribute to a problem, and the potential allies as well as obstacles to its solution. Collecting data collaboratively is an exercise in cooperation, patience, empathy, and mutual understanding that can be generalizable to other community activities. Participatory ethnographic assessment involves all parties directly in observation, interviewing, mapping, and other face-to-face activities that improve interpersonal and crosscultural communication and enhance social solidarity. Group analysis, reflection, and mutual learning are embedded in the entire process. Through participatory assessment community assessors contribute to methodological innovations and knowledge development, and researchers learn new approaches as well as become involved in the first steps in community problem solving. Participatory ethnographic assessment that brings researchers and community assessors together can resolve contradictions and differences in power, authority, and control through joint knowledge development and use.

SUMMARY

This chapter's goal has been to illustrate ways in which ethnography can be included in the repertoire of methods used to assess communities in the context of community-based participatory research in health and other sectors. Ethnographic methods offer readily accessible ways in which academically trained researchers and community researchers can partner to obtain information on an ongoing basis about community life, processes, organizational structures, cultural factors, beliefs, and norms that can help in planning programs of service, intervention, and health promotion. In this chapter we have defined CBPR, ethnography, and community assessment. We have offered an overview of ethnographic methods for community assessment including choice of issue, modeling the problem, causes, and assets and resources to bring to bear on solutions. We have reviewed participatory methodology on the cultural and individual levels. At the cultural level we included mapping, which can be combined with surveys and photography; in-depth interviews with community residents about the issue or assets; and consensus modeling. At the individual level we included semi-structured interviews with people experiencing the problem to understand it more deeply, and ethnographic surveys (built and implemented by local people for local use). Finally, we discussed the triangulation and integration of information to move toward a blueprint for collective action.

The chapter illustrates with an example drawn from the youth action research work of the Institute for Community Research in which a group of Hartford youth identified hustling as a major issue. The ethnographic participatory assessment process we have described provides a rich and rigorous analysis of the multiple factors that contribute to a health problem and the resources available to solve it. Everyone who participates in this process should have a full and clear understanding of the results. If assets and resources are identified through observation, GIS, interviewing, surveys, and elicitation techniques, and are linked to factors contributing to the problem, it should then become possible for community researchers-cum-activists to develop an informed plan to address or reverse a public health problem.

KEY TERMS

Assessment modeling

Assets

Community assessment

Culture

Ethnography

Participatory

DISCUSSION QUESTIONS

1. In what ways, if any, does the use of ethnography enhance community assessment processes in CBPR?

2. How would you apply participatory ethnographic community assessment to a situation in your own community?

3. What are the strengths and potential disadvantages you see in the use of specific ethnographic data collection tools or approaches and methods in participatory community assessment?

REFERENCES

Anyaegbunam, C., Mefalopulos, P., & Moetsabi, T. (2004). *Participatory rural communication appraisal, starting with the people: A handbook* (2nd ed.) Rome, Italy: SADC Centre of Communication for Development, Harare & Food and Agriculture Organization of the United Nations.

Aronson, R. E., Wallis, A. B., O'Campo, P. J., Whitehead, T. L., & Schafer, P. (2007). Ethnographically Informed Community Evaluation: A framework and approach for evaluating community-based initiatives. *Maternal & Child Health Journal*, *11*(2), 97–109.

Bartunek, J., & Louis, M. R. (1996). *Insider Outsider team research* (Vol. 40). Thousand Oaks, CA: Sage.

Berg, M. (2004). Education and advocacy: improving teaching and learning through student participatory action research. *Practicing Anthropology*, *26*(2), 20–24.

Berg, M., & Schensul, J. (2004). Participatory action research with youth. *Practicing Anthropology*, *26*(2) (special issue).

Berg, M., Coman, E., & Schensul, J. (2009). Youth action research for prevention: A multi-level intervention designed to increase efficacy and empowerment among urban youth. *American Journal of Community Psychology*, *43*(3/4), 345–359.

Borgatti, S., & Natick, M. (1998). ANTHROPAC 4.98. Lexington, KY: Analytic Technologies.

Borgatti, S. & Halgin, D. (2012). Elicitation techniques for cultural domain analysis. In J. Schensul & M. LeCompte (Eds.), *Specialized ethnographic methods: Cultural artifacts; using secondary data; mapping culture; spatial data; network research; hidden populations; multimedia techniques and participatory ethnographic video*. Ethnographer's Toolkit Book 4. Lanham, MD: AltaMira Press.

Bronfenbrenner, U. (1989). Ecological systems theory. In R. Vasta (Ed.), *Annals of child development* (Vol. 6, pp. 187–249). Greenwich, CT: JAI Press.

Brydon-Miller, M., Greenwood, D., & Maguire, P. (2003). Why action research. *Action Research*, *1*(1), 9–28.

Catalani, C., & Minkler, M. (2010). Photovoice: A review of the literature in health and public health. *Health Education & Behavior*, *37*(3), 424–451.

Chevalier, J. M., & Buckles, D. J. (2008). *SAS2: A guide to collaborative inquiry and social engagement*. Thousand Oaks: Sage.

Clark, M. J., Cary, S., Diemert, G., Ceballos, R., Sifuentes, M., Atteberry, I., et al. (2003). Involving communities in community assessment. *Public Health Nursing*, *20*(6), 456–463.

Cromley, E., & McLafferty, S. (2002). *GIS and public health*. New York: Guilford Press.

DIFD. (2003). *Tools for Development version 15.1, problem and situational analysis*. London: DIFD: Performance and Effectiveness Department.

Duffy, M. E. (1987). Methodological triangulation: A vehicle for merging quantitative and qualitative research methods. *Journal of Nursing Scholarship*, *19*(3), 130–133.

Fals Borda, O., & Rahman, M. A. (1991). *Action and knowledge: Breaking the monopoly with participatory action research*. New York: Apex.

Fine, M., & Torre, M. E. (2006). Intimate details: Participatory action research in prison. *Action Research*, *4*(3), 253–269.

Fowler, F. J. (2009). *Survey research methods* (4th ed.) (Vol. 1). Thousand Oaks, CA: Sage.

Greenwood, D., & Levin, M. (1998). *Introduction to action research: Social research for social change*. Thousand Oaks: Sage.

Hergenrather, K. C., Rhodes, S. D., Cowan, C. A., Bardhoshi, G., & Pula, S. (2009). Photovoice as community-based participatory research: A qualitative review. *American Journal of Health Behavior, 33*(6), 686–698.

Israel, B. A., Schulz, A. J., Parker, E. A., & Becker, A. B. (1998). Review of community-based research: Assessing partnership approaches to improve public health. *Annual Review of Public Health, 19*, 173–202.

Israel, B., Eng, V., Schulz, A., & Parker, E. (2005). *Methods in community-based participatory research for health*. San Francisco: Jossey-Bass.

Kretzmann, J., & McKnight, J. L. (1993). *Building communities from the inside out: A path toward finding and mobilizing a community's assets*. Evanston, IL: Institute for Policy Research.

Latkin, C., Weeks, M., Glasman, L., Galletly, C., & Albarracin, D. (2010). A dynamic social systems model for considering structural factors in HIV prevention and detection. *AIDS and Behavior, 14*, 222–238.

LaVeist, T. A., Gaskin, D. & Trujillo, A. J. (2011). *Risky places: The effects of racial segregation on health inequalities*. Washington, DC: Joint Center for Economic and Political Studies.

LeCompte, M. D., & Schensul, J. (2010). *Designing and conducting ethnographic research* (Vol. 1). Lanham, MD: AltaMira Press.

Maguire, P. (2006). Uneven ground: Feminisms and action research. In P. Reason & H. Bradbury (Eds.), *Handbook of action research* (pp. 60–71). Thousand Oaks: Sage.

Manderson, L., & Aaby, P. (1992). An epidemic in the field? Rapid assessment procedures and health research. *Social Science & Medicine, 35*(7), 839–850. doi: 10.1016/0277–9536(92)90098-B.

Meinert, L. (2004). Resources for health in Uganda: Bourdieu's concepts of capital and habitus. *Anthropology & Medicine, 11*(1), 11–26.

Merriam, S. B., Johnson-Bailey, J., Lee, M.-Y., Kee, Y., Ntseane, G., & Muhamad, M. (2001). Power and positionality: Negotiating insider/outsider status within and across cultures. doi: 10.1080/02601370120490. *International Journal of Lifelong Education, 20*(5), 405–416.

Minkler, M., & Wallerstein, N. (2008). *Community-based participatory research for health: From process to outcomes* (2nd ed.). San Francisco: Jossey-Bass.

Pelto, P. J., & Pelto, G. H. (1978). *Anthropological research: The structure of inquiry* (2nd ed.). Cambridge: Cambridge University Press.

Reason, P., & Bradbury, H. (Eds.). (2006). *Handbook of action research*. Thousand Oaks: Sage

Schensul, J. (1999). Building research partnerships. In J. Schensul & M. D. LeCompte (Eds.), *Research roles and research partnerships. The ethnographer's toolkit*, Vol. 6 (pp. 85–164). Lanham, MD: Rowman & Littlefield.

Schensul, J. (2005). Strengthening communities through research partnerships for social change: The ICR perspective. In L. Hyland & L. Bennett (Eds.), *Community building in the 21st century*, (pp. 191–218). Santa Fe, NM: SAR Press.

Schensul, J. (2009). Community, culture and sustainability in multilevel dynamic systems intervention science. *American Journal of Community Psychology*, *43*, 241–256.

Schensul, J., Berg, M., Schensul, D., & Sydlo, S. (2004). Core elements of participatory action research for educational empowerment and risk prevention with urban youth. *Practicing Anthropology*, *26*(2), 5–8.

Schensul, J., Berg, M., & Williamson, K. M. (2008). Challenging hegemonies: Advancing collaboration in community-based participatory action research. *Collaborative Anthropologies*, *1*, 102–138.

Schensul, S., Schensul, J., & LeCompte, M. D. (1999). *Essential ethnographic methods* (Vol. 2). Lanham, MD: Altamira Press.

Scrimshaw, S. (1992). *RAP, rapid assessment procedures: Qualitative methodologies for planning and evaluation of health related programmes*. Boston: INFDC.

Skinner, D. (2005). Combining ethnography and GIS technology to examine constructions of developmental opportunities in contexts of poverty and disability. In T. Weisner (Ed.), *Discovering successful pathways in children's development: Mixed methods in the study of childhood and family life*. Chicago: University of Chicago Press.

Smith, G. S. (1989). Development of rapid epidemiologic assessment methods to evaluate health status and delivery of health service. *International Journal of Epidemiology*, *18*(Suppl. 2), S2–S15.

Soo Ah, K. (2008). Moving from complaints to action: Oppositional consciousness and collective action in a political community. *Anthropology & Education Quarterly*, *39*(1), 59–76.

Springgate, B. F., Allen, C., Jones, C., Lovera, S., Meyers, D., Campbell, L., et al. (2009). Rapid community participatory assessment of health care in post-storm New Orleans. *American Journal of Preventive Medicine*, *37*(6), S237–S243.

Sydlo, S., Schensul, J., Schensul, D., Berg, M., Wiley, K., Schensul, S., et al. (2000). *Participatory action research: A curriculum for empowering youth*. Hartford, CT: Institute for Community Research.

Thunhurst, C., & Barker, C. (1999). Using problem structuring methods in strategic planning. *Health Policy and Planning*, *14*(2), 127–124.

Trickett, E. J. (1997). Ecology and primary prevention: Reflections on a meta-analysis. *American Journal of Community Psychology*, *25*(2), 197–205.

Van Willigen, J. (2005). Community assets and the community building process: Historical perspectives. In L. Hyland (Ed.), *Community building in the 21st century* (pp. 25–44). Santa Fe, NM: School for Advanced Research Press.

Viswanathan, M., Ammerman, A., Eng, E., Gartlehner, G., Lohr, K. N., Griffith, D., et al. (2004). *Community-based participatory research: Assessing the evidence.* Research Triangle Park, NC: RTI: University of North Carolina Evidence-Based Practice Center.

Wallerstein, N. B., & Duran, B. (2006). Using community-based participatory research to address health disparities. *Health Promotion Practice, 7*(3), 312–323.

Weller, S. C. (2007). Cultural consensus theory: Applications and frequently asked questions. *Field Methods, 19*(4), 339–368.

Weller, S. C., & Romney, A. K. (1988). *Systematic data collection.* Newbury Park, CA: Sage.

Williams, K. J., Bray, P. G., Shapiro-Mendoza, C. K., Reisz, I., & Peranteau, J. (2009). Modeling the principles of community-based participatory research in a community health assessment conducted by a health foundation. *Health Promotion Practice, 10*(1), 67–75.

Wilson, N., Dasho, S., Martin, A. C., Wallerstein, N., Wang, C. C., & Minkler, M. (2007). Engaging young adolescents in social action through photovoice: The Youth Empowerment Strategies (YES!) Project. *Journal of Early Adolescence, 27*(2), 241–261.

Yosso, T. (2005). Whose culture has capital? A critical race theory discussion of community cultural wealth. *Race, Ethnicity & Education, 8*(1), 69–91.

DEFINE THE ISSUE, DESIGN AND CONDUCT THE RESEARCH

Part Four examines strategies used to define the issue to be addressed within a given community-based participatory research effort. In this phase of the participatory research process, partners work to define the specific issue on which they will work together, building upon the health concerns as well as community histories, resources, and assets identified in the "community assessment" phase. As partners work together to understand in greater depth the factors and processes that contribute to a given issue, and to identify potential points of intervention, they may draw upon a variety of methods for systematic collection and analysis of information. Working collaboratively in this phase of the process not only allows partners to contribute their skills and understandings of the community, but also allows opportunities for partners to learn from each other, continue to build mutual trust, and build their capacity as a partnership, and as individuals and organizations, for identifying, understanding, and creating means to address local health concerns.

Each of the six chapters (Seven through Twelve) in this section describes the application of a particular data collection method within the context of a community-based participatory research effort. The methods described include qualitative (for example, ethnography, focus groups) and quantitative (for example, survey, systematic observation) approaches to data collection. The choice of data collection method is informed by the research questions being asked and, ideally, made collectively by the members of the CBPR partnership. CBPR partnerships may choose to use multiple data collection methods at this phase of the process—for example, survey, focus group, mapping, and systematic observation—in order to address limitations of any one method. Several examples of the use of multiple methods at various stages of a participatory effort, including defining the problem, can be found in Minkler, Vasquez, Chang, Miller, Rubin, Blackwell, et al., (2008) *Promoting Healthy Public Policy Through CBPR Ten Case Studies* (Minkler et al., 2008). Several of the cases highlighted in this publication bring together some combination of ethnography, in-depth interviews, survey and census data, and mapping to conduct in-depth assessments that contribute to policy change efforts on issues ranging from pollutants from industrial hog farming in rural North Carolina, to diesel pollutants as an environmental justice issue in Harlem, New York City, to addressing food insecurity in Bayview Hunter's Point, San Francisco.

The chapters in Part Four illustrate the application of CBPR to collection of data intended to address basic research questions, such as relationships between aspects of the built environment in particular communities and residents' risk of cardiovascular disease, or how economic and social conditions combine with cultural frameworks to influence risk of HIV. Depending on the design and sample size, such data collection can also contribute to basic research questions with relevance beyond the boundaries of the particular community. The chapters in this section also illustrate the use of CBPR to guide intervention research by, for example, identifying how local programs, policies, and new interventions might most effectively support women's efforts to eat a healthy diet and be physically active during and following pregnancy, or the use of surveys as a tool for identifying barriers to and designing interventions to increase participation of Apsáalooke women in screening for cervical cancer. Several of the studies described in these chapters address basic research questions in addition to specific questions designed to inform the development of future interventions, demonstrating the potential for addressing multiple aims.

Together, these chapters illustrate the application of a wide range of data collection methods within the context of community-based participatory research efforts to contribute to understanding community health challenges and to developing their solutions. The chapters also demonstrate a range of partnership approaches and applications of underlying principles associated with CBPR. The mutual understanding that emerges from these processes contributes to the partnership's foundation and capacity to make future decisions about priorities and actions. Despite the wide range of data collection methods and partnership processes described in the following chapters, there are similarities that crosscut these efforts. For example, each chapter describes processes through which community members as well as academically based researchers were engaged in developing measurement instruments, tailoring instruments to local communities and language groups, and interpretation and dissemination of results.

In Chapter Seven, *Community-Based Participation in Survey Design and Implementation: The Healthy Environments Partnership Survey*, Schulz, Zenk, Kannan, Israel, and Stokes describe the application of a population-based community survey within the context of a CBPR effort. The Healthy Environments Partnership, a CBPR effort funded by National Institute of Environmental Health Sciences, examines the contributions of the social and physical environment to cardiovascular risk in Detroit. Surveys, a widely used method of gathering public health information, can be used to describe and document the distribution of particular phenomena, and also to test specific hypotheses or explanations linking, in this case, aspects of the social and physical environment to health outcomes. The survey was conducted to provide the communities involved with the partnerships with data that documented community concerns as well as strengths. This information helped to establish connections between those phenomena and the health of community residents, and provided information to inform specific community-level interventions and policy change efforts.

The authors of this chapter provide a case study that describes the participatory process through which the Healthy Environments Partnership worked together to design, implement, and analyze data from a stratified random sample of Detroit community residents. They describe four mechanisms established to assure community participation and influence in the development and implementation of the community survey: a steering committee made up of representatives from each of the partner organizations; subcommittees with responsibility for specific aspects of the study; focus groups designed to elicit input from community members on specific topics; and pilot tests of data collection instruments with debriefings that engaged community members in resolving concerns. Furthermore, they provide a useful description of challenges encountered in this process, and offer concrete and informative suggestions for both structures and processes that can help to facilitate collaborative working relationships with effective results. Their discussion of the challenge of determining what type of participation, by whom, and in which decisions, at various stages of the process is particularly valuable.

In Chapter Eight, *Using a CBPR Approach to Develop an Interviewer Training Manual with Members of the Apsáalooke Nation,* Christopher, Burhansstipanov, Knows His Gun McCormick, and Watts Simonds focus in detail on one aspect of the process of conducting a community survey—one which, as they argue persuasively, has implications for every other aspect of the survey as well as the broader work of the partnership effort. The authors describe the development of an interviewer training manual for survey interviewers within the context of a CBPR initiative. The project *Messengers for Health* on the Apsáalooke Reservation was designed to decrease barriers to screening for cervical cancer and increase the participation of Apsáalooke women in screening for cervical cancer.

As this CBPR effort emerged, and sought to gather survey information about women's perceptions of and participation in screening for cervical cancer, they found that existing training materials for survey interviewers designed primarily for use within non-Native communities failed to reflect sensitivity to historical inequalities as well as core cultural values such as respect and reciprocity. The description of the CBPR process used to adapt an interviewer training manual designed initially for non-Native communities for use by interviewers on the Apsáalooke Reservation offers a model for partnerships seeking to improve the cultural acceptability of interview protocols, as well as the accuracy and reliability of survey data gathered. The specific modifications to the training process described by the authors include changes in the manner in which participants were recruited, the interview was conducted, the use of language in the context of the interviews, and the dissemination and use of study findings. Each of these modifications was made to convey respect for women in the Apsáalooke community while collecting accurate and valid data to inform efforts to reduce the high rates of cancer of the cervix among Native American women of the Northern Plains. This chapter illustrates the profound implications of historical relations between dominant and dominated groups in shaping contemporary research efforts, and demonstrates both a process and practical strategies through which community-based partnerships may address these factors.

In Chapter Nine, *The Application of Focus Group Methodologies to CBPR,* Kieffer, Salabarría-Peña, Odoms-Young, Willis, Palmisano, and Guzmán describe a multistage process that engaged community residents as well as policymakers in focus groups to define and develop concrete strategies to intervene in challenges faced by women as they sought to maintain healthy diets and physical activity levels during and following pregnancy. This innovative use of focus groups within the context of a community-based participatory research effort offers a model for linking participation and action with research (Israel et al., 1998). As the authors point out in their chapter, the use of focus groups "allows groups and community members to become agents of change by telling their stories, articulating their perspectives regarding health and social issues affecting them, and recommending strategies for addressing these issues that are grounded in the realities of their environment and experience."

By engaging community members first in defining the challenges that they face in attempting to be physically active and to maintain a healthy diet during pregnancy, and then sharing those concerns with policymakers to initiate discussion within a second series of focus groups, decision makers were afforded an opportunity to think together about how they might use resources at their disposal to address some of the women's concerns. Furthermore, focusing discussion on solutions to problems faced by pregnant women in the community also allowed women to provide input into the development of future interventions specifically designed to address those concerns. This is an important chapter offering concrete strategies for building an action-oriented analysis of community factors that contribute to obesity while engaging community women, local organizations, and state decision makers in a problem-solving discussion of future potential action strategies.

In Chapter Ten, *Development, Evolution, and Implementation of a Food Environment Audit for Diverse Neighborhoods*, Zenk, Schulz, Izumi, Sand, Lockett, and Odoms-Young describe a series of participatory approaches used in the design and implementation of systematic observational instruments for documenting food availability, quality, and costs, and linking the information gathered through these observational data collection instruments to dietary-related health outcomes in Detroit. Food audits are of considerable interest to identify differences in neighborhood food environments, examine influences of the neighborhood food environment on health, and evaluate the impact of community change efforts on the neighborhood food environment.

The authors describe how partners based in community-based organizations, health service–providing and academic institutions worked together to design the Healthy Environments Partnerships' food store audit instrument. This instrument built on previous work in Detroit as well as Chicago, where several of the academic and community coauthors have been engaged for over a decade in efforts to understand food environments and their relationship to dietary intakes and ultimately to health outcomes (Izumi, Zenk, Schulz, Mentz, & Wilson, 2011; Zenk, Schulz, Israel, James, Bao, & Wilson 2006; Zenk, Schulz, Kannan, Lachance, Mentz, & Ridella 2009). The HEP food store audit instrument was designed to assess not only food availability and prices but also store characteristics that may serve as potential barriers or facilitators to acquisition of healthy food purchases. The authors provide direct and concrete examples of specific contributions made through this participatory process to the development of this observational tool. They offer a cogent discussion of challenges faced as well as lessons learned in the process of applying a community-based participatory research approach to the design of this food environment observational tool. This is an insightful and instructive chapter for community-based participatory research efforts seeking to apply systematic observation within their efforts to establish links between community contexts and health outcomes.

In Chapter Eleven, *CBPR and Ethnography: The Perfect Union,* Berry, McQuiston, Parrado, and Olmos-Muñiz describe a community-based participatory approach to gathering ethnographic data, with the aim of understanding the social context of health and illness in a population of recent immigrants. Coining the term "community-based ethnographic participatory research" to describe their joint approach to gathering and interpreting ethnographic data, they examine the potential of this process to contribute to an understanding of the factors that contribute to variations in health and illness among recent immigrants. Their focus examines culture as it emerges within local conditions and is influenced by, for example, gender ratios within populations, and conditions of poverty. The process of cultural interpretation that they describe, which emphasizes within-group dialogue about how cultural frameworks and assumptions may influence interpretations, provides a model for conducting collaborative research that is critical and self-reflective.

The authors conclude with a cogent discussion of lessons learned about the conduct of community-based ethnographic participatory research within immigrant communities faced with multiple challenges, including health challenges. Their discussion of the implications of social and economic factors within those communities for health, and the potential for community-based ethnographic participatory research methods to contribute to this understanding, illustrates the joint development of an understanding of community health issues. The skills built by community members in conducting ethnography as well as in understanding research more broadly, the mutual trust and respect that emerged through this process, and the application of the findings to a proposal for intervention funds, illustrate the collective benefit that can emerge from such community-based participatory processes.

In the final chapter in Part Four, Chapter Twelve, *What's with the Wheezing? Methods Used by the Seattle-King County Healthy Homes Project to Assess Exposure to Indoor Asthma Triggers*, Krieger, Allen, and Takaro describe a community-based participatory process used to assess indoor asthma triggers as part of two Healthy Homes interventions designed to reduce household asthma triggers in Seattle, Washington. Application of exposure assessment methods initially developed primarily by industrial hygienists to assess workplace hazards for use in community assessment and intervention efforts is an important development within community health interventions. These applications, however, come with their own set of challenges as they are adapted for use within community settings. The authors describe their efforts to apply exposure assessments within two community-level interventions developed and implemented as part of the Seattle-King County Asthma Program using a community-based participatory process. Their discussion of the application of different methods using a CBPR approach to collect information on exposure to indoor environmental asthma triggers is an important one in illuminating both challenges and contributions made by joining the efforts of epidemiologists, toxicologists, community residents, and community health workers.

The descriptions in this chapter of the partnership's process and evolution over time are particularly useful in identifying challenges that arose, describing the partnership's response as they addressed those challenges, and in understanding the evolution of the partnership over time. The collaborative efforts of the partners as they worked together to address challenges within the project illustrate the emergence of trust and trustworthiness on the part of both the academic researchers and community members involved as they learned to understand and value the contributions that each made to the success of the project. The discussion of lessons learned offers insights for researchers and community members who are seeking to adapt complex and sophisticated technologies for applications to address real public health concerns in real communities.

REFERENCES

Israel, B. A., Schulz, A. J., Parker, E. A., & Becker, A. B. (1998). Review of community-based research: Assessing partnership approaches to improve public health. *Annual Review of Public Health, 19*, 173–202.

Izumi, B., Zenk, S., Schulz, A. J., Mentz, G., & Wilson, C. (2011). Associations between neighborhood availability and individual consumption of dark green and orange vegetables among ethnically diverse adults in Detroit. *Journal of the American Dietary Association, 111*, 274–279.

Minkler, M., Vasquez, V. B., Chang, C., Miller, J., Rubin, V., Blackwell, A. G., et al. (2008). *Promoting healthy public policy through community-based participatory research: Ten case studies.* Berkeley: University of California and PolicyLink.

Zenk, S. N., Schulz, A. J., Israel, B. A., James, S. A., Bao, S., & Wilson, M. L. (2006). Fruit and vegetable access differs by community racial composition and socioeconomic position in Detroit, Michigan. *Ethnicity & Disease, 16*, 275–280.

Zenk, S. N., Schulz, A. J., Kannan, S., Lachance, L., Mentz, G., & Ridella, W. (2009). Neighborhood retail food environment and fruit and vegetable intake in a multiethnic urban population. *American Journal of Health Promotion, 23*, 255–264.

Chapter 7

COMMUNITY-BASED PARTICIPATION IN SURVEY DESIGN AND IMPLEMENTATION

THE HEALTHY ENVIRONMENTS PARTNERSHIP SURVEY

AMY J. SCHULZ

SHANNON N. ZENK

SRIMATHI KANNAN

BARBARA A. ISRAEL

CARMEN STOKES

Population-based community surveys are a primary data collection method for epidemiologists, sociologists, health educators, and others interested in describing and documenting the distribution of health and disease within and across populations. Such surveys are useful for testing hypotheses or explanatory models to establish pathways linking specific risk and protective factors to health outcomes (Fowler, 2008; Groves et al., 2009; Nardi, 2002). Questionnaires used for these purposes generally include a range of closed-ended items that assess health outcomes of interest in addition to a wide range of variables thought to be predictive of health. They are generally administered using a sampling design constructed to allow generalizability of results to a defined population. Furthermore, surveys emphasize consistency of administration, use of standardized items with established reliability (consistency) and validity (the extent to which they measure what they are intended to measure), and a large enough sample size to allow for tests of statistical significance.

Despite the importance of community surveys in research endeavors, there are very few examples in the literature of how to develop and conduct a population-based survey using a community-based participatory research (CBPR) approach. In this chapter, we draw upon the experience of the Healthy Environments Partnership (HEP) to illustrate processes for **collaborative survey development**. Specifically, we describe collaboration among partners from community-based organizations, health service providers, academic institutions, and community residents in jointly developing and implementing two surveys administered to stratified random samples of community residents. We highlight four mechanisms used by this partnership to assure community participation and influence in the development and implementation of the community survey, with particular attention to processes through which representatives from diverse groups were actively engaged, and to varying degrees of **decision-making influence**. We describe the contributions of each of these forms of engagement to the conceptualization, identification of specific areas and items, selection of language/wording, and administration of community surveys, as well as the interpretation of findings and decisions about their use in informing community change to promote cardiovascular health equity. We end with a discussion of challenges, lessons learned, and implications for CBPR partnerships seeking to develop and implement community surveys.

BACKGROUND AND DESCRIPTION: HEALTHY ENVIRONMENTS PARTNERSHIP

HEP is a CBPR partnership that has been working together since 2000 to investigate the contributions of social and physical environments to socioeconomic, racial, and ethnic inequities in cardiovascular disease (CVD) risk, and to develop, implement, and evaluate interventions to promote cardiovascular health in Detroit, Michigan (Schulz et al., 2005; Schulz et al., 2011). Three areas of Detroit (eastside, northwest, and southwest) were selected as focal areas for HEP's work due to variations in cardiovascular risk. There are also differences in socioeconomic characteristics, racial and ethnic composition, air quality, and histories across the three communities. Major hypotheses to be tested in HEP's initial research (the focus of this chapter) examined the contributions of differences in stressors and protective factors associated with local physical and social environments to variations in CVD risk.

HEP was initiated in October 2000 as a part of the National Institute of Environmental Health Science's (NIEHS) "Health Disparities Initiative," and is affiliated with the Detroit Community-Academic Urban Research Center (Detroit URC) (see Chapter Thirteen). The Detroit URC Board, comprised of representatives from community-based organizations, health service and public health institutions, and academic institutions, identified health disparities as a priority, with a particular focus on environmental contributions to those disparities. HEP contributes to this goal by linking aspects of the social and physical environments to health. Our focus in this chapter is on the use of a CBPR approach in the development of a community survey that was a key aspect of the initial HEP study (Schulz et al., 2005). We also briefly describe subsequent etiologic and intervention research that was informed by the community survey described here.

Partners based in academic institutions (University of Michigan), health service organizations (Detroit Department of Health and Wellness Promotion, Henry Ford Health System) and community-based organizations (Butzel Family Center, Detroit Hispanic Development Corporation, Friends of Parkside) affiliated with the Detroit URC initially conceptualized HEP's specific aims and study design.

Because of the comprehensive nature of the study's research questions, HEP employed a wide range of data collection methods (Schulz et al., 2005). In addition to the initial random sample community survey described in this chapter, which included a semi-quantitative food frequency questionnaire, HEP has also: collected biomarker data from survey respondents; analyzed air quality data in the three study communities over a three-year period (data were made available by Community Action Against Asthma, see Chapter Fourteen, this volume; Dvonch et al., 2009; Kannan et al., 2009); collected observational data in neighborhoods in which survey respondents lived (see Chapter Ten; Gravelee et al., 2006; Izumi, Zenk, Schulz, Mentz, & Wilson, 2011; Zenk et al., 2007); gathered information through focus groups and photovoice methods (Israel et al., 2006; Schulz et al., 2011); compiled data from administrative sources (for example, decennial census); and conducted a second-wave survey in 2008. (For a more complete discussion of HEP's overall research design and methods, see Schulz et al., 2005.)

The decision to propose a survey as a component of the initial HEP project was made by members of the Detroit URC Board, who worked together to develop the grant proposal to NIEHS in 1999, to improve understanding of environmental determinants of cardiovascular disease (CVD) in Detroit (Schulz et al., 2005). The HEP Steering Committee (SC) was formally established once that initial grant proposal was funded, and included representatives from the Detroit URC Board involved in putting the proposal together as well as representatives from new partner organizations from southwest, eastside and northwest Detroit. In the following pages, we describe several strategies used once the HEP SC was established to facilitate the engagement of community members, academic partners, and health service providers in the design and implementation of the initial HEP survey. Material for this chapter is drawn primarily from field notes, review of documents (for example, minutes from the HEP SC and HEP Survey Subcommittee meetings), and discussion among members of the SC and the writing team for this chapter.

ROLE OF PARTNERS AND COMMUNITY MEMBERS IN THE DEVELOPMENT, IMPLEMENTATION, AND APPLICATION OF FINDINGS FROM THE HEP COMMUNITY SURVEYS

HEP drew on several key structures and processes to assure input and influence from multiple constituencies as the HEP survey was developed and implemented in 2002/2003. We describe four of these mechanisms in detail in the following pages: (1) the HEP Steering Committee (SC); (2) focus groups with community residents; (3) the HEP Survey Subcommittee; and (4) pretest and discussion of survey instrument with community residents. We give examples of the specific contributions made by each mechanism, and highlight differences in decision-making power or influence across these processes. We then describe the engagement of the SC in the interpretation of findings and in making decisions about how to use those findings to improve cardiovascular health in Detroit communities.

Creating a Framework for Participation and Influence: The Healthy Environments Partnership Steering Committee (HEP SC)

The HEP SC provides a structure and a range of processes through which representatives from diverse organizations, with diverse sets of resources, skills, and perspectives, can not only participate in but also influence the research process (Israel, Schulz, Parker, & Becker, 1998; Israel et al., 2008; Minkler & Wallerstein, 2008). The SC meets monthly to discuss and make decisions about project activities and future priorities.

The HEP SC is guided by a set of CBPR principles adapted from those used by the Detroit URC (see Chapter One of this volume). They were adopted by the HEP SC in November 2001, and are revisited periodically as part of our ongoing self-evaluation processes. To facilitate participation and equitable influence in decision making, at the suggestion of a HEP SC member, HEP also adopted the URC Board's use of the 70% consensus rule (see Chapter Three and Israel et al., 2001). In addition, the HEP SC discussed and adopted a set of guidelines for coauthoring and disseminating presentations and publications of the Partnership's work (see Chapter Fourteen). In sum, the SC structure and agreed-upon processes described here provided the framework for HEP to build a common vision, develop and work toward shared goals, and assure mutual accountability in the process.

Engaging Diverse Community Members: Focus Groups

As the HEP SC developed our initial community survey, we considered variations in local social and physical environments across the study areas. Specifically, in our initial work, we sought to test a set of hypotheses examining relationships between conditions in the physical (for example, air quality) and social (for example, sense of community) environments and their contributions to racial, ethnic, and socioeconomic variations in cardiovascular risk in Detroit.

In 2001, HEP conducted eight focus groups in the study areas to identify stressors and potential protective factors experienced by residents of different neighborhoods, with different racial and ethnic identities, and across genders, to ensure that the survey reflected a comprehensive set of items (focus groups and results are described in greater detail in Israel et al., 2006). The protocol for the focus groups built on prior work with a stress process exercise by members of the Partnership (Israel, Schurman, & House, 1989; Israel et al., 2001; Parker et al., 1998; Schulz, Parker, Israel, & Fisher, 2001). The HEP SC organized focus groups, recruited participants, provided their own community organizations and helped to locate additional community sites—including churches, community or family centers—and housing developments in study communities at which to conduct the focus groups. Each focus group was supported by a team (facilitator, note taker, person handling logistics) comprised of SC representatives from community-based organizations, health service organizations, academic institutions, doctoral students, and community residents, who were matched to focus group participants on gender and primary language spoken (Spanish or English). Facilitators and note takers completed a training sequence on administration of the informed consent statement, facilitation techniques, research ethics (including confidentiality), and strategies for addressing group dynamics issues.

HEP staff summarized themes from the focus groups and presented them for discussion at a Steering Committee meeting. Focus group participants identified multiple stressors that they experienced, several of which were associated with neighborhood contexts (for example, public disorder, neighborhood resources). In addition, participants described a number of things that helped to reduce the negative effects of those stressors on their health (for example, social support). Some issues were raised across multiple groups (for example, safety, concerns about children, schools, city services), whereas others were specific to a subset of groups (for example, in the Spanish-speaking group, stressors associated with language).

The focus groups helped to identify stressors and protective factors that might be associated with health outcomes (Israel et al., 2006). They suggested multiple potential determinants of health within and across the three study areas. The Survey Subcommittee (described in the following section) used themes from the focus groups to help identify topics to be covered in the HEP Community Survey.

Creating a Structure for Focused Collaborative Work: The Survey Subcommittee

Recognizing the challenges involved in having all members of the SC involved in each aspect of the project, HEP decided to divide into subcommittees to work on the various components of the study described earlier: Air Quality, Biomarker, Survey, and (later) Neighborhood Observational Checklist. The Survey Subcommittee was responsible for the development of the survey questionnaire, and was made up of SC representatives from community-based organizations (3), health service organizations (3), and academic institutions (4). The subcommittee also engaged, as needed, several researchers with specific survey expertise who were coinvestigators for HEP, but not active participants in the SC.

The Survey Subcommittee "met" (either face-to-face or via conference call) for over a year, between December 2000 and January 2002. They reviewed results from the focus groups, discussed the literature on CVD risk factors, examined existing scales and measures for a wide range of CVD risk and protective factors, and where no existing scales or items seemed appropriate, developed new items or adapted existing ones. Academic partners contributed knowledge of the peer-reviewed literature and existing measures to this process, while community members and health service providers offered valuable insights into community dynamics and conditions. The subcommittee discussed the intent or purpose of survey sections and language and modified them to facilitate relevance to community respondents. For example, we modified a question asking respondents whether they had ever been tested for diabetes to include commonly used local language: that is, whether they had had a test for "blood sugar." During this development period, the subcommittee reviewed drafts of the entire survey multiple times, as did the full SC at two meetings.

For many topic areas, existing measurement scales or questionnaire items were available that could be used for HEP's survey, sometimes with minor adjustments. For example, the subcommittee used focus group results to modify response options to a scale developed by Williams and colleagues (1997) to assess perceived reasons for discrimination. Specifically, some white focus group participants reported that they experienced employment discrimination as Detroit residents, whereas some Latino respondents reported that limited English language skills and being born outside of the United States were sources of discrimination. Hence, in addition to the response options offered in the original scale (for example, "because of your race" or "because of your age"), we added "because you live in Detroit," "because of your English language skills," and "because you were not born in the United States." When the Survey Subcommittee was unable to identify existing scales and items, they developed, pretested, and piloted new ones. (See Appendix E for a description of measures by survey category included in the final questionnaire.)

Getting Feedback and Fine-Tuning the Survey Questionnaire: Pretesting and Discussion With Community Residents

In October 2001 and January 2002, the SC helped recruit neighborhood residents, and offered community sites to pretest the survey questionnaire. In each pretest, the draft survey was administered to six to twelve community residents, followed by a group debriefing to discuss specific feedback on the survey instrument. We tracked the time required for completing each section of the survey to aid in considering modifications or areas for trimming, and interviewers made notes regarding particular difficulties that arose in the course of the pretest. The mean length of time for completion of the surveys at the second pretest was 1 hour and 20 minutes (not including completion of the informed consent statement and anthropometric measures to be included in the survey). Our goal was an average completion time for the survey of no more than 1½ hours, inclusive of anthropomorphic measures and the informed consent process. The subcommittee reviewed and discussed potential cuts to reduce the length.

The group debriefing with community members who participated in the pretest included discussion of: language used, meanings (or what the respondents were thinking of when they gave their answers), flow and comprehensiveness of survey sections, and clarity and interpretability of questions. Participants' diverse experiences and interpretations of the questions resulted in a number of changes to fine-tune the wording of specific questionnaire items. For example, there was substantial discussion of how to frame and reword questions about police interactions with community residents and groups of youth who are "hanging around" in neighborhoods. Two subsequent pretests were conducted, with similar debriefings and modifications, before the questionnaire was finalized and formal interviewing began. The final version of the questionnaire included 342 psychosocial and health items plus 160 questions specific to frequency and quantity of food intake. Constructs assessed in the questionnaire were categorized along six dimensions: stressors (for example, family stress); neighborhood indicators (for example, perceptions of the physical environment); health-related behaviors (for example, physical activity); social integration and social support (for example, instrumental social support); responses to stressors (for example, hopelessness, anger); and health outcomes (for example, blood pressure).

Steering Committee: Oversight of Field Period

After the Survey Subcommittee held its final meeting in January 2002, several critical discussions and decisions were made by the full SC. For example, several survey items were intended to identify community resources, and SC discussion focused on the definition of neighborhood or community to be used. Initially these items asked about resources (parks, recreation areas, stores) located within a 15-minute drive from the respondents' home. After substantial discussion about the proportion of residents in the survey areas without cars and about different definitions of "neighborhood," the SC modified the question so that it specifically referred to resources within a "half mile" of the respondent's home, and further described a "half mile" as "within a 10–15 minute walk or a 5-minute drive" of their home.

As we prepared to enter the field with the survey, the SC embarked on a series of conversations about subcontracting the administration of the survey to a professional survey firm not affiliated with HEP. Advantages identified included: (1) specific technical expertise in survey administration; (2) availability of staff with experience in survey administration; and (3) availability of infrastructure and resources to conduct a large-scale survey involving face-to-face interviews. Disadvantages raised included the extent to which: (1) the survey would be seen by community residents as conducted by the subcontracted organization, rather than by the local community-based and academic organizations that made up the Healthy Environments Partnership; (2) the subcontracted organization would adhere to HEP's CBPR principles; and (3) community residents would be considered for employment opportunities (for example, hired and trained as interviewers).

Following a series of conversations between the SC and potential sub-contractor, a decision was made to move forward to a subcontract with specific agreed-upon mechanisms to address the SC's concerns. For example, SC members felt strongly that HEP maintain a visible presence and active influence in the administration of the survey, with clear ownership and attribution of the study to HEP and not the subcontracting organization. Toward this end, the subcontract language specified: (1) Detroit community residents would be hired as survey interviewers; (2) interviewers would wear name badges that identified them as HEP interviewers (rather than as employees of the subcontracting organization); (3) study materials and phone lines would identify HEP (rather than the name of the subcontracting organization); (4) study materials and data gathered would be the sole property of HEP; (5) HEP staff would be actively involved in training interviewers; and (6) the survey administrator would attend monthly SC meetings to provide updates on survey progress and discuss survey-related issues. The subcontractor worked closely with HEP staff to assure that all survey decisions were carried out in close communication with the project.

Interviewers were recruited through a variety of mechanisms, including word of mouth, referrals, and distribution of fliers by SC members, and ads placed in local newspapers (for example, *El Centrál*, a local Spanish-language newspaper). Although the subcontractor had primary responsibility for conducting the interviewer training, HEP staff and SC members were actively involved. For example, the HEP project manager, research secretary, research assistants (including community residents, doctoral and master's students), and faculty researchers worked closely with the survey contractor to develop the training manual. HEP staff and students were actively involved in training interviewers, covering such topics as the overall study goals, background on the partnership and the partner organizations, the rationale behind specific survey items, and how to perform anthropomorphic measures (for example, height, weight, hip and waist measurements). Finally, staff from the Detroit Department of Health and Wellness Promotion, a HEP partner organization, provided in-depth training for the interviewers on how to conduct blood pressure readings, which were obtained from survey participants as part of the interview.

As specified in the subcontract, the subcontractor participated in monthly SC meetings for several months prior to the initiation of the survey, and for the entire period that the survey was in the field (April 2002 to March 2003). The subcontractor provided regular updates on survey progress, including issues, questions, and concerns that arose in the course of the field period. The SC was actively involved in problem solving related to survey issues. For example, HEP study communities had been defined based on demographic information available from the 1990 census (2000 census results were not yet available when the sample was drawn). As the field period progressed, it became apparent that some areas of the city had substantially fewer white residents than they had in 1990. This had important implications for the survey's sampling frame and size, which had been designed to provide the statistical power necessary to examine similarities and differences across white, African American, and Hispanic residents of the city. Over a two-month period, the SC embarked on a series of discussions in regularly scheduled meetings and in separate meetings with subgroups of the SC and the sampling expert, who was a part of the HEP research team. During this time, the SC and affiliated researchers considered several potential alternatives, drawing on a number of strategies that had been employed previously by researchers facing similar sampling challenges. All members of the SC felt strongly that the decision reached on this issue should not compromise the scientific merit of the study, emphasizing the importance of findings that would be credible to scientific and policy audiences, as well as useful in informing local interventions.

The SC also considered the technical challenges involved with implementation of each strategy and the sensitivity of the communities involved in the study. Partner organizations were all located in, and members of, the study communities and they, as well as HEP as a whole, expected to continue relationships with the communities over long periods of time. It was a high priority that the solution to this problem be one that would be scientifically sound and acceptable to the communities in which the study was conducted.

Ultimately, the SC decided on a strategy that oversampled census blocks in areas with high proportions of white households, while retaining the random nature of sample selection desired for generalizability of results. This strategy substantially increased the number of white respondents in the sample, and improved statistical power to examine the interplay of race and class in cardiovascular risk.

Results of Survey Implementation

HEP completed 919 valid interviews with residents of the three Detroit communities selected for this study, 92% of the initial goal of 1,000 interviews. Overall, 56% of respondents reported their race as African American, 21% as white, 20% as Hispanic or Latino, and 3% as "other." The proportion of respondents within each of the three racial or ethnic groups of interest in this study varied within each of the three areas of the city, as was expected. On Detroit's eastside, 97% of HEP survey respondents were African American, consistent with the proportion of African American in that area in the 2000 census. As described earlier, we had initially projected that 50% of respondents in northwest Detroit would be white and 50% African American, but found that the proportion of whites in that area of the city had declined considerably between the 1990 and 2000 census. As a result of the strategies already described HEP succeeded in completing 35% of the northwest interviews with white respondents; the majority of the remaining interviews (61%) were conducted with African American residents. In southwest Detroit, the most racially diverse area of the city, 47% of interviews were conducted with Hispanic or Latino residents, 26% with white, and 20% with African American residents. The mean duration of the interviews was 1.57 hours. Participants received a $25 cash incentive for completing the survey, and an additional $50 for completing the optional biomarker component of the study (saliva and blood samples) (Schulz et al., 2005).

As preliminary descriptive data from the 2003 survey became available, they were shared with the SC at regularly scheduled monthly meetings. Analyses addressing specific research questions central to HEP's objectives have yielded a substantial body of work that has been disseminated through peer-reviewed publications, presentations at professional conferences, and presentations in community venues (for greater detail, see: http://www.hepdetroit.org/en/our -documents/publications-a-presentations). Findings from these analyses have established relationships between CVD risk among community residents and aspects of local food environments (Izumi et al., 2011; Zenk et al., 2009a; Zenk et al., 2009b), air quality (Dvonch et al., 2009; Kannan et al., 2010), social environments (Schulz et al., 2008), and economic conditions (Schulz et al., 2008; Schulz et al., 2012). In each case, presentations and manuscripts for peer review have been coauthored by teams of community, health service provider, and academic members of the HEP, providing ongoing structures for engaging in discussions about empirical results, their interpretation, and their potential implications for efforts to reduce cardiovascular risk. These discussions have set the stage for HEP's more recently funded studies, which have included a second wave of the community survey (described briefly in the following section), and the development, implementation, and evaluation of interventions to reduce cardiovascular risk (described briefly in the following section).

Wave 2 Survey, 2008

In 2005, HEP received funding to conduct a second wave of the community survey. Building on preliminary findings from the initial survey described above, and a series of conversations with local groups working to develop greenways or walking trails in Detroit, we jointly identified several areas of mutual interest. The greenway coalitions were interested in documenting the extent to which the new trails were used by area residents and, if possible, the extent to which this use had positive implications for residents' health. They were also very interested in the possibility for programing or activities that would encourage local residents to make use of the greenways as improvements were made (for example, as trails were paved and trees were planted). These areas were consistent with HEP's goal of identifying factors in the social and physical environments that were conducive to cardiovascular health and the development, implementation, and evaluation of multilevel (for example, individual, environmental, policy) change to promote heart health. HEP received funding to conduct a second wave of the survey, and to document changes in physical environmental conditions and health.

In keeping with our interest in assessing change over time, when possible, wave 2 questionnaire items were comparable to those used in the 2002 survey. At the same time, our evolving definition of the problem required several modifications to the questionnaire which, due to limitations of space, are not described in detail here. However, the foundation built through conducting the first survey, and lessons learned in that process (described later in the chapter), substantially informed the development and implementation of the second survey.

Interpretation, Dissemination, and Application of Survey Results

Survey participants received immediate feedback about their blood pressure readings, along with recommendations based on American Heart Association guidelines for follow-up. The SC worked with HEP faculty and students to design personalized Nutrition and Biomarker Feedback forms for each participant, based on results from the nutrition and biomarker data collected, and included recommendations for actions that might be taken to reduce their risk of CVD (see Kannan et al., 2008).

HEP has used a wide variety of mechanisms to disseminate findings from our research to the study communities. These include presentations to community-based organizations, community forums, and local media, including Spanish- and English-language newspapers and newsletters published by local community-based organizations. We have presented findings widely at scientific conferences, and published in peer-reviewed journals. In keeping with the guidelines for disseminating HEP findings (described earlier and in Chapter Fourteen of this volume), analyses have been conducted by teams of academic, community, and health service partners, and presentations have been, whenever possible, copresented by academic and community members of the SC. Working collaboratively to interpret study findings has helped to enhance partners' capacity for collaboration in the dissemination of findings, and the application of those findings to inform interventions to promote greater health equity (see Chapter Fourteen in this volume for further discussion of dissemination within a CBPR project).

In 2005 HEP received funding from the National Center on Minority Health and Health Disparities (now the National Institute on Minority Health and

Health Disparities) to conduct a community assessment and planning process, culminating in the participatory design of interventions to address excess cardio-vascular risk in Detroit. This community planning process was informed by conducting a secondary analysis of the data that had been gathered through the HEP survey described above, to examine the relationships between the food environment, built environment, and air quality environment and cardiovascular risk. HEP engaged community residents, faith-based and secular leadership within local neighborhoods, and citywide formal and informal leaders in this two-year planning process. This was followed by a pilot test of one component of a multilevel intervention that emerged from that process (see Schulz and colleagues, 2011, and Strong et al., 2009 for more detailed descriptions of this process). The multilevel intervention that emerged has been funded, and HEP is midway through implementation and evaluation of that effort.

CHALLENGES, LESSONS LEARNED, AND IMPLICATIONS FOR PRACTICE FROM THE HEP COMMUNITY SURVEYS

As HEP developed and implemented our initial community survey, we encountered a number of challenges and learned (or relearned) a few lessons about using a CBPR approach to design and implement a community survey. We are not the first CBPR partnership to encounter several of these challenges (Green et al., 1995, Krieger et al., 2002), and therefore we focus our discussion on a subset of challenges less commonly described in the literature, and associated lessons learned.

Specifically, HEP faced challenges associated with how to most effectively elicit and synthesize input from multiple groups, including community residents, representatives from community-based organizations, health service providers, and academic researchers from multiple disciplines. These challenges might be briefly summarized as: *whom* to ask for *what* input, *when*, and *how?* Effective participation in survey development and implementation takes time and commitment—both on the part of participants and on the part of staff whose role it is to facilitate and support that participation. Assuring that participation occurs in a manner that minimizes that burden while maximizing informed input and appropriate and shared influence in decision making is an ongoing challenge. A CBPR process that meets that challenge then faces a second: the effective management and synthesize of diverse insights, perspectives, and agendas of participants into a product—in this case, a community survey. That integration requires synergy, willingness to compromise, and the ability to make difficult decisions about priorities. Finally, the HEP survey highlighted challenges related to the importance of establishing mutually agreed-upon objectives, and processes for conducting the survey, and interpreting and disseminating results. In the following paragraphs, we discuss lessons learned with regard to each of these challenges.

Creating Mechanisms for Multiple Forms of Participation from Diverse Groups

Perhaps the most common challenge described among CBPR projects is time, and the HEP survey was no exception. Members of the HEP SC, as well as community members who participated in the development of the survey questionnaire, juggled multiple roles and responsibilities, and time for participation was set aside or negotiated in the context of these other commitments. For example, one member of the HEP Survey Subcommittee was a nurse employed by a large hospital, and had to negotiate her participation within day-to-day responsibilities for management, training, and hospital floor work. Similarly, community residents have critical insights to offer regarding relationships between their environments and health, and a challenge is finding ways to effectively elicit those insights within the context of other roles and responsibilities.

The four mechanisms and strategies described in the preceding sections—SC, focus groups, Survey Subcommittee, and pretest and discussion—reflect HEP's efforts to structure opportunities for different types of participation for people who offered different types of insights, and with varying degrees of involvement with the Partnership. For example, focus group participants were involved for roughly one two-hour period, and influenced the content of the questionnaire items primarily through insights about neighborhood conditions and protective factors. Survey Subcommittee members participated intensively, with multiple meetings and work between meetings, for over a year. They were actively involved in shaping decisions about survey content and presentation, and survey administration. Community residents participating in pretesting were involved for about three hours and helped to identify problematic question wording so that the Survey Subcommittee could use that information in finalizing the questionnaire. SC members have been, and continue to be, involved on a monthly basis over a 12-year period. They have contributed substantially to survey content, administration, sampling, and problem solving. The SC continues to be actively involved with the interpretation, dissemination, and application of findings from HEP research and with the development, implementation and evaluation of interventions informed by that research (see, for example Dvonch et al., 2009; Izumi et al., 2010, Kannan et al., 2010; Schulz et al., 2008, 2011, 2012; Strong et al., 2009, Zenk et al., 2009 a, b).

Addressing Geographic Distance and Difference

Community-based and health service organizations involved with HEP are dispersed widely throughout Detroit, and the University of Michigan's main campus is located an hour's drive from the city. Several strategies facilitate participation in HEP-related meetings. For example, all SC meetings are held at Detroit-based partner organizations, and scheduled well in advance to assure that SC members are able to plan ahead for attendance.

Survey Subcommittee meetings rotated between locations at the University of Michigan and in Detroit, and made use of available technology (for example, conference calls) to facilitate participation while minimizing travel. More recent advances in technological capacity enable videoconferencing between the UM SPH and HEP partner organizations, further facilitating the sharing of information across sites and participation across geographic distance.

Providing Flexible and Organized Support for Participation

Engaging SC members and community residents in processes such as those described here requires flexibility and organization to ensure productive use of participants' time. Strategies for maximizing use of time vary depending on the format. For example, preparation for SC meetings involves crafting agendas, preparing and disseminating background materials necessary for informed participation, appropriate opportunities to influence decisions, and documentation and dissemination of results. For focus groups, a well-organized schedule, trained facilitators, and mechanisms to reduce distractions (for example, child care, room arrangements) help assure that time is well spent and that participants' insights are heard and valued.

Meetings with community residents are most often scheduled on weeknights or weekends. Finding times when all members of ongoing groups, such as the HEP SC or Survey Subcommittee, are available can be a challenge, and sometimes requires alternating meeting days and times to ensure that all members can participate in at least some meetings. Agendas circulated in advance and minutes distributed following meetings provide detailed information to help SC members remain abreast of decisions. Phone calls, conference calls, e-mails, and debriefings with partners unable to attend scheduled meetings facilitate participation and influence in the face of the multiple commitments juggled by SC members.

Substantial time and energy are required from project staff to organize the multiple schedules involved, and to ensure that meetings are well-planned and organized. A full-time project manager, research secretary, and several part-time student research assistants coordinated schedules, arranged meeting locations, speaker phones and conference call lines (see the following section), developed agendas, followed up between meetings, and were responsible for multiple behind-the-scenes tasks essential for progress between meetings and for effective use of meeting time. It is essential to employ a project manager with skills in communication, attention to detail, adeptness at planning ahead on multiple fronts, and a commitment to ensuring that all partners are engaged in major decisions with time for input, discussion, and response.

Recognizing When Participation Is Needed, and from Whom

Recognizing that members have many obligations and responsibilities beyond their participation in HEP also involves judgments about which decisions need participation from whom, and at what point in the process. Too much participation, or poorly coordinated participation, can lead to frustration among all partners, an inability to move forward effectively, and attrition. Conversely, assumptions about which decisions require input and which do not can lead to surprises and, at times, tensions.

We have described multiple mechanisms to facilitate different forms of participation in survey development. Coordinating the roles of these different groups, the timing of their activities, and clarifying which decisions would be made by which group and when, were all challenges that HEP grappled with. For example, a first cut at content for the survey questionnaire was provided by academic partners experienced in cardiovascular health, suggesting the broad content areas to be included in the survey (for example, psychosocial stressors, dietary factors, health indicators). Input from the focus groups suggested additional or revised content for inclusion in the questionnaire. The Survey Subcommittee reviewed and discussed specific questionnaire content, incorporating insights from the focus groups and the pretesting process. Finally, the full SC reviewed the sections and the full questionnaire at several points, contributing comments before it was finalized. Lessons learned in this process included the importance of clarifying the roles of various decision-making bodies, and the importance of effective staff coordination between meetings.

A second, related issue has to do with determining which decisions should be made by project staff, which should be brought to the SC, and when. For example, concerns raised by members of the SC related to the subcontract for administration of the community survey made clear that the SC had a lot to say on this issue. These concerns were addressed through several discussions with individuals, small groups, and in full SC meetings, allowing those insights to be incorporated into the decision-making process. This process led to several important modifications in the survey subcontract, and illustrated the degree to which the SC felt ownership of, and shared responsibility for, the study. More broadly, it served as a reminder of the importance of explicit conversations about which decisions must be brought to the SC for discussion, which require input or insights from outside sources, and which might be made by project staff (Israel et al., 2008).

Recognize Both the Capacities and the Limits of the Partnership

In conducting the first wave of the HEP Community Survey, the Partnership elected to contract with a professional organization with expertise in conducting community surveys. The contract with this organization, however, specified a number of processes that ultimately enabled the Partnership to build its own capacity in conducting surveys. Specifically, trainings were codeveloped and coimplemented by teams that included HEP staff, investigators and members of the SC, as well as staff from the subcontract organizations. Community residents were hired and trained as interviewers, at the request of the SC, and several of those community residents subsequently brought the training and skills they developed through that initial survey to future work as interviewers with subsequent HEP projects. Thus, HEP's capacity, in the form of knowledgeable and trained staff, leadership, and experience in conducting community surveys, increased over time.

Balancing Multiple Priorities

Success in eliciting multiple perspectives and insights carries hand in hand the challenge of what to do with all that input, and all those priorities. In an ideal world, with no limitations of time or funding, all perspectives and priorities might be accommodated. However, the first version of the HEP survey would have taken several hours to administer to each respondent. Given the realities of fixed budgets, participant burden, project time lines, and complex issues, it was essential to prioritize, negotiate, and make difficult decisions about which content would remain and what would be eliminated from the survey questionnaire. The Survey Subcommittee held lengthy conversations about how to contain the length of the survey while retaining the scientific integrity of the data and the usefulness of the results for informing planned community change.

A particular challenge was the tension between capturing issues and concerns that might help explain similarities and differences in CVD risk within and across the involved Detroit communities, and an interest in comparing our local findings with those from regional and national studies. The SC and Survey Subcommittee recognized and discussed at length the relative advantages and disadvantages of using established and validated scales that would allow comparisons with other national studies, but which might be less sensitive to the specifics of Detroit communities. Mechanisms for coming to agreement on such decisions facilitated difficult decision-making processes and helped the group continue to work effectively together. In our case, the 70% consensus rule helped to establish a clear mechanism for decision making. Synthesizing existing literature on cardiovascular risk with results from focus groups, and finding creative ways to integrate contributions from validated scales with community insights, cultures, and perspectives were key.

Demonstrating That Contributions Are Valued

Actively demonstrating that contributions to any CBPR effort are valued is essential, and contributions to a community survey are no exception. In keeping with the multiple forms of participation we have described, such recognition may take many forms. Listening respectfully and honestly to feedback offered and providing concrete support for participation (for example, stipends for time) can demonstrate that participants' time and contributions are valued. Community residents received a small stipend for participation in focus groups and pretests. Focus group participants also received a follow-up packet thanking them for their time and contributions, as well as a summary of focus group results and actions taken based on those results. Public recognition also demonstrated that contributions were valued (for example, expressing appreciation to participants in summaries of focus group results, listing all partner organizations in dissemination materials). SC members have attended and copresented on the study process and results at professional meetings, recognizing their ongoing joint contributions to HEPs work.

Sustaining Mutual Commitment

HEP was the first project affiliated with the Detroit URC that did not include a specific intervention component, due to specifications of our initial funding mechanism. Participating community and public health practitioners invested considerable time and energy in the design and implementation of a research effort with few direct or immediate benefits to the communities. Contributions were made with the understanding that the results would contribute to improved understanding of determinants of heart health in Detroit, and the development of interventions and policies to address these determinants. Now in its twelfth year, HEP has used the data gathered from the 2002 survey and several subsequently funded initiatives to develop, implement, and evaluate multilevel interventions designed to promote cardiovascular health (Schulz et al., 2011). Furthermore, results from HEP analyses have been used to inform community members, organizations, and local, state, and federal policymakers about the health implications of, for example, local transport decisions (Dvonch et al., 2009; Israel et al., 2010; Izumi et al., 2010). The importance of following through on the initial commitment to use data gathered through etiologic research to inform strategies for improvement of heart health has been an essential component of sustained commitment to HEP's work.

The HEP SC established and agreed on CBPR principles for working together, as well as guidelines for the dissemination and application of study findings, early in our work together. These principles specified the Partnership's common goals, and the dissemination guidelines spelled out processes for sharing both responsibility and credit for the Partnership's work. Discussion and mutual agreement regarding these principles made explicit the commitment of all partners to contribute to the development and implementation of the community survey (as well as other data collection and analysis undertaken by HEP), and to the use of findings to address community health concerns. Thus, as discussions were carried out within the SC about the survey questionnaire, items were weighed in terms of their contributions to understanding factors that contribute to CVD, and their potential contributions to understanding opportunities for change.

Establishing Mechanisms to Assure Bidirectional Communication Across Multiple Dimensions

A challenge with which HEP continues to grapple has to do with the richness of the survey data that have been collected, and the large number of investigators, post-doctoral scholars, and students with an interest in analyzing this data and learning to conduct research using a community-based participatory approach. The HEP SC has established a clear process to be followed by individuals who wish to use the HEP database for analyses, including description of how community members will be engaged in the analysis/interpretation, and how findings will be shared with the community to inform community change or promote community health, or both. Even with this mechanism in place, the number of community and academic players engaged in analyses across multiple venues and topics creates challenges for HEP in assuring that findings are used most effectively. Furthermore, our capacity as a partnership to effect change also has limitations—given the breadth of our research, we must prioritize those areas in which we will invest deeply, while limiting efforts in other arenas with clear implications for cardiovascular health. HEP has begun to set aside one full day each year as a "retreat," in which we share and discuss research findings across multiple arenas (for example, relationships between poverty and CVD; food environments and dietary practices), and to encourage greater depth of discussion and analysis.

SUMMARY

Mounting a community survey is a substantial undertaking under any circumstances: doing so using a CBPR process requires commitment and resources to ensure the active engagement of multiple, geographically dispersed partners with diverse perspectives, insights, and priorities. We described four different types of structures and processes that provided opportunities for participation and influence from a wide range of partners in the design and implementation of HEP's 2002 community survey. The *HEP Steering Committee* provided input and oversight for the community survey as well as other aspects of HEP's work prior to, during, and following completion of the initial survey. This role allowed for considerable input, ongoing interaction with project staff, influence and insight in the conduct of the study, as well as long-term follow-up and assurance of accountability. *Community focus groups* provided detailed insights into aspects of the social and physical environments experienced by community residents, their interpretations and meanings, and potential implications for CVD. The *Survey Subcommittee*, made up of SC representatives as well as a broader group of academically based researchers with relevant expertise, provided a mechanism for detailed, ongoing, and intensive input in the design of the questionnaire. And finally, *pretesting and debriefing/discussion with community residents* offered opportunities to test the questionnaire and to gain essential insights into nuances of language, meaning, and experience relevant to finalizing the questionnaire. As members of writing teams, SC members discussed results and implications for interventions. Finally, findings were shared with community residents and leaders through, for example, Town Hall Meetings, Community Forums, and Intervention Planning Teams.

As with any research, a CBPR approach may not always be the most appropriate approach for conducting a community survey. Similarly, a community survey may not always be the most appropriate method for advancing the goals of a CBPR partnership. Each of the mechanisms described here provided opportunities for critical insights into aspects of the social and physical environments in Detroit, and each contributed to understanding environmental variations that might underlie disparities in CVD. Community-based and health service partners facilitated conversations with members of the study communities, contributed a depth of knowledge of community histories, resources, and dynamics, and brought invaluable expertise that helped build HEP's credibility in the community. Academic partners brought in-depth knowledge of specialized literatures in both content (for example, air quality monitoring) and process (for example, CBPR). Creating structures that supported the participation and influence of diverse participants, while recognizing and valuing the insights and expertise each had to offer, enabled HEP to bring to bear a wide array of perspectives and knowledge in the design, implementation, and interpretation of results from community surveys.

The challenges and lessons learned described here are, in many ways, variations on themes or lessons described by other CBPR efforts (Israel et al., 1998; Israel et al., 2008; Minkler & Wallerstein, 2008). Our experience reiterates the importance of the following elements: flexibility and organization; a variety of opportunities for participation; adequate staff support; recognition of partner contributions; patience and commitment to listen to, learn from, and show respect for each other; commitment to equity; and mutually agreed-upon guidelines and procedures for the collective work of the Partnership. All contribute to opportunities for colearning and joint capacity building that can forge a basis for broad community change toward the common goal of health equity.

KEY TERMS

Collaborative survey development

Population-based community survey

Decision-making influence

QUESTIONS FOR DISCUSSION

1. Based on the discussion of designing and implementing a community survey using a CBPR approach presented in this chapter, if you were working as a member of a partnership interested in designing and implementing a survey, in what ways might you begin to structure conversations among the partners regarding priorities for topics to include in the questionnaire?

2. What challenge might you anticipate in ensuring that the insights and contributions of community, practice, and academic researchers were valued in designing a survey questionnaire and data collection process? How might you address those within a partnership of which you were a member to

ensure that all members had opportunities to contribute insights and expertise, and that those insights were valued within the context of the partnership?

3. Anticipating that there may be more interests and priorities among members of a partnership than could be reasonably included in a single community survey, how might you frame a conversation within a partnership about how to prioritize a subset for inclusion in the survey?

REFERENCES

Dvonch, J. T., Kannan, S., Schulz, A. J., Keeler, G. J., Mentz, G., House, J. S., et al. (2009). Acute effects of ambient particulate matter on blood pressure: Differential effects across urban communities. *Hypertension, 53*, 853–859.

Fowler, F. J. (2008). *Survey research methods* (4th ed.). Thousand Oaks, CA: Sage.

Gravelee, C. C., Zenk, S., Woods, S., Rowe, Z., & Schulz, A. J. (2006). Handheld computers for systematic observation of the social and physical environment: The Neighborhood Observational Checklist. *Field Methods, 18*, 382–397.

Green, L. W., George, M. A., Daniel, M., Frankish, C. J., Herbert, C. J., Bowie, W. R., & O'Neill, M. (1995). *Study of participatory research in health promotion*. Vancouver, BC: University of British Columbia, Royal Society of Canada.

Groves, R. M., Fowler, F. J., Jr., Couper, M. P., Lepkowski, J. M., Singer, E., & Tourangeau, R. (2009). *Survey Methodology*. New York: Wiley.

Israel, B. A., Schurman, S. J., & House, J. S. (1989). Action research on occupational stress: Involving workers as researchers. *International Journal of Health Services, 19*, 135–155.

Israel, B. A., Schulz, A. J., Parker, E. A., & Becker, A. B. (1998). Review of community-based research: Assessing partnership approaches to improve public health. *Annual Review of Public Health, 19*, 173–202.

Israel, B. A., Lichtenstein, R., Lantz, P. M., McGranaghan, R. J., Allen, A., Guzman, J. R., et al. (2001). The Detroit Community-Academic Urban Research Center: Development, implementation and evaluation. *Journal of Public Health Management and Practice, 7*(5), 1–19.

Israel, B. A., Schulz, A. J., Estrada-Martinez, L., Zenk, S., Viruell-Fuentes, E., Villarruel, A. M., et al. (2006). Engaging urban residents in assessing neighborhood environments and their implications for health. *Journal of Urban Health, 83*, 523–539.

Israel, B. A., Schulz, A. J., Parker, E. A., Becker, A. B., Allen, A., & Guzman, J. R. (2008). Critical issues in developing and following CBPR principles. In M. Minkler & N. Wallerstein (Eds.), *Community-based participatory research for health: From process to outcomes* (2nd ed., pp. 47–66). San Francisco: Jossey-Bass.

Israel, B. A., Coombe, C. M., Cheezum, R. R., Schulz, A. J., McGranaghan, R., Lichtenstein, R., et al. (2010). Community-based participatory research: A capacity building approach for policy advocacy aimed at eliminating health disparities. *American Journal of Public Health*, *100*, 2094–2102.

Izumi, B., Schulz, A. J., Israel, B. A., Reyes, A., Martin, J., Lichtenstein, R., et al. (2010). The one-pager: A practical policy-advocacy tool for translating community-based participatory research into action. *Progress in Community Health Partnerships*, *4*, 141–147.

Izumi, B., Zenk, S., Schulz, A. J., Mentz, G., & Wilson, C. (2011). Associations between neighborhood availability and individual consumption of dark green and orange vegetables among ethnically diverse adults in Detroit. *Journal of the American Dietetic Association*, *111*, 274–279.

Kannan, S., Schulz, A. J., Israel, B. A., Arya, I., Weir, S., Dvonch, J. T., et al. (2008). A community-based participatory approach to personalized, computer-generated nutrition feedback reports: The Healthy Environments Partnership. *Progress in Community Health Partnerships*, *2*(1), 41–53.

Kannan, S., Arya, I., Wyman, L., Ronita, R., Benjamin, A., Miller, P. T., et al. (2009). *Developing personalized nutrition feedback reports for participants of the community-based Healthy Environments Partnership*. Presented at the American Public Health Association Meetings, San Francisco, California.

Kannan, S., Dvonch, J. T., Schulz, A. J., Israel, B. A., Mentz, G., House, J., et al. (2010). Exposure to fine particulate matter and acute effects on blood pressure: Effect modification by measures of obesity and location. *Journal of Epidemiology and Community Health*, *64*(1), 68–74.

Krieger, J. W., Allen, C., Cheadle, A., Ciske, S., Schier, J. K., Senturia, K. D., et al. (2002). Using community-based participatory research to address social determinants of health: Lessons learned from Seattle Partners for Healthy Communities. *Health Education & Behavior*, *29*, 361–382.

Minkler, M., & Wallerstein, N. (2008). Introduction to CBPR: New issues and emphases. In M. Minkler & N. Wallerstein (Eds.), *Community-based participatory research for health: From process to outcomes* (2nd ed., pp. 5–23). San Francisco: Jossey-Bass.

Nardi, P. M. (2002). *Doing survey research: A guide to quantitative research methods*. Boston: Allyn & Bacon.

Parker, E. A., Schulz, A. J., Israel, B. A., & Hollis, R. (1998). Detroit's east side village health worker partnership: Community-based health advisor intervention in an urban area. *Health Education & Behavior*, *25*, 24–45.

Schulz, A. J., Parker, E. A., Israel, B. A., & Fisher, T. (2001). Social context, stressors and disparities in women's health. *Journal of the American Medical Women's Association*, *56*, 143–149.

Schulz, A. J., Kannan, S., Dvonch, J. T., Israel, B. A., Allen, A., James, S. A., et al. (2005). Social and physical environments and disparities in risk for cardiovascular disease: The Healthy

Environments Partnership conceptual model. *Environmental Health Perspectives, 113,* 1817–1825.

Schulz, A. J., House, J. S., Israel, B. A., Mentz, G., Dvonch, J. T., Miranda, P. Y., et al. (2008). Relational pathways between socioeconomic position and cardiovascular risk in a multiethnic urban sample: complexities and their implications for improving health in economically disadvantaged populations. *Journal of Epidemiology & Community Health, 62,* 638–646.

Schulz, A. J., Israel, B. A., Coombe, C., Gaines, C., Reyes, A., Rowe, Z., et al. (2011). A community-based participatory planning process and multilevel intervention design: Toward eliminating cardiovascular health inequities. *Health Promotion Practice, 12,* 900–911.

Schulz, A. J., Mentz, G., Lachance, L., Johnson, J., Gaines, C., & Israel, B. A. (2012). Associations between socioeconomic status and allostatic load: Effects of neighborhood poverty and mediating pathways. *American Journal of Public Health,* in press.

Strong, L. L., Israel, B. A., Schulz, A. J., Weir, S. S., Reyes, A., Rowe, Z., et al. (2009). Piloting a community intervention within a community-based participatory research framework: Lessons learned from the Health Environments Partnership. *Progress in Community Health Partnerships, 3,* 327–334.

Williams, D. R., Yu, Y., Jackson, J., & Anderson, N. B. (1997). Racial differences in physical and mental health: Socioeconomic status, stress and discrimination. *Journal of Health Psychology, 2,* 335–351.

Zenk, S. N., Schulz, A. J., Mentz, G., House, J. S., Gravelee, C. C., Miranda, P. Y., et al. (2007). Inter-rater and test-retest reliability: Methods and results for the Neighborhood Observational Checklist. *Health & Place, 13,* 452–465.

Zenk, S. N., Schulz, A. J., Kannan, S., Lachance, L., Mentz, G., & Ridella, W. (2009a). Neighborhood retail food environment and fruit and vegetable intake in a multiethnic urban population. *American Journal of Health Promotion, 23,* 255–264.

Zenk, S. N., Schulz, A. J., Lachance, L. L., Mentz, G., Kannan, S., Ridella, W., et al. (2009b). Multilevel correlates of satisfaction with neighborhood availability of fresh fruits and vegetables. *Annals of Behavioral Medicine, 38*(1), 48–59.

Acknowledgments: The Healthy Environments Partnership (HEP) is a community-based participatory research partnership that includes representatives from Brightmoor Community Center, the Detroit Department of Health and Wellness Promotion, Detroit Hispanic Development Corporation, Friends of Parkside, Henry Ford Health System, the University of Michigan School of Public Health, and Warren/Conner Development Coalition (www.hepdetroit.org). The research described in this chapter was partially funded by the National Institute of Environmental Health Sciences, R01 ES10936 and R01 ES14234. HEP is an affiliated partnership of the Detroit Community-Academic Urban Research Center (www.detroiturc.org). We thank the members of the HEP Survey Subcommittee without whom the work presented in this chapter could not have been accomplished: Indira Arya and Paul Max, Detroit Department of Health and Wellness Promotion; Alison Benjamin, Southwest Detroit Environmental Vision; James House, Survey Research Center and Department of Sociology, University of Michigan; Barbara Israel and Amy Schulz, University of Michigan School of Public Health; Sherman James, Duke University; Edie Kieffer, University of Michigan School of Social Work; Srimathi Kannan, University of Massachusetts School of Public Health and Health Sciences; Mary Koch, Brightmoor Community Center; Zachary Rowe, Friends of Parkside; Joan Shields, Henry Ford Health System; Carmen Stokes, University of Detroit Mercy; Antonia Villaruel, University of Michigan School of Nursing; and Shannon Zenk, University of Chicago at Illinois. Finally, we thank Sue Andersen for her assistance with the preparation of this manuscript.

This chapter is dedicated to the memory of Mary A. Koch, HEP Steering Committee and Survey Subcommittee member, and coauthor of the first edition of this chapter. She is greatly missed, and we continue to be grateful for her substantial contributions to the work of the Healthy Environments Partnership.

Chapter 8

USING A CBPR APPROACH TO DEVELOP AN INTERVIEWER TRAINING MANUAL WITH MEMBERS OF THE APSÁALOOKE NATION

SUZANNE CHRISTOPHER

LINDA BURHANSSTIPANOV

ALMA KNOWS HIS GUN McCORMICK

VANESSA WATTS SIMONDS

This chapter will focus on how a **community-based participatory research** (CBPR) approach was used to develop and implement a cancer survey within, and in partnership with, an **American Indian** community (see Chapter Seven for a more detailed discussion of the development of a community survey using a CBPR process). The project Messengers for Health on the Apsáalooke Reservation (MFH) utilized a lay health adviser approach to increase knowledge regarding prevention and screening for cancer of the cervix, decrease barriers to such screening, and increase Apsáalooke women's participation in screenings.

We describe the CBPR process used to conduct a cancer survey with women on the Apsáalooke Reservation. Such an approach reinforces community partnership and investment in the final outcome. Both the cultural acceptability and the accuracy and reliability of survey data are essential for the development of effective efforts to reduce the high rates of cancer of the cervix among Northern Plains Native American women. (The terms "Native American" and "American Indian" are used interchangeably in this chapter except when referring to data.)

COMMUNITY SETTING

The Fort Laramie Treaty established the Apsáalooke Reservation in 1851. Originally 38 million acres, the reservation has been eroded by treaty changes and now stands at approximately 2.25 million acres. Apsáalooke means "children of the large beaked bird," and was communicated in sign language by flapping one's hands as if resembling a bird's wings in flight. White explorers and traders misinterpreted the sign as "Crow," and used that term in reference to the group. Community members asked the research team to use the term Apsáalooke for this project, although the use of the term Crow is ubiquitous on the reservation.

Apsáalooke traditions remain very strong and are part of the Apsáalooke way of life today. Among women who completed the MFH survey (n = 101), 80% reported speaking Apsáalooke at home. In the culture, one's clan, immediate family, and extended family are very close and these ties are extremely important. For example, a cousin is tantamount to one's brother or sister, an aunt is analogous to one's mother, and an uncle to one's father. So, if one's mother were to pass away, other women in the family would take the place as one's mother. These strong clan and family ties form the basis for information networks of communication and support that lie at the core of the MFH project (Bryan, 1995; Four Lodges Technology, 2008; Lowie, 1935; Medicine Crow, 1992).

Although American Indians and Alaska Natives (AIAN) are beginning to experience a decrease in incidence for all cancers combined (Edwards et al., 2010), such decreases are not evident among Northern Plains American Indians (AI) (Espey et al., 2007; Jemal et al. 2004, Wiggins et al., 2008).

According to both Espey and colleagues (2007) and Wiggins (2008), incidence data, and Haverkamp's Indian Health Service (IHS) mortality data (2008), there are significant regional differences for most cancer sites with Alaska typically having the highest rates. However, the Northern and Southern Plains have elevated incidence and mortality rates in comparison to other AIs living in the 48 contiguous states. Such regional differences are not present for non-Hispanic whites (NHW). In addition, AIANs continue to have the poorest five-year relative survival in comparison to all other ethnic and minority groups in the United States ("Cancer Trends," 2010; Clegg, Hankey, Chu, & Edwards, 2002; Edwards, Brown, & Wingo, 2005; Lanier, Holck, Kelly, Smith, & McEvoy, 2001). As shown in Figure 8.1, for all regions except the Pacific Coast, AIs have elevated cancer of the cervix incidence and mortality in comparison with NHW. AIs from the Northern Plains, where the Apsáalooke Reservation is located, have the second highest age-adjusted incidence for cancer of the cervix (Espey, Wu, Swan, Wiggins, Jim, Ward, et al., 2007) and the highest mortality (Haverkamp et al., 2008). Furthermore, AI women are more likely to be diagnosed with later stages (III and IV) of cancer compared with NHWs (Wiggins et al., 2008).

FIGURE 8.1 Cervix Cancer Incidence and Mortality Rates

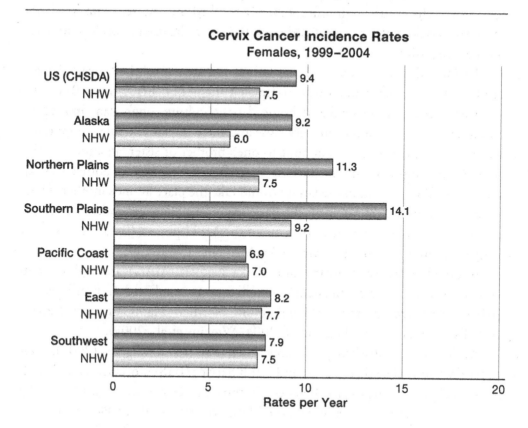

Cervix Cancer Incidence Rates
Females, 1999–2004

- US (CHSDA): 9.4
- NHW: 7.5
- Alaska: 9.2
- NHW: 6.0
- Northern Plains: 11.3
- NHW: 7.5
- Southern Plains: 14.1
- NHW: 9.2
- Pacific Coast: 6.9
- NHW: 7.0
- East: 8.2
- NHW: 7.7
- Southwest: 7.9
- NHW: 7.5

Rates per Year

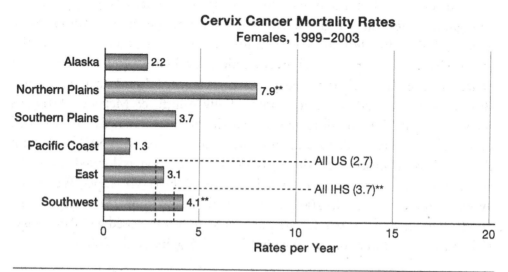

Cervix Cancer Mortality Rates
Females, 1999–2003

- Alaska: 2.2
- Northern Plains: 7.9**
- Southern Plains: 3.7
- Pacific Coast: 1.3
- East: 3.1
- Southwest: 4.1**

All US (2.7)
All IHS (3.7)**

Rates per Year

CBPR PARTNERSHIP BACKGROUND

Alma Knows His Gun McCormick, Apsáalooke tribal member and project coordinator for MFH, and Suzanne Christopher, faculty member at Montana State University and principal investigator on this study, began meeting early in 1996 while working through the Montana Department of Public Health and Human Services (DPHHS) on a CDC-funded National Breast and Cervical Cancer Early Detection Program. Alma and Suzanne met with others over a five-year period to create the MFH project, which was subsequently awarded funding for 10 years.

Most CBPR projects include working with existing community-based organizations (CBOs). While many reservations have few formalized CBOs, there are comparable organized bodies with decision-making and leadership capabilities. On the Apsáalooke Reservation, these groups include the Crow Tribal Legislative Branch, Crow Tribal Executive Branch, the Tobacco Society, and the Crow Tribal Health Board. In addition, tribal members also recognize many individuals as being in positions of leadership. Examples are leaders of traditional groups or organizations (for example, sacred societies), those who have been given the right to lead traditional ceremonies (for example, Sun Dance, sweat lodge, Peyote meetings), leaders of tribal clans, individuals who do traditional healing, and tribal elders. Appropriate protocol for projects is to receive approval and support through a tribal resolution. The Crow legislative branch fully supports the work of MFH through Tribal Resolution LR09–02. The executive branch is also very supportive and offers their assistance and expresses their sincere appreciation to MFH for providing a benefit to the Crow people.

Hence, Native American community partners involved in this project represented a variety of groups and individuals in a variety of leadership positions including the project coordinator, assistant project coordinator, members of the advisory board, lay health advisers, and individuals in leadership roles in the community. The advisory board includes individuals who helped with planning the grant, cancer survivors, tribal elders and leaders, and women who work with or are interested in women's health. During the 10 years of funding for this project, there were two non-Native IHS physicians on the board and the remaining board members were tribal members (see Chapter Two for additional discussion of the development of community partnerships). The number of community partners ranged from eight in the beginning when there were just the project coordinator and board to 45 when there were the same partners plus the lay health advisers. Partners also included the founder and grants director of the Native American Cancer Research Corporation (NACR), an AI CBO that has conducted more than thirty AI community cancer prevention and control interventions, most of which use a CBPR approach (Burhansstipanov et al. 2010a; Burhansstipanov et al., 2010b; Petereit & Burhansstipanov 2008; Burhansstipanov, 2006; Burhansstipanov, Christopher, & Schumacher 2005; Battaglia, Burhansstipanov, Murrell, Dwyer, & Caron, 2011).

Academic partners for the project included the principal investigator and staff from Montana State University, Bozeman (including students who are members of the Apsáalooke Nation and other Native American tribes). There were usually two MSU faculty and up to nine Native American students working on the project at any one time. Community and academic partners are hereafter referred to as the "team."

DEVELOPMENT OF SURVEY RESEARCH PROCESSES

Before processes for conducting the survey could be developed, a survey instrument had to be designed that was culturally, geographically, and scientifically relevant to the Apsáalooke community. The goal of the survey was to gather accurate and comprehensive information to guide the development of a community-based educational intervention to increase cervical cancer knowledge and screening rates. The survey development process included, but was not limited to: the advisory board reviewing community-driven priorities and phrasing, expert (scientific and cultural) panel reviews, and multiple meetings about the phrasing and concepts behind the phrasing. This process required two years and the final tool included 120 items (see Chapter Seven for a description of the development of a survey instrument within the context of a community-based participatory research partnership).

Cochran et al. (2008) emphasized that the research methodology for acquiring knowledge in Indigenous communities are as important as the actual knowledge gained. Indigenous researchers and communities are demanding that research involving Indigenous people use an Indigenous perspective (Christopher, Watts, Knows His Gun McCormick, & Young, 2008; Cochran, Marshall, Garcia-Downing, Kendall, Cook, McCubbin, et al., 2008; Rigney, 1999; Wilson, 2008). According to Wilson (2008), relational accountability is central to **Indigenous**

research methodology and there are three critical concepts to healthy relationships that are also central to an Indigenous methodology: respect, reciprocity, and responsibility.

We sought to integrate these principles in developing and implementing the survey. The concept of *relationality* was integrated throughout our research process. Research builds upon the relationship between ideas and participants (Wilson, 2008). All parts of the research process are related, and the researcher must maintain relationships to the research process and with those in the community. *Respect* can refer to the implementation of the methodology. In addition, respect extends to all those participating in the research and even further to the community as a whole. When developing the survey processes, we integrated respect by ensuring that the methods for gathering information reflected cultural preferences of the community. *Reciprocity* in Indigenous research partly refers to the usefulness of the research. In the past, researchers have extracted information without giving back to the community. Thus, we emphasized with words and followed through with actions that the information gathered directly benefited the community. *Responsibility* refers to our responsibility as researchers to our relationships with our partners, the participants, and the knowledge we are given.

Using methods informed by both Western **survey research** methods and Indigenous ways of knowing can add insight and inventiveness to the research, increasing credibility both in Western terms and cultural terms (Durie, 2004). Although the team was able to locate multiple survey instruments used with Native communities, we were only able to procure one detailed interviewer training manual developed for use with Native communities. The research team determined that that manual was not culturally acceptable for their community (that is, the manual was almost identical to other manuals developed for use with non-Indian populations). Thus, the team used a manual developed for non-Indians as a template, revising the template line by line, discussing the appropriateness of the content, and making changes to increase the cultural acceptability of the survey processes to the local community.

Although every part of the revised interviewer training manual and subsequent survey process had significant changes from the template, due to space limitations, we focus our discussion in this chapter on six areas: (1) the goals of survey research; (2) recruitment and enrollment; (3) the manner of the interviewer; (4) beginning the interview; (5) language use; and (6) dissemination and use of survey findings. In each case, the three key principles of respect, reciprocity, and responsibility emerged as guiding frameworks.

Goals of Survey Research

Most survey research seeks to gain "*accurate, reliable*, and *valid*" answers (Alreck & Settle, 2004, p. 3, italics in original). Collecting valid data was a key component of our study as well. When first discussing the survey, Apsáalooke team members noted the importance of having respect for the women interviewed and for the community as a primary goal. The ability to collect accurate and valid data is dependent on demonstrating respect for the women interviewed. Team members provided examples of disrespect from previous research studies:

- Failing to invite AIs to be involved with research taking place in their community

- Not giving AI community members access to data collected from them

- Failing to provide easy-to-understand findings from the study

- Not involving AIs in data analysis and interpretation, leading to inaccurate conclusions

- Providing benefits primarily for the university researcher's career, promotion, or salary

Thus, the research team needed to implement procedures to avoid similar problems and to demonstrate respect. It was essential for all participants in this study to view their participation as voluntary and as contributing to their community.

Researchers must acknowledge reciprocity, a key Indigenous value, and guarantee that all research is mutually beneficial for both community and researcher (Louis, 2007; Wilson, 2008). Benefits for researchers may include higher response rates and greater follow-up and engagement in subsequent interventions. Community partners emphasize that reciprocity from an Indigenous lens differs from concepts of reciprocity that may come to mind for non-Native researchers. For example, reciprocity is not the concept of repaying someone or owing them a favor. Instead, it is a concept of respectfully acknowledging the gifts that others offer and giving gifts in honor of and with appreciation for others. The team felt strongly that community members, regardless of their direct participation in the survey process, be assured that the information shared in interviews would: (1) remain confidential; (2) be brought to the community (for example, findings made anonymous and shared locally prior to release of information outside of the community); and (3) be used to directly help improve Apsáalooke women's health. Apsáalooke women who worked with the survey process wanted these points shared with the participants to let them know that the intent was to conduct research in a manner different from the past. These concerns and practices are not typical of those addressed as goals of survey research. The research team believed that specifying and implementing such guidelines as part of the survey training manual would increase the likelihood of the project being perceived as trustworthy. Trustworthiness is tied to responsibility, as people who are trustworthy have integrity and will keep their word. This leads to interviewers being welcomed into women's homes and the participants feeling comfortable sharing information.

Recruitment and Enrollment

Standard survey research protocols emphasize the persuasion of potential participants to agree to the interview. Alreck and Settle (2004) suggested keeping "the greeting and introduction by interviewers as short as possible" (p. 233) and that the cardinal rule about interviewer greetings is to "*Never, ever ask permission*" (p. 233, italics in original). They go on to say, "Remember, the sooner respondents start answering, the better" (p. 233).

Tribal members noted that these types of tactics would be detrimental to our study because it is neither appropriate nor acceptable in the Apsáalooke culture to coerce or push someone into doing something. In Apsáalooke, the term "iisáatchuche" literally translates as "bold/hard face." Someone acting this way is being blunt, not taking no for an answer, being bold, or not respecting others. They are regarded as inconsiderate and thinking of themselves rather than thinking of others. Another term to describe someone like this is "baaiilutchichíhletuk," which translates as "bold, self-centered, and inconsiderate." The elders pass on to the younger generations that this is not an appropriate manner in which to behave. Hence, the research team changed the language to read "do not try to persuade her [the potential participant] to complete the interview." This emphasized providing information, rather than coercion and enacts the value of respect.

Interviewers were encouraged to approach potential study participants through a respectful and open dialogue. The team concurred that women would be more likely to want to participate in the study if they fully understood that the purposes of the interview and survey results were to provide information for subsequent interventions in the local community, emphasizing reciprocity with survey results directly applicable and made available to the community. When developing the interview process, elders emphasized that the words we speak are sacred. They said that people should speak to each other using kind words. There is an Apsáalooke term, "baaleéliaitchebaaluúsuuk," which means "it is easy to speak good words." Thus the team determined that a person would be more willing to respond to something said to them when kind and good words were used. Hild (2007) echoed our approach that interviewers use positive terms and speak kindly when talking with participants. This method differs from some literature that suggested a stronger tactic, such as prodding (Suskie, 1996, p. 168). Given the atmosphere of distrust already existing around research, the interviewers were coached not to do any type of prodding. Using this open and respectful dialogue when approaching women to participate in the study, the response rate for the survey was 98%, with only two of the 102 who were invited to participate declining to do so.

Manner of the Interviewer

Usual advice in the literature on survey research processes was to encourage the interviewer to be neutral, distant, and businesslike (Gillham, 2000; Sapsford, 1999; Suskie, 1996) or to practice "conversational neutrality" (Oishi 2003). This attitude is not well received by AIANs. When conducting focus groups to develop interview methods for a survey with Native Hawaiians, Banner and colleagues (1995) found "negative reactions to the standard neutral voice tone and lack of interviewer responsiveness to respondent answers." They altered their methods to reflect Hawaiian cultural norms and interviewers were encouraged to use their normal speech patterns and rhythms. The interviewers in this project established a rapport with women they interviewed by showing compassion and interest in women's stories and answers. Consonant with Apsáalooke culture, interviewers met with women on equal footing, which showed respect for the knowledge they were requesting from the women.

Beginning and Closing the Interview in a Respectful Manner

The team recommended that interviewers proceed at a pace that was comfortable to both the interviewer and the participant. This meant taking time before the interview started to make sure that the participant was comfortable and familiar with the interview process and to describe what would happen with the information she shared. An important Apsáalooke custom guiding when two people come together is to introduce themselves via who each person's family is and where they come from geographically, thus acknowledging the relationships that they have with each other. Apsáalooke team members stated that these behaviors would contribute greatly to trust. In conventional research, most interviewers are discouraged from disclosing personal information.

Oishi recommended that at the close of the interview, the interviewer should "depart expeditiously . . . professionalism can be compromised if the interviewer becomes too chatty" (Oishi, 2003, p. 91). In contrast, Apsáalooke interviewers began and closed the interview with a visit that sometimes included a snack and beverage. Although some non-Native researchers (Suskie, 1996) admonished such practices, others acknowledged that they might be sometimes appropriate (Oakley, 1981; van den Hoonaard, 2005).

The Apsáalooke members of our team viewed the interview as a social situation in which giving and accepting food is an important and traditional way of welcoming someone and revealing a family's generosity. This evolves from the concept of gifting, which is integral to many Native cultures and has been used in health interventions with Native Americans (Dignan et al., 2005). Gifting reflects the principle of reciprocity, resonating with much of the work exploring Indigenous ways of knowing in research. This giving of sustenance happens at clan meetings, after going into the sweat lodge, and whenever people come together. It would, therefore, be disrespectful for the interviewer to refuse a participant's offer of hospitality, with the consequence being responses that are incomplete, guarded, or inaccurate. As one Native woman who participated in another study said, "If they don't trust me enough to visit with me and to eat my food, why should I trust them with my personal knowledge? I told them all kinds of wild stories. They didn't deserve the truth" (NACR, verbatim transcripts, 1996).

Language Use

Crazy Bull (1997b) stated that "language is the medium for the transmission of culture" (p. 21). The usual advice given is that "the research interview should be conducted in the respondent's preferred language" (Keats, 2000, p. 82). As stated previously, 80% of the women interviewed for this study spoke the Apsáalooke language at home and it is the preferred language. This language is mainly oral; most people who speak Apsáalooke are not able to read or write it with the same proficiency. The research team decided that it would not have worked to translate the interview into Apsáalooke nor would it be culturally acceptable to ask the participants to speak only in English. Staff and interviewers discussed the importance of using both the Apsáalooke and English languages to enhance understanding and comfort. Interviewers spoke Apsáalooke and were able to relate any misunderstandings by expanding and clarifying in the language they felt most comfortable. By not imposing language restrictions, we increased the credibility of the information shared while also respecting Apsáalooke culture and social language norms. Others working with Indigenous communities have also followed this method of using both English and the participant's Native language (Smylie, Kaplan-Myrth, & McShane, 2009). The interviewers practiced conducting the interview in this manner during the interviewer training. It appeared to be comfortable and natural as tribal members often speak in this manner in everyday conversation. The project coordinator was familiar with the interviewers and knew that they were all fluent Crow speakers. She observed the interviewers practicing and the interviews were conducted without hesitation and with mutual understanding between the role-played questioner and respondent. This ensured consistency in terminology in both languages.

Some researchers are uncomfortable with real-time translation and clarification of items during survey administration and feel that the exact wording of a question and the alternative responses should be retained (Keats, 2000; Suskie, 1996). The importance of communicating in the Apsáalooke language, and of ensuring that the meaning of the terms was clearly communicated in the absence of a written language, contributed to the teams' decision to use real-time translation and clarification of terms as necessary in this context. Although we did not conduct formal, empirical comparisons of this approach compared to a more standardized approach, project team members felt strongly after observations of practice interviews that it was essential to proceeding through the interview clearly, helping survey participants be at ease, and creating a respectful, comfortable, and nonjudgmental relationship between participant and interviewer.

The interviewers were encouraged to communicate with the interviewee in a manner most comfortable to the participant. For example, the interview question may be first spoken in English and then translated in the Crow language to ensure clearer understanding. We discussed that conversing from English to Crow would take place in a very natural manner. Overall, there was very effective communication between the two parties and the use of the Native language provided an important asset.

Another comment on language regards terms used to describe interviewee responses. Some survey research suggested ways of dealing with "inadequate or irrelevant" responses. Schmidt and Conaway (1999) stated that the "response may be incomplete, or an answer may be irrelevant to the question . . . Sometimes inaccurate information is given" (p. 42). When developing the interview processes, one Apsáalooke woman stated that there was no such thing as an inadequate or irrelevant response and that whatever the participants had to offer was valid and informative. Petereit and Burhansstipanov (2008) encouraged interviewers to listen carefully to the stories the respondent tells because they will frequently provide answers to subsequent interview questions and the stories usually help clarify the responses. Interviewers used probes to receive answers that fit the closed-ended question responses.

When women being interviewed talked about other things, interviewers were patient and courteous, incorporating respect for the women being interviewed into the methodology in a way that is consistent with Apsáalooke practices. Long (1983) noted that among the Apsáalooke people "one does not correct others or indicate that the other's perceptions are incorrect. Tolerance of others is highly valued, and is practiced through silence and nonintrusive behavior" (p. 124). Interviewers used neutral probes if the participant's answer did not fit the question—this allowed for clarification without judgment regarding the response offered. Past practices for interviewers included being advised to say, "What do you mean?" This was felt to be too negative of a response and interviewers used alternatives such as "Could you tell me a little more about . . ." or "I'm not sure I understand what you mean." Interviewers also wrote additional information given in the interview on the side of the questionnaire form in order to include all responses.

Dissemination and Use of Survey Findings

Most research projects consider dissemination and use of survey findings as a task to be addressed after surveys are complete. However, reciprocity (gathering knowledge from participants and ensuring that the knowledge benefits the community) includes sharing findings with the participants. A common and valid complaint in Indian Country is that communities rarely receive survey findings or benefit from surveys performed in their communities. Due to this history, there is resistance to taking part in contemporary surveys. The majority of literature reviewed by this team that discussed dissemination did not discuss dissemination to the community from which the respondents came (Alreck & Settle, 2004; Oishi, 2003) (see Part Six in this volume for further discussion of dissemination within a CBPR approach).

MFH interviewers received information on how previous research had been conducted and the ways in which this project would be different with regard to how findings from this study would be used and shared with the community. MFH updated the community on the progress of the project through multiple community meetings and developed easy-to-understand handouts on the survey results that were widely distributed.

Interviewers gave information on use and dissemination of survey findings to study participants. This included stating that the survey information would be used to help all Apsáalooke women to be healthier and that survey findings would determine: (1) the focus of training of the lay health advisers; (2) information to be emphasized by the lay health advisers during education; and (3) the nature and focus of the community educational materials.

The Interviewers

Hiring and training local community members to conduct the survey demonstrated respect for the community and we believe contributed to the accuracy of the data. Some researchers (Davis, Couper, Janz, Caldwell, & Resnicow, 2010; Singleton & Straits, 2002) suggest that race or gender matching is of limited utility and that few studies have found any association between interviewer demographics and the answers obtained from participants. Other studies suggest that, depending on the topic of study, gender and race and, of course, linguistic matching can have substantial implications (Duncan, Schuman, & Duncan, 1973; and Groves et al., 2009). Finally, some survey experts recommend cultural awareness of the acceptability of matching or not matching on race (Keats, 2000) as well as gender (Burhansstipanov et al., 2010b; Burhansstipanov, Dignan, Wound, Tenney, & Vigil, 2000; Burhansstipanov, 1999a, Burhansstipanov, 1999b). Apsáalooke team members contended that the only way to receive honest and accurate information would be to hire Apsáalooke interviewers. The essential trust to discuss personal health issues would not exist with non-tribal members. Further, they considered it important that the interviewers be female and speak Apsáalooke. Cross-gender taboos exist that would have prohibited male interviewers from being successful in this situation and those working on the project stated that many community members feel more comfortable talking in Apsáalooke than in English. Likewise, there are subtleties of nonverbal communication (for example, proximity to one another and eye contact) that required the interviewer to be intimately familiar with the culture. Thus, the team decided that Apsáalooke women living in and known by the community, who practiced typical Apsáalooke cultural behaviors and norms, would be selected as interviewers.

When hiring local tribal members as interviewers, confidentiality within the tribal nation is of utmost importance. We dealt with confidentiality by choosing interviewers who were known and respected in the community so that interviewees could feel the interviewers were trustworthy and feel comfortable with them. Having interviewers who knew and understood Crow culture was our biggest concern. Furthermore, to ensure confidentiality, interviewer training emphasized confidentiality as an essential component and interviewers signed a confidentiality statement. The statement read:

I [insert name] agree to keep the identity of all persons in the study and any information on these persons that I gain access to as a result of this study completely confidential. I will maintain confidentiality in order to protect the rights and well-being of the women participating in this study. By doing so, I agree to never discuss any information on the women participating in this study with anyone but this research team (including significant others, family, friends, other interviewers, or other women being interviewed), nor will I allow anyone who is not a member of this research team to view interviews, study files, or data.

Interviewers were recruited by a professor at the Little Big Horn College (LBHC), a tribal college on the reservation. They were from all areas of the reservation and ranged in age from late twenties through late fifties. The interviewer training took place over the course of one day at LBHC with a follow-up meeting one week later to discuss progress, questions, and concerns. The training covered the following topics: the purpose and focus of the study, confidentiality and privacy protocols, cervical health and cervical cancer, roles and responsibilities of the interviewer, and interviewing procedures and techniques. Interviewers were trained to conduct interviews in a standardized manner, for example, not varying the order or wording of questions when reading the questions in English. The interviewers also practiced role-playing the interview. Interviewers were paid with project funds at rates agreed to by the study team and support and supervision were provided by the project coordinator.

CHALLENGES

There were a number of challenges that we encountered in the context of developing and implementing a survey for the MFH project. These included challenges associated with cultural dissonances between many readily available survey training manuals and the AI community, as well as challenges associated with the implementation of the interviews themselves. Here we summarize several of these.

The training manuals we drew from and modified were manuals developed for participants from non-Native cultures. Thus, a significant challenge for us was to ensure that essential aspects of Crow culture were infused into all parts of the manual. For example, we were interviewing Crow women and it was important that the interviewer take into consideration the important role a Crow woman plays in her immediate as well as extended family. A model Crow woman is the caregiver and strong pillar of the home. Her time is always in demand. When there is a need, she is the one to whom others turn and this role is important to a Crow woman. She possesses virtuous qualities; attending to the needs of her family takes top priority. An understanding of these responsibilities, and an awareness that we were asking women to set aside their roles to take part in the interviews, was paramount among the interviewers. Because our interviewers were also Crow women, they were aware of this central role and were flexible with scheduling the interviews during a time and location most convenient and comfortable for the interviewee. Taking this into consideration was culturally appropriate and respectful. Information such as this required considerable time to uncover, not due to deliberate attempts to hide information, but because for the local community, as for all of us, this type of information is typically implicit and not immediately accessible to conscious awareness and reporting.

Conducting interviews was also challenging because many times the interview sessions took place later in the evening at the interviewee's home. At these later times, family members would more likely be present and the issue of privacy arose. Often, an alternate private setting had to be used. Some interviews took place in the car, as that was the best place to find privacy. In our interviewer training we encouraged interviewers to be flexible and we discussed the possibility of using the car to ensure privacy.

Finally, due to how close-knit the Crow family and Nation are, when there is a death, it takes precedence. The whole Nation is affected, and all other activities are put aside. For instance, if an interviewer scheduled an interview and the interviewee had a death in the family, then the session would be immediately cancelled. The woman was still interested in participating in the survey, and the interview was rescheduled for a time when she was in a better emotional state during her bereavement. The interview was rescheduled after a length of time that allowed for grieving (at least two weeks or more was allowed before another session was rescheduled). This can be a big challenge because of the extra time and effort provided to complete the interview. The interviewers experienced many episodes of scheduling, cancelling, and rescheduling interview sessions. The interviewer had to overcome these challenges and endure with patience and perseverance to complete the interviews.

Our high response rate demonstrates the extent to which women were comfortable with completing the survey and the manner in which we implemented it. As Crow women, they likely have many responsibilities to their families and communities. However, many of the interviewees really wanted to participate and complete the interview, even going so far as to reschedule their interviews when other priorities arose.

LESSONS LEARNED AND IMPLICATIONS

Using a CBPR approach guided the research team to appreciate and use the Indigenous knowledge in the community to implement the survey in a manner most appropriate for defining, understanding, and addressing local issues (Poupart, Barker, & Red Horse, 2009). We built in three concepts cited in Indigenous research recommendations (Louis, 2007; Wilson, 2008). First, *respect* was essential in all aspects of the survey research process, including respecting cultural norms, respecting our participants and respecting the community. Second, we honored our *responsibilities* to the community throughout the research process. Our community team members often underscored the importance of understanding and respecting all of the relationships that exist throughout the research process. This includes the relationships between researchers and community members, between interviewers and community women, and between each step of the research process. Finally, *reciprocity* was noted throughout our approach to the research. Because the community codeveloped the research strategies, they integrated the core value of reciprocity. Past abuses by researchers made this concept all the more integral to our work in order to establish and maintain trustworthiness. Community team members emphasized that the knowledge shared by the women in the survey must be valued and that we as the research team must make it a priority that the information improve health in the community. Below is a summary of the lessons learned:

Lesson 1. The survey protocols need to reflect local community customs, previous history with research, as well as an understanding of broader historical and contemporary relationships.

Lesson 2. Researchers need to be prepared to spend a considerable amount of time and energy with and in the community with whom they are partnering.

Lesson 3. Researchers need to integrate dissemination of findings with the study participants in a way that does not weaken scientific integrity, yet demonstrates reciprocity and partnership. Community members shared with us stories of researchers who gathered personal and sensitive information from them, never to be heard from again. They did not know what happened to the information, how it was used, and doubted that the information was used to directly help the community.

Lesson 4. Survey findings need to result in beneficial programs or services within the community. Many Native communities, including the Apsáalooke community, are wary about participating in studies of their community's health.

Lesson 5. Researchers and community members are partners in conducting the surveys and need to work honestly and cooperatively with one another.

Lesson 6. Partners need to actively work together on all stages and phases of the research project.

Lesson 7. Survey interview behaviors need to reflect respectful communication styles appropriate for the local community.

Without the use of the CBPR approach, the interviews were unlikely to have addressed the cultural nuances referred to throughout this chapter nor would they have reflected Indigenous values or knowledge that ensured greater success in the implementation of the survey. Because thousands of surveys have been implemented in Indian Country, the team was surprised to learn that no culturally appropriate interviewer manuals or written processes were available to use as a template (that is, the one manual we located that had been used with Native communities had few cultural modifications). The manual created through this process and described in this chapter is available as a downloadable supplement to this book.

SUMMARY

The historical legacy of interactions between Native communities and government officials, health researchers, and health workers has impeded the success of research intended to improve health. Individuals working with Native communities "are likely to be confronted with some of the grief and anger over losses and injustices of the past. They will be better able to deal with these confrontations if they have gained some insight into the events that caused the pain" (Harrison, 2001).

We close with a quotation from Cheryl Crazy Bull (1997a) who eloquently explained a culturally respectful research process. This process is in line with a CBPR approach and was an inspiration for us in developing survey processes that were respectful of the Apsáalooke community and culture.

As we seek our own understanding of tribal research and scholarship, we must remember the people of the community are the source of our profound understanding of tribal life, values, and rituals. We must hear their voices and participate in their stories and ritual in order to attain the wisdom we seek. As we explore the world of scholarship, the everyday people and everyday rituals must form the foundation for the lodges we build. (p. 16)

KEY TERMS

American Indian

Community-based participatory research

Indigenous research methodology

Survey research

DISCUSSION QUESTIONS

1. Discuss the pros and cons of adapting existing material—for example, the authors adapted an existing interviewer training manual using a CBPR approach—versus developing material from scratch using a CBPR approach? Do these pros and cons vary with the community involved? The research participants?

2. In your experience with CBPR or the CBPR case studies you have evaluated, has Indigenous knowledge (meaning knowledge that originates from the community) been incorporated into the methodologies? How so, and in what ways did it have an impact on the project?

REFERENCES

Alreck, P. L., & Settle, R. B. (2004). *The survey research handbook* (3rd ed.) New York: McGraw-Hill Irwin.

Banner, R., DeCambra, H. O., Enos, R., Gotay, C., Hammond, O., Hedlund, N., et al. (1995). A breast and cervical cancer project in a Native Hawaiian community: Wai'anae cancer research project. *Preventive Medicine, 24,* 447–453.

Battaglia, T. A., Burhansstipanov, L., Murrell, S. S., Dwyer, A. J., & Caron, S. E., on behalf of The Prevention and Early Detection Workgroup from the National Patient Navigation Leadership Summit. (2011). Assessing the impact of patient navigation: Prevention and early detection metrics. *Cancer, 117*(Suppl. 15), 3553–3564.

Bryan, W. (1995). *Montana's Indians yesterday and today*. Helena, MT: Farcountry Press.

Burhansstipanov, L. (1999a). Native American community-based cancer projects: Theory versus reality. *Cancer Control: Journal of the Moffitt Cancer Center, 6*(6), 620–626.

Burhansstipanov, L. (1999b). Developing culturally competent community-based interventions. In D. Weiner (Ed.), *Cancer research interventions among the medically underserved* (pp. 167–183). Westport, CT: Greenwood.

Burhansstipanov, L. (2006). American Indian and Alaska Native women and cancer. In Karen Hassey Dow's (ed.) *Nursing care of women and cancer* (Chapter 27) St. Louis, MO: Mosby Elsevier.

Burhansstipanov, L., Christopher, S., & Schumacher, A. (2005). Lessons learned from community-based participatory research in Indian Country. Cancer culture and literacy. *Cancer Control: Journal of the Moffitt Cancer Center, 12*(Suppl. 2), 70–76.

Burhansstipanov, L., Dignan, M. B., Schumacher, A., Krebs, L. U., Alfonsi, G., & Apodaca, C. (2010a). Breast screening navigator programs within three settings that assist underserved women. *Journal of Cancer Education, 25*(2), 247–252.

Burhansstipanov, L., Dignan, M. B., Wound, D. B., Tenney, M., & Vigil, G. (2000). Native American recruitment into breast cancer screening: The NAWWA project. *Journal of Cancer Education, 15*(1), 28–32.

Burhansstipanov, L., Krebs, L. U., Seals, B. F., Bradley, A. A., Kaur, J. S., Iron, P., et al. (2010b). Native American Breast Cancer Survivors' physical conditions and quality of life. *Cancer, 116*(6), 1560–1571.

Cancer Trends Progress Report—2009/2010 Update, (2010). National Cancer Institute, NIH, DHHS, Bethesda, MD. Retrieved April 6, 2011 from http://progressreport.cancer.gov

Christopher, S., Knows His Gun McCormick, A. K., Smith, A., & Christopher, J. C. (2005). Recommendations for conducting successful research with Native Americans. *Journal of Cancer Education, 20*, 47–51.

Christopher, S., Watts, V., Knows His Gun McCormick, A. K., & Young, S. (2008). Building and maintaining trust in a community-based participatory research partnership. *American Journal of Public Health, 98*(8), 1398–1406.

Clegg, L. X., Li, F. P., Hankey, B. F., Chu, K., & Edwards, B. K. (2002). Cancer survival among U.S. whites and minorities: A SEER Program populations-based study. *Archives of Internal Medicine, 162*, 1985–1993.

Cochran, P. A., Marshall, C. A., Garcia-Downing, C., Kendall, E., Cook, D., McCubbin, L., et al. (2008). Indigenous ways of knowing: implications for participatory research and community. *American Journal of Public Health, 98*(1), 22–27.

Crazy Bull, C. (1997a). in the center of the earth i am standing and i am praying as i stand . . . *Tribal College: Journal of American Indian Higher Education, 8*(Summer), 16.

Crazy Bull, C. (1997b). A Native conversation about research and scholarship. *Tribal College: Journal of American Indian Higher Education, 8*(Summer), 17–23.

Davis, R. E., Couper, M. P., Janz, N. K., Caldwell, C. H., & Resnicow, K. (2010). Interviewer effects in public health surveys. *Health Education Research, 25*(1), 14–26.

Dignan, M. B., Burhansstipanov, L., Hariton, J., Harjo, L., Rattler, T., Lee, R., et al. (2005). A comparison of two Native American Navigator formats: Face-to-face and telephone. *Cancer Control, 12*(Suppl. 2), 28–33.

Durie, M. (2004). Understanding health and illness: Research at the interface between science and Indigenous knowledge. *International Journal of Epidemiology, 33*(5), 1138–1143.

Duncan, O. D., Schuman, H., & Duncan, B. (1973). *Social change in a metropolitan community.* New York: Russell Sage.

Edwards, B. K., Brown, M. I., & Wingo, P. A. (2005). Annual report to the nation on the status of cancer 1975–2002, featuring population-based trends in cancer treatment. *Journal of the National Cancer Institute, 97*, 1407–1727.

Edwards, B. K., Ward, E., Kohler, B. A., Eheman, C. E., Zauber, A. G., Anderson, R. N., et al. (2010). Annual report to the nation on the status of cancer, 1975–2006, featuring colorectal cancer trends and impact of interventions to reduce future rates. *Cancer, 116*(3), 544–573.

Espey, D. K., Wu, X., Swan, J., Wiggins, C., Jim, M., Ward, E., et al. (2007). Annual report to the nation on the status of cancer, 1975–2004, featuring cancer in American Indians and Alaska Natives. *Cancer, 110*(10), 2119–2152. doi: 10.1002/cncr.23044

Four Lodges Technology. (2006–2008). *About the Apsáalooke.* Retrieved February 10, 2011, from http://www.crowtribe.com/about.htm

Gillham, B. (2000). *The research interview.* London: Continuum.

Groves, R. M., Fowler Jr., F. J., Couper, M. P., Lepkowski, J. M., Singer, E., & Tourangeau, R. (2009). *Survey methodology.* New York: Wiley.

Harrison, B. (2001). *Collaborative programs in Indigenous communities: From fieldwork to practice.* Walnut Creek, CA: Altamira Press.

Haverkamp, D., Espey, D., Paisano, R., & Cobb, N. (2008). *Cancer mortality among American Indian and Alaska Natives: Regional differences, 1999–2003.* Rockville, MD: Indian Health Service.

Hild, C. M. (2007). *Engaging Inupiaq values in land management for health through an action research appreciative inquiry process.* Saybrook Graduate School and Research Center, San Francisco, California.

Jemal, A., Clegg, L. X., Ward, E., Ries, L. A. G., Wu, X., Jamison, P. M., et al. (2004). Annual report to the nation on the status of cancer, 1975–2001, with a special feature regarding survival. *Cancer, 101*, 3–27.

Keats, D. M. (2000). *Interviewing: A practical guide for students and professionals.* Buckingham: Open University Press.

Lanier, A. P., Holck, P., Kelly, J., Smith, B., & McEvoy, T. (2001). Alaska Native cancer survival. *Alaska Medicine, 43*(3), 61–69, 83.

Long, K. A. (1983). The experience of repeated and traumatic loss among Crow Indian children: Response patterns and intervention strategies. *American Journal of Orthopsychiatry*, *53*(1), 116–126.

Louis, R. P. (2007). Can you hear us now? Voices from the margin: Using Indigenous methodologies in geographic research. *Geographical Research*, *45*(2), 130–139.

Lowie, R. H. (1935). *The Crow Indians*. Lincoln: University of Nebraska Press.

Medicine Crow J. (1992). *From the heart of the Crow Country: The Crow Indians' own stories*. Lincoln: University of Nebraska Press.

Native American Cancer Research. (1996). *Interview transcripts*.

Oakley, A. (1981). Interviewing women: a contradiction in terms. In H. Roberts (Ed.), *Doing feminist research*. London: Routledge & Kegan Paul.

Oishi, S. M. (2003). *How to conduct in-person interviews for surveys (2nd ed.)*. Thousand Oaks, CA: Sage.

Petereit, D. G., & Burhansstipanov, L. (2008). Establishing trusting partnerships for successful recruitment of American Indians to clinical trials. Cancer Culture and Literacy. *Cancer Control: Journal of the Moffitt Cancer Center*, *15*(3), 260–268.

Poupart, M., Barker, L., & Red Horse, J. (2009). Research with American Indian communities: The value of authentic partnerships. *Children and Youth Services Review*, *31*, 1180–1186.

Rigney, L.-I. (1999). Internationalisation of an Indigenous anti-colonial critique of research methodologies. A guide to indigenist research methodology and its principles. *WICAZO SA Review: Journal of Native American Studies*, *14*(2), 109–122.

Sapsford, R. (1999). *Survey research*. London: Sage.

Schmidt, W. V., & Conaway, R. N. (1999). *Results-oriented Interviewing: Principles, practices, and procedures*. Boston: Allyn & Bacon.

Singleton, R. A., & Straits, B. C. (2002). Survey interviewing. In J. F. Gubrium & J. A. Holstein (Eds.), *Handbook of interview research: Context and methods* (pp. 59–82). Thousand Oaks, CA: Sage.

Smylie, J., Kaplan-Myrth, N., & McShane, K. (2009). Indigenous knowledge translation: baseline findings in a qualitative study of the pathways of health knowledge in three Indigenous communities in Canada. *Health Promotion Practice*, *10*(3), 436–446.

Suskie, L. A. (1996). *Questionnaire survey research: What works* (2nd ed.). Tallahassee, FL: Association for Institutional Research.

van den Hoonaard, D. K. (2005). "Am I doing it right?" Older widows as interview participants in qualitative research. *Journal of Aging Studies*, *19*(3), 393–406.

Wiggins, C. L., Espey, D. K., Wingo, P. A., Kaur, J. S., Wilson, R. T., Swan, J., et al. (2008). Cancer among American Indians and Alaska Natives in the United States, 1999–2004. *Cancer*, *113*(Suppl. 5), 1142–1152.

Wilson, S. (2008). *Research is ceremony: Indigenous research methods*. Black Point, Nova Scotia: Fernwood.

Acknowledgments: The support of the American Cancer Society (RSG-01–193–05-CPPB) and the National Institutes of Health National Institute on Minority Health and Health Disparities (R24MD002811) are acknowledged with gratitude. The content is solely the responsibility of the authors and does not necessarily represent the official views of the American Cancer Society, the National Institute on Minority Health and Health Disparities, or the National Institutes of Health.

We also want to thank community members and project staff who codeveloped the survey items and methods, our advisory board, Little Big Horn College staff, and Eugenia Eng, University of North Carolina, Chapel Hill.

Portions of this chapter were adapted from "Development of an interviewer training manual for a cervix health project on the Apsáalooke Reservation" by S. Christopher, A. Knows His Gun McCormick, A. Smith, and J. C. Christopher (2005), *Health Promotion Practice*, 6(4): 414–422. Adapted with permission of the publisher.

Chapter 9

THE APPLICATION OF

FOCUS GROUP

METHODOLOGIES

TO CBPR

EDITH C. KIEFFER

YAMIR SALABARRÍA-PEÑA

ANGELA M. ODOMS-YOUNG

SHARLA K. WILLIS

GLORIA PALMISANO

J. RICARDO GUZMÁN

The *focus group* is a qualitative research method in which a trained moderator facilitates a guided discussion with a small group of people (often six to eight) who have personal or professional experience with the topic being studied (Brown, 1999; Morgan, 1998a). A type of group interview, **focus groups** take advantage of group communication to gain insight into respondents' attitudes, feelings, beliefs, cultural norms, experiences, and reactions regarding a specific topic of interest (Kitzinger, 1995). Although focus groups may be the sole data collection method, they are often triangulated with other qualitative or quantitative methods to enhance credibility, elicit varying or deeper insights, or to verify or confirm results. Focus groups can help researchers understand social experience by answering such questions as: What is going on here? Why and how do things happen the way they seem to? Why and how do people think and behave the way they do? (Denzin & Lincoln, 2005; Morgan, 1998b).

Focus groups are particularly useful for community-based studies and for studies requiring community-level rather than personal information (Hennink, 2007). Through focus groups, community members have participated in identifying problems and needs, studying social change processes, formulating research questions and hypotheses, building knowledge and capacity, analyzing systems of care and barriers to service utilization, and planning, developing, and evaluating programs and policies (Gans et al., 2003; Hennink, 2007; Horowitz et al., 2008; Kieffer, Willis, Arellano, & Guzman, 2002; Kieffer et al., 2004; Morgan, 1998b; Pagdett, 2008; Patton, 2002).

Focus groups offer participants the opportunity to exchange ideas, express opinions, and assert differences and commonalities. Unlike quantitative methods, and among qualitative methods, they have the advantage of stimulating ideas from individual participants that are fostered by the dynamics of the group discussion (Hennink, 2007; Pagdett, 2008). Although focus groups may promote awareness of shared experiences, the goal is not consensus. Ideally, the questions and interactions elicited during focus groups generate rich, diverse stories as participants share experiences in their own words and language. The interactive process may generate responses that are unanticipated by the researcher (Hennink, 2007). The multiple voices, dialogues, and debates among participants may decrease their interaction with the moderator, giving more validation and importance to participants' thoughts and ideas (Hennink, 2007; Kamberelis & Dimitriadis, 2005). This group dynamic may help balance the power between researchers, moderators, and participants because the flow of interactions and opinions empowers participants' voices. Many researchers consider focus groups to be a culturally sensitive research method, reaching those who may feel intimidated by one-on-one interviews and fitting well with cultures and groups that value collectivity (Kamberelis & Dimitriadis, 2005). Holding focus groups in settings familiar to participants may further enhance the participants' influence in the focus group process (Kamberelis & Dimitriadis, 2005).

Focus groups may not be suitable for all research situations. Geographic and socio-demographic characteristics of potential group participants, study goals and objectives, length of study, budget and logistics must all be considered (Peek & Fothergill, 2009). Unless great care is taken during group formation and moderation, the potential for breach of confidentiality, social pressures, hierarchical relationships among participants, and difficulty assembling groups of people who do not know each other well may limit their usefulness in studies with highly sensitive or polarized topics, in stigmatized groups, and in small communities or those with highly structured social relationships organizations (Hennink, 2007; Makosky Daley et al., 2010; Pagdett, 2008).

In this chapter, we concentrate on the use of focus groups in the context of community-based participatory research (CBPR) and related approaches, such as participatory action research, that share an emphasis on participation and action linked with research (Hennink, 2007; Israel, Schulz, Parker, & Becker, 1998; Krueger & Casey, 2009). Community members become change agents by telling their stories, articulating their perspectives on the issues affecting them, and recommending strategies for addressing these issues that are grounded in the realities of their environment and experience. Community and academic partners learn about issues affecting community members. Academic researchers view themselves as members of the team as opposed to being in the position of control (Makosky Daley et al., 2010). Through **colearning**, community and academic partners build mutual capacity to conduct research and take results-based action. We will present a brief description of focus groups conducted in two CBPR projects, and an in-depth discussion of a third, related project. We will summarize capacities developed and lessons learned by our CBPR partnership and their member organizations, through these projects. (For a full description of how to plan and implement focus groups, see Crabtree & Miller, 1999a; Krueger & Casey, 2009; Morgan & Krueger, 1998.) (See Chapter Thirteen in this volume for an examination of the use of in-depth group interviews in the context of CBPR.)

CBPR AND THE PROJECT BACKGROUND

Our CBPR projects are based in the southwest and eastside communities of Detroit, Michigan. At the time of this research, the eastside Detroit community was 89% African American; at least 35% of the ethnically diverse southwest Detroit community was Latino (U.S. Census Bureau, 2000). These communities have experienced the effects of decades of economic decline, including outmigration of employment opportunities, middle-class residents and businesses, and increased concentration of poverty and ethnic segregation, high crime rates, and a decaying and inadequate public infrastructure (Sugrue, 2005). Nonetheless, community-based organizations with long-standing ties to neighborhoods and residents provide social, health, and advocacy services. Several organizations are members of the Detroit Community-Academic Urban Research Center (URC), a partnership of community-based organizations, service providers, and academic institutions. Initiated with funding from the Centers for Disease Control and Prevention (CDC) in 1995, the URC supports interdisciplinary, community-based participatory research that strengthens the ability of its partners to develop, implement, and evaluate health interventions aimed at improving the health and quality of life of families and communities (Israel et al., 2001).

Several URC-affiliated CBPR projects, using community surveys and focus groups, identified diabetes, cardiovascular disease, and their risk factors—including obesity, physical inactivity, and poor diet—as major concerns to community residents and have used these results to plan appropriate interventions (Harvey et al., 2009; Kieffer et al., 2002; Kieffer et al., 2004; Schulz et al., 2002). In one project, a group of Latino women from southwest Detroit participated in three focus groups, two during pregnancy and one postpartum, in an active process that moved from issue identification to data analysis and interpretation to program planning (Kieffer et al., 2002). At the first focus group meeting, women discussed their beliefs about diabetes and factors affecting their risk. During their second meeting, they discussed and extended major ideas that emerged during their first meeting, and identified strategies for reducing barriers to physical activity. During their third meeting, they developed recommendations for a culturally appropriate program to provide group social support and safe opportunities for exercise. This process captured changes in the women's perceptions of themselves, and the barriers in their environment, as they moved through pregnancy and the postpartum period. Their increasingly open discussions and interactions built toward intervention development (Kieffer et al., 2002).

To support the recommended program and other potential diabetes-related interventions, the URC partners formed the REACH Detroit Partnership, which responded to the CDC's Racial and Ethnic Approaches to Community Health (REACH) 2010 initiative to reduce **health disparities**. During its planning year, the REACH Detroit Partnership Steering Committee (SC) invited eastside and southwest Detroit families to participate in intervention planning focus groups (Kieffer et al., 2004). The SC held six gender- and age-specific focus groups in each community that brought together people of all ages to share their perspectives and suggest strategies for reducing barriers to healthy eating, regular physical activity, and diabetes prevention and management. Focus group recommendations resulted in the CDC-funded REACH Detroit Partnership's community, social support group, health system, and family interventions that began in 2000 (CDC grant # U50/CCU517264–01). The grantee was Community Health and Social Services Center, Inc. (CHASS), a federally qualified health center and URC partner organization.

The REACH Detroit Partnership's *community facilitators* and *community health advocates* worked with community organizations and residents to increase awareness of diabetes and its risk factors and to develop resources needed to reduce those risks. Community resident *family health advocates* worked with individuals with diabetes, their families, and health care providers to improve diabetes self-management and health care (Heisler et al., 2009; Rosland et al., 2008; Spencer et al., 2006; Spencer et al., 2011; Two Feathers et al., 2007). This work resulted in consistent and significant improvements in self-management-related knowledge, diabetes-related depressive symptoms, and blood sugar control (Spencer et al., 2011). Enhanced community capacity and resources continued to address community needs after the end of grant funding in 2008. The *family health advocates* continue to help empower community residents to better manage and improve their diabetes control, currently through an NIH-funded randomized clinical trial (R18 DK078558), conducted with a CBPR approach.

In 2000, the URC board and the REACH Detroit Partnership SC also supported the development of *Promoting Healthy Lifestyles Among Women/ Promoviendo Estilos de Vida Saludables Entre Mujeres*, a CBPR project that planned interventions to reduce risk factors for excessive pregnancy weight gain and subsequent obesity and diabetes among Latino and African American women. The CDC's Division of Nutrition and Physical Activity funded the project (U48/CCU522189) from October 2000 to September 2002. The project steering committee (SC) included representatives of URC-affiliated community, service provider, and academic organizations, the Michigan Department of Community Health, and Detroit community resident women of childbearing age, including a pregnant woman. The SC was the research team, participating in all phases of the project, bringing essential ethnic and linguistic backgrounds and skills needed to plan and conduct the methodologies they proposed. Academic team members had experience conducting qualitative research related to nutrition, physical activity, and maternal and child health. Between monthly SC meetings, community and academic members worked in small groups on project activities.

RESEARCH DESIGN AND FOCUS GROUP METHODS

Promoting Healthy Lifestyles Among Women/Promoviendo Estilos de Vida Saludables Entre Mujeres used a multi-method qualitative approach. The project SC planned a three-phase data collection sequence that included in-depth individual interviews and focus groups. The aim of this process was to engage an increasing number and range of community residents and organizations in developing and analyzing the information needed to plan useful, acceptable, and accessible community interventions. During the first phase of data collection, 43 semi-structured, in-depth individual interviews were conducted with pregnant and postpartum African American and Latino women from Eastside and Southwest Detroit, respectively. A person designated by each woman as most likely to influence her beliefs and practices was interviewed separately. The interviews focused on beliefs related to weight, diet, and physical activity and on practices, barriers, and facilitators during and after pregnancy (Thornton et al., 2006). (See Chapters Five, Six, and Thirteen for discussion of the use of in-depth interviews.) The second and third phases of the data collection sequence built upon and extended the results of the first phase through focus groups conducted sequentially—first, with pregnant and postpartum women, and second, with program and policy leaders.

Focus Group Interviews with Pregnant and Postpartum Women

During the second phase of data collection, focus groups were conducted with pregnant and postpartum women in each community (four total). Participants were asked to discuss, confirm, and expand on the key results of the individual interviews and to identify potential intervention strategies.

Development of the Pregnant and Postpartum Women Focus Group Guides

After discussing the individual in-depth interview results, the SC designed four focus group guides that used a common structure to ensure that moderators asked questions that confirmed and extended the results of the individual interviews in a consistent fashion. Within each topic, the guides explored major themes that had arisen from the individual interviews, followed by questions and suggested probes. Each guide was also tailored to probe issues, beliefs, and practices specific to each community, and to pregnant and postpartum women. The final section in each guide focused on women's intervention recommendations, including issues and resources needed to make participation feasible for community women. The Spanish-language guide was translated into English for use by non-Spanish-speaking SC members.

Recruitment and Training of Recruiters, Moderators, and Note Takers

The SC discussed position roles, responsibilities, and selection criteria, and interviewed and selected focus group recruiters, moderators, and note takers. SC members prioritized the moderator as the position that required a trained community resident. Criteria included having experienced pregnancy and the postpartum period, having the same ethnic background as participants, and having some experience facilitating group discussions. SC members nominated women who met the criteria, including a pregnant woman who had joined the SC after participating in an individual interview. Moderators received $250 to compensate for their time and effort. The SC decided that bilingual and bicultural graduate student research assistants and a community resident staff member would serve as recruiters and note takers. These women were familiar with the project's purpose and CBPR principles, and had demonstrated skills in their roles.

Academic SC members conducted two community-specific training workshops for moderators and note takers (see Chapter Six for a discussion of interviewer training). Both workshops were held two weeks before the planned focus group date, hosted by the community organizations that were hosting the focus groups. The workshops built individual and team skills, a shared sense of the focus group purpose, and familiarity with procedures and host settings. The moderators and note takers received a training manual one week prior to the workshop date. Because written Spanish-language material on focus group methodology was scarce, research assistants translated training materials into Spanish under the guidance of an academic SC member. The Southwest trainee workshop was conducted in Spanish, to prepare them in the language spoken by the focus group participants.

The training workshop curriculum covered: introductions; the project background; a focus group definition; moderator and note-taker roles before, during, and after the focus groups; the importance of, and procedures for informed consent, audiotaping, protecting confidentiality; and the purpose, content, and administration of the focus group guide and demographic information sheet; summary report procedures; and role-playing exercises using the focus group guides. All participants in both workshops received certificates of completion. Strengths of the workshop noted by participants in a process evaluation questionnaire included the inherent **capacity building** and the practicality of concepts learned. During the period between the workshop and the focus groups, academic research team members were available to discuss any concerns or questions with the moderators and note takers. (See downloadable supplement for this chapter for the confirmation letter, agenda, and focus group guide that were used for the Eastside and Southwest Detroit moderator training workshops.)

Recruitment of Pregnant and Postpartum Women

SC partner organizations and recruiters distributed flyers advertising the project at community clinics and events for pregnant and postpartum women. Recruiters approached women and described the purpose of the study. The recruiters administered a brief eligibility questionnaire to women who wanted to learn more about participating. Women who requested child care provided the ages and names of their children. Recruiters gave women an information sheet that described project activities and potential benefits, incentives, risks, and protections for participants. To assist with project planning, women who declined to participate were asked to provide their reasons. Interested and eligible women provided contact information so that recruiters could confirm participation, transportation needs, and the focus group date, time, and place. A week before the focus group, project staff mailed a letter to each woman that thanked her for accepting the invitation, reviewed logistics and incentives, and provided a contact number for questions and attendance changes. Given that illness and daily life commitments emerge rapidly, project staff called each woman to confirm attendance and update transportation, child care, and other needs, two to three days before, and again 24 hours prior to the focus group meetings. When possible, the same person who recruited the woman made these calls. Multiple follow-up calls were needed to reach some women; others had disconnected telephones. Of the women who initially agreed to participate, approximately two-thirds confirmed their appointments, and one-half (n = 12) of Southwest and one-third (n = 10) of Eastside women ultimately participated in the focus groups.

Focus Group Implementation and Data Collection

The focus groups were conducted in meeting rooms of SC community partner organizations. A note taker greeted each participant and explained and administered the demographic information and informed consent forms. She addressed questions or concerns and collected the signed forms. She provided the participant with a name tag, introduced mothers and children to the child-care provider, escorted women to the focus group meeting room, and introduced them to the focus group moderator. During this informal period before all of the women had assembled, the focus group moderator welcomed the women, offered refreshments, and conversed with them about daily life activities. This helped the moderator identify possible personalities, such as talkative, quiet, or domineering, and assign seats accordingly. The meetings began with a welcome and an icebreaker exercise, during which the moderator, note taker, and participants introduced themselves. The moderator discussed ground rules, which included guaranteeing confidentiality by identifying participants only by their first names, destroying the audiotapes at the conclusion of the study, and not using identifiers in any reports. Using the focus group guide, the moderator read brief summaries of key themes from the individual interviews for each major topic. The moderator asked women to reflect on, react to, and expand on these themes and to generate and discuss program recommendations. The note taker assigned each participant a position number at the table and used that number as she took detailed field notes, including speaker order and observations of nonverbal cues that added meaning to the discussion. The note taker operated two recorders as a safeguard against equipment failure. The focus groups lasted approximately 90 minutes. At the conclusion, the note taker presented a three-minute summary of key themes, based on her notes, and invited participants to offer additions or corrections (Krueger, 1998). The moderator thanked participants for sharing their time, energy, and ideas, and told them that the SC would mail them a summary report of the focus group results, including recommendations for action. Each participant received $20.

Focus Group Interviews with Policy, Program and Organization Leaders

During the third phase, the SC summarized and shared the results of the first two phases with two community-specific focus groups made up of policy, program, and organization leaders with responsibilities at the community, local, or state level for health, social, or community development services. These focus groups ascertained leaders' perspectives on community-identified issues and potential solutions, and elicited their ideas and investment in identifying the best intervention approaches.

Development of the Organization Leader Focus Group Interview Guide

The organization leader focus groups were designed to engage a variety of individuals and organizations whose interests, responsibilities, and resources could contribute to planning and implementing the ideas and recommendations derived from earlier project phases. The SC discussed summary analyses of key themes and illustrative quotations from the women's focus groups. They created two interview guides with a common structure, tailored to include community-specific themes, with illustrative quotations from the in-depth interviews and women's focus groups, and questions with probes. The SC recommended that focus group participants read each quotation aloud, to facilitate their engagement with the women's experiences.

Recruitment and Training of Moderators

The SC nominated potential moderators who had lived or worked extensively in one of the two communities. The two selected moderators were women from the same ethnic group as the potential population for the planned interventions, including one SC member. Both had extensive experience moderating focus group discussions in similar communities and had played leadership roles in nonprofit organizations similar to the roles of most of the invited participants. The women's focus group note takers filled the note-taking roles. The SC recommended that the REACH Detroit Partnership community facilitators serve as hosts, greeters, and observers. Their strong relationships with local and community organizations made explicit and visible the central role of community organization partners in planning and implementing the focus groups. The REACH Detroit Partnership's objective of promoting diabetes prevention programs for pregnant and postpartum women provided continuity with organization leader participants during subsequent phases of grant writing and program development. Moderators and note takers participated in training workshops similar in goals and methods to those conducted for the women's focus groups and conducted by the same academic SC members. An additional objective was to increase the capacity of all participants to use focus groups for future CBPR activities and to extend their skills to others through similar workshops.

Recruitment of Organization Leaders

The SC and REACH Detroit Partnership community facilitators compiled contact information for organization leaders from programs that directly or indirectly provided services or leadership related to pregnancy, health, social services, community development, safety, food and nutrition, or recreation and physical activity. The SC gave priority to leaders whose organizations' service mandate included Eastside or Southwest Detroit. Using a script designed by project staff, each SC member personally contacted one or more leaders to communicate the focus group purpose, the importance of their participation and to determine their availability. The project principal investigator and the REACH

Detroit Partnership community facilitators signed and mailed formal invitation letters to the leaders or representatives designated during the phone calls. Each SC member, supplemented by staff as needed, made follow-up contacts by telephone or e-mail to confirm participation. A follow-up letter thanked confirmed participants and provided focus group logistics information.

Focus Group Implementation and Data Collection

The SC conducted two community-specific focus groups simultaneously in separate meeting rooms of a SC partner whose building was centrally located between, but not within, the two communities. Participants were assigned to the Eastside or Southwest Detroit group based on their organization's primary service area. Those with broader service areas were distributed between the groups. The REACH Detroit Partnership community facilitators greeted participants. A note taker escorted them to their designated meeting room and administered the demographic information sheet which the SC used to assess the potential influence on the results of participant age, gender, ethnicity, type of organization and organization catchment area. Because this data collection phase involved public sector participants whose identity would be difficult to disguise, the University of Michigan Institutional Review Board ruled that participation demonstrated informed consent so written consent was not administered. Moderators invited participants to share refreshments while waiting for their group to assemble. During this period, the moderator approached several participants to invite them to read one of the selected quotations from the women's interviews that were chosen by the SC as illustrating a major theme. She gave a sheet of paper with a quotation typed in bold text to those who agreed.

The 90-minute focus group interviews began by introducing the moderator and note taker. The moderator reviewed the project background, focus group objective, and ground rules. She asked participants to introduce themselves during a brief icebreaker and presented a review of major themes, during which participants read the selected quotations aloud to the group. The discussion included participants' reactions to what they had heard and their own perspectives about barriers and facilitators to healthy eating and exercise. The moderator asked participants to comment on the feasibility of the women's recommendations, identify factors that might impede or facilitate implementation, and add their own recommendations for planning, implementing, and maintaining interventions, including necessary resources and training, environment, program, and policy components. She encouraged participants to discuss their potential roles in such activities. Moderating, note taking, audio taping, summarizing, thanking, and reporting procedures were similar to those described in the previous section. The moderator told participants that the SC would review the ideas generated in both groups and recommend next steps in the planning process. She invited participants to continue their involvement in planning by contacting the REACH Detroit Partnership community facilitator who had attended their focus group. Participants could complete a form with their name, organization, contact information, and area of interest in follow-up planning. Within two weeks, the SC mailed thank-you letters to participants, and to people who had confirmed but not attended, that described the next steps in the planning process. The SC mailed a summary report to all participants.

DATA ANALYSIS

During each study phase, community members reviewed, gave meaning to, and confirmed, revised, and extended the findings from the previous phase. The SC used summary analysis processes adapted from several used previously in community-based research to facilitate rapid feedback of results to the SC for each phase of planning (Kieffer et al., 2002; Kieffer et al., 2004; Krueger & Casey, 2009; Scrimshaw & Hurtado, 1987). Immediately following each focus group meeting, moderator and note taker pairs met for ten minutes to discuss their overall impressions and key ideas and insights from the interview. Then the moderators, note takers, and observers held a 30-minute debriefing meeting facilitated by an academic SC member. The group members exchanged impressions of the major themes from each focus group and discussed process issues such as interpersonal and environmental factors that may have affected the quality of the data. Academic SC members took notes during this meeting.

Within a week following the focus group meetings, the note takers typed detailed field notes, using the audiotapes to ensure accuracy. Community moderators, note takers, and observers also completed a summary analysis form, an expanded version of the focus group guide, with space for noting new topics that focus group participants had introduced and observations of nonverbal dynamics and selected quotations that allowed the words of participants to illustrate the major themes that they listed. (An abbreviated version of the forms used in Eastside and Southwest Detroit, with examples of questions, is located in Appendix F.) The SC held summary analysis meetings with community moderators, note takers, and observers one week following the focus groups. Each person used his or her summary analysis form to report key themes for each topic until those present agreed that the resulting lists for each focus group represented that group's outcomes. Analysis meeting participants identified overarching themes, those related to specific populations and communities, and the relative importance of items within each theme. The meetings were recorded to provide backup confirmation of written themes, to allow SC members who were not present to listen, and to produce a tool for future training. The SC used oral and typed reports of the summary analysis meeting results at its meetings.

Each focus group audiotape was transcribed verbatim in English or Spanish, as appropriate. Spanish-language transcripts were also translated into English. Each session note taker reviewed and corrected the relevant transcript for accuracy in its original language, integrated the field notes with the transcription to provide a more complete picture of the environment and nonverbal aspects of the focus groups, and identified speakers by seat number to protect participant confidentiality. Procedures described by Krueger & Casey (2009) guided in-depth analysis of the focus group transcripts. The results provided in-depth data for grant proposal and intervention material development. At least two academic SC members read the final transcripts to confirm themes that emerged during the summary analysis and extract additional themes related to target issues. Community SC members' time constraints limited their involvement in these readings. After the initial reading, SC members and several community moderators discussed, confirmed, and refined themes. They expanded a code book developed for analysis of the individual interview data to include new themes derived from the focus groups, so that the widest range of relevant ideas would be available to the SC for intervention planning. The code book included code definitions, inclusion and exclusion criteria, and examples (Crabtree & Miller, 1999b). Two research assistants coded the final transcripts, using Atlas.ti qualitative software, Version 4.1 (Muhr, 2000). Academic SC members reviewed and recoded any text that received less than 80% agreement during intercoder reliability assessment

(Carey, Morgan, & Oxtoby, 1996). The SC selected direct quotations to illustrate major themes.

DATA FEEDBACK, USE OF DATA AND PRODUCTS, AND RESULTING CBPR INTERVENTIONS

Project staff mailed final summary reports to focus group participants, SC members, and other community partners and URC-affiliated projects. One participant from the women's focus groups and two participants from the organization leaders' focus group subsequently joined the SC. The SC used the focus group recommendations to develop two large CBPR projects, tailored to the characteristics, cultural contexts, and needs of the Eastside and Southwest Detroit communities. The Michigan Department of Community Health, an SC partner and active participant in the policy focus groups, funded pilot phases of both projects. Each project involved full collaboration among community, health, and academic partners, guided by project SCs that included several participants from the organization focus groups. The CDC-funded *Promoting Healthy Eating in Detroit (PHED)* (CDC grant # R06/CCR521559–02–01) was a policy- and organization-level intervention designed to increase access to, and demand for, healthy foods in Eastside and Southwest Detroit. Although the primary grantee was the University of Michigan, CHASS, as lead agency for the REACH Detroit Partnership, and the Detroit Department of Health and Wellness Promotion received the majority of implementation funding and project staffing.

Healthy Mothers on the Move (Healthy MOMs) was funded by a grant from the National Institutes of Health-National Institute of Diabetes and Digestive and Kidney Disorders (NIH grant # 5 R18 DK 062344). A prospective randomized controlled clinical trial, Healthy MOMs aimed to demonstrate the effectiveness of a healthy lifestyle intervention tailored to the needs of pregnant and postpartum Latino and African American women in reducing risk factors for type 2 diabetes. The program design, methods, and materials were based directly on the results of the focus groups described in this chapter. The curriculum reflects the women's descriptions of their weight, diet, and physical activity beliefs and practices, and individual, family, social, and community barriers and facilitators to adopting or maintaining healthy lifestyles during and after pregnancy (Thornton et al., 2006). The resulting group program emphasized bringing women together to share, support, and learn from each other about healthy eating and exercise. The focus group participants recommended that the program be led by women "like them," with shared language, cultural, and experiential characteristics. In response, the Healthy MOMs SC placed social support at the heart of its theoretical intervention model. The project was staffed by trained community resident *Women's Health Advocates* and conducted in community settings. The program resulted in significant improvements in life-style practices and reduced depressive symptoms among participants compared to control group participants who received a healthy pregnancy education program as recommended by the SC. Following evaluation focus groups conducted with Healthy MOMs participants, and meetings with community collaborators, a subsequent program, *Mothers Moving to a Healthy Future/Madres Moviendose a un Futuro Saludable* (HRSA/MCHB grant # H59MC07461) extended the Healthy MOMs program through six months postpartum. The Healthy MOMs curriculum and related physical activity promotion video are available in both English and Spanish and are now being disseminated nationally (http://reachdetroit.org).

The SC members and staff of the REACH Detroit Partnership, Healthy MOMs, and other URC-affiliated projects in both communities adopted many of the focus group–related methods and materials developed for this project, including consent forms, training manuals, recruitment protocols, focus group guides, and summary analysis forms. The downloadable supplement for this chapter includes several examples of these materials. The working relationships described in this chapter led to steadily increasing capacities of community and academic partners. The REACH Detroit Partnership community health workers and other staff became very skilled in developing focus group questions, research protocols and procedures, and participant-related materials that are easily under-stood and culturally appropriate. They comfortably use research terms (for example, focus groups, IRB, peer review), participate as coauthors in peer-reviewed publications, and take leading roles in presenting methods and findings at national and local community and professional meetings. Academic partners look to community partners and community health workers to design culturally and linguistically appropriate research materials and to assure that the resulting data are used to benefit the community.

Several coauthors have used the experiences and case study materials described in this chapter for ongoing academic and community-based teaching and research.

For example, because of a lack of material and capacity in this methodology, YSP incorporated her experience and these materials to coach HIV/AIDS program staff in international settings to use focus groups in process and outcome evaluations. The recruitment protocol and script, selection criteria, contact information, and time line helped standardize this process in multisite evaluations using a CBPR approach. YSP also used focus groups for Participatory Evaluation and Empowerment Evaluation in which evaluators teach people to conduct their own evaluations (Fetterman, Kaftarian, & Wandersman, 1996). Involving stakeholders in planning, implementing, and analyzing data from evaluation focus groups has been an asset for stakeholder buy-in and ownership, increased data use for programmatic decision making and improvement, and reduced dependence on external assistance. Another coauthor (AOY) has used the summary analysis approach to develop products for community dissemination (Odoms-Young et al., 2010). All coauthors have used these materials, methods, and lessons learned in CBPR full and short courses and mentoring relationships for university and community-based staff, students, and postdoctoral scholars. We continue to use CBPR approaches to focus groups in our work in communities throughout the United States and internationally.

CHALLENGES AND LIMITATIONS

The success of any CBPR project rests on maintaining the delicate balance between the need for active involvement of community organizations and residents and the effects of this participation on their time and resources. Many organizations and individuals who most represent community interests and needs also face the greatest challenges to participation. Conducting focus groups in the context of CBPR is time-consuming and labor-intensive, considering the time and effort needed to establish partnerships, jointly design methodology, develop materials, organize and conduct training, implement the focus groups, and then analyze and disseminate the results (Makosky Daley et al., 2010). Leaders of small, grassroots community organizations sometimes could not participate to the extent that either they or other SC members had anticipated, because of competing obligations and staff and budget constraints that involved their survival. Some women identified as either prospective SC members or focus group moderators could not assume these roles because of life barriers including competing schedules and responsibilities, language, transportation, and legal status.

Identifying individuals with adequate competencies to serve as moderators, note takers, transcribers, and translators was difficult, even with extensive training available for these roles. A Spanish surname or African American ethnicity did not automatically credential a person as linguistically or culturally competent to interact with focus group participants or to understand the language they used. The SC faced a major challenge in identifying fully bilingual and bicultural individuals and focus group training materials. The SC members and staff of other CBPR projects recommended people with whom they had worked successfully. Nonetheless, it took more time and resources to develop materials and to recruit and train moderators and note takers than had been anticipated in the original grant budget and time line. Focus groups conducted in the context of CBPR may require larger budgets and longer time lines than other focus group research. Academic and community researchers share responsibilities for all stages of focus group planning and implementation. This means giving up *controlling* recruitment procedures, focus group protocols, and data analysis while not abdicating responsibility for contributing their expertise to the process (Makosky Daley et al., 2010). In the context of CBPR, focus group data are most useful for their immediate purpose and context. Triangulation, which is the use of multiple data sources, methods, or theoretical perspectives to address similar questions, is one way to increase the credibility of the focus group results, in the immediate and broader contexts (Gilchrist & Williams, 1999). The SC used a relatively unstructured first data collection phase to explore a broad range of issues that might have affected the beliefs and behaviors of concern. These ideas were discussed with separate groups of individuals with similar backgrounds (women's focus groups) and with groups of others with at least some different characteristics (organization leaders). The SC confirmed most themes and found additional insights during each new phase of data collection.

LESSONS LEARNED AND IMPLICATIONS FOR PRACTICE

The use of focus groups by the REACH Detroit Partnership and Promoting Healthy Lifestyles Among Women built the research capacities of, and trust between, both community and academic partners. Our enduring partnership has learned important lessons that may contribute to similar success for other groups and organizations that seek to conduct CBPR projects.

Involvement of Community Experts in Conducting Focus Groups and Analyzing Results Is Essential

Focus group moderators were either native Detroiters or Latino immigrants living in the city, had the same ethnic background as participants, and had participated either in the in-depth interviews or in facilitating group discussions in their communities. Their recent experiences as pregnant or postpartum women helped them relate to the issues raised by the focus group participants. Their background, experience, skills, and engagement with the entire research process informed the focus group workshop and contributed to their success as moderators. Community partner involvement in planning and conducting the focus groups added contextual information that was vital to understanding what participants expressed during the focus group meetings and, during analyses, to drawing conclusions from the results. All SC partners learned during this process.

Be Intentional About Building Community Capacity and Social Capital in CBPR in Low-Income Communities

The SC was attentive to identifying the potential among community residents. This strengthened the value of the focus groups and addressed the challenge of recruiting individuals knowledgeable about focus groups and communities. In addition to identifying people whom they knew within their organizations, interviewers observed qualities (such as attentive, assertive, able to express succinctly) in interviewees and assessed their potential for being focus group moderators. Including women from the community of identity (Israel et al., 1998) in leadership positions as moderators was a powerful form of capacity building, as they developed or enhanced professional and personal skills and abilities and served as role models for other women in the community. The outcome was a group of community members who proved to be outstanding moderators. Some trainees used their facilitation and observation skills at their jobs, in church-related activities, when communicating with their families, or in other research projects. Several now work in CBPR projects and staff positions in community and health care organizations in Detroit. Moderators and note

---

takers received informal certificates of completion following their training. In the longer term, **community-academic partnerships** should work with formal training entities to develop accredited programs and consulting business opportunities, with individual coaching on qualitative methods (including translation and transcription) for community partners.

Respected Community Organization Partners Are Essential to Building Community Trust

The SC included representatives of respected and committed community organizations whose representatives actively participated in meetings and were strong believers in the project benefits for the communities they served. This connection facilitated the selection of data collection locations and both moderator and participant recruitment. Conducting focus groups in these reputable places provided credibility, dissipated mistrust, and reduced attendance barriers.

Adequate Resources and Logistical Support for Community Experts and Organizations Are Essential

Scheduling focus group training and analysis sessions on weekends in Detroit and providing honoraria enhanced participation of community SC members and moderators. Anticipating and budgeting for hosting-associated expenses also reduce burdens on community partner organizations. The project provided child care, transportation, and translation services to minimize inconvenience to focus group participants. These services facilitated participation by a broader cross-section of community women, including those who were the most isolated, underserved, and often unheard. Offering on-site child care was essential for many women with newborns and young children. Allowing participants to tour the child-care facility and interact with providers helped them to relax and decide to use the services. Because many residents of Detroit and similar cities lack cars or reliable public transportation, the project offered or supported transportation to enhance recruitment and retention of focus group participants. Drivers who knew the communities and could communicate well with participants enhanced participants' trust. Refreshments served as people arrived provided an opportunity for participants to chat and feel at ease, which set a welcoming tone for the focus groups.

Adequate Budgets for Transcription and Translation Services Are Also Essential

Transcription of focus group tapes required special care to distinguish adequately among participants. Translation of project materials and meetings was expensive but essential to project success. The translation service needs far exceeded the budget, and the search for appropriate materials and service providers was a challenge. CBPR projects that use focus groups must adequately budget for such services. Working with linguistically diverse teams during data analysis can greatly enhance project outcomes. Bilingual team (Spanish/English) members provided insights into cultural contexts and appropriate interpretation of terminology and language. It is important to respect and account for the greater pressure and work that these abilities place on some members of the team, as compared to other members.

Participatory Processes Can Affect the Time Line for Focus Groups

Focus groups are often seen as a rapid data collection method. However, using them in the context of CBPR requires a more extended time line. Recruiting moderators and note takers with the aptitudes and time to receive training and conduct the focus groups took four months, resulting in time line delays. Using a participatory data analysis process was also time-consuming. The SC was made up of very committed but busy people who contributed their time and insights during and between meetings and whose tasks included reviewing, discussing, and revising materials. If academic SC members and research assistants had planned and implemented the data collection and analysis to save time, the voice and understanding of community members would have been sacrificed, along with the opportunities and benefits of colearning that occurred.

Ensure Immediate Benefits to the Community from Focus Group Interviews

All phases of the research involved a trust-building process among participants. Staying connected and committed to those project aims that extended beyond data collection and analysis, and that returned results to the community, were essential to maintaining this trust and the success of subsequent activities. Summary reports and presentations were provided to community residents and organizations. Maintaining the SC and extending membership to interested community residents who participated in data collection were also important steps. Collaborative development and implementation of successful grant proposals that addressed community issues and recommendations, and participation by community and academic SC members in other forms of community capacity building are examples of continuing mutual commitments that strengthen and maintain relationships that arise from CBPR.

Be Mindful of Previous and Current CBPR and Other Community Engagement Efforts

With increasing recognition of the benefits of CBPR, funders are requiring researchers to engage community members in the process of developing interventions. Conducting focus groups is a very common response. From a CBPR perspective, this is a great advancement. However, as community engagement gains popularity, there is a risk of overburdening communities and engaging in redundant data collection. Community resentment builds when people repeatedly share their ideas, especially without seeing their recommendations implemented or sustained. Partnerships considering use of focus groups should find out whether similar data are already available and use, and truly build upon, existing data in their planning processes.

SUMMARY

The use of focus groups has become popular in public health research, needs assessment, and program planning. The increased emphasis on addressing social inequities and racial or ethnic disparities in health has encouraged researchers and communities to collaborate on research that emphasizes the importance of community members' knowledge, experiences, and perspectives. The focus group method is ideal for CBPR, in which community members are equal partners in the research process and knowledge translates into action and social change. To develop effective strategies to address risk and protective factors associated with health and disease, community members and organizations recommend strategies for addressing these issues that are grounded in the realities of their environment and experience. Community moderators and focus group participants often develop a common bond based on shared perceptions of health and social issues as well as an investment in solutions that they themselves suggest. Conducting focus groups with organization leaders can actively engage individuals and organizations whose interests, responsibilities, and resources contribute to planning and implementing intervention ideas generated by community residents, and build linkages between them. Although focus group methodologies have specific core features, community partnerships can vary their design sufficiently to target the needs and specific aims of the community, population, and type of intervention under consideration.

Focus groups conducted with a CBPR approach are differentiated from other approaches in a number of ways: (1) their primary purpose and outcomes are aimed at providing both immediate and long-term benefit to the communities in which they are conducted; (2) community experts participate in planning and conducting the focus groups and analyzing the results; (3) community-academic partners intentionally develop and implement opportunities for colearning and capacity building; (4) adequate resources, time, and collaboration methods are allotted to develop and maintain mutual trust, to allow for true participation, and to reduce burden on community partners, as individuals and organizations.

Focus groups, as used in the projects described in this chapter, captured the voice of two communities and translated words into actions. This chapter included examples of a CBPR approach to focus groups conducted with African American and Latino family members of all ages, with pregnant and postpartum women, and with organization leaders. These focus groups identified issues of significance to them, and suggested strategies, programs, and policies. Project members forged expanding and lasting partnerships that built and sustained ongoing CBPR projects. The community and academic capacities, materials and methods developed, and lessons learned, have resulted in significant improvements in health status for many community residents and increased resource availability for organizations in both communities. Our work provides a model for community-academic partnerships in Detroit, elsewhere in Michigan, nationally, and internationally.

KEY TERMS

Capacity building

Colearning

Community-academic partnerships

Focus groups

Health disparities

DISCUSSION QUESTIONS

1. One of the often-cited benefits of focus groups is the ability to gather a large amount of information in a short time. Is this true in the CBPR context? How did the CBPR process used in the chapter affect the time frame between idea inception and data availability? What factors should a CBPR partnership consider in deciding whether to use a focus group approach?

2. In the chapter case study, the project SC was the research team and included members who served as moderators and represented organizations that hosted the focus groups. Discuss the strengths and limitations of this approach.

3. The chapter case study's research design intentionally built community capacity. Provide examples and discuss how capacity building was integrated in each phase of the focus group process. Discuss additional examples and outcomes of colearning described in this chapter.

REFERENCES

Brown, J. B. (1999). The use of focus groups in clinical research. In B. F. Crabtree & W. L. Miller (Eds.), *Doing qualitative research* (2nd ed., pp. 109–124). Thousand Oaks, CA: Sage.

Carey, J. W., Morgan, M., & Oxtoby, M. J. (1996). Intercoder agreement in analysis of responses to open-ended interview questions: Examples from tuberculosis research. *Cultural Anthropology Methods, 8*(3), 1–5.

Crabtree, B. F., & Miller, W. L. (Eds.). (1999a). *Doing qualitative research* (2nd ed.). Thousand Oaks, CA: Sage.

Crabtree, B. F., & Miller, W. L. (1999b). Using codes and code manuals: a template organizing style of interpretation. In B. F. Crabtree & W. L. Miller (Eds.), *Doing qualitative research* (2nd ed., pp. 163–177). Thousand Oaks, CA: Sage.

Denzin, N. K., & Lincoln, Y. S. (2005). The discipline and practice of qualitative research. In N. K. Denzin & Y. S. Lincoln (Eds.), *The SAGE handbook of qualitative research* (3rd ed., pp. 1–41). Thousand Oaks, CA: Sage.

Fetterman, D. M., Kaftarian, S. J., & Wandersman, A. (Eds.). (1996). *Empowerment evaluation: Knowledge and tools for self-assessment.* Thousand Oaks, CA: Sage.

Gans, K. M., Kumanyika, S. K., Lovell, H. J., Risica, P. M., Goldman, R., Odoms-Young, A., et al. (2003). The development of SisterTalk: a cable TV-delivered weight control program for black women. *Preventive Medicine, 37*(6), 654–667.

Gilchrist, V. J., & Williams, R. L. (1999). Key informant interviews. In B. F. Crabtree & W. L. Miller (Eds.), *Doing qualitative research* (2nd ed., pp. 82). Thousand Oaks, CA: Sage.

Harvey, I. S., Schulz, A. J., Israel, B. A., Sand, S., Myrie, D., Lockett, M. P., et al. (2009). The Healthy Connections project: A community-based participatory research project involving women at risk for diabetes and hypertension. *Progress in Community Health Partnerships, 3*(4), 273–274.

Heisler, M., Spencer, M., Forman, J., Robinson, C., Shultz, C., Palmisano, G., et al. (2009). Participants' assessments of the effects of a community health worker intervention on their diabetes self-management and interactions with healthcare providers. *American Journal of Preventive Medicine, 37*(6 Suppl 1), S270–279.

Hennink, M. M. (2007). *International Focus Group Research: A handbook for the health and social sciences.* Cambridge, UK: Cambridge University Press.

Horowitz, C. R., Goldfinger, J. Z., Muller, S. E., Pulichino, R. S., Vance, T. L., Arniella, G., et al. (2008). A model for using community-based participatory research to address the diabetes epidemic in East Harlem. *Mt. Sinai Journal of Medicine, 75*(1), 13–21.

Israel, B. A., Lichtenstein, R., Lantz, P., McGranaghan, R., Allen, A., Guzman, J. R., et al. (2001). The Detroit Community-Academic Urban Research Center: Development, implementation, and evaluation. *Journal of Public Health Management & Practice, 7*(5), 1–19.

Israel, B. A., Schulz, A. J., Parker, E. A., & Becker, A. B. (1998). Review of community-based research: Assessing partnership approaches to improve public health. *Annual Review of Public Health, 19*, 173–202.

Kamberelis, G., & Dimitriadis, G. (2005). Focus groups: Strategic articulations of pedagogy, politics, and inquiry. In N. K. Denzin & Y. S. Lincoln (Eds.), *The SAGE handbook of qualitative research* (3rd ed., pp. 887–907). Thousand Oaks, CA: Sage.

Kieffer, E. C., Willis, S. K., Arellano, N., & Guzman, R. (2002). Perspectives of pregnant and postpartum Latino women on diabetes, physical activity, and health. *Health Education & Behavior, 29*(5), 542–556.

Kieffer, E. C., Willis, S. K., Odoms-Young, A. M., Guzman, J. R., Allen, A. J., Two Feathers, J., et al. (2004). Reducing disparities in diabetes among African American and Latino residents of Detroit: The essential role of community planning focus groups. *Ethnicity & Disease, 14*(3 Suppl 1), S27–37.

Kitzinger, J. (1995). Qualitative research. Introducing focus groups. *British Medical Journal, 311*(7000), 299–302.

Krueger, R. A. (1998). Analyzing and reporting focus group results. In D. L. Morgan & R. A. Krueger (Eds.), *The focus group kit* (Vol. 6). Thousand Oaks, CA: Sage.

Krueger, R. A., & Casey, M. A. (Eds.). (2009). *Focus groups: A practical guide for applied research* (4th ed.). Thousand Oaks, CA: Sage.

Makosky Daley, C., James, A. S., Ulrey, E., Joseph, S., Talawyma, A., Choi, W. S., et al. (2010). Using focus groups in community-based participatory research: Challenges and resolutions. *Qualitative Health Research, 20*(5), 697–706.

Morgan, D. L. (1998a). What focus groups are (and are not). In D. L. Morgan & R. A. Krueger (Eds.), *The focus group kit* (Vol. 1, pp. 29–35). Thousand Oaks, CA: Sage.

Morgan, D. L. (1998b). Why should you use focus groups? In D. L. Morgan & R. A. Krueger (Eds.), *The focus group kit* (Vol. 1, pp. 9–15). Thousand Oaks, CA: Sage.

Morgan, D. L., & Krueger, R. A. (Eds.). (1998). *The focus group kit.* Thousand Oaks, CA: Sage.

Muhr, T. (2000). Atlas.ti, Version 4.1: Scientific Software Development, Berlin.

Odoms-Young, A., Zenk, S., Holland, L., Watkins, A., Wroten, J., Oji-Njideka, N., et al. (2010). *Family food access report: "When we have better, we can do better."* Chicago: University of Illinois at Chicago and Chicago Department of Public Health Englewood Neighborhood Health Center.

Pagdett, D. K. (2008). *Qualitative methods in social work research* (2nd ed.). Thousand Oaks, CA: Sage.

Patton, M. Q. (2002). *Qualitative research and evaluation methods* (3rd ed.). Thousand Oaks, CA: Sage.

Peek, L., & Fothergill, A. (2009). Using focus groups: Lessons from studying daycare centers, 9/11, and Hurricane Katrina. *Qualitative Research, 9*(1), 31–59.

Rosland, A. M., Kieffer, E., Israel, B., Cofield, M., Palmisano, G., Sinco, B., et al. (2008). When is social support important? The association of family support and professional support with specific diabetes self-management behaviors. *Journal of General Internal Medicine, 23*(12), 1992–1999.

Schulz, A. J., Parker, E. A., Israel, B. A., Allen, A., Decarlo, M., & Lockett, M. (2002). Addressing social determinants of health through community-based participatory research: The East Side Village Health Worker Partnership. *Health Education & Behavior, 29*(3), 326–341.

Scrimshaw, S., & Hurtado, E. (Eds.). (1987). *Rapid assessment procedures for nutrition and primary health care: Anthropological approaches to improving programme effectiveness* (Vol. 11). Tokyo: The United Nations University.

Spencer, M. S., Kieffer, E. C., Sinco, B. R., Palmisano, G., Guzman, J. R., James, S. A., et al. (2006). Diabetes-specific emotional distress among African Americans and Hispanics with type 2 diabetes. *Journal of Health Care for the Poor and Underserved, 17*(2 Suppl), 88–105.

Spencer, M. S., Rosland, A. M., Kieffer, E. C., Sinco, B. R., Valerio, M. A., Palmisano, G., et al. (2011). Effectiveness of a community health worker intervention among African American and Latino adults with type 2 diabetes: A randomized controlled trial. *American Journal of Public Health*, *101*(12):2253–2260. http://dx.doi.org/10.2105/AJPH.2010.300106

Sugrue, T. J. (2005). *The origins of the urban crisis: Race and inequality in postwar Detroit*. Princeton, NJ: Princeton University Press.

Thornton, P. L., Kieffer, E. C., Salabarría-Peña, Y., Odoms-Young, A., Willis, S. K., Kim, H., et al. (2006). Weight, diet, and physical activity-related beliefs and practices among pregnant and postpartum Latino women: The role of social support. *Maternal and Child Health Journal*, *10*(1), 95–104.

Two Feathers, J. T., Kieffer, E. C., Palmisano, G., Anderson, M., Janz, N., Spencer, M. S., et al. (2007). The development, implementation, and process evaluation of the REACH Detroit Partnership's Diabetes Lifestyle Intervention. *Diabetes Education*, *33*(3), 509–520.

U.S. Census Bureau. (2000). *American FactFinder—Census 2000*. Retrieved June 13, 2011, from http://factfinder.census.gov

Acknowledgments: The project described in this chapter was conducted in collaboration with the Detroit Community-Academic Urban Research Center, whose members provide unfailing guidance in conducting community-based participatory research. The authors thank the Promoting Healthy Lifestyles Among Women Steering Committee, whose continual efforts and dedication to the well-being of Detroit residents made this work possible. Committee members included Butzel Family Center, Community Health and Social Services Center (CHASS), the Detroit Department of Health and Wellness Promotion, Friends of Parkside, Henry Ford Health System, Kettering/Butzel Health Initiative, Latino Family Services, the Michigan Department of Community Health, the REACH Detroit Partnership, and University of Michigan Schools of Public Health and Nursing. The authors also thank the community focus group moderators, the host sites, and project staff and students for their contributions and commitment to the project and the focus group participants for sharing their time and ideas. This project was supported by the Centers for Disease Control and Prevention, Division of Nutrition and Physical Activity (grant U48/CCUSI577S-/SIP 10), with additional support from the REACH Detroit Partnership (grant USO/ CCU522189) and the W.K. Kellogg Foundation–funded Community Health Scholars Program. This chapter was coauthored by Yamir Salabarría-Peña in her private capacity. No official support or endorsement by the CDC is intended or should be inferred.

Chapter 10

DEVELOPMENT, EVOLUTION, AND IMPLEMENTATION OF A FOOD ENVIRONMENT AUDIT FOR DIVERSE NEIGHBORHOODS

SHANNON N. ZENK

AMY J. SCHULZ

BETTY T. IZUMI

SHARON SAND

MURLISA LOCKETT

ANGELA ODOMS-YOUNG

Interest in the contributions of **food environments** to health outcomes has grown exponentially over the past decade (Cummins & Macintyre, 2006; Larson, Story, & Nelson, 2009; Morland, Wing, & Diez Roux, 2002). While there are numerous conceptualizations (McKinnon, Reedy, Morrissette, Lytle, & Yaroch, 2009), food environments often include macro-level environments (for example, food marketing, agricultural policies, food assistance programs, food distribution systems) and more micro-level environments or settings (for example, homes, organizations and institutions such as child-care facilities, schools, churches, and worksites and neighborhoods) and their interrelationships (Story, Kaphingst, Robinson-O'Brien, & Glanz, 2008). The neighborhood food environment, specifically, has been of particular interest to researchers, practitioners, advocates, and policymakers. It includes the number, type, location, and accessibility of food outlets, as well as elements that consumers encounter within and around retail food outlets, for example, food availability, prices, quality, promotion, and placement (Glanz, Sallis, Saelens, & Frank, 2005). Research on the neighborhood food environment has found, for example, that economically disadvantaged and African American neighborhoods have fewer supermarkets than more advantaged neighborhoods and that living in closer proximity to a supermarket is associated with better dietary quality and lower risk of obesity (Larson et al., 2009). The distribution of food outlets has been the focus of the majority of research on neighborhood food environments to date, in part due to ready access to secondary data from commercial (for example, Dun & Bradstreet) and public (departments of public health) sources. However, research on food availability and, to a lesser extent, food prices and quality, which involves more detailed data, is increasing (Larson, et al., 2009).

A variety of methodologies are used to study neighborhood food environments, including geographic analysis, nutrient analysis, surveys (self-report or perceptual measures), and qualitative interviews (Matthews, Moudon, & Daniel, 2009; McKinnon et al., 2009; Moore, Diez Roux, Nettleton, & Jacobs, 2008; Zenk et al., 2011). One increasingly popular method is **food audits.** In this chapter, we describe how the Healthy Environments Partnership (HEP), a CBPR partnership involving community-based organizations, health services organizations, and academic institutions, designed and implemented a food audit. Called the Food Environment Audit for Diverse Neighborhoods (FEAD-N), it was an assessment of food stores in eastside, southwest, and northwest Detroit for the purpose of examining relationships between the food environment and dietary intakes and weight status of local residents and identifying environmental targets for interventions. We begin with a brief overview of food audits and HEP. We then describe the development and implementation of the HEP Food Environment Audit for Diverse-Neighborhoods (FEAD-N), and conclude with a discussion of challenges and lessons learned.

WHAT IS A FOOD AUDIT?

A food audit involves **direct observation** by trained observers systematically documenting predefined aspects of food outlets (for example, stores, restaurants) using a standardized instrument. Numerous standardized audit instruments for food outlets have now been developed

(McKinnon et al., 2009; National Cancer Institute, 2011). Food audit instruments can generally be classified into one of three types based on their predominant approach: checklists (based on indicator foods), market baskets (based on foods representing the total diet), and inventories (reporting of all foods) (McKinnon et al., 2009). As reviewed by McKinnon and colleagues (2009), checklists include foods based on predetermined criteria (for example, foods that are consistent or inconsistent with current dietary recommendations), while market baskets include foods that represent an adequate total diet (for example, healthy and unhealthy foods frequently consumed by the population) or reflect a standardized diet plan (for example, USDA's Thrifty Food Plan). Instruments are typically designed for stores or restaurants (and thus are often referred to as "store audits" or "restaurant audits") and are focused on food availability, but many include food prices and some incorporate food quality as well. Food audit instruments are often implemented using paper forms, and may also be loaded onto handheld computers or other electronic devices for data collection.

Food audits serve a variety of purposes. They have been used to: document characteristics of neighborhood food environments; test for differences in the food environment by neighborhood economic characteristics, racial/ethnic composition, and urbanicity; and identify contributions of the neighborhood food environment to variations and disparities in dietary behaviors, obesity risk, and related health outcomes (Franco, Diez Roux, Glass, Caballero, & Brancati, 2008; Larson et al., 2009; Rose et al., 2009). They can also be used to identify points of intervention and to evaluate the effects of such interventions. In addition, data generated from food audits can be valuable in policy advocacy. Although there is interest in common measures so that findings can be compared across contexts, the content of food audit instruments may also vary depending on the study purpose, population of interest, and context (Gittelsohn & Sharma, 2009; Larson et al., 2009; Odoms-Young, Zenk, & Mason, 2009; Sharkey, 2009).

OVERVIEW OF THE HEALTHY ENVIRONMENTS PARTNERSHIP (HEP)

The Healthy Environments Partnership (HEP), affiliated with the Detroit Community-Academic Urban Research Center (Detroit URC) (Israel et al., 2001), was established in October 2000 as part of the National Institute of

Environmental Health Sciences' Health Disparities Initiative (Schulz, Kannan, et al., 2005) (R01ES10936). HEP is comprised of community-based organizations (Brightmoor Community Center, Detroit Hispanic Development Corporation, Friends of Parkside, Warren/Conner Development Coalition), health services organizations (Detroit Department of Health and Wellness Promotion, Henry Ford Health System), and academic institutions (University of Michigan). Representatives of these partner organizations make up the HEP Steering Committee, which meets monthly and is involved in all aspects of the research process, consistent with CBPR principles adopted by HEP in 2001 (Israel, Schulz, Parker, & Becker, 1998). Additional academic researchers and students also contribute to HEP's work, though they are not Steering Committee members (Schulz, Kannan, et al., 2005). HEP's overarching goal is to examine and address aspects of the neighborhood social and physical environment that contribute to **urban health**, specifically, cardiovascular disease risk among adults in three Detroit neighborhoods (eastside, southwest, and northwest).

DEVELOPMENT OF FOOD STORE AUDIT

The HEP Food Environment Audit for Diverse Neighborhoods (FEAD-N), a food store audit that was ultimately implemented in 2008, emerged from over a decade of CBPR work in Detroit and Chicago, with multiple projects ultimately shaping its content.

Origins and Evolution of the Food Store Audit

Interest in the neighborhood food environment initially emerged from community members' concerns over lack of high-quality, affordable fresh produce, which were raised as part of the work of the East Side Village Health Worker Partnership (ESVHWP) (Schulz et al., 2001). Many of the partners involved in the ESVHWP later became involved in HEP.

East Side Village Health Worker Partnership (ESVHWP)

The ESVHWP was a CBPR partnership affiliated with the Detroit URC (1995–2003) and focused on identifying and addressing social determinants of women's health in eastside Detroit (Schulz et al., 2001), a low-income, predominately African American community. Lay health workers (known as "village health workers") and community representatives involved in the ESVHWP identified diabetes as a priority in 1999 and developed a pilot project to prevent diabetes in 2000–2001: Healthy Eating and Exercising to reduce Diabetes (HEED) (Schulz, Zenk, Odoms-Young, et al., 2005). In conversations among those involved in this project, eastside Detroit residents identified a shortage of super-markets in the city and an abundance of liquor stores. They described fresh fruits and vegetables as scarce, of poor quality, or overpriced at local stores. In response, the ESVHWP initiated a variety of action strategies including monthly fruit and vegetable "minimarkets" at readily accessible community sites.

Based on these activities, in 2001, the ESVHWP added items to a survey of African American women living in eastside Detroit. Results of analyses using those data suggested that women with higher incomes were more likely to shop at suburban supermarkets than other food stores and that the type of food store to which women had access and the selection and quality of fresh produce for sale may have influenced their fruit and vegetable consumption (Zenk, Schulz, Hollis-Neely et al., 2005). Conversations about these results among members of the ESVHWP encouraged efforts to expand activities and research to understand the neighborhood food environment. (See Zenk, Schulz, Odoms-Young, & Lockett, 2009 for more detail on the growth of interest in the food environment through the ESVHWP and HEP.)

Early Observations of Food Stores in Detroit

In the early 2000s, a public health doctoral student working with the ESVHWP and HEP (and first author of this chapter, SNZ) had general interests in nutri-tion and the role of neighborhood environments in health disparities. As part of her dissertation research, she and other members of the ESVHWP and HEP mapped the locations of supermarkets in metropolitan Detroit (Zenk, Schulz, Israel et al., 2005). In addition, this team conducted food store audits in fall 2002 in four Detroit area communities (three of which corresponded with those involved with HEP), with different racial/ethnic and socioeconomic characteris-tics to examine variations in the availability, quality, and price of fresh fruits and vegetables across neighborhoods (Zenk et al., 2006).

The content of the instrument and data collection protocol were informed by the discussions taking place through the ESVHWP and HEED. Adapted in part from a checklist of "powerhouse" produce being utilized in a CBPR project in Saint Louis, Missouri (Baker, Schootman, Barnidge, & Kelly, 2006), the instrument was designed, for example, to include fruits and vegetables that were popular among the three predominant racial/ethnic groups in the study communities (African Americans, Latinos, non-Hispanic Whites). Because poor quality was a major concern expressed by community members, measures of fruit and vegetable quality were developed. Ultimately, the instrument assessed availability for 80 fresh fruits and vegetables and price and quality for a subset of 20 items. Local residents' observations about prevalent liquor stores in the community led to the inclusion of liquor stores, in addition to grocery stores, convenience stores, and specialty markets (meat, fruit and vegetable), as part of the audit. A team made up of the doctoral student, a resident of eastside Detroit, and another graduate student assessed 304 food stores across the four communities. Findings from analysis of these data indicated that eastside Detroit had the poorest quality of fresh produce of the four study neighborhoods, and found no differences in fruit and vegetable availability or prices across the four communities (Zenk et al., 2006).

Informal observations at stores and conversations among the data collectors as part of this data collection effort provided additional insights. We found, for example, that: (1) our instrument did not include many fruits and vegetables that were common in Latino neighborhoods (for example, tomatillo, mango) (Zenk, Schulz, Odoms-Young, & Lockett, 2009); (2) besides fresh produce, stores commonly lacked other healthy food options (for example, low-fat dairy, whole grains), but stocked many energy-dense, nutrient-poor foods and beverages; and (3) physical and social environments of some stores presented additional barriers to food acquisition, including: lack of cleanliness, security features (for example, plexiglass security barriers at checkout, shopping cart rails), tensions between African American clientele and non–African American (for example, Middle Eastern) owners and employees, loitering outside stores, and alcohol availability and promotion.

These aspects of the food environment were not systematically observed in the first food audit conducted by this team. However, as the HEP Steering Committee and other partnership members continued to analyze data from these early observations, to talk with residents about their neighborhoods and health (Schulz & Lempert, 2004), and shop at neighborhood stores, the range of questions about aspects of the food environment and their potential implications for dietary behaviors and health of neighborhood residents continued to grow.

Contributions of CBPR Work in Chicago

In 2004, the doctoral student working with HEP who initiated the food environment audit completed her degree and relocated to Chicago, where she became involved with studies of the food environment in that city. Based on experiences in Detroit and drawing on food store audit instruments that had recently become available (Glanz, Sallis, Saelens, & Frank, 2007; Sloane et al., 2003), she collaborated with community partners affiliated with the Illinois Prevention Research Center in Chicago to develop an expanded food store audit instrument (Zenk, Grigsby-Toussaint, Curry, Berbaum, & Schneider, 2010). Working within predominantly African American and Latino communities in southwest Chicago, the food audit instrument was modified to include: (1) additional fresh fruits and vegetables consistent with food preferences of Latinos (Grigsby-Touissant, Zenk, Odoms-Young, & Ruggerio, 2010); (2) canned and frozen fruits and vegetables, in order to capture more fully those available in neighborhood stores; (3) healthy and less healthy indicator foods from the other food groups: grains, meat and beans, and dairy; and (4) environmental measures, including tobacco and alcohol advertisements, store cleanliness, and acceptance of food assistance program benefits (for example, Special Supplemental Nutrition Program for Women, Infants, and Children [WIC]).

Around this same time, the Chicago-based member of HEP and another researcher (AOY) who had previously worked with the ESVHWP as a postdoctoral fellow also became engaged in a CBPR effort with service providers at a neighborhood health center to improve food access in a low-income, predominately African American community in Chicago. To better understand food access challenges from the perspective of local residents, thirty African American women were interviewed in 2006–2007 about their perceptions of the neighborhood food environment, process used to obtain food, environmental barriers and facilitators to food acquisition, and retail food outlet preferences and concerns. These interviews further highlighted food acquisition barriers in urban areas related to the physical and social environments of retail stores (for example, loitering, panhandling, poor upkeep, security guards, unfair treatment) (Zenk et al., 2011).

In summary, these diverse CBPR efforts across two cities were instrumental in shaping the content of HEP's 2008 food store audit instrument, the focus of this chapter. Each effort built on what was learned in the previous one, and engaged community members using different mechanisms (for example, data collection, in-depth interviews, structured discussions). Though each was informed by distinct local contexts, the dialogue across communities and over time allowed cross-fertilization and mutual learning, with development and adaptations over time.

Overview of the HEP Food Environment Audit for Diverse Neighborhoods (FEAD-N)

In 2005, HEP received additional financial support from the National Institute of Environmental Health Sciences (R01ES14234). The Lean & Green in Motown project expanded HEP's work to examine in greater depth relationships between the neighborhood built environment, including the food environment, and obesity risk. The project included a second food store audit designed to enable the partnership to examine change in the food environment over a six-year period, as well as additional aspects of the food environment not assessed in 2002.

The HEP FEAD-N was designed to not only assess food availability and prices, but also store characteristics that may serve as potential barriers or facilitators to food acquisition or healthy food purchases. Items fell into eight broad categories: fruits (fresh, canned, frozen, juice); vegetables (fresh, canned, frozen, juice); meat; beans (canned, dried); grains; dairy; fats and added sugars; and store environment (physical, social). The list of foods included more and less healthy items (for example, whole milk and skim milk) commonly consumed in the United States, as well as culturally specific foods often consumed within African American (for example, collard greens, okra) and Latino (for example, tomatillo, mango) populations. The FEAD-N also included foods that corresponded with the Spanish version of the Block 2005 food frequency questionnaire, which was administered to local residents in HEP's 2008 community survey (see Chapter Seven in this volume). The FEAD-N allowed observers to assess *availability* of each food item by documenting whether an item was present in the store. *Price* was recorded for a sample of foods as the lowest priced item (sale or regular price) of a pre-specified size (for example 24-ounce loaf of 100% whole wheat bread, 14–16 ounce can of sweet peas). *Food store environment* included physical and social aspects of the store that may influence the accessibility of the store or that may hinder (for example, candy or gum at checkout) or promote (for example, health promotion signs) healthy food purchases. In the following section, Table 10.1 shows the items included in the FEAD-N. (See the downloadable supplement for this chapter for a copy of the audit instrument.)

IMPLEMENTATION OF FOOD STORE AUDIT

Community members played an integral role not only in the development of the HEP FEAD-N, but also in its implementation.

Recruitment, Hiring, and Training of Community Members as Observers

Recruitment and Hiring

Consistent with HEP's CBPR approach, community members were recruited, hired, and trained as observers to conduct the food store audits. We advertised the positions by dropping off job fliers to community organizations and recreation centers for inclusion in their resource tables and by forwarding the job posting to the student employment offices at local colleges. We also distributed the job posting to HEP's community partners and asked them to disseminate it through their networks. Requested qualifications included a valid driver's license with access to a reliable and insured automobile, excellent interpersonal skills, good organizational skills, ability to do basic math calculations using a calculator, and ability to read a street map. This recruitment effort yielded twenty applicants, of which we interviewed nine. The interviews involved the HEP project manager (SS), a community partner (ML), and an academic researcher (SNZ) who jointly developed the interview questions. The questions included prior experiences and perceptions of local stores, a hypothetical label reading exercise, role-playing of interactions with store owners, and practice scenarios for calculating prices of different foods. After checking professional references, the three interviewers jointly decided to offer training to five of the applicants.

TABLE 10.1 Items from the Healthy Environments Partnership's Food Environment Audit for Diverse Neighborhoods (FEAD-N)

Category	Subcategory	# Items	Examples of Items
Fruits	Fresh	44[a]	Apples, banana, cherimoya, cherries, grapefruit, grapes, kiwi, mango, watermelon, oranges, strawberries
	Frozen	6[b]	Blueberries, mangos, peaches, mixed berries, raspberries, strawberries
	Canned	6[b]	Apricots, mangos, oranges, peaches, pear, pineapple
	Juice	1[b]	100% orange juice (fresh)
Vegetables	Fresh	86[a]	Avocado, green bell pepper, broccoli, carrot, chard, collard greens, green cabbage, tomatillo, tomato
	Frozen	7[b]	Broccoli, carrots, collard greens, corn, green beans, spinach, sweet peas
	Canned	6[b]	Carrots, corn, green beans, sweet peas, spinach, tomatoes
	Juice	1[b]	100% tomato or V-8 juice
Meat	Fresh	7[b]	Boneless skinless chicken breast, split chicken breast with skin, extra lean ground beef, regular ground beef, extra lean ground turkey, lean ground turkey, ground turkey
	Processed	4	Regular hotdogs, low-fat hotdogs, regular lunch meats, turkey or low-fat lunch meats
Beans	Canned	6[b]	Black beans, black-eyed peas, garbanzo beans, red or white kidney beans, pinto beans, red beans
	Dried	6[b]	Black beans, black-eyed peas, garbanzo beans, red or white kidney beans, pinto beans, red beans
Grains	—	14[c]	100% whole wheat bread, white bread, high fiber bread, brown rice, white rice, 100% whole wheat pasta, white pasta, whole wheat or whole grain "blend" pasta, 100% whole wheat tortilla, corn tortilla, flour tortilla, high fiber cereal, sweetened cereal, other cold cereal
Dairy	—	9[d]	Skim milk, 1% milk, whole milk, low-fat yogurt, regular yogurt, low-fat cheese, regular cheese, low-fat soy milk or Lactaid, regular soy milk or Lactaid

(Continued)

TABLE 10.1 (Continued)

Category	Subcategory	# Items	Examples of Items
Fats and added sugars	—	10	Diet soda; regular soda; low-fat salad dressing; regular salad dressing; low-fat snack chips or pretzels; regular snack chips; low-fat breakfast bars, regular breakfast bars, cereal bars or granola bars; low-fat cookies; regular cookies
Store environment	Physical	34	Infrastructure (store type, parking lot available, number of operational cash registers, store signs in languages other than English); services (bakery, butcher, deli section, pharmacist, gas station, sign for jitney); products (primary product for sale, fresh produce section, fresh meat or poultry section, alcohol available, carry-out food/fast food, most food prepackaged or ready-to-eat/heat items); marketing (5-A-Day, nutritional information, Food Guide Pyramid, Fruits and Veggies—More Matters, ads for alcoholic beverages on storefront, ads for tobacco products on storefront, liquor largest sign on storefront, candy or gum at checkout); government assistance program participation (WIC, Food Stamps/SNAP); disorder outside (broken glass, graffiti, visible trash/debris); disorder inside (foul odor, dirty floors, visible trash/debris, store cleanliness)
	Social	20	Security features (security guard, security camera, security bars on doors or windows, bullet-proof glass at checkout, enclosed checkout counter with turnstile, security mirror, elevated area/office for store management, shopping cart guard rails); disorder inside (people "hanging out" or loitering, panhandling); disorder outside (people "hanging out" or loitering, panhandling); behaviors of owner or employees (swearing/cursing, joking around/talking loudly, smoking); race/ethnicity of employees and owners (white, African-American, Latino/Hispanic, Asian, Middle Eastern)

a. Price assessed for subset of 6 items.
b. Price assessed for all items.
c. Price assessed for subset of 12 items.
d. Price assessed for a subset of 7 items.

Training

The five Detroit residents completed 25 hours of paid training (classroom and field work) in the fall of 2008 to prepare them for conducting observations using the FEAD-N. The trainers were HEP research team members, the HEP project manager, and a HEP staff member who was also a community resident. The classroom component of the training included instructions on field procedures, review of operational definitions, information on safety while collecting data, and guidance for interactions with store owners and employees. Field work was essential for developing observers' skills in conducting the food store audit. We were committed to achieving high consistency across observers in their ratings (inter-rater reliability) using the audit instrument, in order to ensure that any differences found across stores were not due to variations in implementation among observers. Therefore, as done previously by HEP in training community members to conduct systematic ratings of neighborhood environments (Zenk, Schulz, House, Benjamin, & Kannan, 2005; Zenk et al., 2007), several recognized strategies for promoting inter-rater reliability were used during training (Izumi et al., 2012).

First, to ensure easy reference for the observers, the instrument included detailed instructions, a color photograph of each fresh fruit and vegetable, and operational definitions of more ambiguous items (for example, store cleanliness).

Second, observers audited five practice stores as a group, in pairs, or individually. After each practice store, group debriefings were held to review results and to allow observers to ask questions about items and operational definitions. When group debriefings were held in the store, discrepancies among observers were resolved immediately by, for example, reassessing the availability or price of the item in question.

Third, oral and written feedback was provided to observers based on computed inter-rater reliability results from the practice stores. Inter-rater reliability scores (percent agreement) for the group and for each individual observer compared with a post-doctoral fellow working with HEP (BTI; the "gold standard") were computed and shared with observers on an ongoing basis. The post-doctoral fellow, who also was a registered dietitian, served as the gold standard throughout the training period given her food and nutrition expertise. Inter-rater reliability results were discussed with observers during subsequent training sessions. For group results, items with low levels of agreement were highlighted and feedback from observers was elicited to determine reasons for low inter-rater reliability. Observers were encouraged to use this feedback to improve their performance.

Fourth, observers were certified to conduct the food store audit based on their individual inter-rater reliability results. At the end of their training, observers were certified and hired if they achieved the certification criterion of 80% agreement as compared to the gold standard on each section of the food store audit instrument at a test store located outside of the study communities. Observers had the opportunity to attempt up to three test stores for certification. Following each certification attempt, individual feedback was provided on the individual's performance compared with the gold standard. Three observers met the certification requirement on their first attempt; one met the requirement on her second attempt; and one did not meet the certification requirement.

Contributions to Instrument Content and Formatting

The training also provided an opportunity to seek and incorporate additional input from community members working as observers on the audit instrument's content and formatting. With respect to what was rated, for example, observers suggested adding an item to document the presence or absence of an enclosed, elevated area found in some area stores, in which store personnel stand to monitor shoppers. Other contributions made by observers included suggestions to: make changes in the tortilla and frozen fruit package sizes assessed for price to best reflect sizes most commonly available in the community; add spaces to indicate grams of fat or percentage of fat for fresh meats, as this information was not routinely included on packaging in many stores; assess prices only of fresh produce that was not marked down in separate discounted produce section; use descriptive language whenever possible (for example, half gallon) rather than numbers (for example, 64 ounces); and list fresh produce items in alphabetical order rather than separating fruits from vegetables, in order to facilitate data collection. These and other concrete suggestions helped improve the local relevance of the food store audit instrument, avoided distortions in documentation of pricing that may have occurred through recording of discounted prices on produce that was past its prime, and helped to improve the inter-rater reliability of audits through improved layout.

Data Collection

To conduct the food store audit, we obtained a list of stores that sold food in Detroit from the Michigan Department of Agriculture. The list included all grocery stores, convenience stores, liquor stores, specialty food stores, pharmacies, and dollar stores in Detroit. Through a review of the list and using a geographic information system (GIS), we identified all stores with ZIP codes that intersected the study communities. Before going into the field, we mailed a letter to each of these stores, describing the study and requesting their participation. We used a ground-truthing procedure (Sharkey & Horel, 2008; Ward et al., 2005) in which community members systematically drove along every street in the study communities to confirm that the stores included on the Michigan Department of Agriculture list had not permanently closed and to identify any additional stores that sold food in the communities of interest. Institutional Review Board (IRB) approval was not required because the research did not involve human subjects.

Upon arriving at a store, observers generally introduced themselves to the store manager or owner and obtained permission to conduct the audit. In small stores, at least one observer found that it was easiest to complete the audit (because they did not carry many of the items) without approaching the store manager or owner. Due to the relatively sensitive nature of some items assessed (for example, race/ethnicity of store employees and owners, security features, store cleanliness), observers were instructed to leave the last page of the instrument which included these items in their vehicle and take notes relevant to each item while in the store. Immediately after conducting the audit, observers completed these items in their vehicles. The average length of time to conduct the audit was 26.6 minutes with a range of 15 minutes for small stores (such as a convenience store) to 60 minutes for large stores (such as a grocery store). A HEP staff member who was also a community resident supervised the data collection.

Of the 170 stores on the original list from the Michigan Department of Agriculture across the three study communities, sixteen stores were out of business, three residential homes were misclassified as food stores. Four additional stores were identified through the ground-truthing procedure. Thus, a total of 155 stores were identified across the three study communities. Of these stores, three refused to participate in the audits and one store was inaccessible due to construction. In-store observations were completed at all remaining 151 stores over a 10-week period between October and December 2008. To assess inter-rater reliability, two data collectors independently visited, on the same day, a random subset of 44 food stores over the course of the data collection period.

Inter-Rater Reliability Results

Overall, data collectors achieved high consistency in their observations of food stores as evidenced by the inter-rater reliability results for the instrument (Izumi et al., 2012). With the exception of price, items on the instrument were categorical. For kappa statistics, 0.80–1.00 is considered almost perfect agreement, 0.60–0.79 substantial agreement, 0.40–0.59 moderate agreement, 0.20–0.39 fair agreement, 0–0.19 slight agreement, and <0 poor agreement (Landis & Koch, 1977). Overall, more than 75% of the 267 categorical items on the instrument had almost perfect agreement, 21% substantial agreement, 2% moderate agreement, and one item fair agreement (Izumi et al., 2012). Inter-rater reliability of items assessing food price also was high; the concordance correlation coefficient for almost 85% of the 71 price items ranged from 0.70 to 1.00 (Izumi et al., 2012).

CHALLENGES AND LIMITATIONS

We encountered several challenges in the design and implementation of the food store audit described here. Many of these challenges stemmed from the tension between a positivist scientific paradigm, in which food audits are rooted, and the local knowledge of community members (Cochran et al., 2008; Schensul, 2002). Some of these challenges are discussed in this section.

Food Audits Are Based on a Common Rubric

Food audit instruments are standardized, requiring data collectors to document predefined aspects of retail food outlets using common operational definitions. If reliably implemented, an advantage of food audits is that they allow comparison of data across observers and places and over time. To do so, however, they do not allow observers, in this case community members, to bring to bear their prior experience or their subjective assessments of what is desirable in the process. Observers are asked to set aside their historical and contextual experiences and to rate outlet characteristics solely on what they see at the time of the audit and according to the prespecified definitions. Thus, food audits do not capture, for example, community members' previous experiences in the stores that they are auditing. During the design stage, engaging community members in the process of identifying and defining relevant items for the audit can help to assure that the instrument reflects their knowledge and experiences (for example, how to operationalize fruit and vegetable quality, environmental features that make them feel more or less safe in a store) and thus enhance construct validity. During training and the field period, we found that modifying the instrument and data collection protocol, to the extent possible, based on additional input from community members trained as observers also incorporated local knowledge. In addition, emphasizing the reasons that it was important to conduct observations according to the instrument's definitions (for example, comparability of data across observers and over time) and recognizing the limitations of this approach was helpful for training observers.

Food Audit Was Cross-Sectional

A related challenge is that food audits are typically a snapshot of food outlets at one point in time. Although research has shown that food availability, prices, and quality at urban stores are generally stable over a very short time period (that is, two weeks) (Zenk, Grigsby-Toussaint, et al., 2010), this may not be the case over longer time periods; hence the results may not adequately reflect the food environment, including community members' experiences with food stores that often span several years. In addition to the challenges associated with training community members to conduct the audit related to this methodological limitation, it is important to recognize that results based on food audits have limitations. For example, it is possible for an audit to show that a particular store has fresh fruits and vegetables, but based on the history of the store, community members do not utilize it for fresh produce because it has not consistently carried these foods in the past or for a variety of other reasons.

Limits on How Much Data Can Be Reliably Collected Due to Financial and Time Constraints

Financial and time constraints are common and very real in most research efforts. HEP had a limited amount of resources to conduct the food audit and ultimately faced time pressures to get into the field so that the audit could be conducted during the same season as the 2002 fruit and vegetable audit, in order to maximize comparability of data. The scope of the FEAD-N (for example, based on the relatively large number of food categories of interest) required fairly intensive training of observers, including time for practice stores and subsequent review of their work. This process required more time than we had anticipated, in order for observers to achieve the levels of proficiency and consistency in their ratings that were considered desirable. Ultimately, to meet our time line for getting into the field, we decided to reduce the number of items and complexity of the instrument. For example, in order to begin data collection on time, we eliminated the fresh fruit and vegetable quality assessment. This required more training time than we had in the end to achieve the desired proficiency and inter-rater reliability.

Balance Between Data Comparability and Local Relevance

In the academic literature, use of common measures and methods across various contexts is viewed as essential for advancing science on the neighborhood food environment. Though important, failure to consider the appropriateness of measures for local contexts and populations may limit our understanding. For example, measures that do not consider the local context and population may miss culturally specific foods. Due to the role of food in maintaining cultural traditions and affirming group identity, this may limit our understanding of the degree to which the neighborhood food environment is supportive for diverse groups. Thus, another challenge we found in conducting a food store audit was balancing the use of common measures with those that were relevant for our study communities. Our general approach was to use common measures when possible and to include additional measures that were relevant for our context and populations of interest based on a decade of working with and input from our community partners in Detroit and Chicago. Although this lengthened the instrument, we believe that the additional items enhanced the instrument's validity.

LESSONS LEARNED AND IMPLICATIONS FOR PRACTICE

In addition to those previously highlighted, we learned several lessons in conducting the HEP food audit that have implications for practice.

Invest in Training and Supervision of Community Members

First, while we faced constraints that led to trade-offs in the content of our instrument, we found that investing in training and supervision of observers was essential. We dedicated a fair amount of time to training because we wanted to achieve high consistency in ratings across observers (inter-rater reliability), viewed as important for ensuring data accuracy and publishing the food audit findings in academic literature. Not all projects will include this goal. Some projects, for example, may utilize food audits primarily to increase dialogue in the community about the neighborhood food environment and to develop action strategies. In these cases, it may be less important to achieve high inter-rater reliability and more important to provide opportunities to systematically observe food outlets, converse with store owners, and move forward a dialogue for change. Projects proposing food audits, especially those with a goal of disseminating results in academic literature, need to factor in time and resources for training, including multiple practice opportunities and subsequent discussions. Further, we found that supervision of observers, including spot-checking their work, was invaluable for providing observers with occasions to discuss their experiences in the field and for identifying potential problems (for example, missing data, unclear responses). That the HEP staff member providing the supervision was also from the community was particularly advantageous due to her familiarity with many of the stores in the community. Thus, we recommend building in time and resources for training and adequate supervision and support, ideally by a community member.

Complement with Other Research Methods that Engage Community Members

As discussed, food audits have limitations, including that they may miss valuable information in terms of community members' prior shopping experience and local knowledge of stores. Thus, we recommend the use of food audits in conjunction with other research methods and engaged dialogue with CBPR partners and other community leaders. Focus groups and in-depth interviews with community members revealed additional aspects of food stores, particularly with regard to the physical and social environment, that influenced where community members shopped for food and which foods they purchased. These insights were essential for broadening elements of the food environments that we examined, though it was still not possible to capture some aspects of store environments (for example, unfair treatment) well through audits (Izumi et al., in press). We also used participant observation as part of regular partnership activities not related to the food audits. For example, in purchasing food for meetings and training, traveling, and spending time in the communities, HEP partners were exposed to and had opportunities to observe neighborhood food environments. This included academic partners who were not from Detroit and community partners who attended partnership activities in communities different from their own. These exposures enhanced understanding and dialogue around the neighborhood food environment. In addition, the two surveys of community residents conducted by HEP included questions on their perceptions of the neighborhood food environment and food shopping behaviors (Schulz, Zenk, et al., 2005; also see Chapter Seven in this volume), providing opportunities to examine, for example, relationships between residents' perceptions of food environments and the observational measures obtained through the food audits and the independent and joint contributions of perceived and observed food environments to dietary practices and health outcomes (Izumi, Zenk, Schulz, Mentz, & Wilson, 2011; Zenk, Lachance, et al., 2009; Zenk, Schulz, Lachance, et al., 2009). Finally, members of the HEP Steering Committee and other community leaders have engaged in discussions of findings from the food audits, jointly developed recommendations for local, state, and national policies, and continue to work closely with community groups and coalitions to ensure that findings are integrated into ongoing efforts to improve aspects of the food environment in Detroit.

Create Synergies Between Action and Research and Among CBPR Projects

A key principle of CBPR is the use of a cyclical, iterative process that includes community assessment, problem definition, development of research methodologies, data collection and analysis, dissemination, and action (Israel et al., 1998). We encountered challenges in pursuing this approach, including both community and academic partners' frustration with the slow pace of data collection and analysis and desire for faster action (Zenk, Schulz, Odoms-Young et al., 2009). Balancing research and action is a well-recognized goal and challenge in CBPR (Israel et al., 1998). Nonetheless, the work in Detroit, spanning two partnerships, exemplified this approach. As described earlier, based on the identification of this issue by Village Health Workers in the late 1990s, members of the ESVHWP and HEP systematically documented how food environments vary across areas of the city and contribute to inequalities in dietary intakes, and ultimately, inequalities in cardiovascular disease incidence and mortality. HEP has applied the generated knowledge in subsequent planning processes to design interventions to reduce health disparities in Detroit, including efforts to influence policy decisions to promote more equitable access to healthy foods (Schulz et al., 2011). Furthermore, HEP's initial work informed CBPR efforts using food audits in Chicago and, in turn, benefited from these different projects for the 2008 food store audit. By taking advantage of synergies among all these efforts, the food store audit instrument, the data collection protocols, and intervention efforts in both Chicago and Detroit have been informed by both the process and the results. Thus, we recommend that ongoing attention needs to be paid to the role of all partners in not only the data collection and analysis phase of a food audit, but also in deciding how the knowledge gained will be used to inform action to bring about change in the food environment.

Promote Colearning and Benefits for All Partners in Keeping with CBPR Principles

Colearning and mutual benefits for all partners are well-recognized principles of CBPR (Israel et al., 1998). Both community and academic partners, as well as the partnership as a whole, benefited from working together on the food audits. Community members who conducted the food audits gained observational skills that can be applied to a variety of settings. Some indicated that it influenced their awareness of the food environment in their neighborhoods as well as their own food choices. Through joint participation in these food audits, and the findings produced through this systematic research, HEP has been able to document associations between the neighborhood food environment and dietary practices and health of local residents (Izumi et al., 2011; Zenk, Lachance, et al., 2009). Community and academic members of HEP have used these findings to inform policymakers of the implications of policy decisions at both the state and federal level that influence food availability for dietary intakes and cardiovascular health of Detroit residents (Izumi et al., 2010). This systematic research has also enabled the partnership as a whole to continue to develop this important line of research and action through continued grant funding, which has brought additional resources into Detroit neighborhoods as well as additional funding for intervention research to reduce racial and socioeconomic health inequities. We suggest that CBPR partnerships work to ensure colearning and mutual benefits throughout their efforts, attending to both process methods and outcomes. (See chapters in Part Two for specific strategies on how to accomplish this.)

SUMMARY

Food audits are of considerable interest to identify differences in neighborhood food environments, examine influences of the neighborhood food environment on health, and evaluate the impact of community change efforts on the neighborhood food environment. In this chapter, we described how the Healthy Environments Partnership used a CBPR process to design and implement a food store audit. The food store audit described here emerged from and was informed by over a decade of CBPR efforts in Detroit and elsewhere. It originated almost ten years earlier in community concerns over lack of high-quality, affordable fresh produce in the community, raised as part of the work of the ESVHWP. It evolved through interventions to address inadequate access to fresh produce, an audit of fresh fruits and vegetables conducted in 2002, structured conversations with community members over time and in multiple contexts, and food audits conducted as part of CBPR efforts in Chicago. Based on what was learned, FEAD-N was designed to assess not only food availability and prices but also store characteristics that may serve as potential barriers or facilitators to food acquisition or healthy food purchases. Community members were trained to conduct the food store audit and ultimately observed 167 food stores across three Detroit communities. They collected high-quality data, as demonstrated by the generally high inter-rater reliability results.

We encountered several challenges in the design and implementation of the food store audit, many of which stemmed from the tension between positivist scientific paradigms, in which food store audits are rooted, and local knowledge of community members. The challenges were related to the common rubric used for food audits that attempt to systematize data collection, minimize subjectivity, and emphasize cross-sectional data. Challenges also include limits on how much data can be reliably collected and the balance between data comparability across time and space and tailoring for local relevance, and the tension between the time involved in collecting and analyzing data compared to the urgency of addressing local food environments to promote health equity. We learned several lessons that have implications for future efforts utilizing food audits. In general, we recommend that CBPR partnerships conducting food audits need to: invest in training and supervision; complement food audits with other research methodologies; recognize the value of multiple data collection methods that capture different aspects of food environments (for example, observed and perceived environments); create synergies between action and research and among CBPR projects; and promote colearning and mutual benefits for all partners consistent with the principles of community-based participatory research.

KEY TERMS

Direct observation

Food audit

Food environment

Urban health

DISCUSSION QUESTIONS

1. How did community members contribute to the origination, design, and implementation of the food store audit?

2. What challenges arose in designing and implementing the food store audit related to the tension between a positivist scientific paradigm and local knowledge?

3. Based on the lessons learned, what are the implications for future food store audits?

REFERENCES

Baker, E. A., Schootman, M., Barnidge, E., & Kelly, C. (2006). The role of race and poverty in access to foods that enable individuals to adhere to dietary guidelines. *Preventing Chronic Disease, 3*(3), A76.

Cochran, P. A. L., Marshall, C. A., Garcia-Downing, C., Kendall, E., Cook, D., McCubbin, L., et al. (2008). Indigenous ways of knowing: Implications for participatory research and community. *American Journal of Public Health, 98*(1), 22–27.

Cummins, S., & Macintyre, S. (2006). Food environments and obesity—neighborhood or nation? *International Journal of Epidemiology, 35*, 100–104.

Franco, M., Diez Roux, A. V., Glass, T. A., Caballero, B., & Brancati, F. L. (2008). Neighborhood characteristics and availability of healthy foods in Baltimore. *American Journal of Preventive Medicine, 35*(6), 561–567.

Gittelsohn, J., & Sharma, S. (2009). Physical, consumer, and social aspects of measuring the food environment among diverse low-income populations. *American Journal of Preventive Medicine, 36*(4), S161–S165.

Glanz, K., Sallis, J. F., Saelens, B. E., & Frank, L. D. (2005). Healthy nutrition environments: Concepts and measures. *American Journal of Health Promotion, 19*(5), 330–333.

Glanz, K., Sallis, J. F., Saelens, B. E., & Frank, L. D. (2007). Nutrition environment measures survey in stores (NEMS-S): Development and evaluation. *American Journal of Preventive Medicine, 32*(4), 282–289.

Grigsby-Touissant, D., Zenk, S. N., Odoms-Young, A., & Ruggerio, L. (2010). Availability of commonly consumed and culturally specific fruits and vegetables in African-American and Latino neighborhoods. *Journal of the American Dietetic Association, 110*(5), 746–752.

Israel, B. A., Schulz, A. J., Parker, E. A., & Becker, A. B. (1998). Review of community-based research: Assessing partnership approaches to improve public health. *Annual Review of Public Health, 19*(1), 173–202.

Israel, B., Lichtenstein, R., Lantz, P., McGranaghan, R., Allen, A., Guzman, R., et al. (2001). The Detroit Community-Academic Urban Research Center: Lessons learned in the development, implementation and evaluation of a community-based participatory research partnership. *Journal of Public Health Management and Practice, 7*, 1–19.

Izumi, B. T., Zenk, S. N., Schulz, A. J., Mentz, G., Sand, S. L., de Majo, R., et al. (2012). Inter-rater reliability of the food environment audit for diverse neighborhoods (FEAD-N). *Journal of Urban Health, 89*, 486–499.

Izumi, B. T., Zenk, S. N., Schulz, A. J., Mentz, G., & Wilson, G. (2011). Associations between neighborhood availability and individual consumption of dark green and orange vegetables among ethnically diverse adults in Detroit. *Journal of the American Dietetic Association, 111*(2), 274–279.

Izumi, B. T., Schulz, A. J., Israel, B. A., Reyes, A. G., Martin, J., Lichtenstein, R. L., et al. (2010). The one-pager: A practical policy advocacy tool for translating community-based participatory research into action. *Progress in Community Health Partnerships, 4*(2), 141–147.

Landis, J. R., & Koch, G. G. (1977). The measurement of observer agreement for categorical data. *Biometrics*, *33*(1), 159–174.

Larson, N. I., Story, M. T., & Nelson, M. C. (2009). Neighborhood environments disparities in access to healthy foods in the U.S. *American Journal of Preventive Medicine*, *36*(1), 74–81.

Matthews, S. A., Moudon, A. V., & Daniel, M. (2009). Work group II: Using geographic information systems for enhancing research relevant to policy on diet, physical activity, and weight. *American Journal of Preventive Medicine*, *36*(4), S171–S176.

McKinnon, R. A., Reedy, J., Morrissette, M. A., Lytle, L. A., & Yaroch, A. L. (2009). Measures of the food environment: A compilation of the literature, 1990–2007. *American Journal of Preventive Medicine*, *36*(4), S124–S133.

Moore, L. V., Diez Roux, A. V., Nettleton, J. A., & Jacobs, D. R., Jr. (2008). Associations of the local food environment with diet quality—a comparison of assessments based on surveys and geographic information systems: The multi-ethnic study of atherosclerosis. *American Journal of Epidemiology*, *167*(8), 917–924.

Morland, K., Wing, S., Diez Roux, A. V. (2002). The contextual effect of the local food environment on residents' diets: The atherosclerosis risk in communities study. *American Journal of Public Health*, *92*, 1761–1767.

National Cancer Institute. *Risk factor monitoring and methods*, 2011, from https://riskfactor.cancer.gov/mfe/instruments/

Odoms-Young, A. M., Zenk, S., & Mason, M. (2009). Measuring food availability and access in African-American communities: Implications for intervention and policy. *American Journal of Preventive Medicine*, *36*(4S), 145–150.

Rose, D., Hutchinson, P. L., Bodor, N., Swalm, C. M., Farley, T. A., Cohen, D. A., et al. (2009). Neighborhood food environments and body mass index: The importance of in-store contents. *American Journal of Preventive Medicine*, *37*(3), 214–219.

Schensul, J. J. (2002). Democratizing science through social science research partnerships. *Bulletin of Science, Technology & Society*, *22*(3), 190–202.

Schulz, A. J., Israel, B. A., Parker, E. A., Lockett, M., Hill, Y., & Wills, R. (2001). The east side village health worker partnership: Integrating research with action to reduce health disparities. *Public Health Reports*, *116*(6), 548–558.

Schulz, A. J., Israel, B. A., Coombe, C., Gaines, C., Reyes, A., Rowe, Z., Sand, S., Strong, L., Weir, S. (2011). A community-based participatory planning process and multilevel intervention design: Toward eliminating cardiovascular health inequities. *Health Promotion Practice*, *12*(6), 900–911.

Schulz, A. J., Kannan, S., Dvonch, J. T., Israel, B. A., Allen III, A., James, S. A., et al. (2005). Social and physical environments and disparities in risk for cardiovascular disease: The healthy environments partnership conceptual model. *Environmental Health Perspectives*, *113*(12), 1817–1825.

Schulz, A. J., & Lempert, L. B. (2004). Being part of the world: Detroit women's perceptions of health and the social environment. *Journal of Contemporary Ethnography*, *33*(4), 437–465.

Schulz, A. J., Zenk, S., Odoms-Young, A., Hollis-Neely, T., Nwankwo, R., Lockett, M., et al. (2005). Healthy Eating and Exercising to Reduce Diabetes (HEED): Exploring the potential of social determinants of health frameworks within the context of community-based participatory diabetes prevention. *American Journal of Public Health, 95,* 645–651.

Schulz, A. J., Zenk, S. N., Kannan, S., Israel, B. A., Koch, M., & Stokes, C. (2005). Community-based participation in survey design and implementation: The healthy environments partnership. In B. A. Israel, E. Eng, A. J. Schulz, & E. Parker (Eds.), *Methods for conducting community-based participatory research for health* (pp. 107–127). San Francisco: Jossey-Bass.

Sharkey, J. R. (2009). Measuring potential access to food stores and food-service places in rural areas in the U.S. *American Journal of Preventive Medicine, 36*(4), S151–S155.

Sharkey, J. R., & Horel, S. (2008). Neighborhood socioeconomic deprivation and minority composition are associated with better potential spatial access to the ground-truthed food environment in a large rural area. *Journal of Nutrition, 138,* 620–627.

Sloane, D. C., Diamant, A. L., Lewis, L. V. B., Yancey, A. K., Flynn, G., Nascimento, L. M., et al. (2003). Improving the nutritional resource environment for healthy living through community-based participatory research. *Journal of General Internal Medicine, 18*(7), 568–575.

Story, M., Kaphingst, K. M., Robinson-O'Brien, R., & Glanz, K. (2008). Creating healthy food and eating environments: Policy and environmental approaches. *Annual Review of Public Health, 29,* 253–272.

Ward, M. H., Nuckols, J. R., Giglierano, J., Bonner, M., Wolter, C., Airola, M., et al. (2005). Positional accuracy of two methods of geocoding. *Epidemiology, 16,* 542–547.

Zenk, S. N., Odoms-Young, A., Dallas, C., Hardy, E., Watkins, A., Wroten, J., et al. (2011). "You have to hunt for the fruits, the vegetables": Environmental barriers and adaptive strategies to acquire food in a low-income African-American community. *Health Education & Behavior, 38,* 282–292.

Zenk, S. N., Schulz, A. J., House, J. S., Benjamin, A., & Kannan, S. (2005). Application of community-based participatory research in the design of an observational tool: The neighborhood observational checklist. In B. A. Israel, E. Eng, A. J. Schulz, & E. Parker (Eds.), *Methods for conducting community-based participatory research for health* (pp. 167–187). San Francisco: Jossey-Bass.

Zenk, S. N., Grigsby-Toussaint, D. S., Curry, S. J., Berbaum, M., & Schneider, L. (2010). Short-term temporal stability in observed retail food characteristics. *Journal of Nutrition Education and Behavior, 42,* 26–32.

Zenk, S. N., Schulz, A. J., Lachance, L. L., Mentz, G., Kannan, S., Ridella, W., et al. (2009). Multilevel correlates of satisfaction with neighborhood availability of fresh fruits and vegetables. *Annals of Behavioral Medicine, 38*(1), 48–59.

Zenk, S. N., Schulz, A. J., Odoms-Young, A., & Lockett, M. (2009). Interdisciplinary, participatory research to understand urban retail food environments and dietary behaviors. In N.

Freudenberg, S. Saegert & S. Klitzman (Eds.), *Urban health and society: Interdisciplinary approaches to research and practice* (pp. 45–62). San Francisco: Jossey Bass.

Zenk, S. N., Lachance, L. L., Schulz, A. J., Mentz, G., Kannan, S., & Ridella, W. (2009). Neighborhood retail food environment and fruit and vegetable intake in a multiethnic urban population. *American Journal of Health Promotion, 23,* 255–264.

Zenk, S. N., Schulz, A. J., Hollis-Neely, T., Campbell, R. T., Holmes, N., Watkins, G., et al. (2005). Fruit and vegetable intake in African Americans: Income and store characteristics. *American Journal of Preventive Medicine, 29*(1), 1–9.

Zenk, S. N., Schulz, A. J., Israel, B. A., James, S. A., Bao, S., & Wilson, M. L. (2005). Neighborhood racial composition, neighborhood poverty, and the spatial accessibility of supermarkets in metropolitan Detroit. *American Journal of Public Health, 95*(4), 660–667.

Zenk, S. N., Schulz, A. J., Israel, B. A., James, S. A., Bao, S., & Wilson, M. L. (2006). Fruit and vegetable access differs by community racial composition and socioeconomic position in Detroit, Michigan. *Ethnicity & Disease, 16*(1), 275–280.

Zenk, S. N., Schulz, A. J., Mentz, G., House, J. S., Gravelee, C. C., Miranda, P. Y., et al. (2007). Inter-rater and test-retest reliability: Methods and results for the neighborhood observational checklist. *Health & Place, 13,* 452–465.

Acknowledgments: The Healthy Environments Partnership (HEP) (www.hepdetroit.org) is an affiliated partnership of the Detroit Community-Academic Urban Research Center (www.detroiturc.org). We thank the members of the HEP Steering Committee for their contributions to the work presented here, including representatives from Brightmoor Community Center, Detroit Department of Health and Wellness Promotion, Detroit Hispanic Development Corporation, Friends of Parkside, Henry Ford Health System, Warren/Conner Development Coalition, and University of Michigan School of Public Health. HEP is supported by the National Institute of Environmental Health Sciences (NIEHS) (R01ES10936, R01ES014234). We also would like to acknowledge the contributions of Chicago collaborators: Englewood Neighborhood Health Center and Illinois Prevention Research Center. The results presented here are solely the responsibility of the authors and do not necessarily represent the views of NIEHS.

Chapter 11

CBPR AND

ETHNOGRAPHY

THE PERFECT UNION

NICOLE S. BERRY

CHRIS McQUISTON

EMILIO A. PARRADO

JULIO CÉSAR OLMOS-MUÑIZ

Racial and ethnic disparities in health are well documented, yet they are not explained merely by lack of health insurance or income (Flaskerud & Kim, 1999; Weinick, Zuvekas, & Cohen, 2000; D. Williams & Mohammed, 2009; D. R. Williams & Sternthal, 2010). In places like the "new south" in the Southeastern United States, where the demographics have radically changed in response to new global patterns of migration (Furuseth & Smith, 2006; Mohl, 2003; Vásquez, Seales, & Marquardt, 2008), research into health disparities must explore the multiple and complex issues related to migration, culture, and ethnicity in newly established communities (Flaskerud & Winslow, 1998; Weinick et al., 2000). Working in such marginalized immigrant communities challenges researchers to move beyond "matching" their methodology to their research question (McQuiston, Larson, Parrado, & Flaskerud, 2002) to consider the ethics and sustainability of useful research.

One response to the necessity for health disparities research within ethnic (and often marginalized) communities has been a turn toward collaborative processes of engagement, such as **community-based participatory research (CBPR)** (Wallerstein & Duran, 2006). CBPR approaches bring important safeguards for all involved partners, including a shift toward shared power, attention to the importance of the health and well-being of the community (rather than just individual research participants), and attention to action or knowledge translation as well as data collection (Israel, Schulz, Parker, & Becker, 1998). It also provides the distinct advantage of incorporating community members' knowledge of their own lived experiences into the design of the research (Mosavel, Simon, van Stade, & Buchbinder, 2005). Nevertheless, as CBPR offers an approach for collaborative research processes but does not dictate methods, engaged scholars are exploring the effects and possibilities of marrying diverse traditional research methods to CBPR (Farquhar et al., 2010).

This chapter takes up this latter point and explores how the CBPR process can guide a collaborative approach to **ethnography** that helps bolster the fit of a research project to one particular cultural context. This combination, which we call **community-based ethnographic participatory research (CBEPR)**, explicitly blends community engagement and ethnographic knowledge generation, focuses on culture and cultural **interpretation**, and utilizes a CBPR process. We begin with an introduction to ethnography and a combined look at ethnography and CBPR followed by a case study, which engaged community partners in designing an ethnographically informed survey, participant observation, as well as in analyzing and interpreting data on gender, migration, and HIV risks among Mexican migrants living in Durham, North Carolina. We conclude with lessons learned and implications for CBEPR.

A GENERAL DESCRIPTION OF ETHNOGRAPHY

Ethnography refers to both a particular type of inquiry and the products that result from that inquiry. Doing ethnography may take various forms, for example, semi-structured or unstructured interviews, surveys, or other elicitation techniques (Tedlock, 2000). A consistent theme, however, is that ethnography is "always informed by a concept of culture" (Boyle, 1994, p.160) and involves rigorous observation and communication in the "field" to insure accuracy of data (LeCompte & Schensul, 1999; Vidich & Lyman, 1994). In other words, ethnography demands that the production of knowledge about a particular context (aka "the field") be immersed in that context. The sense that ethnographers seek to make of the world is predicated on a view of culture as a "complex whole" (Tylor, 1871, p. 1) that pushes one to explore more than just the ostensible subject of research. More recently, ethnography has been cast as an interpretative project that "attempt[s] to come to terms with the diversity of the ways human beings construct their lives in the act of leading them" (Geertz, 1983, p. 16).

Interpreting culture is facilitated by participant observation in the field (where people live, work, attend events, and so forth). Participant observation may vary in terms of how much the ethnographer actually participates (for example, going to a health fair or actually helping to organize it). However, regardless of the approach to participant observation, the record of the event, referred to as *field notes*, is a contextualized and systematic description (LeCompte & Schensul, 1999). For the purpose of the study described here, we define *ethnography* as research based on participant observation of life in a natural setting utilizing the researcher as a major instrument of the research (LeCompte & Schensul, 1999).

Traditional ethnography focuses on obtaining knowledge, often resulting in a book developed solely by the ethnographer (Chambers, 2000). Many ethnographers have chosen to embrace a more collaborative model, which lends itself to participatory research. Terms describing this type of ethnography include: collaborative, community-based, narrative, reciprocal, and dialogic (Austin, 2003; Lassiter, 2000; Stringer, 1997; Tedlock & Mannheim, 1995). These labels represent an approach to a more egalitarian type of research with the participants providing ongoing dialogue about the emerging ethnographic text. The approaches to accomplish this goal may differ and some may be more collaborative than others, but there is a common theme among collaborative models of ethnography. In general, the hierarchical approach in which the researcher as a participant-observer authors alone an account (an ethnography) of the "other" (Schensul, Weeks, & Singer, 1999) has been replaced by a model marked by a coproduction of analysis, interpretation, and in some cases, text. Studies that combine ethnography and CBPR may be carried out, for example, by partnerships established as community-university-agency partnerships (Austin, 2003), or as university–Native American (tribal) relationships (Chrisman, Strickland, Powell, Squeochs, & Yallup, 1999; Jacklin, 2009; Menzies, 2001). University faculty may also be joined by graduate students in such studies (Stringer, 1997; Trujillo, Melendez,

& Owen, 2007). A common thread in these studies is the desire and attempt to fully include nonacademics in multiple levels of the ethnographic study and to collectively work on real-life problems (Lamphere, 2003).

METHODS WITHIN METHODS

From an ethnographic perspective, community-based participatory research offers an approach to conducting "culturally compelling" (Panter-Brick, Clarke, Lomas, Pinder, & Lindsay, 2006) research based on the cultural interpretation of research findings with community members as researchers (Meleis, 1996; Sawyer, et al., 1995). CBPR includes community members as researchers in all aspects of the research process including the development of research concepts, the conduct of the research, and the interpretation of the findings (Israel, et al., 2003). Community-based ethnographic participatory research (CBEPR) seeks to close the gap between ethnography and community engagement. Whereas in collaborative ethnography community members help with interpretation, (Rhodes, et al., 2010; Savage, et al., 2006; Silverstein, Reid, DePeau, Lamberto, & Beardslee, 2010) CBEPR takes us one step further and trains community members as ethnographers, fully involved with the systematic collection and interpretation of cultural knowledge that constitutes the research process. The goal of this study was to explain how Latino experiences and perceptions are shaped by the cultural background and structural position of Latino immigrants in U.S. society. Because the ethnographer is interested in the cultural interpretation (Schwandt, 1994) of the data, working with community members as research colleagues allows for sustained collective debate about data and what these data mean within the context of the culture of the group participating in the study.

In the following section we describe a CBEPR project undertaken to provide information for the development of culture-specific interventions, and to produce data for model and theory development (see Chapters Five, Six, and Seven for further discussion of community-based participatory approaches to the development of conceptual models and community assessments). We triangulate multiple methods, including a survey of sexual practices that was tailored to this particular context (what we refer to as the *"ethnosexual survey"*), participant observation, the taking of field notes, and the analysis of qualitative data derived from structured discussions during team meetings.

COMMUNITY ETHNOGRAPHERS

The purpose of this discussion is to demonstrate the use of CBEPR methods by describing three separate stages of *Gender, Migration, and HIV Risks Among Mexicans*, a study funded by the National Institute of Nursing Research (NINR). Each stage used different methods to implement a CBEPR approach. In the first stage, community and academic team members developed the conceptual basis of a grant proposal. Preliminary ethnographic data were gathered and used to write the background and significance sections and part of the preliminary studies sections of the grant proposal. In Stage Two, community and academic team members, or more specifically, ethnographers, developed and refined the ethno-sexual survey to be used in the larger study, and community team members were formally trained in ethnographic methods and conducted the surveys. In Stage Three, community participants interpreted and analyzed research findings

Study Background

Latino community members and academics worked collaboratively on all components of the Gender, Migration, and HIV Risks Among Mexicans study that aimed to compare prevalent sexual behaviors among Mexican men and women in Durham, North Carolina, and four sending communities in Mexico, and to identify and describe the impact of migration on the gender structures of labor, power (imbalances within relationships), and gender-specific norms among the Mexican population (McQuiston, Parrado, Martínez, & Uribe, 2005; Parrado & Flippen, 2005; Parrado, Flippen, & McQuiston, 2005). The specific objectives for the community members of the research team were to increase capacity on the individual, group, organizational, and community levels as they collectively developed an understanding of community needs and strengths related to gender, migration, and HIV risk. These objectives mirrored the mission statement of El Centro Hispano (ECH), the Latino advocacy agency that was a key institutional partner in this CBEPR effort.

Study Setting

Community members were engaged from and this study was conducted in Durham County, North Carolina, an urban area with a strong economy and numerous construction, hotel, restaurant, and landscaping jobs. These jobs often require minimal or no English language skills and draw Latinos to the area. According to U.S. Census data available from http://www.census.gov, the Latino immigrant population in Durham grew exponentially from 2,054 in 1990 to an estimated 32,900 in 2009 (about 12.2% of the total population). In addition, in 2000, when this project began, Durham had the most unbalanced sex ratio among immigrant Latinos, age 20–29 years, of any metropolitan area in the country (Suro, Singer, & Center, 2002), with approximately 2.5 men for every woman. New arrivals to the area typically had few resources, worked low-level entry jobs without health insurance, and many lived in crowded substandard housing (Uribe, 2007). The combination of migratory stress, limited resources, and predominately male migration put these immigrants at increased risk for HIV/AIDS (Hondagneu-Sotelo, 2003; McQuiston & Uribe, 2001).

CBEPR Partnership

Eight community members from Mexico and Honduras and two staff members at ECH were involved in the Stage One of the project (discussed in the following section) along with four academic members of the team. Two of the academic team members were from the United States, one from Colombia, and one from Argentina. The full team met bimonthly for three months to develop a research-based grant proposal. Working in this partnership was a new experience for ECH, as it required them to make space for a project that was not directly tied to an intervention. Initially, ECH had some difficulty visualizing how research could lead to interventions. As the project progressed, however, ECH viewed it as a valuable resource and requested data from the project to inform ECH's grant proposal writing for subsequent programs.

It was helpful that the community participants knew the academic researchers from collaborating on a previous HIV prevention project. Four of the community participants had been trained as lay health advisors (LHAs) for the project *"Protegiendo Nuestra Comunidad"* (Protecting Our Community) and the other four had attended additional community training for HIV prevention facilitated by trained LHAs and academics (McQuiston, Choi-Hevel, & Clawson, 2001; McQuiston, et al., 2002; McQuiston & Uribe, 2001). They viewed research examining HIV/AIDS in the context of migration and gender as a priority. Their awareness and experiences with the academic team members over a five-year period greatly facilitated the CBEPR process.

Although the team was intentionally kept small to develop the grant proposal, once funding was secured the team felt that expanding the diversity of views would help make sure the project was on the right track. Accordingly, four additional women and two men, recommended by ECH and the existing community team members, were invited to participate in Stages Two and Three, bringing the final total of community members on the research team to 14. Community members engaged in Stages Two and Three were from Mexico (ten), Honduras (one), Peru (two), and Colombia (one). This group named itself *Horizonte Latino* (Latinos Moving Forward). The relationship of Horizonte Latino with ECH was fluid, with academic team members serving on ECH committees, and ECH staff and board members participating in Horizonte Latino.

The roles and responsibilities, philosophy, purpose, and process of collaboration were agreed upon among the initial research team during Stage One, but then were reviewed when new community members were invited to join. The team embraced an empowerment philosophy and methodology (looking, critically reflecting, and acting), based on the works of Paulo Freire (Freire, 1970, 1973). This philosophy assumed that community team members' lived experience brought important insights to the research that their academic partners may not have (Averill, 2005; McQuiston, et al., 2002). Community team members lived in the neighborhoods in which research took place, and in the case of *Horizonte Latino*, also experienced migration and the numerous challenges it holds, including the interface of their own culture with that of the dominant U.S. culture. They had observed and experienced the influence of the dominant culture on their own values, beliefs, behaviors, and relationships and observed the effects of "settling in" to the United States on community members around them.

THE CBEPR PROCESS EXEMPLIFIED

There were three stages involved in our CBEPR process: proposal development (Stage One), from concept to process (Stage Two), and analyzing the findings (Stage Three).

Stage One: Developing the Proposal

The conceptual development of the grant proposal was accomplished through research team meetings, conducted in Spanish, in which academic facilitators asked community team members to identify root causes of HIV/AIDS in their community (Hope, Timmel, & Hodzi, 1995). The first step in the process consisted of dividing the team into two (sometimes three) small groups, often by gender if sensitive topics were to be discussed. Each small group identified a community member facilitator who kept the group on track. This facilitator was given a task (by the academic facilitator), for example, to ask the group to define HIV in the Latino community, or to describe what contributes to the problem and what results from the problem. A scribe was asked to write the "findings" on a flip chart, and a presenter was asked to present the small group's results to the entire group (Arnold, Burke, James, Mardint, & Thomas, 1995). After the small groups had finished their discussion, the presenters posted their findings and summarized the discussions. Many of the concerns the groups shared were related to the process of migration, and participants frequently grounded these discussions in both time and place. For example, when discussing values and beliefs—specifically, issues of gender roles for men and women—the participants would frequently talk about "here" (the United States) or "there" (Mexico). Roles "here" and roles "there" signaled changes in gender roles as part of the migration experience.

The second step to developing the grant proposal involved the whole research team examining the flip chart notes to identify common themes that emerged from the small-group sessions. Typically, team members readily agreed on common themes. Yet when themes arose that were not agreed upon, team members had to make decisions about whether to keep them or leave them out. Ultimately, discussion continued until consensus could be reached. At times the academic facilitator would help to summarize what the group had agreed on or disagreed on up to that point. Once there was final agreement, the concepts were included in the grant proposal. Thus, the concepts for the study came from community members. The academic team members then pulled the concepts together to create a potential study design, which was presented to the community team members for approval.

Substantively, the major causes of HIV, identified by the research team over the course of six two-hour meetings, included: sexual behavior (the availability and use of commercial sex workers); alcohol or other drug use; lack of education or information about HIV and resources; migration (including limited opportunities available to migrants owing to their concentration in low wage, poorly paid work); gender roles; and cultural beliefs and values. The group had identified both structural and cultural causes of HIV risk and the interface between the two. For example, they suggested that the uneven sex ratio (more men than women immigrants) and availability of commercial sex workers (CSWs) and a culture that does not always condemn marital infidelity among men could increase HIV risk in their community.

Stage Two: Moving from Concept to Process

In this stage, the research team prepared the ethnosexual survey, trained community team members in ethnographic and survey interview methods, and administered the survey.

Ethnosexual Survey

In Stage Two, the academic team members applied the findings from Stage One on root causes of HIV in the Latino community to develop a draft of an ethnographically informed, culture-specific survey instrument, which we refer to as the ethnosexual survey (Schensul, et al., 1999). For example, use of CSWs was a concern within the context of alcohol use and *tiempo libre* (free time where you have nothing to do and can get into trouble). The community team members also thought that men were more vulnerable to CSWs because of depression resulting from migration and social isolation. Therefore, all these concepts were included in the ethnosexual survey using both closed- and open-ended questions. (See Chapters Seven and Thirteen for a discussion of the development and implementation of closed-ended survey questionnaires within the context of CBPR projects.) Questions were anchored in time and place by asking the same questions in the context of Mexico and then again in the context of the United States, to address the "here" and "there" issues raised in Stage One.

Once the draft survey was developed, team members met weekly in small groups to scrutinize it. Survey questions were read out loud, discussed, reflected upon, and evaluated for cultural and linguistic fit. Comments from the small groups were then presented to the entire group. Further discussion and decisions regarding which questions to include in the survey ensued.

Community team members expressed concern about the wording of several items and were especially sensitive to the potential of various interpretations of a question or phrase based on the respondent's country or place (for example rural or urban) of origin. In several cases the wording was changed as a result of these discussions. In other cases, alternative words for the same concept were included so that when the team's community members functioned as ethnographers they would have multiple alternative words readily available as they conducted the interviews. Additionally, community team members were concerned about the sensitive nature of some of the questions, which they felt needed to be introduced in a general manner. Questions about particularly sensitive issues, such as homosexuality and drug use, were deemed too "alarming" to ask directly and were introduced as hypothetical scenarios. These numerous suggestions and insights were used to revise the ethnosexual survey.

Ethnographic Training

After finalizing the survey, academic team members trained the community team members in ethnographic techniques, including interviews, participant observation, and taking field notes. The center of the interviewer training focused on how to follow a respondent's story line, using a conversational narrative approach, whereby the interviewer moves back and forth in the guide as the respondent's story evolves (Parrado, McQuiston, & Flippen, 2005). For example, a respondent might tell the interviewer that she initially followed her boyfriend to Texas and that she lived and worked there cleaning houses. Later she might say she moved to Durham with her husband. Following the conversational approach, the interviewer would need to remember the boyfriend in Texas and say something like, "Is the husband you came to Durham with the same as the boyfriend you went to be with in Texas?" The interviewer would follow the story line that resulted from the respondent's answer to this question. In this process, there could be several more moves and another boyfriend might be "discovered." All this would take place in a normal conversational manner, rather than a predetermined sequential format more typical of conventional interviews. The community team members used role playing to practice interviewing and discussed potential problems related to both asking questions and documenting responses (the interviews conducted in the field were not taped).

A significant part of the ethnographic training involved how to observe the environment where the ethnographers worked, and what to record in the field notes. A field notes guide was originated for the purpose of organizing observations and field notes. (See Appendix G for a copy of the Field Notes Guide.) At a minimum, the guide was used after each interview to debrief the experience, including the reflections and observations of the interviewer.

Administering the Survey

Through field work around the city of Durham, the research team identified 13 apartment complexes that housed predominantly Latino residents. The team then constructed a census of all housing units in these complexes to serve as a sampling frame, and from this list of over 2,000 apartments drew an independent random sample. The community team members, who were now fully functioning as community ethnographers, were given a list of the apartments selected and instructed to administer the ethnosexual survey with the person that answered the door if he or she was Latino, between the ages of 18 and 45, and the same sex as the ethnographer. In cases where the person who answered the door did not correspond to the target population, the ethnographer asked if someone with such characteristics lived in the apartment and interviewed the first person suggested by the individual answering the door. Dwellings without residents who met the study criteria were excluded.

Checking in with the Ethnographers

Two academic team members went to ECH once a week to meet with the ethnographers and debrief the completed ethnosexual surveys with the person who had done the interviewing. In this way, the academic team member checked each survey for consistency and accuracy of information. Community ethnographers would often point out questions or areas of the survey where the respondent contradicted him- or herself, struggled with questions, or provided a particularly detailed response.

Once the academic team member and the community ethnographer finished reviewing the survey for consistency and accuracy, they reviewed field notes taken about the outing. Community ethnographers took different approaches to field notes. Some were particularly detailed in their observations of the physical conditions of the apartment and the complex, providing specifics on the parking lots, amounts of litter, noting whether there were areas for recreation, and what the respondent's apartment looked like on the inside. Others focused more on the life story and experience of the respondent. Any verbal observations made by the community ethnographer that were not included in the field notes were jotted down by the academic team member on the survey at the time of the meeting.

These meetings were important because errors could be caught almost immediately and corrected before the next interview, and the academic team member could provide the community ethnographers with additional training if needed. It was also a good opportunity for community ethnographers to reflect on their experience with particular informants while the interview was still fresh in their minds. In addition to these one-on-one meetings, the research team met monthly to discuss insights, problems, and begin an initial analysis of what it was seeing and experiencing. At this point in the process, information was going back and forth to ECH and *Horizonte Latino* and the tension experienced during the initial meetings concerning the relevance of the research to ECH was replaced with a sense that *Horizonte Latino* had become institutionalized at ECH.

Stage Three: Analyzing the Findings

Ongoing iterative presentation and discussion of the findings allowed the team to assess the study results, reconsider preliminary expectations, provide a cultural understanding of specific findings, and identify new lines of research and intervention. Central to the CBEPR approach used in this study was the critical reflection of cultural values of the group members. Viewing findings within the context of culture as well as social structures allowed *Horizonte Latino* to build a collective ethnographic account of the community that was not just the sum of personal experiences, but the product of community ethnographers looking into themselves and discussing their own experiences and ideas in relation to those of the community respondents.

One example of this process was an exploration of the data pertaining to the relationship between migration and women's power. The prevailing image of gender roles in Mexico was that of submissive women and chauvinistic, *machista* men. Prior to data collection and group discussion, community and academic team members alike believed that migrant women are, to some extent, liberated when they come to the United States, as the ethos of egalitarianism (real or imagined) prevalent in the United States comes into conflict with the more traditional, patriarchal gender ideologies brought from communities of origin. Current academic literature recognizes the complexity and limits of gender change resulting from immigration (Parrado & Flippen, 2005), but tends to frame it in positive terms akin to liberation (Hondagneu-Sotelo, 2003).

Through a process of critical reflection, the group reexamined the root causes of gender role change with migration within the context of the survey data and personal and collective experiences. As a result of this reflection, community and academic ethnographers began to take a more varied view, recognizing both positive and negative aspects of the greater freedom offered by life in the United States.

The third author conducted a preliminary analysis of the quantitative findings from the ethnosexual survey related to gender roles and migration: comparing labor force participation, the division of household responsibilities (housework and family finances), relationship control, and gender attitudes among married Mexican women in Durham, North Carolina, and in Mexico. Prior to presenting the findings to the group, the academic team members explained the statistics needed to understand the data and then presented research questions followed by a table with empty cells representing numbers and percentages of survey responses to specific questions. Each community ethnographer gave his or her "guess" estimate of the results of each research question and an explanation of that estimate. There was often group discussion about the community ethnographers' varying perspectives of the community. The women shared their experiences interviewing women in the community and the men shared their experiences interviewing male informants. Therefore, their perspective and data collection experiences varied and were debated among group members. After the group guesses were recorded on a flip chart, academic facilitators presented and explained the survey results. Group discussion followed about the differences between the community ethnographers' perceptions of the community as informed by their experiences with data collection, and the data presented. The academic team members used three questions to guide the group discussion of survey results: What is happening here? Why is it happening? What program does the community need to address this issue? These questions are based on Freire's problem-posing approach to critical reflection (Hope, Timmel, & Hodzi, 1984).

For example, the academic team members asked the group to guess the percentage of married women working and the percentage of husbands sharing household work in the United States and Mexico. To illustrate how these guesses related to findings, Table 11.1 presents selected guess estimates with data from the ethnosexual surveys for the gendered household division of labor. What is striking about the information in Table 11.1 is that, in many cases, community ethnographers overestimated the traditional orientation of Mexican women in Mexico, and underestimated traditional gender orientations in Durham. Specifically, they tended to think a greater percentage of women worked in the United States than was actually the case, and they tended to grossly underestimate the share of men who assist with housework in both Mexico and Durham.

In elaborating on the lack of correspondence between expectations and estimates, the research team provided an ethnographic account of the processes at play, grounding the immigrant experience within the structural context of the community in the United States. Even though employment opportunities are more plentiful in the United States than in Mexico, community members of the research team suggested that the constraints imposed by family life might be stronger as the kin-provided child care common in Mexico is not available. Some women in the group also suggested that the poor quality of jobs available to immigrant women in the United States restricts their employment. The majority of jobs open to these women, who generally lack legal authorization to work and have limited English language ability, are in domestic and other low-skilled service occupations that pay very poorly.

Similar considerations applied to the interpretation of the estimates for the proportion of men assisting with household work. Although most of the group held a view of Mexican men as being *machista* and very unlikely to assist with household chores, they believed men were considerably more likely to do so in the United States than in Mexico. The ethnosexual survey results showed very little differences across contexts, however, with close to 37% of husbands assisting with household work in both Mexico and the United States (Parrado, Flippen, & McQuiston, 2004; Parrado, Flippen, & McQuiston, 2005).

The group suggested that differences in men's work environments in Mexico and the United States might explain why men do not become more involved in

TABLE 11.1 Community Ethnographers' Predictions and Results from the Ethnosexual Survey for Household Division of Labor in Mexico and the United States

| | CBPR Predictions | | | | Observed Through Ethnosexual |
| | # of participants guessing each percentage | | | | |
	1 Ethnographer	2 Ethnographers	3 Ethnographers	4 Ethnographers	Survey
Married women working					
Mexico	30%	20%	10%	5%	25%
U.S.	60	70	90	80	51
Husbands sharing household work					
Mexico[a]	1	0	5	—	36
U.S.	10–20	15	10	0	37

a. The numbers of guesses do not add up to ten for this item because not all group members offered a guess.

housework in Durham, especially given that many more women work outside the house in Durham than do in Mexico. The types of jobs that men worked in Durham usually involved long shifts and manual labor, construction being a typical example. After migrating to the United States, women sometimes feel that it is unreasonable to ask their husbands returning from such demanding jobs to do work around the house.

This example illustrates the importance of reflection in the design of CBEPR, including the centrality of group discussions and collective understanding to interpret the findings. Once presented with survey findings, community ethnographers were confronted with unexpected patterns that led them to examine their own preconceptions and draw from their participant observation in the community to help explain the survey results. This process not only gave depth and context to the quantitative analysis, but also broadened the whole group's understanding of the community. The end product of the reciprocal questioning of findings, assumptions, and experiences was a collective ethnographic account of the findings as well as the group's critical reflections.

CHALLENGES AND LIMITATIONS

Combining ethnography and CBPR added an additional level to an already complex and time-consuming process. However, much of what the community ethnographers learned, they learned from each other in collaborative meetings. Therefore, what might be viewed as a time-consuming challenge produced the shared learning that allowed for collective insight and problem solving. However, there are always additional challenges. Differences in educational levels and style meant that some of the community ethnographers wrote little and verbally relayed stories they gathered to the academic team members, who wrote them down. These differences in approaches meant that the project has a wealth of data, but there are some inconsistencies in the type of data recorded for each interview. The academic team members also had to learn and recognize the strengths of the ethnographers to support them.

The team meetings to discuss data and work on analysis and cultural and structural interpretation were sometimes a challenge because the ethnographers had such compelling stories to tell about their field experiences. The group had to balance staying on task with allowing members to share their stories.

Facilitators became skillful at keeping the group on task while respecting the members' needs to tell stories.

LESSONS LEARNED

This section is divided into how team members learned, what they learned, and how the development of skills translated into a new understanding of HIV in the migrant Latino community. Sometimes a statement from a team member is supplied to give the reader a better understanding of the lessons presented. Many statements represent colearning and are a melding of insights by both the academic and community team members.

How Team Members Learned

Pedagogical styles are certainly important in facilitating learning among diverse groups (Bryan, Kreuter, & Brownson, 2009; Pheiffer, Andrew, Green, & Holley, 2003). However, we found that aspects of how this process was structured also was important to learning.

Group Structure

The academic team members learned that, when dealing with culturally sensitive topics, splitting the large group by gender facilitated discussions. The community team members said that they felt more comfortable discussing in their small groups even though sensitive topics would later be shared with the large group.

Ownership

Participating in the research process both from its inception and in all of its aspects was very important for community team members to build a sense of ownership over the process. They particularly valued designing the ethnosexual survey. For example, Consuelo said, "I have learned so many lessons . . . the main one is having had the possibility to participate from the beginning, starting from the design of the survey."

What Team Members Learned

Activities of *Horizonte Latino* certainly led to an increased understanding of issues concerning migrant Hispanics in Durham. Nevertheless, participating in this process resulted in wider learning opportunities.

Building an Understanding of Ethnographic Methods

The academic team members learned that the community ethnographers more easily understood difficult concepts if they were presented in a context relevant to the group's life experiences. Community team members learned that sharing some of their own stories helped respondents feel more at ease when discussing sensitive topics such as migration.

Immigrants Interviewing Immigrants

The community team members learned that sharing their own stories of migration helped build a relationship with the respondents and encouraged openness. As Adriana said, "You need to build a relationship first, a conversation, a shared feeling that we are both going through the same experiences, that we are both immigrants."

Building on Capacity at the Individual and Organizational Levels

Inviting LHAs trained in our earlier programs allowed the group to build on existing capacity. This saved the academic team members' time and energy and increased the project's likelihood of being successful. Including ECH staff in the group facilitated the flow of information between the ECH and *Horizonte Latino* and allowed for direct application of skills to ECH. Blanca reported, "I like the way the group is organized because I can use it as a model for my work at El Centro Hispano."

Carrying out CBEPR in a Context of Marginalization

The academic team members felt that the group could not have successfully conducted its research with recently arrived and often fearful immigrants nor could it have fully understood the meaning of much of the data without the community team members. The ethnographic approach the academics took with their community colleagues enriched the experience and facilitated an in-depth cultural and structural interpretation of data.

Taking Action

There are many spin-offs from this research, things that were never planned or even thought about. Motivation for action comes through this work. Julio told the group:

> One of the most rewarding experiences for me was my presentation at the CBPR conference (Julio is referring to his role in the following presentation: McQuiston, C., Uribe, L., Olmos-Muñiz., J., & Parrado, E., March 2003. *Horizonte Latino: Participatory Action Research with Latino Community Members*. Paper presented at Building Connections for Community Health: Best Practices for Promoting Health Through Participatory Methods in the Workplace and Community, CDC sponsored. Chapel Hill, North Carolina). This was the first time that I ever gave a presentation and I did it in English. I did not feel very comfortable, but I took it as a challenge. I felt very good that the audience had a lot of questions and comments for me. This experience helped me to realize what I had learned, it was like suddenly realizing "here I am" . . . to collect all the ideas that I ever had as I realized that people in the audience had an interest in listening to them. It was like "open your eyes" and "oh! this is what I have to do." From the day after the conference I felt motivated to reach out and talk to men in the community. We founded a group so men would have something to do with their free time. One of the participants from the community had experience in a soccer league so we decided to create one in Durham. Our initial group of 8 has grown to 27 soccer teams. This is something that makes me feel good, because I always thought that we needed alternatives for the use of free time among Latinos, but it was only until after I gave that presentation that I took action.

Skills and Understandings

Ultimately, the CBEPR team members wanted to gain additional understanding regarding the types of intervention(s) the community needed as well as how best to deliver each intervention in this context. *Horizonte Latino* identified an initial list of intervention ideas, including the following:

- Programs targeting men at the work site;
- A men's group at ECH;
- Multiple LHA groups to target large Latino apartment complexes; and
- Activities for Latinos to do in their free time.

These interventions were still targeted at HIV/AIDS, but in a very broad context including migration, gender, social isolation, alcohol use, and perhaps domestic violence.

In addition to the broader picture, *Horizonte Latino* members learned multiple research skills such as:

- Human subjects training
- Research 101 including random sampling techniques
- Structured and semistructured interviewing skills
- Participant observation and recording field notes
- Group facilitation and organizational skills
- Group process and critical reflection
- Cultural analysis and interpretation

One community team member described the value of the experience as follows:

The story of the group is like a long journey . . . we began brainstorming, then planned the ethnosexual survey. We designed the survey ourselves, discussed each question including which words to use and which words not to use. We decided which questions were good and which were not. Then we went back and checked the survey again, added a few new questions and discarded others. Finally, we went to the apartments to find people, to observe how they live, what the apartments and the surroundings looked like. We learned so many things by going to the apartments. Then we came back to the group meetings and discussed our experiences, what it was like to do the surveys. Many of us were surprised by what we were finding because we witnessed so many things while doing the surveys. We liked this fieldwork and think it was a great idea that the same people who developed the questions for the survey would then reach out and visit the apartments and do the surveys and then come back and discuss our experiences. We could see how the questions we helped to design worked in real life.

ECH staff, who were also members of *Horizonte Latino*, commented on how their dual roles basically cross-fertilized each other and how skills learned in each role were used in both ECH and *Horizonte Latino*. Academic team members had similar experiences, as some were members of multiple ECH committees in addition to their roles as *Horizonte* members.

Moreover, existing community resources that had contributed to the CBEPR project were also enhanced as a result. Many of the community team members involved in this project continue to work on health issues in their community—through volunteer roles, as lay health advisors, or in conjunction with ECH. For others, *Hortizonte Latino* was a proving ground for learning about challenges to the new immigrant community—one that inspired them to look for solutions and resources available in Durham. As such, these members have become leaders of the community who are sought out by others for advice and guidance.

Building Knowledge About Health Disparities in Diverse Communities

The collaboration described in the preceding pages was ethnographic in its reliance on interpretation to make meaning in this particular context. The theory that drove the development of the ethnosexual survey developed from a dialogue about the particulars of everyday life for Latino immigrants. As a result, which questions were included and what aspects of people's lives were discussed were specifically tailored to community members' understandings of migration, and the structural and individual challenges and opportunities that it creates. Later in the project, when we analyzed the results of the survey, we privileged meanings that community team members had derived—both from their experiences as ethnographers who collected the data and again as their experiences as individuals who had also migrated and settled in Durham. Indeed community members' field notes reflecting on their experiences and transcripts of dialogues from our own team meetings were immeasurably valuable sources of data.

A second important aspect of this project that made it ethnographic was the focus on holism. Rather than predefining and restricting the areas that we considered relevant to the migration and HIV in Durham, in this project we collected data on all aspects of people's lives. Accordingly, the project was based on ethnographic methods including participant observation, interviews, and field notes, which lend themselves to exploring holism. This broad approach ultimately enabled us to understand connections between things we never expected, such as the relationship between living conditions and risk behaviors for HIV (Parrado, Flippen, & Uribe, 2009). It also changed our approach to how we would intervene in the problem. For example, team members agreed that one conclusion of this process was that it would be more productive to focus on free time as a preventative measure rather than just trying to intervene when members of the migrant community were already engaging in risky behavior (for example, increasing condom use).

Finally, reflective of both ethnography and other critical traditions, researchers were considered instruments of research and, as such, every team member reflected on his or her own subject position, particularly in relation to the research. In the example discussed earlier where community team members guessed the results of the ethnosexual survey, we all realized that we brought perspectives and biases to the group. A deeper understanding of HIV risk in the migrant community dictated that we be willing to reflect upon and discuss how our position affected the research, both advantageously as well as disadvantageously.

Taking these steps to combine CBPR and ethnography therefore resulted in a process that adapted well to the particular cultural and contextual environment. Initially, we set out to match our methods to a cultural group (Flaskerud & Nyamathi, 2000; McQuiston & Uribe, 2001): our choice was driven by finding methods that would allow, ensure, and hinge on community participation. Ethnography was an excellent fit as the premium placed on interpretation of cultural facts from an emic perspective allowed *Horizonte Latino* to be about developing theories that accounted for gender and migration experiences and related these experiences to HIV risk in Durham.

IMPLICATIONS FOR PRACTICE

Our experience of marrying ethnography and CBPR brought to the fore some aspects of partnership that need to be in place in order to successfully do CBEPR. First, CBEPR dictates a particular composition of the research team: there must be substantial representation of team members based in the community. For us this meant including both community members at large and those who were on the team as affiliates of our institutional partner, ECH. Ultimately the balance of community team members to academic team members was 14 to 4. The reluctance of Holkup and colleagues (Holkup, Tripp-Reimer, Salois, & Weinert, 2004) to attempt to employ ethnographic methods in a CBPR project in a Native American community with just one team member who was Native further highlights how ethnography might not be useful or appropriate in these circumstances. They cite team members "discomfort" with the potential dangers of (mis) representation that can result when predominantly noncommunity members are to be ethnographers (Holkup et al., 2004, p. 168).

Another important aspect of CBEPR is that it hinges not just on *using* community members to collect data and but it relies on them as important *instruments of research*. A number of CBPR projects have used ethnography to inform the process, but frequently academic team members are the only ethnographers (Anthony, Lee, Barry, & Kappesser, 2010; Averill, 2005; Moodie, Tsui, & Silbergeld, 2010; Savage, Anthony, Lee, Kappesser, & Rose, 2007). The example of *Horizonte Latino* and CBEPR pushes this boundary by making community team members the most important ethnographers in the process. Training the community team members in systematic observation and centering theory making on dialogic processes primes community members to become expert interpreters and creators of knowledge. Both *Horizonte Latino* as well as Van Sluys's experience (2010) of working with eighth graders, show that educational level need not be a barrier to full inclusion.

SUMMARY

Cross-cultural research on health disparities is a challenge for everyone. Applying a community-based participatory approach in conducting ethnographic research —which we describe here as CBEPR—creates a context that considers cultural values, beliefs, and behaviors, as well as shared experiences and structures that shape everyday life. This CBPR approach to ethnography is particularly important for studies of immigrants and facilitates a view of both the positive and negative effects of migration. In this case, engaging community partners as ethnographers in participant observation and the dialogic approach to the ethnosexual survey allowed the research team to learn about the respondents' stories and to see how they live in the community. Their involvement in participant observation was critical to providing a context for analysis of the data as well as for grant proposal writing efforts. The CBEPR approach reinforced the authors' belief that any culturally competent program or research project with immigrants must be informed by the immigration experience and the cultural values that are in flux as a result of that experience.

In this study, time spent in the community allowed both academic and community ethnographers to see firsthand the crowded and sometimes dangerous conditions of the apartment complexes. It also allowed them to see that for some the challenges of migration brought great creativity and capabilities to think beyond boundaries and to face adversity with ingenuity. The stories heard reflected courage and strength as Latinos learned to value their homeland, to gain a wider perspective on world issues, and to develop skills to adapt to adversity and challenges. Eventually, these skills will result in less vulnerability and more self-confidence. CBEPR provides an opportunity for deep understanding and identification of the needs and capacity of the community and can lead to action to address the issues identified.

KEY TERMS

CBEPR	Ethnosexual survey
CBPR	Field notes
Ethnography	Interpretation

DISCUSSION QUESTIONS

1. The authors present CBEPR as a unique process that is different from CBPR alone. How do they describe these differences? How do they distinguish CBEPR from other CBPR projects that use ethnography to inform their process?

2. What strengths do the authors claim that CBEPR can offer over using CBPR alone? What circumstances are best suited to CBEPR? What weaknesses, challenges, or limitations might you face in employing CBEPR rather than CBPR?

3. The article offers a number of examples of the particular context of the new immigrant experience of Latinos in Durham that shaped both risk for HIV and potential interventions to mitigate that risk. Describe one such example.

REFERENCES

Anthony, J. S., Lee, R. C., Barry, D. G., & Kappesser, M. (2010). Recruiting and keeping African American women in an ethnographic study of pregnancy: The community-based partnership model. *Field Methods, 22*(2), 125–132.

Arnold, R., Burke, B., James, C., Mardint, D., & Thomas, B. (1995). *Educating for change* (4th ed.). Toronto: Between the Lines.

Austin, D. (2003). Community-based collaborative team ethnography: A community-university-agency partnership. *Human Organization, 62*(2), 143–152.

Averill, J. B. (2005). Studies of rural elderly individuals: Merging critical ethnography with community-based action research. *Journal of Gerontological Nursing, 31*(12), 11.

Boyle, J. (1994). Styles of ethnography. In J. M. Morse (Ed.), *Critical issues in qualitative research methods* (pp. 159–185). Thousand Oaks, CA: Sage.

Bryan, R. L., Kreuter, M. W., & Brownson, R. C. (2009). Integrating adult learning principles into training for public health practice. *Health Promotion Practice, 10*(4), 557–563.

Chambers, E. (2000). Applied ethnography. In N. K. Denzin & Y. S. Lincoln (Eds.), *Handbook of qualitative research* (pp. 851–869). Thousand Oaks, CA: Sage.

Chrisman, N., Strickland, C., Powell, K., Squeochs, M., & Yallup, M. (1999). Community partnership research with the Yakama Indian nation. *Human Organization, 58*(2), 134–141.

Farquhar, S., Celaya-Alston, R., Centurion, L., Maldonado, J., Gregg, J., & Aguillon, R. (2010). Interpretations of interpretations: Combining community-based participatory research and interpretive inquiry to improve health. *Progress in Community Health Partnerships: Research, Education, and Action, 4*(2), 149–154.

Flaskerud, J., & Kim, S. (1999). Health problems of Asian and Latino immigrants. *The Nursing Clinics of North America, 34*(2), 359.

Flaskerud, J., & Nyamathi, A. (2000). Collaborative inquiry with low-income Latina women. *Journal of Health Care for the Poor and Underserved, 11*(3), 326–342.

Flaskerud, J., & Winslow, B. (1998). Conceptualizing vulnerable populations health-related research. *Nursing Research, 47*(2), 69.

Freire, P. (1970). *Pedagogy of the oppressed.* New York: Herder and Herder.

Freire, P. (1973). *Education for critical consciousness* ([1st American] ed.). New York: Seabury Press.

Furuseth, O. J., & Smith, H. A. (2006). From Winn-Dixie to tiendas: The remaking of the New South. *Latinos in the new South: transformations of place,* 1–17.

Geertz, C. (1983). *Local knowledge: Further essays in interpretive anthropology.* New York: Basic Books.

Holkup, P. A., Tripp-Reimer, T., Salois, E. M., & Weinert, C. (2004). Community-based participatory research: an approach to intervention research with a Native American community. *Advances in Nursing Science, 27*(3), 162.

Hondagneu-Sotelo, P. (2003). *Gender and U.S. immigration: Contemporary trends.* Berkeley: University of California Press.

Hope, A., Timmel, S., & Hodzi, C. (1984). *Training for transformation: A handbook for community workers.* Zimbabwe: Mambo Press Gweru.

Hope, A., Timmel, S., & Hodzi, C. (1995). *Training for transformation: A handbook for community workers* (rev. ed.). Zimbabwe: Mambo Press Gweru.

Israel, B., Schulz, A., Parker, E., & Becker, A. (1998). Review of community-based research: Assessing partnership approaches to improve public health. *Annual Review of Public Health, 19,* 173–202.

Israel, B., Schulz, A., Parker, E., Becker, A., Allen, A., & Guzman, J. (2003). Critical issues in developing and following community based participatory research principles. In M. Minkler & N. Wallerstein (Eds.), *Community-based participatory research for health,* San Francisco: Jossey-Bass, 56–73.

Jacklin, K. (2009). Diversity within: Deconstructing Aboriginal community health in Wikwemikong Unceded Indian Reserve. *Social Science & Medicine 68*(5), 980–989.

Lamphere, L. (2003). The perils and prospects for an engaged anthropology: A view from the United States. *Social Anthropology, 11*(02), 153–168.

Lassiter, L. (2000). Authoritative texts, collaborative ethnography, and Native American studies. *The American Indian Quarterly, 24*(4), 601–614.

LeCompte, M., & Schensul, J. (1999). Designing and conducting ethnographic research. In M. LeCompte & J. Schensul (Eds.), *Ethnographer's toolkit* (Vol. 1). Walnut Creek, CA: Altamira Press.

McQuiston, C., Choi-Hevel, S., & Clawson, M. (2001). Protegiendo nuestra comunidad: Empowerment participatory education for HIV prevention. *Journal of Transcultural Nursing, 12*(4), 275.

McQuiston, C., Larson, K., Parrado, E., & Flaskerud, J. (2002). AIDS knowledge and measurement considerations with unacculturated Latinos. *Western Journal of Nursing Research, 24*(4), 354.

McQuiston, C., Parrado, E. A., Martínez, A. P., & Uribe, L. (2005). Community-based participatory research with Latino community members: Horizonte Latino. *Journal of Professional Nursing, 21*(4), 210–215.

McQuiston, C., & Uribe, L. (2001). Latino immigrants: Latino recruitment and retention strategies: Community-based HIV prevention. *Journal of Immigrant Health, 3*(2), 97–105.

Meleis, A. (1996). Culturally competent scholarship: Substance and rigor. *Advances in Nursing Science, 19*(2), 1.

Menzies, C. R. (2001). Reflections on research with, for, and among Indigenous peoples. *Canadian Journal of Native Education, 25*(1), 19–36.

Mohl, R. A. (2003). Globalization, latinization, and the nuevo New South. *Journal of American Ethnic History, 22*(4), 31–66.

Moodie, S. M., Tsui, E. K., & Silbergeld, E. K. (2010). Community- and family-level factors influence care-giver choice to screen blood lead levels of children in a mining community. *Environmental Research, 110*(5), 484–496.

Mosavel, M., Simon, C., van Stade, D., & Buchbinder, M. (2005). Community-based participatory research (CBPR) in South Africa: Engaging multiple constituents to shape the research question. *Social Science & Medicine, 61*(12), 2577–2587.

Panter-Brick, C., Clarke, S. E., Lomas, H., Pinder, M., & Lindsay, S. W. (2006). Culturally compelling strategies for behaviour change: A social ecology model and case study in malaria prevention. *Social Science & Medicine, 62*(11), 2810–2825.

Parrado, E., Flippen, C., & McQuiston, C. (2004). Use of commercial sex workers among Hispanic migrants in North Carolina: Implications for the spread of HIV. *Perspectives on Sexual and Reproductive Health, 36*(4), 150–156.

Parrado, E. A., & Flippen, C. A. (2005). Migration and gender among Mexican women. *American Sociological Review, 70*(4), 606.

Parrado, E. A., Flippen, C. A., & McQuiston, C. (2005). Migration and relationship power among Mexican women. *Demography, 42*(2), 347–372.

Parrado, E. A., Flippen, C. A., & Uribe, L. (2009). Concentrated disadvantages. In F. Thomas, M. Haour-Knipe, & P. Aggleton (Eds.), *Mobility, Sexuality and AIDS* (p. 40). New York: Routledge.

Parrado, E. A., McQuiston, C., & Flippen, C. A. (2005). Participatory survey research—Integrating community collaboration and quantitative methods for the study of gender and HIV risks among Hispanic migrants. *Sociological Methods & Research, 34*(2), 204–239.

Pheiffer, G., Andrew, D., Green, M., & Holley, D. (2003). The role of learning styles in integrating and empowering learners. *Investigations in University Teaching and Learning, 1*(2).

Rhodes, S. D., Hergenrather, K. C., Aronson, R. E., Bloom, F. R., Felizzola, J., Wolfson, M., et al. (2010). Latino men who have sex with men and HIV in the rural south-eastern USA: findings from ethnographic in-depth interviews. *Culture Health & Sexuality, 12*(7), 797–812.

Savage, C. L., Anthony, J., Lee, R., Kappesser, M. L., & Rose, B. (2007). The culture of pregnancy and infant care in African American women: An ethnographic study. *Journal of Transcultural Nursing, 18*(3), 215–223.

Savage, C. L., Xu, Y., Lee, R., Rose, B. L., Kappesser, M., & Anthony, J. S. (2006). A case study in the use of community-based participatory research in public health nursing. *Public Health Nursing, 23*(5), 472–478.

Sawyer, L., Regev, H., Proctor, S., Nelson, M., Messias, D., Barnes, D., et al. (1995). Matching versus cultural competence in research: Methodological considerations. *Research in Nursing & Health, 18*(6), 557–567.

Schensul, J., Weeks, M., & Singer, M. (1999). Building research partnerships. In M. LeCompte (Ed.), *Researcher roles and research partnerships* (pp. 85–164). Walnut Creek, CA: Altamira Press.

Schwandt, T. (1994). Constructivist, interpretivist approaches to human inquiry. In N. K. Denzin & Y. S. Lincoln (Eds.), *Handbook of qualitative research* (pp. 118–137). Thousand Oaks, CA: Sage.

Silverstein, M., Reid, S., DePeau, K., Lamberto, J., & Beardslee, W. (2010). Functional interpretations of sadness, stress and demoralization among an urban population of low-income mothers. *Maternal and Child Health Journal, 14*(2), 245–253.

Stringer, E. (1997). *Community-based ethnography: Breaking traditional boundaries of research, teaching, and learning.* Hillsdale, NJ: Erlbaum.

Suro, R., Singer, A., & Center, P. (2002). *Latino growth in metropolitan America: Changing patterns, new locations*: Brookings Institution, Center on Urban and Metropolitan Policy in collaboration with the Pew Hispanic Center.

Tedlock, B. (2000). Ethnography and ethnographic representation. In N. K. Denzin & Y. S. Lincoln (Eds.), *Handbook of qualitative research* (2nd ed., pp. 455–486). Thousand Oaks, CA: Sage.

Tedlock, D., & Mannheim, B. (1995). *The dialogic emergence of culture.* Urbana: University of Illinois Press.

Trujillo, F., Melendez, G., & Owen, G. (2007). Community perspectives on building partnerships with university students. *Practicing Anthropology, 29*(3), 9–13.

Tylor, E. B. (1871). *Primitive culture: researches into the development of mythology, philosophy, religion, art, and custom.* London: J. Murray.

Uribe, L. (2007). *Social isolation and sexual risk behavior among recently arrived male Hispanic migrants in Durham, North Carolina.* Unpublished doctoral dissertation. The University of North Carolina, Chapel Hill, NC.

Van Sluys, K. (2010). Trying on and trying out: Participatory action research as a tool for literacy and identity work in middle grades classrooms. *American Journal of Community Psychology*, *46*(1), 139–151.

Vásquez, M. A., Seales, C. E., & Marquardt, M. F. (2008). New Latino destinations. In H. Rodríguez, R. Saenz, & C. Menjívar (Eds.), *Latinas/os in the United States: Changing the face of America* (pp. 19–35). New York: Springer.

Vidich, A., & Lyman, S. (1994). Qualitative methods: Their history in sociology and anthropology. In N. Denzin & Y. Lincoln (Eds.), *Handbook of qualitative research* (Vol. 1, pp. 23–59). Thousand Oaks, CA: Sage.

Wallerstein, N. B., & Duran, B. (2006). Using community-based participatory research to address health disparities. *Health Promotion Practice*, *7*(3), 312.

Weinick, R., Zuvekas, S., & Cohen, J. (2000). Racial and ethnic differences in access to and use of health care services, 1977 to 1996. *Medical Care Research and Review*, *57*(suppl 1), 36.

Williams, D., & Mohammed, S. (2009). Discrimination and racial disparities in health: Evidence and needed research. *Journal of Behavioral Medicine*, *32*(1), 20–47.

Williams, D. R., & Sternthal, M. (2010). Understanding racial-ethnic disparities in health. *Journal of Health and Social Behavior*, *51*(1 suppl), S15–S27.

Acknowledgments: This research was funded by the National Institute of Nursing Research NR08052–03 and NR08052–02S2. The authors would like to thank Amanda Phillips Martínez and Leonardo Uribe for all their help in the community and with translation and transcription, and would like to thank Alejandro Mukhtar Bustillo for his contributions to the first version of this manuscript. We would also like to thank El Centro Hispano, Horizonte Latino, the Latino community in Durham, North Carolina, and the Center for Innovation in Health Disparities Research P 20NR08369.

Chapter 12

WHAT'S WITH THE WHEEZING?

METHODS USED BY THE SEATTLE-KING COUNTY HEALTHY HOMES PROJECT TO ASSESS EXPOSURE TO INDOOR ASTHMA TRIGGERS

JAMES KRIEGER

CAROL A. ALLEN

TIM K. TAKARO

Exposure to harmful substances in the environment is associated with many adverse health effects. Allergens and irritating chemicals can worsen **asthma** (Institute of Medicine, 2000). Lead can decrease IQ and cause elevated blood pressure (Needleman & Gatsonis, 1990). Air pollution can induce respiratory problems and worsen heart disease (Holgate, Samet, Koren, & Maynard, 1999). Pesticides are often neurotoxic, can disrupt hormonal functions, and can cause cancer (Rom & Markowitz, 2007).

Assessment of harmful environmental exposures is crucial to understanding and preventing environmentally linked disease. Numerous exposure assessment methods are applicable to community-based participatory research (CBPR). These methods have arisen primarily from techniques developed by industrial hygienists to assess hazards in the workplace. The requirements of sampling design, sample collection, laboratory detection and quantification methods, and time-space analysis require the integration of multiple disciplines, including toxicology, physical science, chemistry, engineering, biostatistics, and medicine.

The techniques developed for measuring specific workplace exposures have been applied in the community setting to some of the same hazards, although adapted for assessing lower levels of exposure. For example, the outdoor area monitors used by the U.S. Environmental Protection Agency (EPA) to identify pollution airsheds had their origins in the workplace as particulate monitors. Methods of measuring exposures include air, dust, water, and soil sampling and biomarker measurements. Air samplers allow quantification of levels of ozone, sulfur dioxide, oxides of nitrogen, particulates, volatile organic compounds, biohazards such as fungi, endotoxins, and allergens along with other pollutants. Dust samples collected from inside the home are used to determine levels of allergens, lead, pesticides and other persistent organic compounds, endotoxins, and fungi. Water and soil samples are assessed for heavy metals such as lead or arsenic, persistent organic compounds, and carcinogens. Biomarkers measure levels in bodily fluids of toxic substances such as heavy metals, organic compounds, and antibodies to allergens; they can also assess markers of the body's own inflammatory response to toxicants (American Conference of Governmental Industrial Hygienists, 2010).

Sampling techniques for measuring exposures to environmental hazards may be burdensome and require a high degree of study participant cooperation. Therefore a community-based participatory research (CBPR) approach may be especially useful in fostering collaboration between outside researchers and community members to design sampling methods that are acceptable to participants. In this chapter, we describe the application of CBPR to collecting information on exposure to indoor environmental **asthma triggers**.

ENVIRONMENTAL EXPOSURE ASSESSMENT METHODS AND ASTHMA

Asthma is a common environmental disease triggered by airborne allergens and respiratory irritants. Asthma affects 25 million Americans (8.2% of the population) (Zahran, Bailey, & Garbe 2011). Asthma prevalence and morbidity among children in the United States have increased dramatically in the past three decades and remain high. The causes of increased asthma prevalence are not well understood (Eder, Ege, & Mutius, 2006, Greenwood, 2011). However, a large body of evidence suggests that exposure to respiratory irritants and sensitization to allergens found in the indoor environment are major factors in the development and exacerbation of asthma; these allergens and irritants include dust mite allergens, pet danders, tobacco smoke, dampness and molds, cockroach antigens, rodent urine, endotoxins, and viruses (Ahluwalia & Matsui, 2011; DiFranza, Aligne, & Weitzman, 2004; Eder, Ege, & von Mutius, 2006; Illi et al., 2006; Institute of Medicine, 2000; Phipatanakul, 2006; Wegienka, Johnson, Havstad, Ownby, & Zoratti, 2010).

Given the widespread prevalence of indoor asthma triggers (Salo et al., 2008), decreasing exposure to them is an important strategy for reducing asthma morbidity. Reduction of exposure to specific triggers in the home, such as dust mite antigen or tobacco smoke, can reduce asthma morbidity (Diette, McCormack, Hansel, Breysse, & Matsui, 2008; Shapiro et al., 1999; Wilson et al., 2001). Other chemical exposures are also of interest such as oxides of nitrogen, diesel, and other particulates, plasticizers, and semi-volatile compounds (Breysse et al., 2010; Sandel et al., 2010). Socially marginalized populations often live in substandard housing and experience high levels of asthma morbidity and exposure to asthma triggers (Aligne, Auinger, Byrd, & Weitzman, 2000; Krieger et al., 2002; Matsui et al., 2008).

In recent years the **Healthy Homes model** has emerged as an evidence-based approach for reducing exposure to multiple asthma triggers and improving indoor environmental quality (Community Guide to Preventive Services, 2008; Crocker, Kinyota, Dumitru, Ligon, Herman, Ferdinands, et al., 2011; Environmental Health Watch, 2011; Krieger, Song, Takaro, & Weaver, 2005; Krieger, Takaro, Song, Beaudet, & Edwards, 2009; Krieger, 2010; Krieger et al., 2010; Morgan et al., 2004; Morley & Tohn, 2008; Nurmagambetov et al., 2011; Takaro, Krieger, Song, Sharify, & Beaudet, 2011). The model includes auditing the home environment, addressing multiple exposures, motivating participants to take low-cost actions, offering advice and tools to reduce exposures, and providing advocacy. We—the Seattle-King County Asthma Project—along with others, have developed and tested the effectiveness of the Healthy Homes model for reducing asthma morbidity among low-income children with asthma. More recent work has expanded the model to include construction of new, asthma-friendly homes (Takaro et al., 2011).

Reduction of exposure to indoor asthma triggers is a major intermediate outcome that can be used for assessing the impact of home interventions on asthma. The most common approach for assessing exposure to allergens (usually dust mite, cat, dog, roach, and rodent) is to measure allergen concentrations in house dust, using a vacuum to collect surface dust from floors and/or bedding, and then employing immunological methods to determine the concentration of allergens (Chapman, Aalberse, Brown, & Platts-Mills, 1988; Luczynska et al., 1989; Vojta et al., 2002). Specialized vacuums can collect dust quantitatively from measured surface areas, allowing the determination of surface dust loading. *Loading* is a measure of the amount of allergen per unit of area, which may be a more accurate measure of exposure than simply reporting the concentration of allergen in dust, which is a measure of a trigger per gram of dust (Roberts et al. 2009; Takaro, Krieger, Song, & Beaudet, 2004). Measurement of surface dust, however, may convey only a partial picture of exposure to toxicants contained in dust. Roberts and colleagues suggest that dust deeply embedded in carpet serves as a reservoir for surface dust, continually recharging the surface component (Roberts et al., 2009).

Methods to assess exposure to tobacco smoke include self-reported smoking behavior, observation of evidence of smoking in the home, air sampling for nicotine, and measurement of nicotine metabolites in urine or saliva. Self-reported tobacco use correlates well with ambient nicotine levels as a measure of environmental tobacco smoke (Hovell, Zakarian, Wahlgren, Matt, & Emmons, 2000).

Measurement of indoor mold levels presents special challenges. There is no agreed-upon standard method to assess the hazard. Visible mold is assessed by observing the density and area of mold-covered surfaces in the home, using a standardized rating system (Miller, Haisley, & Reinhardt, 2000; Reponen et al., 2010). Mold in settled dust can be measured with assays that determine fungal biomass (for example ergosterol or beta-D-glucan) (Bush & Portnoy, 2001; Iossifova et al., 2007).

The presence of pests such as rodents and roaches is assessed by observational methods, such as setting roach traps to count the number of active roaches or observing for evidence of roach or rodent presence in the home (for example, eggs, feces, surface staining) or asking study participants if they have seen any of these pests, as well as measurement of allergen in dust.

Myriad indoor chemical exposures have caught the interest of public health based in part on findings from Scandinavia that several semivolatile plasticizers known as phthalates have been linked to asthma and allergy in population studies (Jaakkola & Knight, 2008). In addition to tobacco smoke and oxides of nitrogen, other chemicals of interest include aldehydes, and infiltrated traffic-related pollutants, and other products of combustion. These exposures are routinely assessed through questionnaires and house dust sampling and sometimes air sampling (Arrandale et al., 2011). Novel assessment methods including window film wipes and absorbent passive samplers are under development for a wide range of indoor chemical compounds (Bohlin, Jones, & Strandberg, 2007).

SEATTLE-KING COUNTY ASTHMA PROGRAM

The Seattle-King County Asthma Program (SKC-AP) employs **community health workers** (CHWs) to reduce asthma morbidity among children with asthma living in ethnically diverse, low-income communities. The program began in 1997 as a research project called Healthy Homes-I (HH-I) that assessed the efficacy of a CHW home visit intervention for improving control of asthma among low-income children by reducing exposure to asthma triggers in the home. SKC-AP has grown over the years to include several follow-up projects that have built on HH-I. HH-II, completed in 2008, added support for self-management of the medical aspects of asthma control to the trigger reduction support of HH-I. We are currently testing the effectiveness of the HH approach for adults and implementing a translational research project to adapt the research intervention for use in real-world settings and assess the effectiveness of the adapted approach (Krieger, Allen, et al., 2002; Krieger et al., 2005, Krieger et al., 2009). Our Web site contains further information on these projects. (http://www.kingcounty.gov/healthservices/health/chronic/asthma.aspx). This chapter will focus on the exposure assessment activities in the two HH projects.

Community health workers (CHWs) are well suited to implementing the HH approach in these communities (Butz et al., 1994; Swider, 2002). They are members of the community who promote health through education, social support, and advocacy. CHWs have been increasingly involved in environmental exposure reduction projects in marginalized communities in the past decade.

In both HH projects, project staff recruited children with symptoms of asthma and their families for the projects from community and public health clinics, local hospitals, and emergency departments and also through referrals from community residents and agencies. A CHW made an initial home visit to each participant, in which the CHW and the home resident conducted a structured home environmental assessment. Each finding from the assessment was used to generate specific actions for the resident and the CHW. The CHW and the resident then prioritized the actions to prepare an action plan. The CHW made an average of three to four additional visits over a year to provide education and social support, encouragement of participant actions, resources to reduce exposures (allergy control pillow and mattress encasements, low-emission vacuums with dirt finders, commercial-quality doormats, cleaning kits, referrals to smoking cessation counseling, roach bait, rodent traps), assistance with roach and rodent eradication, and advocacy for improved housing conditions. (For more details about the program, see Krieger, Takaro, et al., 2002; Krieger, et al., 2005; Krieger, et al., 2009; Public Health-Seattle & King County, 2011.)

The SKC-AP evaluated the HH projects with a randomized, controlled trial (RCT) design. The RCT, widely used in clinical research, is well suited for measuring the health effects of a carefully defined, individual-level intervention. It permits direct assessment of the intervention effect while minimizing threats to internal validity (such as confounding and bias in measurement of outcomes) and removes the effects of external temporal trends. RCTs rarely incorporate a CBPR approach. The SCK-AP found the application of a CBPR approach to be quite helpful, if not essential, in conducting an RCT of the HH interventions.

We designed the organizational structure of the two HH projects to formalize participation by involved agencies, parents, staff, and researchers and to promote implementation of the CBPR principles developed by Seattle Partners for Healthy Communities (Krieger, Takaro, et al., 2002; Sullivan et al., 2001). Seattle Partners (a CDC-funded Urban Research Center that comprises community agencies, community activists, public health professionals, academics, and health providers) provided high-level project oversight and guidance for the first HH project (Krieger, Allen, et al., 2002). The King County Asthma Forum (the local asthma coalition, with community participation from people with asthma, their families, and 21 agencies) played a similar role for the second project. These partnerships participated in the development of the initial protocol and approved any major deviations from protocols and budget.

Once each of the HH projects was funded, the SKC-AP developed a project steering committee consisting of CHWs, community partners (for example, community health providers, community-based organizations), and researchers for each project. Some committee participants were also members of Seattle Partners or the King County Asthma Forum, whereas others were associated only with the HH projects. The committee met monthly during the start-up phase, semiannually during implementation, and every two months during the data analysis process. The committee participated in the development and approval of project protocols and evaluation methods, approved key project staff hires, monitored project progress, suggested questions for analysis, and reviewed and interpreted evaluation results. Committee members made decisions by consensus, and the principal investigator facilitated committee meetings. An operations team from Public Health-Seattle & King County, the fiscal agent, had responsibility for day-to-day operations.

We also formed the HH Parent Advisory Group for each project, consisting of parent representatives of project enrollees. This group reviewed participant recruitment strategies, evaluation tools, intervention protocols, project implementation, and evaluation findings. The steering committee and operations team valued the advice they received from the advisory group and, in nearly every case, adopted it. A CHW coordinated the group and represented it on the steering committee. The steering committee experimented with having two parents as committee members but found this was not particularly effective in gaining participant input. Parents were more vocal when they had a separate forum.

The HH interventions significantly reduced asthma-related symptoms and urgent health services utilization and improved caregiver quality of life (Krieger et al., 2005, Krieger et al., 2009). We observed an increase in participant actions to reduce exposures, and decreases in floor dust loading, excessive moisture, roach activity, and a composite measure of exposure to asthma triggers (Krieger et al., 2005; Krieger et al., 2009; Takaro et al., 2004).

HOME ENVIRONMENTAL ASSESSMENT IN THE HEALTHY HOMES PROJECTS

The home environmental assessment component of Healthy Homes had two goals. The first was to identify exposures in the home in order to develop a home action plan. The second was to collect research data to describe the effect of the intervention on exposures. As described in the following sections, the partners involved in the HH projects engaged in a number of activities related to this environmental assessment (for example, deciding what to measure and determining measurement protocols).

Deciding What to Measure

The researchers brought scientific knowledge of indoor asthma triggers and the underlying housing conditions that increase trigger levels. They also offered knowledge of methods of assessing exposure to triggers.

Community members (CHWs, partner agency representatives, and parents of children with asthma) knew which exposures were common in their communities. Their insights were useful in prioritizing the exposures to measure. For example, although the researchers initially believed that roaches were not common in the Seattle climate zone, community members knew otherwise and encouraged more extensive roach exposure assessment. The subsequently collected exposure data substantiated the community members' knowledge: 18% of the homes had roaches.

Local experts in exposure assessment also helped identify measures of exposure. The Washington chapter of the American Lung Association had developed the Home Environmental Assessment List (HEAL) for use by community volunteers in assessing indoor environmental quality (Dickey, 1998). Working with community environmental activists, the Lung Association, and community residents, researchers modified the HEAL so that it included more information about asthma triggers and was more culturally appropriate for the HH participants (Krieger, Takaro, et al., 2002).

We recently have further modified the checklist to adapt the HH research-derived tool for use in real-world community practice. Local experts in exposure assessment and building science reviewed the research checklist and selected items most likely to yield actionable information to guide home interventions. Program managers and CHWs reviewed the tool with an eye toward streamlining it and making it easier to use, as well as omitting less useful information.

Exposure Measures

The researchers synthesized the input from community members and local experts and proposed a set of exposure measures for research use in HH-I. The project steering committee reviewed the proposal and agreed to measure the following: floor surface dust loading (Roberts et al., 2009); dust mite allergen level (Luczynska et al., 1989); tobacco use in the home (self-report and visual observation); ergosterol (a measure of fungal contamination) (Miller & Young, 1997);

visible mold (Miller, Haisley, & Reinhardt, 2000); visual evidence of roaches and rodents (Mollet et al., 1997); and home dampness (assessed visually and with a surface moisture probe) (Dales, 1991; Pasanen et al., 2000) (see Table 12.1). The researchers developed technical protocols to collect data for these measures.

In addition to assessing the exposures themselves, HH-I assessed the underlying conditions that affect exposure levels, including dust-control behaviors

TABLE 12.1 Healthy Homes I Exposure Assessment Measures

Exposure	Measure	Reference
Floor surface dust loading	μg of fine dust per m²	Roberts, Clifford, Glass, & Hummer, 1999
Carpet deep dust loading	Three-spot dirt sensor test (seconds)	Roberts, Glass, & Mickelson, 2004
Dust mites	ELISA (μg of allergen per g dust, μg per m²)	Luczynska et al., 1989
Fungi in settled dust	Ergosterol (μg per g dust, μg per m²)	Axelsson, Saraf, & Larsson, 1995; Miller & Young, 1997; Saraf, Larsson, Burge, & Milton, 1997
Fungi in settled dust	beta-d-glucan	Foto et al., 2004; Rylander & Lin 2000
Visual mold	Cm² covered; mold intensity scale	Miller, Haisley, & Reinhardt, 2000
Surface Moisture	Surface moisture probe (percentage)	
Home dampness	Presence of visible mold, water damage, or condensation	Dales, 1991; Dales, Burnett, & Zwanenburg, 1991; Pasanen et al., 2000; Strachan, 1988
Global moisture score	Observer-rated moisture using 1–10 Likert scale	
Roaches	MaxForce traps (number of roaches trapped); participant and community health worker observation; ELISA (μg of allergen per g dust, μg per m²)	Mollet et al., 1997; Pollart et al., 1991
Pets	Self-report and observation: pets in home, access to child's bedroom; ELISA (μg of allergen per g dust, μg per m²)	Chapman, Aalberse, Brown, & Platts-Mills, 1988; de Groot, Goei, van Swieten, & Aalberse, 1991

TABLE 12.1 *(Continued)*

Exposure	Measure	Reference
Tobacco use: caregiver	Self-report of use: frequency/quantity; site(s) of smoking; use of smoking jacket	Glasgow et al., 1998; Coghlin, Hammond, & Gann, 1989
Tobacco use: others in household	Self-report of use: frequency/quantity; site(s) of smoking; use of smoking jacket	
Viral respiratory infections	Symptoms by self-report	
Toxic products in home/brought home from work	Inventory by interview and observation; work history	U.S. Department of Health and Human Services, 1995
Global indoor environment appearance	Observer rating using 1–10 Likert scale	

(controlling track-in, vacuuming and cleaning, using allergen-control bedding covers), mold and moisture problems and contributing "structural" factors (condensation, water infiltration and damage, leaks), ventilation (windows, fans, appliances, weatherization, heating, insulation, vapor barriers), structural conditions (carpeting, building age, condition of paint, structural deficits, recent remodeling), food debris and storage, trash, clutter, heating system filters and ducts, heating and cooking sources, location of garage, use and storage of hazardous and toxic products, and tap and washing machine water temperature. These measures were identified through a participatory process similar to that already described in the "deciding what to measure section."

In subsequent projects, where we have emphasized application of the HH approach to real-world settings, we have simplified exposure assessment. We have retained most of these measures, added others, and discarded a few. We no longer assess dust loading and dust allergen concentrations because of the cost and logistical complexity of collection. Use of a moisture probe did not add to visual inspection, so we do not use one. We now assess the subjective presence of strong odors (for example, from cleaners, fragrances, incense, and other chemicals) and rodents.

In all projects, we also assess the presence of home environmental features that increase exposure to asthma triggers, such as moisture intrusion, deteriorated carpeting, and inadequate ventilation (Public Health-Seattle & King County, 2011).

Data Collection Methods

The two HH projects collected exposure data by completing a home environmental audit, collecting dust samples, and measuring deep carpet dust with the three-spot test. Subsequent projects have used only the audit.

Home Environmental Checklist

The CHWs have used the **Home Environmental Checklist** (HEC) to obtain data for many exposure measures. The HEC is a structured audit of the indoor environment. Involving CHWs and participants in development of the original HEC was important for ensuring its feasibility, and soliciting feedback over the years has led to further improvements. Drawing from the Home Environmental Assessment List mentioned previously, researchers developed an initial draft of the HEC and revised it based on comments from CHWs and steering committee members. For example, a community partner pointed out that renters might lack the knowledge to answer some questions about their homes (for example, whether vapor barriers were present in crawl spaces) and suggested that it would be better to rely on data collectors' observations for these variables. The CHWs then pilot-tested the draft HEC in each other's homes and reported their suggestions to the researchers, who made further modifications. Then the CHWs tested the next draft in the homes of five parent advisory group members and gave further feedback to the researchers. For example, some parents found the wording of the question, "Have you had roaches in your home?" offensive and were more comfortable when the question was reworded as, "Have you had any problems with roaches in your home?"—a small change, but one the parents felt placed less blame on the participant. Parents also suggested prefacing collection of data on pet exposure with the statement that any information about pets in the home would be kept confidential, because the parents knew that many pets were in violation of the terms of a rental agreement. In addition, the CHWs suggested changing the format and item order of the HEC to coordinate the flow of data collection with the sequence of inspection during the home visit (for example, assessing outdoor features before indoor features). CHW input was collected during regular staff meetings held every two weeks attended by CHWs, researchers, and project managers, and during special meetings to review drafts.

Once the English version was finalized, the researchers contracted for translation of the HEC into Spanish and Vietnamese, followed by back translation and then a review by a local native speaker of the translated HEC to ensure accuracy and cultural equivalence of the document. CHWs then pilot-tested the translated versions, and researchers made additional refinements based on the pilot test results.

The HEC was completed jointly by the participant and the CHW as they walked through the home at the first visit. Discussions at staff and parent advisory group meetings revealed several benefits of including the participants in the data collection process: participants were able to observe and learn about adverse exposures, the awkwardness of having an "inspector" walk around the home unattended was avoided, and CHWs and participants agreed about the presence of exposures. (The HEC is available at http://www.kingcounty.gov/healthservices/health/chronic/asthma/resources/tools.aspx.)

Dust Sampling

Community data collectors learned how to collect dust samples. The researchers made modifications in response to comments from the data collectors as they gained experience in the field (for example, it was decided to discontinue the use of metric numbers in the data collection and to create pre-sized sampling templates to replace measuring and taping of the sampling area). The data collectors also provided feedback to project engineers on how the dust-sampling vacuum could be improved. The engineers used this information when they redesigned the vacuum to improve ease of use.

Data Collectors

Project partners had lively discussions about who could best collect data. Advantages that may accrue when professional, experienced research staff collect data include fewer missing data, less bias and more neutrality in posing questions, less need for training and monitoring, and greater adherence to collection protocols. However, community members who collect data may obtain more accurate and honest responses and greater engagement by respondents. Community data collectors may be particularly successful in collecting data in marginalized communities because they share community, culture, and life experiences with the participants and are readily welcomed into the home (Swider, 2002). Ultimately, HH used community members (both CHWs and others) to collect exposure data. (See Chapter Eight for a discussion of the development of an interviewer training manual for community members.)

IMPROVING EXPOSURE ASSESSMENT WITH A CBPR APPROACH

Using a CBPR approach improved exposure assessment in a number of arenas: cross-cultural issues, quantity and complexity of data, and data collection.

Cross-Cultural Issues

SKC-AP participants have come from diverse cultural groups. When collecting data, the CHWs have found that different groups have different boundaries of privacy that affect what they are comfortable discussing or showing about their homes. It has been best to ask directly about certain stigmatizing exposures (for example, roaches or tobacco use) with some groups and best to rely on observation with other groups. Members of some groups have been more likely to "clean house" before the exposure assessment visit, which can affect the assessment. The CHWs have learned how to explain to participants the importance of not engaging in more intensive cleaning, because of its impact on the assessment.

To address these differences across cultural groups, the CHWs have performed their work with cultural competence (Kleinman, Eisenberg, & Good, 1978; Manson, 1988), and the researchers have needed to accept some flexibility in implementing data collection protocols. When possible, the projects have matched the ethnicities of CHWs (African American, Latino, and Vietnamese) and participants (for example, 54% of the participants in HH-I shared ethnicity with their CHWs). In addition, all the CHWs have lived in the projects' targeted geographical areas. CHWs have communicated in the primary language of nearly all participants and have used interpreters for the few who needed this service.

When educational materials have not been available in the participant's language, the CHWs have participated in developing "homegrown" resources. Regardless of ethnicity, all CHWs participated in training about the variety of cultures among all clients. We observed that CHWs learned much about cultures other than their own through formal and informal interactions with each other.

The ability of the CHWs to connect with participants through shared culture and ethnicity has facilitated development of trust, which in turn has made participants more willing to engage in data collection. When a CHW works with a participant whose culture differed from hers, it has been especially valuable to talk person-to-person about neutral subjects (for example kids, food, weather) before moving into collecting data. The added communication has helped build trust and cooperation.

Quantity and Complexity of Data

The SKC-AP has experienced tension between the researchers' desire for more data and more complex data collection methods and the participants' and CHWs' desires for a simpler approach. The researchers' interest in collecting comprehensive data covering multiple domains led to long initial versions of the HEC. The CHWs and participants pointed out that if the HEC were too long, participants would grow weary and not respond reliably to questions. The data collectors were uncomfortable in asking too much of the participants. Eventually, compromises on both sides resulted in a shorter HH-I HEC that still satisfied researcher needs for collecting what they perceived as the most valuable data. We have continued to simplify and shorten the HEC in subsequent projects based on CHW and participant feedback.

The participatory approach led the project to the use of exposure measurement methods that relied on simple types of observation and data collection in addition to the more traditional, complex quantitative sampling methods used by many research studies. We wanted methods that could be used by CHWs and participants for developing action plans in the home. The researchers felt comfortable with this approach because some but not all evidence suggests that interviews and visual inspection can provide valid measures of home environmental conditions when compared with quantitative assessments (Dharmage et al., 1999; Loo et al., 2010).

Data Collection

The project staff has found that frequent review and reinforcement of protocols and field observation were valuable for ensuring the quality of the data collected by community staff. For example, researchers found dust samples improperly stored on shelves or among project paperwork, which potentially affected the accuracy of the samples. Regular training and field observations addressed this issue. The principal investigator met regularly with the CHWs to review cases and protocols. The research coordinator performed quarterly quality-control field visits to observe dust collection, give feedback, and answer questions.

In the early stages of this work, Public Health-Seattle & King County (the project's administrative and fiscal sponsor) had contracted out the data collection and CHW components of HH-I to a community-based organization. However, difficulties arose with coordination of field and research activities and with the quality of data collection. A concerted effort to resolve these issues did not succeed, and the steering committee decided to transfer these activities to the public health department in order to meet project goals.

After the first two HH projects, we assessed whether using university clinical research nurses to obtain questionnaire data would result in more efficient and reliable data collection. We also wished to obtain data on lung function (spirometry) and assumed nurses would be more appropriate than CHWs for collecting such information. However, we learned that requiring participants to travel to the university created logistical and cultural/linguistic barriers for participation and that the nurses were not as invested in the projects as were the CHWs and therefore were actually less meticulous in collecting data. We have returned to using CHWs as data collectors, and have found that they can reliably collect not only questionnaire and observational data but also perform spirometry.

CHALLENGES, LESSONS LEARNED, AND IMPLICATIONS FOR PRACTICE

The application of a CBPR approach in the context of two randomized, controlled trials resulted in projects that were well adapted to community values and realities. The perspectives of the community partners, staff, and participants have led to data collection methods that are practical and culturally appropriate. The benefits in terms of logistics and participant satisfaction have been evident. Field staff reported that after data collection protocols were modified based on their suggestions, data collection took less time and participants were pleased with a shorter visit. Whether there were additional benefits in the form of improved data quality was difficult to ascertain, although this appears to be the case. For example, we observed that after dust collection protocols were modified based on field staff suggestions, adherence to the protocols increased. After revising the HEC to incorporate parent and staff feedback, data completeness increased.

Each community-based participatory research project comes with its unique set of challenges and rewards (Krieger, Collier, Song, & Martin, 1999; Krieger, Castorina, Walls, Weaver, & Ciske, 2000; Krieger, Allen, et al., 2002). Much depends on the styles and attitudes of partners, how relationships develop, available time and resources, and the degree of congruence in vision and goals. There is always a need for mutual learning and accommodation. (See Chapter Three for a discussion of group processes appropriate for fostering partnership maintenance.) What we have experienced in the SKC-AP has been similar to what we have encountered across all our CBPR projects. The following paragraphs summarize these lessons learned and their implications for practice.

Striking a Balance Between Scientific Rigor and Practicality Is Healthy

Researchers need to contain their zeal for collecting detailed data across every conceivable domain. In most cases excessive data do not contribute to the final analyses, burden respondents unnecessarily, and waste staff time. Measures that require overly complex data collection methods can result in poor-quality data.

Community members provide a valuable perspective on what data are feasible and useful to collect. For example, in HH-I, the community staff pointed out that baseline data collection was taking over two hours and that both staff and participants were becoming fatigued. The researchers initially resisted shortening data collection protocols and instruments. They believed that with training and experience, the staff would become more proficient or that more skilled staff would have to be found. However, with time the researchers saw that it was the complexity of the data collection process that was the cause of the fatigue. The researchers simplified procedures and gained more respect for the skills of the staff.

However, community members do not always know what is needed to establish the scientific validity of an evaluation. They may not be aware of the information that policymakers and funders value as evidence of effectiveness. One of the benefits of our work has been the increased capacity of community partners to understand how "research" works, enabling them to become more active participants in the process.

It is common practice in exposure assessment research to adhere to the initially established data collection protocols throughout the study. This maximizes the consistency of data collected over time. However, most traditional exposure assessment research takes place in predictable, controlled environments. The community context is much more heterogeneous and fluid. As a result, researchers must be flexible. Protocols, and even data collection instruments, may need to be modified before the data collection is completed to reflect new knowledge acquired during study implementation. For example, the CHWs observed that participants were guessing, not paying close attention, or answering inconsistently when responding to questions requiring recall over a defined time period. Researchers added prompts and began using visual cues (for example, calendars with pictures of seasons) to assist participants in answering. In addition, the questions initially used to assess exposure to environmental tobacco smoke did not appear to be determining exposure accurately, despite prior pilot testing. The CHWs observed that the questions were not sufficiently sensitive for detecting smoking by others in the household. Following this observation, the questions were revised. Any loss in the ability to make "pure" baseline and exit comparisons may be outweighed by the higher quality of the exit data.

An Inclusive, Participatory Process Has Value but Is Time-Consuming

The participatory process is iterative, requires much communication and negotiation among partners, and is affected by personalities and relationships. Yet, as relationships deepen over the years, they become easier to maintain as community partners and researchers build trust and get to know each other. For example, the CHWs and researchers negotiated many of the details of the way the CHWs would collect kitchen dust samples. Initially, the researchers wanted to collect dust from multiple locations, including behind the refrigerator. The CHWs found this too difficult, so this location was dropped, and dust was sampled from other locations in the kitchen. As data collection proceeded, the researchers noticed that the amount of dust collected from the kitchen was too small for analysis. The CHWs suggested additional sites that were relatively easy to access (such as under the sink and near trash receptacles), and the researchers agreed to include them.

Another instance of negotiation involved redesign of the specialized vacuum cleaners used to collect dust samples. In the HH-I Project, the vacuum was awkward to carry, complicated to clean, and broke easily. The researchers' insistence on using it nearly led to a revolt among staff; due to the vacuum, they identified dust collection as the least desirable part of their job. Working with feedback from the CHWs, a new version of the vacuum was developed that was easier to use.

All of our projects have engaged community partners from start to finish, including the design phase, implementation monitoring and mid-course review, interpretation of findings, and planning for sustainability. However, the degree of community participation has varied across projects. Earlier projects such as HH-I and HH-II included a higher degree of participation in study and intervention design as we were developing protocols de novo and learning about implementation. As we gained experience in the field and collected feedback from hundreds of exiting participants, there was less need to review the protocols of subsequent projects with community partners. Issues had been identified and addressed and our approach became better established. All our projects include a steering committee made up of researchers, project staff and community partners, and a participant advisory committee; the frequency of meeting and intensity of discussion in the groups have decreased in later projects.

A Participatory Process Facilitates Recruitment

Exposure assessment is often burdensome and invasive for study participants, making it challenging to recruit them. We would not have been able to identify the hundreds of households eligible for participation in the projects without community collaborators. Community organizations will refer potential participants to research projects they believe have value. Potential participants are more likely to enroll when they learn of the research project from a trusted source. The ability of a CBPR approach to facilitate recruitment may enhance participation in other exposure assessment research projects.

Mutual Accountability Is Necessary

Researchers and community partners must agree on standards for productivity and quality in data collection and do their best to meet them. This can be tricky, especially when partners have not worked together before and discover their expectations are not the same. The HH-I project ran into difficulties collecting dust samples early in its life when the research coordinator noticed that the sampling vacuum was not being adequately cleaned between samples (allowing cross-contamination) and that samples were not being properly labeled and stored. Researchers had not adequately explained the importance of these steps in dust collection, and the community partner organization responsible for collecting samples did not maintain adequate quality assurance mechanisms. The steering committee learned that it was simpler and more reliable to have samples collected by community staff under the direct supervision of researchers rather than to have the supervision come from a community partner organization with limited experience in environmental sampling.

Environmental Exposure Assessment Methods Can Be Burdensome and Invasive and Have the Potential to Cause Labeling and Embarrassment

Some community partners raised concerns that potential participants would decline participation or spread the word that HH was a project to avoid if data collection were too burdensome, embarrassing, or disrespectful of privacy. Given that collecting data involved going into the home and seeing how much dust was on the floors, looking into cabinets for roaches, and asking if people exposed a child with asthma to secondhand smoke, potential participants might have refused to permit environmental sampling or might have cleaned up their home prior to an assessment visit to avoid embarrassment.

The CBPR approach made exposure assessment more acceptable. The ability of community staff to establish rapport with participants and engage in nonjudgmental relationships helped to overcome these concerns. For example, the CHWs learned that "having tea" with Vietnamese participants prior to collecting data facilitated the data collection process. In addition, including community members in the design of environmental sampling methods made these methods more likely to meet community standards of acceptability. Among those eligible to enroll, 70–84% currently choose to do so.

Extensive Quality Control and Frequent Reinforcement of Protocols Is Required When Using Community Members as Data Collectors

Collecting exposure assessment data in a standard, rigorous manner is a learned skill, especially when it involves technical skills and requires precision. The SKC-AP staff have become increasingly proficient in collecting data. However, their lack of prior experience required research staff to provide more initial and ongoing training than might have been the case had professionals been employed. Likewise, researchers have had to invest more time in reviewing the quality of data as it was collected and provide more intensive feedback to staff. At times the data collectors have been frustrated with the researchers' insistence on adherence to protocols and consistent documentation. Explaining the rationale behind the protocols to the collectors on several occasions has helped convince them that standardization and consistency are important. This process has paid off with more complete and reliable data. And as CHWs have seen how the researchers have used the data to build the case for sustaining their program, they have become more motivated to collect complete data.

When researchers shared data from HH-I with community staff, these staff members saw the impact of missing data on the analysis. Some staff obtained more complete data in HH-II, an example of a benefit arising from applying the CBPR principle of sharing data and analysis with community members. Mutual benefits also accrued, as the data collectors developed a new set of marketable skills and the researchers obtained better data.

Training Community Members Leads to Long-Term Jobs and Opportunities

Staff hired from the community gained living-wage jobs with benefits along with specialized skills and knowledge. They have been able to transition to new projects as funding for earlier ones ended and some have progressed to higher-level jobs within the health department or externally. Researchers have benefited by having a skilled and motivated group of staff with whom to work.

Hiring Community Members as Project Staff Strengthens Community Participation in Research

A theme running across many of these lessons is the valuable role played by community staff (data collectors and CHWs) in representing community perspectives on exposure assessment. Community staff, like other community partners, are knowledgeable about their communities. Yet they also have firsthand experience in conducting assessment activities, allowing them to provide insights about exposure assessment not available from other partners. They can also participate in project decision making more regularly because they have daily contact with research staff.

Incentives Are Important to Successful Recruitment

Both monetary and resource incentives have proved highly useful for encouraging enrollment in SKC-AP projects and participation in the time-intensive data collection process. Participants have received $25 gift cards for groceries upon completion of data collection and kept the vacuums and other resources mentioned earlier. SKC-AP is known as the "asthma vacuum program" among community members. Another incentive reported by parent advisory group members is the satisfaction they feel in seeing their actions benefit their children and in knowing that other families benefit from the research. Providing benefits to the participants and communities involved is another principle of CBPR.

Community Participation Helps in the Application of Generalized Scientific Knowledge to the Needs of a Specific Community

Knowledge derived from scientific literature and nationally developed guidelines might not apply in a local context. Some scientific knowledge is generalizable and some is not. The knowledge of community members is critical when deciding how to apply and adapt this general information to the local community.

SUMMARY

In summary, an approach to exposure assessment developed through a participatory process involving community members, local experts, and researchers led to exposure data that were collected in a culturally competent manner and were of increasing quality over time. These data provide support for the Healthy Homes approach (Krieger et al., 2005; Takaro et al., 2004, Krieger et al., 2009) and are proving useful in advocating for more widespread recognition of the important role that community health workers can play in interventions to reduce indoor triggers for asthma. Although conducting an exposure assessment using a CBPR approach has been challenging at times, we believe that the use of a CBPR approach has improved the overall research design as well as the accuracy of the data and findings.

KEY TERMS

Asthma

Asthma triggers

Community Health Worker

Healthy Homes model

Home Environmental Checklist

DISCUSSION QUESTIONS

1. How did researchers and community partners differ in their perceptions of how to collect environmental exposure data?

2. How did researcher-community collaboration result in more appropriate data collection?

3. What are three methods for collecting environmental exposure data?

REFERENCES

Ahluwalia, S. K., & Matsui, E. C. (2011). The indoor environment and its effects on childhood asthma. *Current Opinion in Allergy and Clinical Immunology, 11*(2), 137–143.

Aligne, C. A., Auinger, P., Byrd, R. S., & Weitzman, M. (2000). Risk factors for pediatric asthma: Contributions of poverty, race, and urban residence. *American Journal of Respiratory and Critical Care Medicine, 162*, 873–877.

American Conference of Governmental Industrial Hygienists. (2010). *Documentation of the TLVs® and BEls® with other worldwide occupational exposure values* [CD-ROM]. Cincinnati: Author.

Arrandale, V. H., Brauer, M., Brook, J. R., Brunekreef, B., Gold, D. R., London, S. J., et al. (2011). Exposure assessment in cohort studies of childhood asthma. *Environmental Health Perspectives, 119*(5), 591–597.

Axelsson, B. O., Saraf, A., & Larsson, L. (1995). Determination of ergosterol in organic dust by gas chromatography-mass spectrometry. *Journal of Chromatography B: Biomedical Sciences and Applications, 7*(666), 77–84.

Bohlin, P., Jones, K. C., & Strandberg, B. (2007). Occupational and indoor air exposure to persistent organic pollutants: A review of passive sampling techniques and needs. Journal of Environmental Monitoring, *9*(6), 501–509.

Breysse, P. N., Diette, G. B., Matsui, E. C., Butz, A. M., Hansel, N. N., McCormack, M. C. (2010). Indoor air pollution and asthma in children. *Proceedings of the American Thoracic Society, 7*(2), 102–106.

Bush, R. K., & Portnoy, J. M. (2001). The role and abatement of fungal allergens in allergic disease. *Journal of Allergy and Clinical Immunology, 107*(Suppl.), 430–440.

Butz, A. M., Malveaux, F. J., Eggleston, P., Thompson, L., Schneider, S., Weeks, K., et al. (1994). Use of community health workers with inner-city children who have asthma. *Clinical Pediatrics, 33*, 135–141.

Chapman, M. D., Aalberse, R. C., Brown, M. J., & Platts-Mills, T. A. (1988). Monoclonal antibodies to the major feline allergen Fel d I. II: Single step affinity purification of Fel d I, N-terminal sequence analysis, and development of a sensitive two-site immunoassay to assess Fel d I exposure. *Journal of Immunology, 140*, 812–818.

Coghlin, J., Hammond, S. K., & Gann, P. H. (1989). Development of epidemiologic tools for measuring environmental tobacco smoke exposure. *American Journal of Epidemiology, 130*, 696–704.

Community Guide to Preventive Services. (2008). Asthma control: Home-based multi-trigger, multicomponent environmental interventions. Retrieved May 7, 2011, from http://www.thecommunityguide.org/asthma/multicomponent.html

Crocker, D. D., Kinyota, S., Dumitru, G. G., Ligon, C. B., Herman, E. J., Ferdinands, J. M., Hopkins, D. P., Lawrence, B. M., & Sipe, T. A. (2011). Task Force on Community Preventive Services. Effectiveness of home-based, multi-trigger, multicomponent interventions with an environmental focus for reducing asthma morbidity a community guide systematic review. *American Journal of Preventive Medicine, 41*(2 Suppl 1), S5–S32.

Dales, R. E. (1991). Respiratory health effects of home dampness and molds among Canadian children. *American Journal of Epidemiology, 134*, 196–203.

Dales, R. E., Burnett, R., & Zwanenburg, H. (1991). Adverse health effects among adults exposed to home dampness and molds. *American Review of Respiratory Disease, 143*, 505–509.

de Groot, H., Goei, K. G., van Swieten, P., & Aalberse, R. C. (1991). Affinity purification of a major and a minor allergen from dog extract: Serologic activity of affinity-purified *Can f*I and of *Can f*I-depleted extract. *Journal of Allergy and Clinical Immunology, 87*, 1056–1065.

Dharmage, S., Bailey, M., Raven, J., Cheng, A., Thien, F., Rolland, J., et al. (1999). A reliable and valid home visit report for studies of asthma in young adults. *Indoor Air, 9*, 188–192.

Dickey, P. (Ed.). (1998). *Master Home Environmentalist training manual.* Seattle: American Lung Association of Washington.

Diette, G. B., McCormack, M. C., Hansel, N. N., Breysse, P. N., & Matsui, E. C. (2008). Environmental issues in managing asthma. *Respiratory Care, 53*(5), 602–615; discussion 616–617.

DiFranza, J. R., Aligne, C. A., & Weitzman, M. (2004). Prenatal and postnatal environmental tobacco smoke exposure and children's health. *Pediatrics, 113*(4 Suppl), 1007–1015.

Eder, W., Ege, M. J., & von Mutius, E. (2006). The asthma epidemic. *New England Journal of Medicine, 355*, 2226–2235.

Environmental Health Watch. (2011). *Healthy green housing.* Retrieved May 6, 2011, from http://www.ehw.org/healthy-green-housing/

Foto, M., Plett, J., Berghout, J., & Miller, J. D. (2004). Modification of the Limulus amebocyte lysate assay for the analysis of glucan in indoor environments. *Analytical and Bioanalytical Chemistry 379*, 156–162.

Glasgow, R. E., Foster, L. S., Lee, M. E., Hammond, S. K., Lichtenstein, E., & Andrews, J. A. (1998). Developing a brief measure of smoking in the home: Description and preliminary evaluation. *Addictive Behaviors, 23*, 567–571.

Greenwood, V. (April 2011). Why are asthma rates soaring? *Scientific American.* Retrieved May 6, 2011, from http://www.scientificamerican.com/article.cfm?id=why-are-asthma-rates-soaring.

Holgate, S. T., Samet, J. M., Koren, H. S., & Maynard, R. L. (Eds.). (1999). *Air pollution and health.* San Diego: Academic Press.

Hovell, M. F., Zakarian, J. M., Wahlgren, D. R., Matt, G. E., & Emmons, K. M. (2000). Reported measures of environmental tobacco smoke exposure: Trials and tribulations. *Tobacco Control, 9*(Suppl. 3), 22–28.

Illi, S., von Mutius, E., Lau, S., Niggemann, B., Gruber, C., Wahn, U., & Multicentre Allergy Study (MAS) group. (2006). Perennial allergen sensitisation early in life and chronic asthma in children: A birth cohort study. *Lancet, 368*(9537), 763–770.

Institute of Medicine. (2000). *Clearing the air: Asthma and indoor air exposures.* Washington, DC: National Academies Press.

Iossifova, Y. Y., Reponen, T., Bernstein, D. I., Levin, L., Kalra, H., Campo, P., & LeMasters, G. (2007). House dust (1–3)-beta-D-glucan and wheezing in infants. *Allergy, 62*(5), 504–513.

Jaakkola, J. J., & Knight, T. L. (2008). The role of exposure to phthalates from polyvinyl chloride products in the development of asthma and allergies: A systematic review and meta-analysis. *Environmental Health Perspectives, 116*, 845–853. doi: org/10.1289/ehp.10846

Kleinman, A., Eisenberg, L., & Good, B. (1978). Culture, illness, and care: Clinical lessons from anthropologic and cross-cultural research. *Annals of Internal Medicine, 88,* 251–258.

Krieger, J. W., Allen, C., Cheadle, A., Higgins, D., Schier, J., Senturia, K., et al. (2002). Using community-based participatory research to address social determinants of health: Lessons learned from Seattle Partners for Healthy Communities. *Health Education & Behavior, 29,* 361–381.

Krieger, J. W., Castorina, J., Walls, M., Weaver, M., & Ciske, S., (2000). Increasing influenza and pneumococcal immunization rates: A randomized controlled study of a senior center-based intervention. *American Journal of Preventive Medicine, 18,* 123–131.

Krieger, J. W., Collier, C., Song, L., & Martin, D. (1999). Linking community-based blood pressure measurement to clinical care: A randomized controlled trial of outreach and tracking by community health workers. *American Journal of Public Health, 89,* 856–861.

Krieger, J. W., Song, L., Takaro, T., & Weaver, M. (2005). The Seattle-King County Healthy Homes Project: A randomized, controlled trial of a community health worker intervention to decrease exposure to indoor asthma triggers among low-income children. *American Journal of Public Health, 95,* 652–659.

Krieger, J. W., Takaro, T. K., Allen, C., Song, L., Weaver, M., Chai, S., et al. (2002). The Seattle-King County Healthy Homes Project: Implementation of a comprehensive approach to improving indoor environmental quality for low-income children with asthma. *Environmental Health Perspectives, 110*(Suppl 2), 311–322.

Krieger, J. W., Takaro, T., Song, L., Beaudet, N., & Edwards, K. (2009). The Seattle-King County Healthy Homes II Project: A randomized controlled trial of asthma self-management support comparing clinic-based nurses and in-home community health workers. *Archives of Pediatrics & Adolescent Medicine, 163,* 141–149.

Krieger, J. W. (2010). Home is where the triggers are: Increasing asthma control by improving the home environment. *Pediatric Allergy, Immunology, & Pulmonology, 23,* 139–145.

Krieger, J. W., Jacobs, D.E., Ashley, P. J., Baeder, A., Chew, G., Dearborn, D., Hynes, H. P., Miller, J. D., Morely, R., & Rabito, F. (2010). Housing interventions and control of indoor biologic agents: A review of the evidence. *Journal Public Health Management and Practice, 16*(E-Suppl), S75–S78.

Loo, C. K., Foty, R. G., Wheeler, A. J., Miller, J. D., Evans, G., Stieb, D. M., & Dell, S. D. (2010). Do questions reflecting indoor air pollutant exposure from a questionnaire predict direct measure of exposure in owner-occupied houses? *International Journal of Environmental Research in Public Health, 7,* 3270–3297.

Luczynska, C. M., Arruda, L. K., Platts-Mills, T. A., Miller, J. D., Lopez, M., & Chapman, M. D. (1989). A two-site monoclonal antibody ELISA for the quantification of the major Dermatophagoides spp. allergens, Der p I and Der f l. *Journal of Immunological Methods, 118,* 227–235.

Manson, A. (1988). Language concordance as a determinant of patient compliance and emergency room use in patients with asthma. *Medical Care, 26,* 1119–1128.

Matsui, E. C., Hansel, N. N., McCormack, M. C., Rusher, R., Breysse, P. N., & Diette, G. B. (2008). Asthma in the inner city and the indoor environment. *Immunology & Allergy Clinics of North America, 28*(3), 665–686.

Miller, J. D., Haisley, P. D., & Reinhardt, J. H. (2000). Air sampling results in relation to extent of fungal colonization of building materials in some water-damaged buildings. *Indoor Air, 10*(3), 146–151.

Miller, J. D., & Young, J. C. (1997). The use of ergosterol to measure exposure to fungal propagules in indoor air. *American Industrial Hygiene Association Journal, 58*(1), 39–43.

Mollet, J. A., Vailes, L. D., Avner, D. B., Perzanowski, M. S., Arruda, L. K., Chapman, M. D., et al. (1997). Evaluation of German cockroach (Orthoptera: Blattellidae) allergen and seasonal variation in low-income housing. *Journal of Medical Entomology, 34*(3), 307–311.

Morgan, W. J., Crain, E. F., Gruchalla, R. S., O'Connor, G. T., Kattan, M., Evans, R., III, et al. (2004). Results of a home-based environmental intervention among urban children with asthma. *New England Journal of Medicine, 351*, 1068–1080.

Morley R., & Tohn, E. (2008). *How healthy are national green building programs*. Columbia, MD: National Center for Healthy Housing.

Needleman, H. L., & Gatsonis, C. A. (1990). Low-level lead exposure and the IQ of children: A meta-analysis of modern studies. *Journal of the American Medical Association, 263*, 673–678.

Nurmagambetov, T. A., Barnett, S. B., Jacob, V., Chattopadhyay, S. K, Hopkins, D. P., Crocker, D. D., Dumitru, G. G., Kinyota, S., Task Force on Community Preventive Services. (2011). Economic value of home-based, multi-trigger, multicomponent interventions with an environmental focus for reducing asthma morbidity: A community guide systematic review. *American Journal of Preventive Medicine, 41*(2 Suppl 1), S33–S47.

Pasanen, A. L., Rautiala, S., Kasanen, J. P., Raunio, P., Rantamaki, J., & Kalliokoski, P. (2000). The relationship between measured moisture conditions and fungal concentrations in water-damaged building materials. *Indoor Air, 11*, 111–120.

Phipatanakul, W. (2006). Environmental factors and childhood asthma. *Pediatric Annals, 35*, 646–656.

Pollart, S. M., Smith, T. F., Morris, E. C., Gelber, L. E., Platts-Mills, T. A., & Chapman, M. D. (1991). Environmental exposure to cockroach allergens: Analysis with monoclonal antibody-based enzyme immunoassays. *Journal of Allergy and Clinical Immunology, 87*, 505–510.

Public Health-Seattle & King County (2011). King County Asthma Program. Retrieved May 2011, from http://www.kingcounty.gov/healthservices/health/chronic/asthma.aspx

Reponen, T., Singh, U., Schaffer, C., Vesper, S., Johansson, E., Adhikari, A., & Lemasters, G. (2010). Visually observed mold and moldy odor versus quantitatively measured microbial exposure in homes. *The Science of the Total Environment, 408*(22), 5565–5574.

Roberts, J. W., Clifford, W. S., Glass, G., & Hummer, P. G. (1999). Reducing dust, lead, dust mites, bacteria, and fungi in carpets by vacuuming. *Archives of Environmental Contamination and Toxicology, 36*, 477–484.

Roberts, J. W., Glass, G., & Mickelson, L. (2004). A pilot study of the measurement and control of deep dust, surface dust, and lead in ten old carpets using the 3-spot test while vacuuming. *Archives of Environmental Contamination and Toxicology, 48,* 16–23.

Roberts, J. W., Wallace, L. A., Camann, D. E., Dickey, P., Gilbert, S. G., Lewis, R. G., & Takaro, T. K. (2009). Monitoring and reducing exposure of infants to pollutants in house dust. *Reviews of Environmental Contamination and Toxicology, 201,* 1–39. doi:10.1007/978–1 –4419–0032–6_1

Rom, W. N., & Markowitz, S. B. (Eds.). (2007). *Environmental and occupational medicine* (4th ed.). Philadelphia: Wolters Kluwer/Lippincott Williams & Wilkins.

Rylander, R., & Lin, R. H. (2000). Beta-(1,3)-d-glucan—relationship to indoor air-related symptoms allergy and asthma. *Toxicology, 152,* 47–52.

Sandel, M., Baeder, A., Bradman, A., Hughes, J., Mitchell, C., Shaughnessy, R., & Jacobs, D. E. (2010). Housing interventions and control of health-related chemical agents: A review of the evidence. *Journal of Public Health Management & Practice, 16*(5 Suppl), S24–S33.

Saraf, A., Larsson, L., Burge, H., & Milton, D. (1997). Quantification of ergosterol and 3-hydroxy fatty acids in settled house dust by gas chromatography-mass spectrometry: Comparison with fungal culture and determination of endotoxin by a limulus amebocyte lysate assay. *Applied and Environmental Microbiology, 63,* 2554–2559.

Shapiro, G. G., Wighton, T. G., Chinn, T., Zuckrman, J., Eliassen, A. H., Picciano, J. F., et al. (1999). House dust mite avoidance for children with asthma in homes of low-income families. *Journal of Allergy & Clinical Immunology, 103,* 1069–1074.

Salo, P. M., Arbes, S. J., Jr., Crockett, P. W., Thorne, P. S., Cohn, R. D., & Zeldin, D. C. (2008). Exposure to multiple indoor allergens in U.S. homes and its relationship to asthma. *Journal of Allergy & Clinical Immunology, 121,* 678–684.

Strachan, D. P. (1988). Damp housing and childhood asthma: Validation of reporting of symptoms. *British Medical Journal, 297,* 1223–1226.

Sullivan, M., Kane, A., Senturia, K. D., Chrisman, N. J., Ciske, S. J., & Krieger, J. W. (2001). Researcher and researched-community perspectives: Toward bridging the gap. *Health Education & Behavior, 28*(2), 130–149.

Swider, S. M. (2002). Outcome effectiveness of community health workers: An integrative literature review. *Public Health Nursing, 19,* 11–20.

Takaro, T., Krieger, J. W., Song, L., & Beaudet, N. (2004). Effect of environmental interventions to reduce asthma triggers in homes of low-income children in Seattle. *Journal of Exposure Analysis and Environmental Epidemiology, 14*(Suppl. 1), S133–S143.

Takaro, T. K., Krieger, J., Song, L., Sharify, D., & Beaudet, N. (2011). The breathe-easy home: The impact of asthma-friendly home construction on clinical outcomes and trigger exposure. *American Journal of Public Health, 101*(1), 55–62.

U.S. Department of Health and Human Services. (1995). *Report to Congress on Workers' Home Contamination Study, conducted under the Workers' Family Protection Act* (29 U.S.C. 671a). Retrieved March 2005, from http://www.cdc.gov/niosh/contamin.html

Vojta, P. J., Friedman, W., Marker, D. A., Clickner, R., Rogers, J. W., Viet, S. M., & Zeldin, D. C. (2002). First national survey of lead and allergens in housing: Survey design and methods for the allergen and endotoxin components. *Environmental Health Perspectives*, *110*(5), 527–532.

Wegienka, G., Johnson, C. C., Havstad, S., Ownby, D. R., & Zoratti, E. M. (2010). Indoor pet exposure and the outcomes of total IgE and sensitization at age 18 years. *The Journal of Allergy and Clinical Immunology*, *126*(2), 274–9, 279.e1–5.

Wilson, S. R., Yamada, E. G., Sudhakar, R., Roberto, L., Mannino, D., Mejia, C., et al. (2001). A controlled trial of an environmental tobacco smoke reduction intervention in low-income children with asthma. *Chest*, *120*, 1709–1722.

Zahran, H. S., Bailey, C., & Garbe, P. (2011). Vital signs: Asthma prevalence, disease characteristics, and self-management education—United States, 2001–2009. *Morbidity and Mortality Weekly Reports*, *60* (17), 547–552.

Acknowledgments: Primary funding for the work discussed in this chapter was provided by National Institute of Environmental Health Sciences (NIEHS) grants 1 R21 ES09095, 1 R01 ES11378 and 1 R01 ES014583; U.S. Department of Housing and Urban Development WALHH0115; Centers for Disease Control grants U58/CCU023330, U48/CCU009654–07, and 5R18EH000537; the Nesholm Foundation, the Seattle Foundation; and the Robert Wood Johnson Foundation Allies Against Asthma Initiative. Many community health workers—Carol Allen, Michelle DiMiscio, Zhoni Gilbert, Jean Jackson, Cindy Mai, Maria Martinez, Margarita Mendoza, Nilsa Nicholson, Matthew Nguyen, and LaTanya Wilson—have worked devotedly with their clients. Carol Allen, Georgiana Arnold, Marissa Brooks, Kristine Edwards, Miriam Philby, Lisa Ross, and Diana Vinh have coordinated field and research operations.

DOCUMENTATION AND EVALUATION OF PARTNERSHIPS

In Part Five, we focus on the CBPR phase of documenting and evaluating, on an ongoing basis, the progress of the partnership toward achieving a collaborative process. Given the fundamental importance of partnership formation and maintenance to CBPR, as illustrated by the chapters in Part Two of this book, it is essential to document and evaluate the effectiveness of the process methods used by a partnership (Butterfoss, 2009; Cheadle et al., 2008; Israel et al., 2008; Plumb, Collins, Cordeiro, & Kavanaugh-Lynch, 2008; Schulz, Israel, & Lantz, 2003; Wallerstein et al., 2008).

By using a partnership's CBPR principles as a guide, an evaluation can determine intermediate outcomes to be used by the partnership to refine and improve their progress toward achieving an effective collaborative process, and ultimately, to accomplish long-term outcomes (King et al., 2009; Lantz, Viruell-Fuentes, Israel, Softley, & Guzman, 2001; Plumb et al., 2008; Rossi, Lipsey, & Freeman, 2004; Schulz, Israel, & Lantz, 2003). Examples of intermediate outcomes can be found in the chapters for Part Two, *Partnership Formation and Maintenance*, and include the following: fosters colearning and capacity building; involves equitable participation, sharing of influence and power among all partners; and achieves balance between knowledge generation and action. Although the emphasis in Part Five is on assessing a partnership's attainment of intermediate outcomes, it is important to recognize that evaluating the long-term outcomes of a

CBPR partnership, such as achieving intervention objectives, is another critical aspect of the evaluation phase. Numerous methods are appropriate for documenting progress toward attainment of both intermediate and long-term outcomes (for example, survey, focus group interview). In Part Five, the methods of in-depth, semistructured interview and closed-ended survey questionnaire are examined.

In Chapter Thirteen, *Documentation and Evaluation of CBPR Partnerships*, Israel, Lantz, McGranaghan, Guzmán, Lichtenstein, and Rowe present a conceptual framework for evaluating the process and impact of CBPR partnerships, and the application of the framework by the Detroit Community-Academic Urban Research Center. Their conceptual framework identifies the role of several dimensions that have an impact on the extent to which a partnership achieves its ultimate outcomes. Particular emphasis is placed on assessing the dimensions of "Structural Characteristics," "Group Dynamics Characteristics," and "Intermediate Measures of Partnership Effectiveness." To document and monitor change in these dimensions, they used two data collection methods: in-depth, semistructured interviews and closed-ended survey questionnaires. The authors provide insightful details on the structures and procedures used to engage academic and community partners in evaluating the process and impact of their CBPR partnership. They give particular attention to the participatory process of designing and conducting the evaluation, feeding back and interpreting findings, and applying the results to refine and improve the partnership's adherence to CBPR principles. The authors examine the challenges and limitations, lessons learned, and implications for the use of these methods, which are applicable to documenting and evaluating both partnership formation and maintenance and the more long-term outcomes of a CBPR effort.

REFERENCES

Butterfoss, F. D. (2009). Evaluating partnerships to prevent and manage chronic disease. *Preventing Chronic Disease, 6*(2), A64.

Cheadle, A., Hsu, C., Schwartz, P. M., Pearson, D., Greenwald, H. P., Beery, W. L., et al. (2008). Involving local health departments in community health partnerships: Evaluation results from the partnership for the public's health initiative. *Journal of Urban Health, 85*(2), 162–177.

Israel, B. A., Schulz, A. J., Parker, E. A., Becker, A. B., Allen, A., & Guzman, J. R. (2008). Critical issues in developing and following community-based participatory research principles. In M. Minkler & N. Wallerstein (Eds.), *Community-based participatory research for health* (2nd ed., pp. 47–66). San Francisco: Jossey-Bass.

King, G., Servais, M., Kertoy, M., Specht, J., Currie, M., Rosenbaum, P., et al. (2009). A measure of community members' perceptions of the impacts of research partnerships in health and social services. *Evaluation and Program Planning, 32*(3), 289–299.

Lantz, P., Viruell-Fuentes, E., Israel, B. A., Softley, D., & Guzman, J. R. (2001). Can communities and academia work together on public health research? Evaluation results from a community-based participatory research partnership in Detroit. *Journal of Urban Health, 78*(3), 495–507.

Plumb, M., Collins, N., Cordeiro, J. N., & Kavanaugh-Lynch, M. (2008). Assessing process and outcomes: Evaluating community-based participatory research. *Progress in Community Health Partnerships, 2*(2), 85–97.

Rossi, P. H., Lipsey, M. W., & Freeman, H. E. (2004). Tailoring evaluations: The nature of the evaluator stakeholder relationship. In P. H. Rossi, M. W. Lipsey, & H. E. Freeman (Eds.), *Evaluation: A systematic approach* (7th ed., pp. 48–52). Thousand Oaks, CA: Sage.

Schulz, A. J., Israel, B. A., & Lantz, P. (2003). Instrument for evaluating dimensions of group dynamics within community-based participatory research partnerships. *Evaluation and Program Planning, 26*, 249–262.

Wallerstein, N., Oetzel, J., Duran, B., Tafoya, G., Belone, L., & Rae, R. (2008). What predicts outcomes in CBPR? In M. Minkler & N. Wallerstein (Eds.), *Community-based participatory research for health* (2nd ed., pp. 371–394). San Francisco: Jossey-Bass.

Chapter 13

DOCUMENTATION AND

EVALUATION OF CBPR

PARTNERSHIPS

THE USE OF IN-DEPTH INTERVIEWS AND CLOSED-ENDED QUESTIONNAIRES

BARBARA A. ISRAEL

PAULA M. LANTZ

ROBERT McGRANAGHAN

J. RICARDO GUZMÁN

RICHARD LICHTENSTEIN

ZACHARY ROWE

The number of research and intervention partnerships that address the complex set of determinants associated with public health problems, particularly health inequities, has grown substantially in the past two decades. These partnerships have identified numerous challenges, facilitating factors, and benefits associated with the collaborative approach to public health research (Brooks, 2010; Cheadle et al., 2008; Israel, Schulz, Parker, & Becker, 1998; Johnson, Hayden, et al., 2009; Kegler, Hall, & Kiser, 2010; Minkler & Wallerstein, 2008; Plumb, Collins, Cordeiro, & Kavanaugh-Lynch, 2008). Specifically, such partnerships have gained an enhanced understanding of the time needed to develop and maintain partnerships and to show an impact on health outcomes (Brooks, 2010; Cheadle et al., 2008; Israel et al., 1998; Kegler et al., 2010; Weiss, Anderson, & Lasker, 2002). Therefore it is particularly important that partnerships document and evaluate early on the extent to which and the ways in which their partnership process is effective in adhering to key principles of collaboration (Brooks, 2010; Butterfoss, 2009; Cheadle et al., 2008; Israel et al., 2008; Lasker, Weiss, & Miller, 2001; Plumb et al., 2008; Schulz, Israel, & Lantz, 2003; Sofaer, 2000; Tolma, Cheney, Troup, & Hann, 2009; Wallerstein et al., 2008; Weiss, Anderson & Lasker, 2002) and is having an impact on intended outcomes (Butterfoss, 2009; Curie et al., 2005; King, et al., 2009; Plumb et al., 2008; Schulz, et al., 2003; Wallerstein et al., 2008).

A determination of whether and how effectively a partnership is collaborative and participatory, and whether and how effectively it achieves its intermediate or impact objectives, can occur long before it is possible to assess the partnership's impact on health (Butterfoss, 2009; Cheadle et al., 2008; King et al., 2009; Rossi, Freeman, & Lipsey, 2004; Schulz et al., 2003; Wallerstein et al., 2008). Such documentation and evaluation information can be used by the partnership to improve its actions and in turn the achievement of its ultimate goals (Brooks, 2010; Butterfoss, 2009; Lantz, Viruell-Fuentes, Israel, Softley, & Guzman, 2001; Schulz et al., 2003; Wallerstein et al., 2008; Weiss et al., 2002).

There are many different types of evaluation—such as process, impact, outcome, participatory, formative, and summative (Butterfoss, 2009; Israel et al., 1995; Patton, 2002; Plumb et al., 2008; Springett & Wallerstein, 2008; Tolma et al., 2009)—and multiple data collection methods—quantitative and qualitative—that can be used for evaluating partnerships (Butterfoss, 2009; Cheadle et al., 2008; Patton, 2002; Schulz et al., 2003; Tolma, et al., 2009; Weiss et al., 2002). The purpose of this chapter is to examine the use of two data collection methods, **in-depth, semistructured interviews** and **closed-ended survey questionnaires**, for assessing the process and impact of (CBPR) partnerships on the different phases of their research process. We will present a conceptual framework for assessing CBPR partnerships and a brief description of each of these two data collection methods. The application of these methods by the Detroit Community-Academic Urban Research Center (Detroit URC) will be presented as a case example. Emphasis will be placed on the participatory process used in designing and conducting these methods and in feeding back and interpreting the data collected for an evaluation of a CBPR partnership. We will examine the challenges and limitations, lessons learned, and implications for the use of these methods.

CONCEPTUAL FRAMEWORK FOR
ASSESSING CBPR PARTNERSHIPS

There are a number of theoretical and conceptual models that provide useful frameworks for understanding and assessing how partnerships operate and their impacts and outcomes (Butterfoss & Kegler, 2009; Curie et al., 2005; Johnson et al., 2009; Lasker & Weiss, 2003; Schulz et al., 2003; Sofaer, 2000; Wallerstein et al., 2008). In our own work we have placed particular emphasis on the importance of a given partnership's adhering to the principles of CBPR—for example, displaying a collaborative, equitable partnership in all phases of the process (see Chapter One in this volume and Israel et al., 1998, 2008)—and the recognition that success in following these principles and achieving long-term outcomes is dependent on the effectiveness of the group in using its resources and satisfying the needs of group members (Johnson & Johnson, 2008; Schulz et al., 2003; Plumb et al., 2008; Wallerstein et al., 2008). Therefore the development of the evaluation instruments discussed here was based on an extensive review of the group process literature at the time in which the initial tools were developed in 1985 (Johnson & Johnson, 1982; Shaw, 1981) as part of another participatory action research project (Israel, Schurman, & House, 1989). We selected the priority aspects of groups to assess (such as shared leadership; open, two-way communication; and high levels of trust) based on the characteristics of effective groups delineated by Johnson & Johnson (1982). (See Chapter Three for a discussion of group facilitation strategies that can be used to foster the achievement of these characteristics.)

As shown in Figure 13.1, these characteristics of effective groups have been placed in the context of a conceptual framework for understanding and assessing partnerships (adapted from Sofaer, 2000; Schulz et al., 2003; with additional points from Lasker & Weiss, 2003). (Portions of this section of this chapter were adapted from Schulz et al., 2003.) Briefly, the extent to which a partnership achieves its ultimate outcomes or outputs (for example, improved community health) is influenced by intermediate measures or characteristics of partnership effectiveness (for example, extent of member involvement) that are determined by the partnership's programs and interventions. In turn, these are shaped by the group dynamics of the partnership (for example, communication, conflict resolution), which are also influenced by structural characteristics of the partnership (for example, membership). All these factors in the framework are shaped by

FIGURE 13.1 Conceptual Framework for Understanding and Assessing the Effectiveness of the CBPR Partnership Process

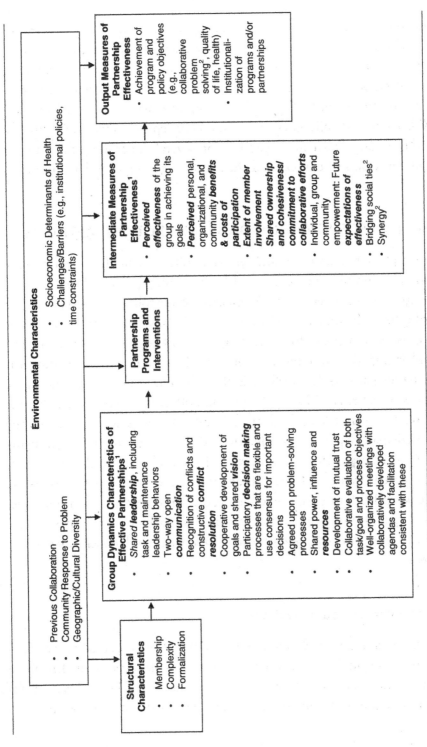

1. As presented in Schulz et al., 2003, italicized and bolded items were derived from Johnson and Johnson (1982, 1997) and also included in Sofaer, 2000. Other items were derived from Johnson and Johnson and not included in Sofaer's model.

2. Derived from Lasker and Weiss, 2003.

Source: Adapted from Lasker and Weiss, 2003; Schulz et al., 2003; Sofaer, 2000. Portions reprinted from Schulz, A. J., Israel, B. A., and Lantz, P. M. (2003), Instrument for evaluating dimensions of group dynamics within community-based participatory research partnerships: *Evaluation and program planning,* 26(3), 249–262. Copyright 2003, with permission from Elsevier.

environmental characteristics (for example, geographical and cultural diversity). The items included in the closed-ended survey questionnaire and the in-depth interview protocol that will be presented here were informed by this framework, with particular emphasis on assessing the dimensions of "structural characteristics," "group dynamics characteristics," and "intermediate measures." (See the work of Wallerstein and colleagues [2008] for a conceptual model of CBPR that was adapted from our model and expands upon several dimensions, for example, the different constructs of context and their influence on group dynamics.)

GENERAL DESCRIPTION OF DATA COLLECTION METHODS

A number of qualitative and quantitative data collection methods can be used to gather information to evaluate the CBPR partnership process (Brooks, 2010; Butterfoss, 2009; Cheadle et al., 2008; Denzin & Lincoln, 2011; Kegler et al., 2010; Nardi, 2006; Patton, 2002; Tolma et al., 2009). The integration of the two methods is recommended for increasing the knowledge gained from any one method, enhancing the comprehensiveness of the results, and increasing the acceptance by all partners (Butterfoss, 2009; Cheadle et al., 2008; Denzin & Lincoln, 2011; Israel et al., 1995; Tolma et al., 2009). It is our premise that the evaluation questions and specific data collection methods selected (identified through a participatory process) are determined by the type of evaluation being conducted (that is, evaluating the process and impact of a CBPR partnership) and the conceptual framework that guides the assessment of the partnership. Given the conceptual framework described earlier and the evaluation objectives that have emerged in our work, we have relied primarily on two types of data collection methods: *in-depth, semistructured interviews* and *closed-ended survey questionnaires.*

In-Depth, Semistructured Interviews

There are a number of approaches to the design of one-on-one, qualitative interviews, and different authors use different terms and definitions in describing them, such as *informal conversational interview* and standardized *open-ended interview* (Patton, 2002). Among the areas in which key distinctions occur across these approaches are the comparative degree of formality or informality, the decision to use fully specified questions or to use topic guidelines, and the degree of flexibility in phrasing questions (asking all respondents the same questions or employing some variation). One of the strengths of all these approaches is the emphasis on asking open-ended questions, with follow-up probes, as necessary, that allow the respondent to provide an in-depth explanation of the issues being addressed (Patton, 2002). In addition to the way the questions are asked, such aspects as whom to interview, where to conduct the interview, note taking, tape recording, informed consent and confidentiality, cross-cultural dimensions, and data analysis approaches (Patton, 2002) have to be considered in conducting qualitative interviews. The focus of this chapter is on the use of the qualitative in-depth, semistructured interview, which is aimed at gaining an in-depth understanding of a given phenomenon without imposing any categorization of responses that might limit the inquiry (Fontana & Frey, 2000). (See Chapter Five for a discussion of the use of in-depth key informant interviews.) In-depth, semistructured interviews use a standard set of pre-specified, open-ended questions, with follow-up probes to obtain the desired depth of understanding, and allow questions to be asked somewhat differently, if necessary.

Closed-Ended Survey Questionnaires

The closed-ended survey questionnaire is one of the most frequently used methods for gathering information in a systematic and quantitative fashion (Fowler, 2008; Nardi, 2006). Although questions may be asked in different ways, with different response categories, the key dimensions are the use of a predetermined set of questions that are asked of all respondents and the provision of a set of specified response categories into which the respondents' answers have to fit (Fowler, 2008; Nardi, 2006). In addition to the questions themselves, a number of other dimensions of survey questionnaires have to be considered: whom to interview and how the individuals are selected, use of face-to-face or self-administered modes, informed consent and confidentiality, language and translations, number of respondents needed for purposes of statistical power, and use of a cross-sectional or longitudinal approach (Fowler, 2008; Nardi, 2006). (See Chapter Seven for an examination of a random sample survey conducted using a CBPR approach.)

APPLICATION OF METHODS TO DETROIT COMMUNITY-ACADEMIC URBAN RESEARCH CENTER

In this section we present a case example, involving the Detroit Community-Academic Urban Research Center (Detroit URC). The partnership's background, goals and objectives for the partnership evaluation, design issues, and implementation steps are described.

Partnership Background

The Detroit URC is a CBPR partnership of community-based organizations, public health and health care institutions, and academia (see the Acknowledgments at the end of the chapter for a list of the organizations). The Detroit URC began in 1995, with core funding from the Centers for Disease Control and Prevention (CDC), and since 2004, has received funding from the W.K. Kellogg Foundation, The Skillman Foundation, the University of Michigan, and the National Institute on Minority Health and Health Disparities. The Detroit URC operates primarily in selected neighborhoods, initially in east and southwest Detroit in which approximately 100,000 community members reside. The east-side is predominantly African American (approximately 95%) and the southwest area of the city is where the largest percentage of Latinos reside (approximately 60% of the residents). Since 2005 the Detroit URC has expanded its efforts into five other neighborhoods in the city (Israel et al., 2010).

The overall goal of the Detroit URC is to examine and address the social and physical environmental determinants of health aimed at eliminating health inequities. Specific objectives include: to develop and conduct CBPR projects in Detroit as identified by the partner organizations; to increase knowledge and capacity to apply CBPR principles and processes; to enhance the capacity of academic researchers, health professionals, community-based organization members, and community residents to impact policy change; and to educate policymakers and funders on the public health policy implications of the knowledge gained through CBPR projects.

The Detroit URC is governed by a board, comprised of representatives from each of the partner organizations, that meets monthly. During the first two years of its existence, the board adopted a set of CBPR principles that would guide its work, and it determined the partnership's mission, goals and objectives, operating norms and values, and the public health priorities it would address (Israel et al., 2001). At the first meeting of the board, members discussed and adopted operating norms, including: mutual respect, everyone participates, shared leadership, conflicts are brought up and discussed, everyone listens, meetings not dominated by a few members, members agree to disagree, and decisions are made by consensus (Israel et al., 2001). These norms were distributed in print at a subsequent board meeting, periodically reviewed, and used to guide the design and methods of the Detroit URC's evaluation of its partnership.

Evaluation Design and Role of the Evaluation Subcommittee

The overall research design for the Detroit URC evaluation is the case study. A case study design provides an in-depth analysis of the different aspects of a program and is an appropriate design for assessing an ongoing, complex phenomenon in its real-life context (Yin, 1984). The URC uses both a **participatory evaluation** and **formative evaluation** approach (Israel et al., 2001; Lantz et al., 2001), involving program participants and staff in multiple components of the evaluation process (Springett & Wallerstein, 2008). Members of the Detroit URC board have played a critical role in the design, implementation, interpretation, and dissemination of the evaluation results. Thus this evaluation approach adheres to the partnership's CBPR principles (Israel et al., 2001, 2008).

In 1995, board members participated in the selection of the person who was to serve as the initial evaluator. The person selected, a University of Michigan School of Public Health (SPH) faculty member, started attending board meetings in the middle of the first year. After attending two meetings, the evaluator presented to the board some ideas regarding different directions that an evaluation could take and proposed that an evaluation subcommittee be established. The overarching purpose of the subcommittee was to create a mechanism through which some of the board members would participate outside the monthly meetings in the development of an evaluation plan, which would subsequently be recommended to the entire board. The intent was that subcommittee members would meet in person and by conference call in order to discuss potential evaluation questions and strategies, assist the evaluator in crafting an evaluation proposal, review draft documents and data collection instruments, and help lead discussion of proposed evaluation efforts at full board meetings.

Although board members were committed to evaluation and believed it to be important, given the other demands and constraints on their time, no nonacademic partners volunteered initially to participate on the evaluation subcommittee when the evaluator solicited volunteers at two different board meetings. Subsequently, the evaluator contacted two board members representing community-based organizations and asked them individually if they would be willing to join the subcommittee, and they both agreed. They had prior experience with evaluation research in their organizations and were vocal, active members of the board. Thus, during the Detroit URC's first year, the evaluation subcommittee was established, made up of representatives from academia (the evaluator, another SPH faculty member on the board, and a graduate student research assistant), one representative from a community-based organization in eastside Detroit, and one from southwest Detroit. After several years, as the board became more established, the subcommittee was less involved as a separate entity, and the evaluator brought evaluation issues to the entire board for discussion and resolution.

In addition to being participatory, the evaluation design is formative, which means that the results of the evaluation have been shared with the board members on an ongoing basis, for the purpose of using the findings to improve how the board operates and what it accomplishes, and the board members have been involved in the interpretation and application of the evaluation findings to enhance how the board works (Patton, 2002; Rossi, Freeman, & Lipsey, 2004). The evaluation approach also applies both process and impact evaluation (Butterfoss, 2009; Israel et al., 1995; Patton, 2002; Tolma, et al., 2009). As is typical in case studies (Denzin & Lincoln, 2011; Patton, 2002; Yin, 1984), multiple methods for data collection (quantitative and qualitative) and multiple sources of information have been used to understand the process by which the Detroit URC has developed and worked toward meeting its objectives, to provide feedback on an ongoing basis to board members, and to assess the impact of the partnership. As suggested by Yin (1984), three principles of data collection for case studies have been used in evaluating the Detroit URC:

1. Use multiple sources of evidence, also referred to as *triangulation*;

2. Develop a well-organized database; and

3. Maintain a chain of evidence that is consistent with the conceptual framework for the partnership (see Figure 13.1).

The set of data sources that have been used includes in-depth, semistructured interviews; closed-ended survey questionnaires; field notes of URC board meetings; documents and correspondence generated by the URC; and minutes from board and subcommittee meetings (Lantz et al., 2001).

In-Depth, Semistructured Interviews

In the remainder of this section we describe our collaborative approach to the development of the interview protocol, data collection and analysis, data feedback, interpretation, and discussion. We then provide an example of how the results from the in-depth interviews were used to guide changes in the Detroit URC.

Development of Interview Protocol

During the first year of the board's operation (1996), the evaluation subcommittee met two times outside of monthly board meetings to discuss evaluation design issues. The subcommittee decided that it wanted to obtain in-depth information from board members and that individual, face-to-face interviews would be the most effective way to do so. The subcommittee members discussed the advantages and disadvantages of the use of in-depth, semistructured interviews and decided that this was the approach they wanted to use. They decided that a standard set of open-ended questions would be identified, with appropriate follow-up probes, with the understanding that the evaluator would be flexible in the actual asking of the questions, changing wording as appropriate and eliminating questions if necessary.

The evaluator shared with the evaluation subcommittee members a draft of questions based on their discussions of topics that they wanted to be included and the characteristics of partnerships as outlined in the literature (as depicted in Figure 13.1). These draft questions were discussed and then revised based on the guidance of the subcommittee. For example, subcommittee members wanted a clear distinction between benefits gained by individuals and those gained by organizations when gathering information regarding perceived benefits of participating in the partnership, and questions were added accordingly. The topics that were covered in the interview questions included expectations and hopes for the first year and whether they were met; major accomplishments, barriers, and challenges and recommendations for meeting them; personal knowledge or skills gained; tangible benefits from an organization's affiliation with the URC; and examples of exchanges of information or assistance or support between partner organizations (see Appendix H for the interview protocol).

These in-depth interviews were conducted with members of the Detroit URC board originally in 1996 and again in 1999 and 2002. Many of the same questions were asked, and in 1999, based on discussions with the evaluation subcommittee and the board as a whole, questions were added to address several topics of particular interest. The new topics covered included factors that facilitated accomplishments, establishment of new relationships among partner organizations, and recommendations to other partnerships on what went well and what to do differently (see Appendix H). Some of these topics were added because the Detroit URC was participating with the CDC and two other Urban Research Center sites in a cross-site evaluation that year (Metzler et al., 2003). In 2002, only one of these "new" topics (factors that facilitated accomplishments) was retained in the interview protocol, and several other topics were added, based on discussions with the board, that were especially germane to members at that time. These topics addressed benefits of the Detroit URC to the community and ways to improve benefits, costs to or problems for an individual or an organization because of affiliation with the partnership, and considerations if funding were to end and options for future funding (see Appendix H).

Data Collection

The first set of interviews was conducted in late 1996 with current board members (n = 15), former board members (n = 3), and staff (n = 5), for a 100% response rate (Lantz et al., 2001). The second set was conducted in late 1999 with current board members (n = 15) and staff (n = 3), for a 100% response rate (Lantz et al., 2001). The third set was conducted in 2002 with 16 board members and staff, for an 84% response rate.

The interviews were conducted by the evaluator with a graduate student assistant and were documented through verbatim field notes that they each took. The interviews conducted in 2002 were also tape-recorded. The interviews averaged one hour in length and for board members were carried out most frequently in the member's place of work. The interviewees signed a consent form and were guaranteed confidentiality.

Data Analysis

The two sets of written notes taken at each interview were reconciled and then transcribed (Lantz et al., 2001). In 2002, audiotapes were used as a backup to supplement the handwritten notes taken during the interview. Using a qualitative data analysis approach of *open coding* (Corbin & Strauss, 2008), the transcripts were reviewed systematically by the evaluator and her assistant, and categories that captured embedded concepts or meanings were identified from within the interviews as a whole as the data were reviewed (not beforehand) and then compared across the interviews (Patton, 2002). The results of the qualitative data analysis were also stratified by subgroup (university-based and Detroit-based board members) to identify similarities and differences in responses. Due to the small numbers and issues of confidentiality, the results were not further subdivided, for example, by responses from Detroit-based community-based organization partners and health service provider partners.

Data Feedback, Interpretation, and Discussion

Several months after the completion of the first set of interviews, the evaluator presented the results to the evaluation subcommittee members for their review and comment. Using their input, the evaluator developed a six-page report of evaluation results that she presented to the entire board at one of its monthly meetings. The findings were organized according to the topics covered in the interview protocol, for example, expectations, accomplishments, and challenges and barriers. The results were presented for all of the interviews combined, except where there were meaningful differences in the ways university-based and Detroit-based board members responded. For example, several university respondents reported that their main expectations for the first year of the partnership related to the goals of establishing a common agenda and developing processes and infrastructure for the board. However, only two Detroit partners expressed similar expectations; the majority of Detroit-based partners stated that their primary expectation was to see new CBPR projects implemented during the first year, particularly in southwest Detroit.

The results of the interviews conducted in 1999 and 2002 were organized by question and presented by the evaluator to the board, using a PowerPoint presentation format. In addition, from her overall analysis of the data the evaluator identified a set of "issues for ongoing discussion" that were highlighted and discussed by the board. For example, an issue addressed in both 1999 and 2002 was the degree to which people believed resources were fairly distributed among organizations participating in the Detroit URC. During the data collection process for the evaluation, a number of respondents raised concerns regarding perceived inequities in financial and other benefits of Detroit URC participation, with the main concern being that the academic partner seemed to be benefiting disproportionately when compared to the community partners. Information regarding this concern was presented to the board and became a starting point for ongoing discussions and action on a number of related issues (Lantz et al., 2001).

Program Changes Based on In-Depth Interview Results

Although the focus of this chapter is on the data collection methods themselves and their application within the context of CBPR, given the important formative evaluation dimension of this approach, an example is provided here of how the results of the in-depth interviews were used to guide changes in the Detroit URC. One finding from the first set of interviews was a suggestion by several of the Detroit partners that they would like to see the partnership expand to include a broader range of community partners. When this was reported to the board, it was decided that this issue should be considered in more depth. Over several meetings the board discussed the potential benefits and disadvantages of adding new community partners and reached a consensus that it did not want to do so at that time but that it wanted to revisit the issue a year later. In the subsequent wave of interviews, this topic was again identified, and at that point the board decided it wanted to add new community-based organizations to the partnership.

Closed-Ended Survey Questionnaire

In the remainder of this section we describe our collaborative approach to the development of the survey questionnaire, data collection and analysis, data feedback, interpretation, and discussion. We then present a number of program changes that have been made over the years based on the results of the closed-ended survey questionnaires.

Development of Survey Questionnaire

At the end of the Detroit URC's first year, subcommittee members decided that in addition to the semistructured, in-depth interviews, they also wanted to use a closed-ended survey questionnaire with the board members. The purpose of the survey was to assess, in a standardized fashion, the partners' impressions about and attitudes toward different aspects of the partnership's efforts (Lantz et al., 2001). Drawing on the operating norms generated and adopted by the board from characteristics of effective groups (described earlier), on the literature on partnership effectiveness factors (as discussed and depicted in Figure 13.1), and on the CBPR principles and specific objectives of the Detroit URC, and building on a questionnaire initially developed and revised in the context of two other participatory research efforts (Israel et al., 1989; Schulz et al., 2003), the evaluator drafted a questionnaire that was initially reviewed and revised by members of the evaluation subcommittee. (See Appendix I for the survey questionnaire.) The questionnaire uses mostly Likert scale response categories (for example, ranging from "strongly agree" to "strongly disagree") and, in accordance with Figure 13.1, includes items related to:

- Structural characteristics, such as meeting organization, facilitation, and staffing;

- Group dynamics characteristics, such as leadership and open communication; and

- Intermediate measures of partnership effectiveness, such as effectiveness in achieving the group's goals, general satisfaction, benefits of participation, and sense of ownership or belonging to the group (Schulz et al., 2003).

During 1997–2002, when the initial evaluator was working with the board, the survey questionnaire was administered at four different times (1997, 1999, 2001, 2002), with each version including all the items on the original questionnaire. Additional items were included in subsequent years to assess more specifically levels of trust, decision-making procedures, the degree to which CBPR principles are followed, role of the funder, and accomplishments or impact of the group. When core funding from CDC ended in 2004, the role of the initial evaluator concluded. In 2007, a post-doctoral scholar at the University of Michigan, involved in the

W.K. Kellogg Foundation–funded Community Health Scholars Program, became involved as the evaluator to administer the closed-ended questionnaire. In working with the board as a whole, decisions were made to delete some questions which were no longer relevant, and to add others that would better assess aspects of and changes over time in what was now a long-standing partnership. Additional items addressed more specifically levels of participation, board capacity and operations, communication, benefits/challenges/limitations of involvement, results of strategic planning process, and policy impact (see Appendix I).

Data Collection

The survey questionnaire was mailed to all board members, along with a postage-paid return envelope, in 1997, 1999, 2001, 2002, and 2007 and response rates were 100%, 100%, 95%, 86%, and 94% respectively. Across the years the board numbered approximately twenty individuals, representing 10 organizations and institutions. The self-administered questionnaire took about 15 to 25 minutes to complete.

Data Analysis

The analysis of the data from the survey questionnaires was carried out by the evaluator and involved descriptive statistics (that is, frequency distributions and comparison of means). For each of the surveys the data were analyzed for the entire sample and for the two main subgroups: university-based board members and Detroit-based board members. Given that the total number of board members is so small (n = 20), no statistical tests of significance were computed when comparing results across the subgroups. Rather, the results were examined to identify any patterns that were different across the two main partner groups. Similarly, comparisons of the frequency distributions for all respondents for the same questionnaire items were made across the years that the surveys were conducted.

Data Feedback, Interpretation, and Discussion

The results of the analysis of both the initial survey administration and the initial in-depth interviews were included when the evaluator shared the evaluation findings with the evaluation subcommittee and developed the first feedback report (described earlier) and subsequently presented the findings to the board. At this presentation, the frequency distributions for all the questionnaire items were provided, along with a verbal summary of the key findings. In subsequent years, at a regularly scheduled board meeting, the evaluator provided the frequency distributions for all the items and presented PowerPoint slides of key findings across major question categories (for example, perceptions of trust, decision making, general satisfaction, and perceived impact). Major differences that were found over time and between the university partners and the Detroit partners were highlighted. For example, in 1999, 53% of the board members agreed with the statement, "I have adequate knowledge of the URC budget, URC resources, and how resources are allocated," and in 2001, 70% agreed. In further examination by subgroup in 2001, it was noted that 100% of the university respondents agreed, whereas only 43% of the Detroit partners agreed. The board engaged in a series of discussions following the presentation of these results. One result of these discussions was the decision to present budget and other financial information to board members on a more regular schedule and in a manner that is transparent and allows time for discussion.

Program Changes Based on Survey Questionnaire Results

A number of program changes have been made over the years based on the results of the closed-ended survey questionnaires (Lantz et al., 2001). For example, the questionnaire asked whether (1) "certain individuals' opinions get weighed more than they should" and whether (2) "one person or group dominates at URC board meetings." In 1997 and 1999, the responses of those who agreed or strongly agreed with the first statement were 50% and 53%, respectively. In 1997 and 1999, the same responses to the second statement came from 28% and 42% of the group, respectively. There was no clear pattern regarding the person or group thought to dominate, but in discussion of these results at the board meeting, concern was expressed that changes needed to be made and that everyone needed to pay attention to fostering more equitable levels of participation. The facilitator of the board meetings tried consciously to encourage all members to participate actively at these meetings. In 2001 and 2002, the responses to the first statement were considerably lower (18% and 13%, respectively), as were the responses to the second statement (24% and 19%, respectively). In 2007, a new item was added to the questionnaire to assess satisfaction with visibility of the URC within Detroit. Only 28% of the board members indicated that they agreed or strongly agreed that they were satisfied with the URC's visibility. The board discussed this finding over several meetings and decided to take a number of steps to increase visibility, for example, developed a Detroit URC logo, and upgraded the URC Web site.

CHALLENGES AND LIMITATIONS

In the course of our evaluation activities, we have identified challenges and limitations in the use of both in-depth interviews and closed-ended questionnaires. Although in-depth interviews provide rich information that can contribute to an enhanced understanding of the phenomenon being investigated, they are extremely labor and time intensive, which necessitates extensive resources, and they require considerable skill on the part of the evaluator. The time needed to conduct the analysis often means the results may not be presented until several months after the data have been collected, which can be frustrating for the partners waiting for the results and because changes can occur over that time period that might make the results less relevant. Several of the difficulties related to the use of closed-ended questionnaires are associated with the method itself. First, the use of closed-ended questions limits both the responses that can be provided and the issues that can be addressed (Schulz et al., 2003). Furthermore, the wording and interpretation of the questions themselves can be problematic. It is likely that not everyone interprets each question or the response categories in the same way. As one community member emphasized at a board meeting, some people are not going to indicate the best or most positive response category for most items simply because they believe "there is always room for improvement. This doesn't mean, however, that we have big problems."

Given the small number of members in most partnerships and the turnover that occurs, several challenges and limitations arise in the data analysis of closed-ended questionnaires. First, only simple descriptive statistics can be used, and it is not possible to apply tests of statistical significance to assess whether there have been any changes over time (Schulz et al., 2003). Second, we chose to assess change in the group as a whole over time by aggregating the results across respondents at two points in time, rather than tracking change in individual respondents over time. Although such an approach is useful for capturing what is occurring within the group over time, if there are any changes it is not possible to determine whether they are due to changes in group membership or events that have happened in the group or events that may have had an impact on some members of the group but not others (Schulz et al., 2003).

Another challenge, the inability to analyze the data by many different subgroupings, relates to partnership size and data analysis and applies to the use of interviews as well as questionnaires. It is critically important to guarantee confidentiality, and the analysis of data by small subgroups would run the risk of exposing the responses of individual group members (Schulz et al., 2003). Hence, although we were able to analyze the data for two categories, university-based and Detroit-based partners, we were not able to further examine the data by Detroit-based health providers and Detroit-based community-based organizations. There might have been some important differences there that we were not able to identify.

An additional challenge, and one that also applies to the participatory evaluation process and both data collection methods, is the time constraints on the partners involved. Participating in the evaluation subcommittee and the in-depth interviews in particular, but also completing the closed-ended questionnaire, can place time pressures on the partners' already busy schedules. This can cause additional strain on the evaluator, who may have to be persistent with members in order to obtain their input and collect the data, which can in turn create tension in the relationships between the evaluator and the members.

Another specific area of concern was the subcommittee's and the board's lack of involvement in the data analysis. Although the evaluator certainly considers it "appropriate" for the community partners to be involved in the data analysis, a decision was made not to do so in this instance due to the confidential nature of the responses. Given the small number of respondents for both the closed-ended questionnaire and the in-depth, semistructured interviews, it would not have been possible for community partners to review and analyze the data without identifying who the respondents were, and this would have violated confidentiality. Importantly, as described earlier, the evaluation subcommittee and board members were actively involved in a number of meetings in which the results of the data were fed back and the members engaged in discussions to interpret the findings.

A further potential limitation is that although these two data collection methods have provided a wealth of information for assessing the URC partnership process, there may be important dimensions that they do not measure. For example, as indicated in Figure 13.1, drawing on the work of Lasker and colleagues (Lasker & Weiss, 2003; Lasker et al., 2001), we consider *synergy*, defined as the actions and products that a partnership can create when its members combine their skills and resources, to be an intermediate measure of partnership effectiveness. However, to date, we have not directly measured this concept with either the interview protocol or the survey questionnaire.

An additional set of challenges inherent in the evaluation of CBPR partnerships involves decisions regarding who is going to lead the partnership evaluation efforts and the degree to which the evaluation process is participatory. Should the evaluation be led by an individual or team external to and ostensibly without a vested interest in the partnership, or should it be led by a member or member organization of the partnership? In addition, to what degree should the members of a CBPR partnership have input into the design, implementation, and interpretation of its evaluation? One can think of these questions as a 2 × 2 matrix, with an internal versus external evaluator on one dimension, and a participatory versus nonparticipatory process on the other. Challenges arise in that there are four possible general approaches here, with of course great variation in the actual implementation of a selected approach.

Debates about the pros and cons of internal versus external evaluators have long been addressed in the evaluation research literature (Conley-Tyler, 2005; Cronbach et al., 1981). Advantages to external evaluators include that they are more likely to: be viewed as having less of a vested interest and thus being more objective; have relevant evaluation experience; collect honest information from participants; and offer criticism that will lead to program improvement (Conley-Tyler, 2005; Rossi, Freeman, & Lipsey, 2004). In contrast, advantages to internal evaluators include: a deeper knowledge of the program and its context; an increased ability to collect certain types of information given the level of trust that is likely to exist; and increased likelihood of collecting useful evaluation results (Conley-Tyler, 2005; Patton, 1997). Challenges in the evaluation of CBPR partnerships arise in the tension between the desire for an "objective" and valid evaluation approach with the need to ensure a process that all members of a partnership trust and believe will reflect their unique perspective and voice. Challenges also arise in the tension between the desire to follow the participatory principles of a CBPR partnership in all activities—including its evaluation—and the desire to avoid appearances that a partnership is "evaluating itself" and thus not engaging in an objective or rigorous process.

LESSONS LEARNED AND IMPLICATIONS FOR PRACTICE

Given the strengths and limitations of the evaluation approach presented here, we recommend, as have others, the use of multiple methods (for example, both closed-ended survey questionnaires and in-depth, semistructured interviews) as a way to complement and enhance the knowledge gained from any one method and to increase the acceptance of the findings by all partners (Butterfoss, 2009; Cheadle et al., 2008; Denzin & Lincoln, 2011; Israel et al., 1995; Tolma et al., 2009). It is often suggested that these methods can be used sequentially, for example, qualitative interviews may be conducted first and used to inform the development of closed-ended survey questionnaires, or qualitative interviews may be conducted after a survey is administered to assist in explaining the meaning of the quantitative data (Denzin & Lincoln, 2011; Israel et al., 1995). It is also frequently suggested that these methods can be used simultaneously, allowing triangulation with the results of both methods to assess convergence as well as differences in the findings (Denzin & Lincoln, 2011; Israel et al., 1995). With the evaluation of the Detroit URC board, the initial interviews and questionnaires were conducted within several months of each other (1996/1997), and the data were analyzed and the results presented at the same time. The two methods were used nearly a year apart in subsequent years (through 2002). This approach was beneficial in that there was an assessment annually that obtained useful information, using one method or the other, and it was not as demanding on everyone's time as annual in-depth interviews would have been. Furthermore, the closed-ended survey questionnaires provided standardized data, which could be compared over the years, including the subsequent survey administration carried out in 2007. The use of in-depth interviews during the early phases of partnership formation and development was particularly valuable in that it allowed for issues that were not covered in the initial survey questionnaire to be identified and discussed, some of which were subsequently added to the questionnaire. As depicted in Figure 13.1, and in other conceptual models (for example, Wallerstein et al., 2008), a general set of issues is applicable across partnerships, and these issues can guide the development of interview protocols and survey questionnaires. It is important that a partnership develop its own conceptual framework or logic model, and the specific questions asked need to be tailored to the context and the culture of the partnership. For example, with the Detroit URC board, the collectively determined operating norms that grew out of group members' experiences with effective groups suggested many of the questions initially included in the closed-ended questionnaire (Israel et al., 2001). This joint process also served to enhance the partners' buy-in and sense of ownership when it came to the evaluation (Schulz et al., 2003). It is also necessary to recognize that the measurement instruments used and the questions asked in a partnership evaluation are part of an iterative process, with revisions and additions made over time as the partnership evolves. Partnerships go through different phases or stages and some of the dimensions that need to be evaluated also change over time (Tolma et al., 2009). For example, with the Detroit URC, during the early phases of partnership formation emphasis was placed on assessing issues such as trust, relationship building, and communication. Although these areas remained important, as the partnership evolved into a long-term working entity the evaluation has evolved to also address dimensions of benefits and costs of participation, impact of the partnership, and sustainability.

This tailoring of the evaluation to the specific partnership is particularly critical for partnerships that include members from diverse communities and ethnic groups. Given the long-standing inequities that exist and the understandable mistrust of research in communities of color (Israel et al., 1998), an assessment of the partnership process needs to examine, for example, the extent to which community partners are engaged on an equal power basis (Wallerstein, 1999), the reasons and incentives for members to "come around the table," how and why diverse interests work together for common goals, and the challenges and opportunities provided by the partnership for serving different interests in diverse communities.

The use of an evaluation approach that is participatory is particularly important in the context of a CBPR partnership. The active involvement of all partners in the evaluation is consistent with the core principles of CBPR. Every partnership needs to decide how it wants this participatory process to occur. For example, it may be decided that an evaluation subcommittee is needed to work closely with the evaluator or that the entire partnership will serve in that capacity.

Furthermore, a partnership may decide that it is interested primarily in influencing and being involved in the data collection, interpretation, and dissemination activities but not in data entry and data analysis per se. What is critical here is that the partnership as a whole makes these decisions, rather than the evaluator or academic partners.

As part of this participatory process, a key decision that CBPR partnerships need to make is whether to engage an evaluator who is internal or external to the partner organizations involved. Based on the experience of the Detroit URC, there are several lessons that can be learned from exploring why we chose to have an internal evaluator. First, it is important to note that the lead evaluator (there have been two to date), although from the University of Michigan, was in the first instance only involved in the role of partnership evaluator, and in the second instance was primarily in the evaluator role. This reduces some of the concerns about objectivity and conflict of interest, since the evaluators were not directly involved in the interventions or activities as long-term members of the partnership. Second, it is not necessarily the case that external evaluators are always more objective than internal ones (Mathison, 1994). All evaluators, whether internal or external, struggle with how best to gather information about a program or intervention that is objective, valid, and useful (Patton, 1997). As Cronbach and colleagues argue, what is essential is that the evaluator has some degree of separation from the project/partnership, not that they have no relationship or "intimacy" (Cronbach et al., 1981). It is the evaluation approach or methods implemented that determine the degree of objectivity and validity, not simply whether the evaluator is internal or external. Third, the key elements of trust and shared understanding in a successful CBPR partnership also apply to its evaluation. In a CBPR model, the evaluator must have trust and buy-in, a deep understanding of the partnership, its history and goals, and its dynamics to fully engage the partnership in the evaluation activities, to achieve high response rates, and to elicit honest and frank responses. This is most likely to be someone from a member organization.

The formative component of the evaluation, with its emphasis on ongoing feedback and group interpretation of the data, for the purpose of improving the partnership, is particularly germane when evaluating a CBPR partnership. This feedback and interpretation, and any subsequent actions based on the results, need to occur in a timely manner. Given the volume of data collected, it is necessary to be selective in presenting and discussing results in meetings with the partnership as a whole. Here again, the evaluator needs to work with a subcommittee or the entire partnership to determine what criteria to use in selecting the findings to present (for example, identify issues in which substantial changes have occurred or not over time, choose differences across subgroups) (Schulz et al., 2003).

The evaluation of a CBPR partnership's process and impact needs to begin as soon as possible and continue throughout the duration of the partnership. It is important to recognize that the collection of baseline data, in the traditional sense, is not possible because by the time of the first data collection point, a partnership may well have been working together for a year or more. Therefore it is valuable to begin documenting the efforts of the partnership (for example, through field notes of meetings) as soon as possible. In addition, the first major data collection point (for example, in-depth interviews or a survey questionnaire) becomes a key time with which all subsequent data results can be compared. The ongoing collection of data using similar methods then provides beneficial information for assessing the partnership's progress over time. With the Detroit URC board, we have now been able to compare the responses to closed-ended questions over five points in time. In addition, the first time that the in-depth interviews were conducted, one of the major "challenges" identified was bringing the southwest and eastside communities together for a common purpose. When the interviews were conducted subsequently, one of the major "strengths" identified was that the Latino community (southwest Detroit) and the African American community (eastside Detroit) were working together on common issues for the first time in the history of the city. Thus, the use of these data collection methods needs to extend beyond capturing only a snapshot at one point in time to capturing multiple points in order to assess the dynamic, evolving partnership process and its impact.

The application of these two data collection methods requires an investment in time and resources on the part of the partnership. Where external funding is involved, some of the costs of conducting an evaluation need to be budgeted up front. Although this might be seen as taking resources away from other program functions of the partnership, the knowledge gained and changes made can contribute greatly to the effectiveness of the partnership. We suggest, as have others (Butterfoss, 2009), that it is better to evaluate some aspects of the partnership in some small way even if the funds are not available to implement a more comprehensive evaluation using the data collection methods discussed here. For example, there are three basic questions that can be used to assess a specific meeting or the partnership more generally; these can either be discussed as a group at a regular meeting of the partnership, or members can be asked to write down their responses and then the results can be summarized and shared, as appropriate. These questions are: (1) What did/do you value most about the meeting/partnership?; (2) What did/do you value least about the meeting/partnership?; and (3) What suggestions do you have for how to improve the meeting/partnership? Here again, the extensiveness and resources put into a partnership evaluation need to be discussed openly by the partners. Furthermore, given that the resources needed often involve the group members' time, the partnership needs to decide the extent to which and the ways in which this time commitment can be managed and members compensated for it.

SUMMARY

Given the growing emphasis on the use of partnership approaches, particularly CBPR, to address health problems and eliminate health inequities, the evaluation of the partnership process is critical for improving partnership functioning and enhancing the likelihood of partnership success. In this chapter we have examined the use of two methods for these purposes, in-depth interviews and closed-ended survey questionnaires, using the Detroit Community-Academic Urban Research Center as a case example. There are a number of useful resources, measurement instruments, workbooks, and Web-based materials available for partnership evaluation purposes (see the downloadable supplement for this chapter for examples). The critical component is that all members of the partnership are actively engaged in the evaluation process (for example, design, implementation, interpretation, dissemination), and that the methods used are developed in accordance with the local context, culture, and goals of the partnership. As more such evaluations are conducted, assessing the partnership process, its impact, and the association between the two, researchers and communities will gain an increased understanding of the factors that contribute to effective community-based participatory research partnerships, and the strategies for affecting these factors in ways that contribute to improved health and quality of life.

KEY TERMS

Closed-ended survey questionnaires

Formative evaluation

In-depth, semistructured interviews

Participatory evaluation

DISCUSSION QUESTIONS

1. Based on the conceptual framework described here (Figure 13.1), the in-depth semistructured interview protocol (Appendix H), and your understanding of the literature, in what ways might you revise and/or add to the interview questions? Why? Why not?

2. Based on the conceptual framework described here (Figure 13.1), the closed-ended survey questionnaire presented (Appendix I), and your understanding of the literature, in what ways might you revise and/or add to the survey questions? Why? Why not?

3. You are part of a CBPR partnership that is designing an evaluation of the partnership process. Based on the experience and lessons learned from the Detroit URC, what methods and strategies would you incorporate (for example, use of multiple methods, formative, participatory, internal or external evaluator)?

REFERENCES

Brooks, P. E. (2010). Ethnographic evaluation of a research partnership between two African American communities and a university. *Ethnicity & Disease*, *20*(1 Suppl 2), S2–21–29.

Butterfoss, F. D. (2009). Evaluating partnerships to prevent and manage chronic disease. *Preventing Chronic Disease*, *6*(2), A64.

Butterfoss, F. D., & Kegler, M. (2009). The community coalition action theory. In R. J. DiClemente, R. A. Crosby, & M. C. Kegler (Eds.), *Emerging theories in health promotion practice and research: Strategies for improving public health* (2nd ed., pp. 237–276). San Francisco: Jossey-Bass.

Cheadle, A., Hsu, C., Schwartz, P. M., Pearson, D., Greenwald, H. P., Beery, W. L., et al. (2008). Involving local health departments in community health partnerships: Evaluation results from the partnership for the public's health initiative. *Journal of Urban Health*, *85*(2), 162–177.

Conley-Tyler, M. (2005). A fundamental choice: Internal or external evaluation? *Evaluation Journal of Australasia*, 4(1–2), 3–11.

Corbin, J., & Strauss, A. (2008). *Basics of qualitative research* (3rd ed.). Thousand Oaks, CA: Sage.

Cronbach, L. J., Ambron, S. R., Dornbusch, S. M., Hess, R. D., Hornik, R. C., Phillips, D. C., Walker, D. F., & Weiner, S. S. (1981). *Towards reform of program evaluation: Aims, methods and institutional arrangements*. San Francisco: Jossey-Bass.

Curie, M., King, G., Rosenbaum, P., Law, M., Kertoy, M., & Specht, J. (2005). A model of impacts of research partnerships in health and social services. *Evaluation and Program Planning, 28*, 400–412.

Denzin, N. K., & Lincoln, Y. S. (Eds.). (2011). *The Sage handbook of qualitative research* (4th ed.). Thousand Oaks, CA: Sage.

Fontana, A., & Frey, J. H. (2000). Interviewing: The art of science. In N. K. Denzin & Y. S. Lincoln (Eds.), *Handbook of qualitative research* (pp. 361–376). Thousand Oaks, CA: Sage.

Fowler, F. J. (2008). *Survey research methods* (4th ed.). Thousand Oaks, CA: Sage.

Israel, B. A., Cummings, K. M., Dignan, M. B., Heaney, C. A., Perales, D. P., Simons-Morton, B. G., et al. (1995). Evaluation of health education programs: Current assessment and future directions. *Health Education Quarterly, 22*(2), 364–389.

Israel, B. A., Lichtenstein, R., Lantz, P. M., McGranaghan, R. J., Allen, A., Guzman, J. R., et al. (2001). The Detroit Community-Academic Urban Research Center: Development, implementation and evaluation. *Journal of Public Health Management and Practice, 7*(5), 1–19.

Israel, B. A., Schulz, A. J., Parker, E. A., & Becker, A. B. (1998). Review of community-based research: Assessing partnership approaches to improve public health. *Annual Review of Public Health, 19*, 173–202.

Israel, B. A., Schulz, A. J., Parker, E. A., Becker, A. B., Allen, A., & Guzman, J. R. (2008). Critical issues in developing and following community-based participatory research principles. In M. Minkler & N. Wallerstein (Eds.), *Community-based participatory research for health: From process to outcomes* (2nd ed., pp. 47–66). San Francisco: Jossey-Bass.

Israel, B. A., Schurman, S. J., & House, J. S. (1989). Action research on occupational stress: Involving workers as researchers. *International Journal of Health Services, 19*(1), 135–155.

Israel, B. A., Coombe, C. M., Cheezum, R. R., Schulz, A. J., McGranaghan, R., Lichtenstein, R., et al. (2010). Community-based participatory research: A capacity building approach for policy advocacy aimed at eliminating health disparities. *American Journal of Public Health, 100*, 2094–2102.

Johnson, D. W., & Johnson, F. P. (1982). *Joining together: Group theory and group skills* (2nd ed.). Upper Saddle River, NJ: Prentice Hall.

Johnson, D. W., & Johnson, F. P. (1997). *Joining Together: Group theory and group skills* (6th ed.). Needham Heights, MA: Allyn & Bacon.

Johnson, D. W., & Johnson, F. P. (2008). *Joining together: Group theory and group skills* (10th ed.). Needham Heights, MA: Allyn & Bacon.

Johnson, J. C., Hayden, U. T., Thomas, N., Groce-Martin, J., Henry, T., Guerra, T., et al. (2009). Building community participatory research coalitions from the ground up: The Philadelphia area research community coalition. *Progress in Community Health Partnerships, 3*(1), 61–72.

Kegler, M. C., Hall, S. M., & Kiser, M. (2010). Facilitators, challenges, and collaborative activities in faith and health partnerships to address health disparities. *Health Education & Behavior, 37*(5), 665–679.

King, G., Servais, M., Kertoy, M., Specht, J., Currie, M., Rosenbaum, P., et al. (2009). A measure of community members' perceptions of the impacts of research partnerships in health and social services. *Evaluation and Program Planning, 32*(3), 289–299.

Lantz, P. M., Viruell-Fuentes, E., Israel, B. A., Softley, D., & Guzman, J. R. (2001). Can communities and academia work together on public health research? Evaluation results from a community-based participatory research partnership in Detroit. *Journal of Urban Health, 78*(3), 495–507.

Lasker, R. D., & Weiss, E. S. (2003). Broadening participation in community problem solving: A multidisciplinary model to support collaborative practice and research. *Journal of Urban Health, 80*(1), 14–60.

Lasker, R. D., Weiss, E. S., & Miller, R. (2001). Partnership synergy: A practical framework for studying and strengthening the collaborative advantage. *Milbank Quarterly, 79*(2), 179–205.

Mathison, S. (1994). Rethinking the evaluator role: Partnerships between organizations and evaluators. *Evaluation and Program Planning, 17*(3), 299–304.

Metzler, M. M., Higgins, D. L., Beeker, C. G., Freudenberg, N., Lantz, P. M., Senturia, K. D. et al. (2003). Addressing urban health in Detroit, New York, and Seattle through community-based participatory research partnerships. *American Journal of Public Health, 93*(5), 803–811.

Minkler, M., & Wallerstein, N. (Eds.). (2008). *Community-based participatory research for health: From process to outcomes* (2nd ed.) San Francisco: Jossey-Bass.

Nardi, P. M. (2006). *Doing survey research: A guide to quantitative research methods* (2nd ed.). Boston: Pearson Allyn & Bacon.

Patton, M. Q. (1997). *Utilization-focused evaluation* (3rd ed., pp. 138–143). Thousand Oaks, CA: Sage.

Patton, M. Q. (2002). *Qualitative evaluation and research methods* (3rd ed.). Thousand Oaks, CA: Sage.

Plumb, M., Collins, N., Cordeiro, J. N., & Kavanaugh-Lynch, M. (2008). Assessing process and outcomes: Evaluating community-based participatory research. *Progress in Community Health Partnerships, 2*(2), 85–97.

Rossi, P. H., Freeman, H. E., & Lipsey, M. W. (2004). *Evaluation: A systematic approach* (7th ed.). Thousand Oaks, CA: Sage.

Schulz, A. J., Israel, B. A., & Lantz, P. M. (2003). Instrument for evaluating dimensions of group dynamics within community-based participatory research partnerships. *Evaluation and Program Planning, 26,* 249–262.

Shaw, M. E. (1981). *Group dynamics: The psychology of small group behavior* (3rd ed.). New York: McGraw-Hill.

Sofaer, S. (2000). *Working together, moving ahead: A manual to support effective community health coalitions.* New York: Baruch College School of Public Affairs.

Springett, J., & Wallerstein, N. (2008). Issues in participatory evaluation. In M. Minkler & N. Wallerstein (Eds.), *Community-based participatory research for health: From process to outcomes* (2nd ed., pp. 199–220). San Francisco: Jossey-Bass.

Tolma, E. L., Cheney, M. K., Troup, P., & Hann, N. (2009). Designing the process evaluation for the collaborative planning of a local turning point partnership. *Health Promotion Practice, 10*(4), 537–548.

Wallerstein, N. (1999). Power between evaluator and community: Research relationships within New Mexico's healthier communities. *Social Science & Medicine, 49*(1), 39–53.

Wallerstein, N., Oetzel, J., Duran, B., Tafoya, G., Belone, L., & Rae, R. (2008). What predicts outcomes in CBPR? In M. Minkler & N. Wallerstein (Eds.), *Community-based participatory research for health: From process to outcomes* (2nd ed., pp. 371–394). San Francisco: Jossey-Bass.

Weiss, E. S., Anderson, R. M., & Lasker, R. D. (2002). Making the most of collaboration: Exploring the relationship between partnership synergy and partnership functioning. *Health Education & Behavior, 29*(6), 683–698.

Yin, R. K. (1984). *Case study research: Design and methods.* Thousand Oaks, CA: Sage.

Acknowledgments: The authors appreciate the involvement of all of the partners involved in the Detroit Community-Academic Urban Research Center since it was established in 1995, who have contributed greatly to the success of the partnership described in this chapter and to enhancing the authors' understanding of CBPR and research methods for evaluating CBPR (Butzel Family Center, Community Health and Social Services Center, Inc., Community In Schools, Detroit Department of Health and Wellness Promotion, Detroit Hispanic Development Corporation, Detroiters Working for Environmental Justice, Friends of Parkside, Henry Ford Health System, Kettering/Butzel Health Initiative, Latino Family Services, Neighborhood Service Organization, Southwest Counseling and Development Services, University of Michigan Schools of Public Health, Nursing and Social Work, and Warren/Conner Development Coalition). (See www .detroiturc.org for more details.) We acknowledge the contribution of Shawn Kimmel, postdoctoral scholar funded by the W.K. Kellogg Foundation, for his role in the Detroit URC's partnership evaluation conducted in 2007–2008. The authors also thank Sue Andersen for her assistance in preparing the manuscript.

FEEDBACK, INTERPRETATION, DISSEMINATION, AND APPLICATION OF RESULTS

Part Six focuses on four components of the two "final" phases of the CBPR process, as presented in Chapter One, Figure 1.1: feedback and interpretation of research findings, and dissemination and translation/application of research findings to guide the development of interventions and policy formation. Feedback and interpretation of findings involves all research partners and participants in reviewing results from data analysis to share their reactions and possible corrections, as well as their interpretation of what the results may mean in the context of their community (Brenner & Manice, 2011; Horowitz, Robinson, & Seifer, 2009). As Stoecker (2003) noted, although it is optimal for data analysis to be done collaboratively by all research partners, at the very least, data analysis should be done with strict accountability to the community. Such accountability can be ensured by feeding back results to the community to engage them in reacting to the findings, including correcting findings, and offering their interpretation of what these findings mean for their community.

Equally important to the CBPR process is the dissemination of findings to all research partners and communities through multiple venues and in ways that are understandable, respectful, and useful (Boyer, Mohatt, Pasker, Drew, & McGlone, 2007; Israel, Schulz, Parker, & Becker, 1998; Pufall, Jones, McEwen, Lyall, Peregrine, & Edge, 2011). Moreover, dissemination of results is an increasing requirement of funding agencies (Ammerman et al., 2003; Green et al., 2003; Pufall et al., 2011) and an expectation of study participants and their communities (Lopez, Parker, Edgren, & Brakefield-Caldwell, 2005). Nonetheless, broad dissemination activities can be challenging for academic partners, who may have to go beyond the usual bounds of scientific journals and audiences (Chavez, Duran, Baker, Avila, & Wallerstein, 2008; Flaskerud & Anderson, 1999). Dissemination can also be challenging for community members, who may have little time, training, or both to develop guidelines for, plan, and conduct dissemination activities.

Finally, the translation and application of research findings for intervention development and policy formation is a crucial link to CBPR's commitment to action (Ahmed & Palermo, 2010; Cook, 2008). As noted by Themba and Minkler (2003), one of the critical differences between CBPR and other research approaches is CBPR's commitment to action and helping to foster social changes as an integral part of the research process.

In Part Six, the six chapters collectively illustrate the four elements of data feedback, interpretation, dissemination, and translation/application of research findings. They show how various data collection methods used within CBPR relate to these four elements. The data collection methods used include, for example: community forums, photo-elicitation, photovoice, document review, mapping, survey questionnaire, elicitation dialogues, focus group interview, and secondary data analysis. These chapters also describe process methods that were used to ensure active participation of all partners in the activities of this phase.

In Chapter Fourteen, Parker, Robins, Israel, Brakefield-Caldwell, Edgren, O'Toole, Wilkins, Batterman, and Lewis describe the development and application of guidelines for the dissemination of results from the Community Action Against Asthma partnership in Detroit, Michigan. The authors offer valuable detail on how and why the partnership decided that they needed guidelines for dissemination and created a structure to develop both the guidelines and procedures for disseminating results. The guidelines provide a useful template for other partnerships to consider and adopt. The authors present concrete examples of procedures and mechanisms to feed back specific components of the research findings to project participants, build in structured time for participants to interpret these findings, and share the results more broadly with community members. The authors also highlight both the successes and challenges of implementing the dissemination guidelines, and the lessons learned throughout the process.

In Chapter Fifteen, a new chapter for this edition, Baker, Motton, Barnidge, and Rose focus on the use of multiple methods in their Men on the Move CBPR project to assess individual, environmental, and social determinants of cardiovascular disease in rural Southeast Missouri. They provide a cogent and compelling description of how their partnership used community forums, economic assessment, and photo-elicitation to provide the different types of data which together led to a better understanding of the factors contributing to health disparities and informed the development of effective interventions to address those factors.

In Chapter Sixteen, another new chapter in this volume, Corburn, Lee, Imara, and Swanston describe the use of map making as a tool for CBPR partnerships to highlight health equity issues in their neighborhoods. Two case studies are presented—one from East Oakland, California, and one from Brooklyn, New York—both of which provide compelling examples of challenges, strengths, and lessons learned from creating and using maps to generate visual representations of community and professional knowledge and how that knowledge can be used effectively to inform action for health equity.

In Chapter Seventeen, López, Robinson, and Eng describe the use of photovoice, which was the principal method for a CBPR project with African American women breast cancer survivors in rural eastern North Carolina. Photovoice is a participatory method in which community members use cameras to take photos that represent and communicate to others their experiences (Wang & Burris, 1994). The authors present a brief overview of photovoice, including the origins and previous applications of this method. Their case example is the Inspirational Images project, an academic-community partnership formed to enable breast cancer survivors to explore and voice their survivorship concerns so that appropriate interventions could be developed to address them. The authors' description of how they conducted photovoice and disseminated their findings, using a CBPR process, offers unique insights into combining research with empowerment education methods. Their examination of challenges and lessons learned is also most instructive.

In Chapter Eighteen, another new chapter in this volume, Tsui, Cho, and Freudenberg describe community-based participatory policy work (CBPPW), which is an approach to policy activism that combines community-based participatory research and community-based policy advocacy. The authors describe methods used in three different collaborative efforts in New York City to change food-related policies, including literature reviews, surveys, elicitation dialogues, and participatory mapping. The methods are particularly useful to CBPPW practitioners interested in food policy work to be able to elicit data on experiences of current policies, collect and/or analyze data on food environments, policy scanning and analysis, and eliciting views on policy opportunities. The authors end the chapter with a thoughtful discussion of limitations and challenges and lessons learned through their experiences conducting CBPPW.

In Chapter Nineteen, the final chapter of Part Six, Morello-Frosch, Pastor, Sadd, Prichard, and Matsuoka describe how the Los Angeles Collaborative for Environmental Health and Justice (the Collaborative) used the method of secondary data analysis to identify and change policies that adversely affect communities. The authors offer valuable detail on how the Collaborative collectively developed research projects, interpreted data, disseminated study findings, and leveraged the results of secondary data by linking research with community organizing and advocacy activities to promote policy change. They conclude with insights on the challenges and limitations of using secondary data analysis in a CBPR project and the lessons learned by the Collaborative.

REFERENCES

Ammerman, A., Corbie-Smith, G., St. George, D. M. M., Washington, C., Weathers, B., & Jackson-Christian, B. (2003). Research expectations among African-American church leaders in the PRAISE! Project: A randomized trial guided by community-based participatory research. *American Journal of Public Health, 93,* 1720–1727.

Ahmed, S. M., & Palermo, A. G. (2010). Community engagement in research: Frameworks for education and peer review. *American Journal of Public Health, 100,* 1380–1385.

Boyer, B. B., Mohatt, G. V., Pasker, R. L., Drew, E. M., & McGlone, K. K. (2007). Sharing results from complex disease genetics studies: A community-based participatory research approach. *International Journal of Circumpolar Health, 66,* 19–30.

Brenner, B. L., & Manice, M. P. (2011). Community engagement in children's environmental health research. *Mt. Sinai Journal of Medicine, 78,* 85–97.

Chavez, V., Duran, B. M., Baker, Q. E., Avila, M. M., & Wallerstein, N. (2008). The dance of race and privilege in community-based participatory research. In M. Minkler & N. Wallerstein (Eds.), *Community-based participatory research for health: From process to outcomes* (2nd ed., pp. 81–97). San Francisco: Jossey-Bass.

Cook, W. K. (2008). Integrating research and action: A systematic review of community-based participatory research to address health disparities in environmental and occupational health in the USA. *Journal of Epidemiology & Community Health, 62*, 668–676.

Flaskerud, J. H., & Anderson, N. (1999). Disseminating the results of participant-focused research. *Journal of Transcultural Nursing, 10*, 340–349.

Green, L. W., George, M. A., Daniel, M., Frankish, C. J., Herbert, C. J., Bowie, W. R., et al. (2003). Guidelines for participatory research in health promotion. In M. Minkler & N. Wallerstein (Eds.), *Community-based participatory research for health* (pp. 27–52). San Francisco: Jossey-Bass.

Horowitz, C. R., Robinson, M., & Seifer, S. (2009). Community-based participatory research from the margin to the mainstream—Are researchers prepared? *Circulation, 119*, 2633–2642.

Israel, B. A., Schulz, A. J., Parker, E. A., & Becker, A. B. (1998). Review of community-based research: Assessing partnership approaches to improve public health. *Annual Review of Public Health, 19*, 173–202.

López, E. D. S, Parker, E. A., Edgren, K. K., & Brakefield-Caldwell, W. (2005). Lessons learned while using a CBPR approach to plan and conduct forums to disseminate research findings back to partnering communities: A case study from Community Action Against Asthma, Detroit, Michigan. *Metropolitan Universities Journal, 16*, 57–76.

Pufall, E. L., Jones, A. Q., McEwen, S. A., Lyall, C., Peregrine, A. S., & Edge, V. L. (2011). Community-derived research dissemination strategies in an Inuit community. *International Journal of Circumpolar Health, 70*, 532–541.

Stoecker, R. (2003). Are academics irrelevant? Approaches and roles for scholars in community-based participatory research. In M. Minkler & N. Wallerstein (Eds.), *Community-based participatory research for health* (pp. 98–112). San Francisco: Jossey-Bass.

Themba, M. K., & Minkler, M. (2003). Influencing policy through community-based participatory research. In M. Minkler & N. Wallerstein (Eds.), *Community-based participatory research for health* (pp. 349–370). San Francisco: Jossey-Bass.

Wang, C. C., & Burris, M. A. (1994) Empowerment through photo novella: Portraits of participation. *Health Education Quarterly, 21*(2), 171–186.

Chapter 15

COLLABORATIVE DATA COLLECTION, INTERPRETATION, AND ACTION PLANNING IN A RURAL AFRICAN AMERICAN COMMUNITY: MEN ON THE MOVE

ELIZABETH A. BAKER

FREDA MOTTON

ELLEN BARNIDGE

FRANK ROSE III

Although cardiovascular disease (CVD) rates in the United States have been declining overall (Harper, Lynch, & Davey-Smith, 2011), the differences in the rates of decline across race and socioeconomic position have contributed to significant health disparities. Data show that **African Americans** have higher CVD mortality rates than whites and those of lower socioeconomic position (SEP) are at greater risk than those of higher SEP (Harper, Lynch, & Davey-Smith, 2011; Mensah, Mokdad, Ford, Greenlund, & Croft, 2005; Wong, Shapiro, Boscardin, & Ettner, 2002).

Inequitable distribution of **social determinants** such as money, power, and resources across various populations is a significant contributor to persistent and pervasive health disparities, such as those related to CVD (Baker, Metzler, & Galea, 2005; Braveman & Gruskin, 2003; Commission on Social Determinants of Health, 2008; Dahlgren & Whitehead, 1992; Daniels, Kennedy, & Kawachi, 2003; Link, Phelan, Meich, & Westin, 2008; Robert Wood Johnson Foundation, 2008, Wilkinson & Marmot, 2003; Woodward & Kawachi, 2000). Some estimate that social determinants (for example, education, income, employment, housing) and environmental conditions account for approximately 20% of deaths in the United States (McGinnis, Williams-Russo, & Knickman, 2002; Williams, 2005). For example, living in disadvantaged circumstances (for example, poverty) as well as having little control over one's life choices puts individuals at greater risk of **cardiovascular disease** (Wilkinson & Marmot, 2003). Our expanding knowledge of disease etiology has established that individual, environmental, and social determinants act synergistically to contribute to health problems such as cardiovascular disease, through direct effects, as well as their effects on risky health behaviors and other pathways linked to heart health (such as stress, exposure to environmental toxins) (Frieden, 2010; Schulz, et al., 2005).

These findings suggest that traditional interventions to reduce CVD risk that focus on behavioral determinants such as nutrition and physical activity (Lloyd-Jones, et al., 2010) are insufficient. Interventions that address multiple levels of the ecological framework are more likely to successfully reduce CVD risk because they address broader social and structural factors in addition to individual ones, and hence benefit all individuals exposed to the social and physical environment, rather than focusing on improving the health of one person at a time (Economos et al., 2001; Glanz et al., 1995; Schulz et al., 2005).

Previous research shows that to create changes at multiple ecological levels it is important to utilize approaches that incorporate community members in all phases of the research process (Warnecke et al., 2008). Community-based participatory research (CBPR) is one such approach. CBPR not only strengthens the research process by incorporating local knowledge and expertise but it also increases the likelihood that interventions are culturally appropriate, relevant, and feasible (Israel, Schulz, Parker, & Becker, 1998). Further, the use of multiple data collection methods provides different types of data and answers different types of questions (Patton, 2002) which together enhance understanding of the complex set of factors that contribute to health disparities. Such nuanced, in-depth understandings are essential for the development of viable, appropriate, and effective intervention strategies. This chapter describes how Men on the Move, a CBPR project, used multiple methods to assess individual, environmental, and social determinants of CVD in a rural community in Southeast Missouri. The chapter also describes the impact of collaboration on the development of tools, data collection, and interpretation, and the influence of our findings on subsequent action planning.

OVERVIEW OF MEN ON THE MOVE

To **better** understand the nature of the problem, in this section we provide an overview of some of the contextual factors influencing Men on the Move.

Statement of Problem

Pemiscot County is a rural community located in the Bootheel Region of Southeast Missouri. Unlike other rural communities in Missouri, Pemiscot County has a large African American population constituting 25% of the 20,047 residents (U.S. Census Bureau, 2011). Compared to Pemiscot County residents as a whole, as well as the state of Missouri, a greater percentage of African Americans have less than a high school education and are living in poverty, while a lower percentage of African Americans are in the labor force (U.S. Census Bureau, 2011; see Table 15.1). Pemiscot County has one of the highest rates of heart disease in the state (Missouri Department of Health and Senior Services [MDHSS], 2008). In 2006, this rate was nearly 70% higher than the national rate (MDHSS, 2008; National Center for Vital Statistics, 2006). While Pemiscot County as a whole experiences higher heart disease morbidity than the state and nation, the heart disease morbidity rate for African Americans in Pemiscot County is two times higher than the state rate (MDHSS, 2008).

Despite these economic and health-related challenges, Pemiscot County has a number of strengths and resources. African American community leaders within Pemiscot County have a strong sense of what is happening within their community and the synergistic effects of these multiple factors. They attempt to

TABLE 15.1 Demographics for African Americans in Pemiscot County, All Residents in Pemiscot County and Missouri (U.S. Census Bureau, 2011)

	African American Men and Women in Pemiscot County	Adults in Pemiscot County: All Races	Missouri: All Races
Median Age	22	34	36
Less than high school education	55%	41%	23%
Individuals below poverty	56%	30%	11%
% in labor force	28%	40%	50%

maximize on the positive potential of the community by building local leaders and, where possible, strengthening structures within the community. A result of their consciousness and attitudes is a current generation of strong community advocates. This chapter focuses on the work that this current generation of community advocates is doing to continue to improve community health.

Evolution of Partnership

This section provides a description of the overall evolution of the **partnership**, followed by an examination of the specific data collection methods used by the partnership during this evolution. In 1989, academics from Saint Louis University began developing heart health coalitions in regions of Missouri with high rates of heart disease. Initially, strategies to address heart health were designed by academics to have an impact on individual determinants of nutrition and physical activity and were implemented by volunteer community members as part of a Prevention Research Center of the Centers for Disease Control and Prevention (Brownson et al., 1996). Over time, the academic and community members incorporated environmental changes such as the development of walking trails (Brownson et al., 2000, Brownson et al., 2004). As the relationship between academic and community members evolved, another important shift occurred. What started as academically defined programs that were implemented in community settings (community-placed research) moved to programs that enabled

FIGURE 15.1 Multi-Method Sequence for the Development of Men on the Move Phases I and II

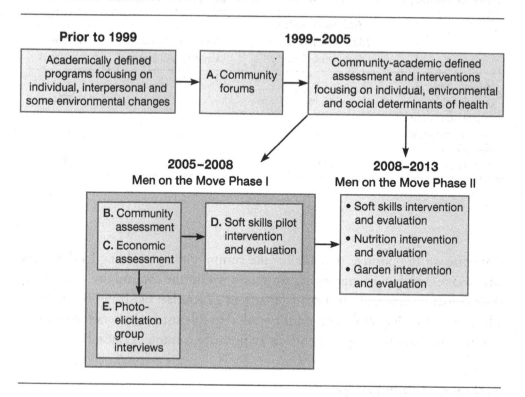

community members to have some input in terms of a restricted menu of choices (community-based research).

Subsequently, as illustrated in Figure 15.1, the efforts moved toward a community-based participatory research (CBPR) approach where the community and academic partners jointly define issues, implement and evaluate the initiative, and disseminate findings (Minkler & Wallerstein, 2008). There were a number of factors that contributed to the shift toward a CBPR approach, including: (1) hiring a community member as a community liaison, and (2) conducting a series of community forums. A long-term, respected community resident was hired to facilitate the implementation and evaluation of activities, to actively engage community members as partners in the research process, and to identify ways to build on community partners' local knowledge and experience. The community liaison opened up the process for community partners to share their experience and perspective, enhancing relationships between community and academic partners. As shown in Figure 15.1, community forums were held to enable academic partners and staff to listen to the community. Within this context, community partners shared their perspective that a focus on individual behaviors alone, such as nutrition and physical activity, was insufficient to reduce CVD and improve community health. This transition to a CBPR approach resulted in a shift in understanding of the determinants affecting heart health in Pemiscot County and a subsequent shift in the strategies to address them. Namely the partnership placed increased emphasis on addressing individual, environmental, and social determinants to improve CVD. The following sections describe multiple methods used to identify these determinants and to develop, implement, and evaluate Men on the Move Phase I (assessment and pilot intervention) and Phase II (multiple interventions) that address these determinants.

Methods for Partner Engagement, Multilevel Assessment, and Findings and Action Steps

Partner Engagement

During the course of our project academic and community partners engaged in the development and implementation of a variety of assessment methods that were used to inform and evaluate activities. A small group of what will be referred to as *core partners* was involved throughout the process. These core partners included four community and two academic partners, (including coauthors of this chapter) who met monthly in person, with intermittent conference calls. Other community and academic partners provided specific expertise when needed. Core partners worked jointly to: develop a common understanding of the purpose of the assessment; discuss the advantages and challenges of the assessment method from their perspectives; develop the tools needed for each assessment; collect and analyze the data; and interpret findings and move to action planning.

Multilevel Assessment

The core partners used five approaches to gather information, allowing for the collection of different types of data addressing different types of questions

(Patton, 2002). The sequence and timing of these data collection methods, in the context of the partnership's transition from academically driven to community driven, is illustrated in Figure 15.1. One method was used prior to Phase I, and four methods were used to gather information as part of *Men on the Move* in this phase. Together these data helped inform the Phase II Men on the Move intervention. A brief summary of each method is provided in Table 15.2, along with the research question to be addressed. Following the table, we describe each data collection method, specific partner engagement, findings, and action steps.

Community Forums

A series of five community forums were held to better understand community members' perspectives on community health (see Figure 15.1, item A). Each forum was held in a local church and attended by approximately 15–20 African American adult community members. Participants included employees of community-based or faith-based organizations, individuals who worked with the community in less formal ways, and community members interested in learning more about the project. The forums were used to identify: (1) key community health issues and determinants; and (2) strengths, assets, or capacities that contribute to overcoming the health issues and minimizing the impact of the determinants. The five community forums are briefly outlined below (see Baker & Motton, 2005, for a more detailed description).

- **Community Forum One**: Community participants worked in small groups to create a poster that visually represented the health of the community.

- **Community Forum Two**: Academic partners provided statistical information on the issues identified in the first forum. URL links were provided to guide community participants and partners to additional information (for example, high school graduation rates, rates of CVD).

- **Community Forum Three**: Community participants and core partners watched a video of a community development project, followed by discussion of the ways that communities have addressed issues in the past and possibilities for the future.

TABLE 15.2   Methods Used to Understand the Social and Environmental Factors That Influence Health in Pemiscot County and to Inform Action Planning

Method	Description	Research question
A. Community forums	Public meetings to discuss factors that influence health in the African American community in Pemiscot County.	What factors influence health in your community?
B. Community-wide assessment	Quantitative surveys with 125 African American men in Pemiscot County to assess the factors (behavioral, social, and environmental) that influence health.	What factors influence African American male health in Pemiscot County? What are the social determinants of health within this community?
C. Economic assessment	Review of publicly available data to assess economic strengths, weaknesses, opportunities and threats in Pemiscot County.	What are the strengths, weaknesses, opportunities, and threats to the economy in Pemiscot County?
D. Soft skills class evaluation	Pre- and post-intervention survey conducted with 100 African American men attending a soft skills course (i.e., skills critical to developing a viable workforce, such as, communications, time management, team building).	Did the soft skills intervention change participants' beliefs or behaviors in the domains covered in the intervention (e.g., hope, stress, communication, conflict management, team building)?
E. Photo-elicitation focus groups	Focus groups using photographs as an additional prompt for dialogue with 24 African Americans in Pemiscot County to assess structural factors affecting health.	What are the assets, institutional practices, and policies that affect education, employment, and community health in Pemiscot County?

- **Community Forum Four**: Community participants were asked to describe the strengths and challenges they face in changing determinants of health.

- **Community Forum Five**: Academics presented the community partners and participants with summaries from the previous forum (and how this related to previous literature) and worked with local community participants to determine the accuracy of the findings (member checking) (Baker & Motton, 2005).

Partner Engagement in Community Forums

Community engagement during this process allowed for academic and community partners to develop a common understanding of the issues facing the community and alternative strategies for addressing these issues. This process engaged more community members in defining issues than had occurred with the initial heart health coalitions. The challenges, however, were that the community forums were fairly large, participants changed over time, and individuals had diverse reasons for attending. In the latter instance, for example, not all participants were interested in working on initiatives to create change, and those who were interested had a fairly wide range of ideas on where to begin. In addition, the relationships between many of the community participants and the core community partners were often superficial, and the relationships between the broader community participants and academic partners were typically nonexistent. This, coupled with the newness of the relationship among the core partners, led to issues being articulated (such as racism) but not fully explored (Baker & Motton, 2005).

Findings and Action Steps Taken Based on Community Forums

Two findings from this process were of particular importance to the development of Men on the Move (MOTM), Phase I. First, the posters developed in Community Forum One showed that an absence of employment and educational opportunities was seen as a key determinant of physical health (diabetes and CVD) and mental health (stress, hope, substance abuse), especially for African American men. In the fourth forum, the community participants identified several aspects of community capacity present in their community. During this forum the academic partners presented and community partners reviewed the definitions of community capacity provided in the literature and the operationalization of these constructs. Community partners stated that while some of the capacities they identified had been previously identified in other research as important (for example, history, community values) (Baker & Motton, 2005; Goodman et al., 1998) other capacities had not. One newly expressed aspect of community capacity is best described as the community's ability to work within partnerships to name issues of privilege and oppression including racism and classism, and to work on strategies for change that minimize the impact of these issues on interventions and community health. Community participants saw an ability to discuss individual and institutional racism within partnerships, not just among community members, as a dimension of community capacity that affects community health directly and indirectly [for example, through enhanced access to connections and power outside the African American community, that is, vertical social capital (Kawachi, Kennedy, & Glass, 1999)]. The findings from this assessment led to the development of *MOTM*, an intervention focusing on the individual, environmental, and *social* determinants of cardiovascular disease, capacity building, and African American men.

COMMUNITY-WIDE ASSESSMENT

The community forums challenged the partners to look specifically at African American men's health in Pemiscot County. Funding was obtained from the National Center on Minority Health and Health Disparities (R24-MD001590) to conduct a community action planning process including a community assessment and pilot test of an intervention designed on the basis of that assessment (Figure 15.1, item B). A survey was conducted to assess factors that influence African American male health in Pemiscot County. The survey's intent was a quantitative assessment of factors influencing educational and economic development and current educational and occupational status of African American men in Pemiscot County. One hundred and twenty-five African American men between the ages of 18 and 55, or roughly 20% of the African American male population in Pemiscot County, completed the survey. Factors assessed by the questionnaire included: motivation to achieve, coping strategies, sense of hope, communication skills, experiences of discrimination, social capital, anxiety, and depressive symptoms. Also, health behavior and health status questions were included to provide an initial assessment of the association between education, economics, and health behaviors and health status.

Partner Engagement in Community-Wide Assessment

A multidisciplinary team of core partners and additional academic and community partners brainstormed constructs to include, identified and reviewed existing tools, and worked together to identify specific questions to assess each construct. Community partners pilot-tested survey items with a small sample of African American men before finalizing the survey instrument. Cognitive response testing was used to assess the extent to which respondents understood the questions in the same way that was intended by the core partners. This involved asking respondents to "think out loud" as they read the questions. Participants were asked to describe what they thought the question was asking and identify changes in question wording (Damaio & Rothgeb, 1996). Academic partners worked with community partners to develop protocols to administer the survey. Community partners completed university-sanctioned institutional review board certification, recruited participants, and conducted the survey with men not involved in earlier cognitive response testing. Academic partners worked with community partners to build a data entry system and community partners entered survey data. Academic partners analyzed the data and all partners worked together to interpret the results.

Findings and Action Steps Taken Based on Community-Wide Assessment

Surveys were completed with 125 African American men. Mean age was 28, slightly older than the average age of 22 among African Americans in the county as a whole.

Seventy percent of survey participants reported household incomes of less than $20,000; 40% were out of work (not including those indicating they were unable to work); and 30% reported less than a high school education, compared to 55% for African Americans generally in the county. Sixty percent of the men had low or very low food security; 60% were overweight or obese; 50% indicated that they currently smoked and 50% that they consumed more than five drinks in one sitting during the last 30 days. Seventy-five percent indicated that they had experienced at least one type of discriminatory event in their lifetime (for example, unfairly fired or denied a promotion, not hired, threatened by police, discouraged by a teacher, prevented from moving into a neighborhood). In spite of these findings, 80% reported very good or excellent general health, and a low mean number of depressive and anxiety symptoms. These assessment findings helped to frame the soft skills classes that were developed (described later in the chapter). For example, as a result of these data the classes focused on improved education and employment skills among African American men, included information about specific health issues, and discussed how discriminatory experiences influenced intent to apply for a job.

ECONOMIC ASSESSMENT

Findings from the community-wide assessment survey identified factors that were dependent on broader environmental and social structures (see Figure 15.1, item B). To identify and understand these broader determinants, especially those related to economic factors, the partnership decided to conduct a "2,000-foot view" analysis of Pemiscot County (see Figure 15.1, item C). This analysis used a search of existing data to assess strengths, weaknesses, opportunities, and threats (SWOT) to economic development within Pemiscot County. Pemiscot County and the names of specific towns within the county (for example, Caruthersville, Hayti, Steele, and Hayti Heights) were used as place identifiers. This information was combined with an array of search terms culled from prior research on community competitiveness including employment rates, education, recreation, natural resources, highway systems, and other indicators of economic strength. Data sources included newspaper and popular articles, technical reports, government documents, and public use statistical information (such as U.S. Census data) from a 15-year period from 1991 to 2006.

Partner Engagement in Economic Assessment

The core partners invited a nationally recognized business consultant to conduct this assessment and present the findings back to the community. The core partners had a conference call with the consultant to share our goals and interest and to learn about his process. From an early summary of the "2,000-foot view" findings, the core partners realized the information would be helpful to others in the community. The partners set up a meeting with key community members and civic leaders (such as mayors, city council members) and business leaders (such as bankers, economic developers) to plan a larger dissemination meeting. Engaging a diverse group of people in the dissemination of findings ensured that the information would be heard by a variety of sectors within the community. Core partners had a second conference call with the consultant to identify any challenges and arrange for a meeting with local community organizations. Core partners discussed the results of the report within the partnership as well as in this larger gathering to determine how to incorporate findings into program design.

Findings and Action Steps Taken Based on Economic Assessment

The economic assessment identified a number of regional strengths, including a vocational school in the region that provides educational opportunities for local residents. It also identified weaknesses and threats, such as high school drop-out rates, limited creation of new jobs, few entertainment and recreational facilities, and poor health indicators, including high rates of obesity.

The report was instrumental in identifying opportunities for change, for example, opportunities to improve school performance and decrease drop-out rates. One key recommendation was the creation of opportunities to strengthen "soft skills." These skills (for example, communication, time management, conflict management, team building) are seen as critical to the development of a viable workforce and can often make the difference in terms of obtaining and keeping a job. This finding reinforced the partnership's intent to develop a soft skills class for men. The report also encouraged the development of strategies to keep young people from leaving Pemiscot County and to attract new people through job creation. The report suggested utilizing available resources—agriculture, river, trains, and interstate highways—within the county. Used strategically, these resources positioned the county as a logistics and distribution hub. County-level economic developers used this data to support the development of a rail spur in the region. The core partners used this data to develop small-scale production gardens, which increased access to produce and local jobs, as part of MOTM Phase II. The initial engagement of this broader range of partners has continued to enhance our work. For example, the mayor of the county seat and economic developer for the region attend MOTM quarterly meetings to learn about our activities and provide tangible support (for example, free storage of MOTM farm equipment in the winter).

SOFT SKILLS CLASS EVALUATION

Based on initial community forums, the community-wide assessment, and the economic analysis, core partners developed the MOTM Phase I pilot intervention. This intervention consisted of a one-week soft skills class for African American men in Pemiscot County (see Figure 15.1, item D). The core partners worked together to determine the content of the modules, and reviewed and finalized the material for each module. African American male community partners were trained to conduct the modules. This training included the opportunity to pilot the modules and obtain feedback on how to improve presentation and approach.

The one-week soft skills class was offered multiple times over the course of a year. Five to ten men participated in each session, and 100 men completed the class the first year. During each one-week class, one or two modules were reviewed each day (taking approximately four hours per day). The core partners created pre- and posttests to evaluate the impact of the course and ascertain the extent to which, for example, the intervention influenced participants' beliefs and behaviors related to stress, communication, hope, and healthy or risky behaviors. The core partners also conducted qualitative interviews with some of the participants to get a more in-depth understanding of what they liked about the program and what they would change. These data were used to modify the modules.

Partner Engagement in Soft Skills Class Evaluation

Community and academic partners worked together to develop and evaluate the classes. Academic partners took the lead in identifying evaluation tools that had been used in previous studies. The core partners reviewed the measures to determine fit with program needs. Academic partners trained community partners to administer the pre- and posttest evaluation surveys. Community partners entered the data and academic partners analyzed the data. The qualitative interview protocol was created jointly with academic and community partners. Community partners conducted the interviews and academic partners transcribed and analyzed the interview data. All partners reviewed the qualitative data. All partners interpreted the results and worked to disseminate findings in both written and oral presentations.

Findings and Action Steps Taken Based on Soft Skills Class Evaluation

One hundred African American men completed the soft skills classes. One-third of the participants had less than a high school education and nearly half were out of work at enrollment. The pre-post assessment found increases in sense of hope, particularly sense of direction in life, and significant decreases in the use of smoking as a way to cope with life stressors among participants. After completing the course the participants indicated that it was less difficult to talk to people and they were more likely to report that people understood their feelings. A majority of the men (86%) set short-term goals (for example, job readiness, stress reduction, time management, communication, smoking cessation, physical activity) for change and reported feeling confident that they could meet these goals.

The qualitative interviews found that the participants liked the participatory format of the course and found it easy to relate to the instructor. The men appreciated the opportunity for self-reflection and self-evaluation, as well as the opportunity to speak with other men about how to make themselves and the community better. They saw themselves as better able to be role models for others and to take part in group and community activities. They indicated a more positive outlook and hope that they had a better chance to do what they wanted in life. The participants felt that as a result of the course they were better able to express themselves, more prepared for a job interview, and had the skills needed to complete a job application. They also noted that they felt support from other class participants, which would help them cope with rejection if or when it came. Over 10% of the men who completed the soft skills course found jobs after being part of the program, which was impressive, given the overall economic state of the area.

In terms of suggestions for changes, participants wanted to have more opportunities to be together and they did not want the program to end. Several men noted that they were unable to obtain employment because they did not have the documents required for employment (such as state identification, birth certificate, social security card). As a result, several modifications to the modules were made. Booster sessions were added to provide additional support for the men involved, and the program started to provide the transportation and funding necessary for men to obtain the legal documents needed for employment.

PHOTO-ELICITATION GROUP INTERVIEWS

In addition to the soft skills recommendation, the economic assessment identified structural changes that needed to be addressed (for example, improvement of the educational system). Core partners voiced a need to better understand how social structures affect African American experiences. Core partners decided that photo-elicitation interviews would be a viable method for this purpose. Photo-elicitation interviews are qualitative group interviews conducted using photographs as a prompt for dialogue (Figure 15.1, item E; Wang & Pies, 2008). These interviews were guided by the Sustainable Livelihood Framework (Department for International Development [DFID], 1999). This framework suggests that the ways of making a living in a community are shaped by community assets and institutional practices and policies. Together these factors influence community health and well-being. Group interviews were used to determine how economic conditions and educational opportunities influenced access to jobs in Pemiscot County and general community health outcomes (Barnidge, Baker, Motton, Rose, & Fitzgerald, 2010). Two group sessions, one addressing economic conditions and the other educational opportunities, were conducted, involving both men and women in Pemiscot County.

Partner Engagement in Photo-Elicitation Group Interviews

Core partners discussed the elements of the Sustainable Livelihoods Framework (DFID, 1999) and the fit for Pemiscot County, as well as photo elicitation as a method prior to initiating the data collection. Once there was agreement on using the framework and method, core partners brainstormed a list of ideas for photographs. Core partners determined the photographic content while a trained photographer determined the specific angles and photographic perspectives of the pictures.

Core partners played unique roles. Academic partners conducted the photo-elicitation group interviews. Community partners participated in the interviews. Academic partners did initial data analysis while all core partners participated in analysis review at multiple stages. All core partners interpreted the findings and determined how to incorporate findings into program components. Together the partners disseminated the findings in oral and written forms.

Findings and Action Steps Taken Based on Photo-Elicitation Group Interviews

The photo-elicitation data both validated findings from other methods previously discussed and added to our understanding of the structural factors affecting community health. For example, the photo-elicitation participants identified the lack of business development in the county. As noted, the economic assessment identified Pemiscot County as an ideal distribution and logistics hub that could stimulate business development. Participants echoed this in the photo elicitation interviews as well. The photo-elicitation interviews also uncovered specific barriers that African Americans face when trying to capitalize on business development opportunities not uncovered in the economic assessment. For example, photo-elicitation participants highlighted the importance of self-employment in the community, noting that people find ways to make a living. Despite this entrepreneurial spirit, they noted institutional racism manifested through discriminatory lending practices as a significant barrier to new business development. Participants also noted challenges faced by African American business owners related to limited support from African Americans. The participants connected the difficulties developing businesses and "doing things for themselves" as factors detrimental to health (Barnidge, Baker, Motton, Rose, & Fitzgerald, 2011).

Photo-elicitation findings helped to support and develop interventions in Phase I and Phase II. The data clarified barriers for African American men in both educational and economic sectors. This information was used to enhance the soft skills classes in Phase I. The findings stirred the idea of developing small-scale production gardens through a community food system that has resulted in MOTM, Phase II (see Figure 15.1). Our community food system provides employment opportunities for African American men and builds social capital among African Americans as well as between African Americans and whites in Pemiscot County. The findings also suggest that some barriers to local food production are a function of history and the current state of the community. Core partners engaged local politicians from the outset to ensure their continued support. They also took steps to develop relationships across traditional barriers. For example, core partners sought support for storing MOTM equipment at a traditionally white community site as a way to begin to build relationships, and help the white community see the African American community as a source of resource enhancement.

CHALLENGES

A key challenge was the time it took to engage in the CBPR process. For example, colearning about survey items took additional time, including the time it took the partnership to discuss the pros and cons of asking questions in different ways. It took time to find the balance between relying on existing items to enhance reliability and validity and reframing the questions to enhance the likelihood of community understanding. The length of time this took was frustrating for some academic and community partners. Time was also an issue in terms of relationship building. Many of our processes required a certain level of trust to be effective, and the willingness to work through difficult conversations. For example, partners differed in their tolerance for conversations about many things including racism, and how to present information about the community in ways that are accurate and not judgmental. Last but not least, core academic and community partners are 3 to 3½ hours away from each other. Travel time between locations poses a significant challenge.

A second challenge was around formal procedures required by "outside" entities. For example, survey administration procedures needed to adhere to IRB and grant regulations. Although it was ultimately understood to be important, there was frustration among the partners about the level of organization required for survey administration (for example, tracking incentives).

An additional challenge speaks to the longevity of our partnership. Although a core group of partners has been working on this project for nearly a decade, other members have transitioned in and out during that time. Often, there is a learning curve for new partners. At first, there may be confusion about our approach and the ways that community as well as academic partners are involved.

Another challenge was the ability to integrate our work with that being done in other parts of the community so that it could best inform action. For example, we were not very successful in integrating our findings from the economic development assessment with the other economic development activities in the county. Although we have significant engagement from the economic development specialist in our work (for example, attends quarterly meetings, assists us with local businesses), our core community partners have not been regularly invited to local economic development meetings.

LESSONS LEARNED AND IMPLICATIONS FOR PRACTICE

As presented below, we have learned several key lessons about using a CBPR approach to conduct multiple research methods to inform an action planning process.

Recognizing the Benefit of a CBPR Approach

As described above, a CBPR approach takes a significant investment of time, including the time it takes to develop and maintain relationships to build a truly collaborative partnership. We believe that the return on time invested is multi-faceted and the benefits outweigh the costs. For example, benefits of using a CBPR approach when conducting multiple data collection methods as presented here include that it: fosters the selection of highest priority research questions; allows community and academic partners to develop a common understanding of issues facing the community and alternative strategies for addressing them; increases the quality of data collected by enhancing the appropriateness of items used on data collection instruments; provides an opportunity for collective reflection by all partners on the findings, enabling them to challenge preconceived ideas of the community; and presents results in a way that all partners can use for their own purposes. Recognizing such benefits is important for engaging in a CBPR approach.

Readiness Is Important for Determining Utility of Various Methods

Different assessment and intervention methods may be appropriate at different times, with each building on and enhancing understanding of the findings. Readiness, on the part of both community and academic partners, is important in determining the potential utility of various assessment and intervention methods. In each of the methods described here the approach that core partners used to engage the wider community varied. Core partners discussed whether a method was appropriate given what was known about readiness (academic and community). The community forums, which occurred several years after the community and university partners had been working together, are a good example. In the forums, community participants identified a need to increase the ability to openly discuss privilege and oppression on the basis of race and class. The community participants identified an ability to confront these issues constructively as an essential capacity for developing change strategies to have a positive impact on community health. Although the community identified a desire to discuss these issues, our readiness to address these issues as a multiracial, multiclass community-academic partnership required more time. The actual work the core partners have done in discussing and addressing institutional racism (for example, being able to obtain land, access to water, being part of local political and economic decision making) has taken several years, with additional learning from both the economic and photo-elicitation assessments. Academic partners, who do not live in the community, have had to learn to listen to community partners about community readiness to address an issue, rather than push for change when, as outsiders, they do not have to live with the consequences.

Methods and Tools May Not Accurately Capture Information Desired

Even with an enhanced community-academic relationship the methods and tools employed may not accurately capture the information desired. For example, we believe that our finding of low levels of depressive symptoms as measured by standard tools may not accurately represent the experience of depression within this population. Based on the results of our assessments, we found that the men's experience might be better defined as an absence of hope than the presence of depression. As our partnership develops deeper social cohesion and trust we hope to develop better methods for capturing, understanding, and developing appropriate interventions.

CBPR Approach Can Enhance Collection and Interpretation of Data

Using a CBPR approach can enhance collection and interpretation of data because the inclusion of both community and academic lenses can lead to the development of more appropriate interventions. Our collaborative processes enabled us to interpret data, and use the information to develop multilevel interventions that address the determinants of health most pressing to the community. For example, we made the choice to have academic partners facilitate the group interviews of community members for our photo-elicitation process. Our past experience suggested that when community partners facilitated interviews within their community there was a level of assumed cultural knowledge that was not articulated. While the presence of community partners created a safe environment, the academic partners facilitated the dialogue in a valued way that challenged the participants to articulate cultural connections more explicitly.

Engaging Participants from Outside Core Partnership Can Increase Skills and Credibility

Engaging participants from outside the core partnership can increase skills available to the community as well as enhance project credibility. One example of this in our work was inviting the outside consultant to conduct the economic assessment. The consultant provided an objective outsider view of Pemiscot County that was consistent with what outside businesses would see, rather than from the perspective of those within the county. His "outsider status" allowed him to frame his comments in ways that businessmen, politicians, and community groups found useful for their own purposes. In addition, at that time, there was not an economic developer, or anyone with such skills, working specifically for the county. Moreover, his credentials created interest from a wider range of community leaders, including the mayor, whose personal invitation to other community leaders created more involvement than we would have otherwise received. As a result, we were able to engage members of the community who, traditionally, may have declined an invitation because they did not see how their work connected with the work of Men on the Move. The mayor's invitation was an indicator of the community's openness to this type of outside assistance. The presentation increased awareness not only about the economic conditions in the county but also about the value that our project brought to the community.

Not All Aspects of Community Represented in Any Given CBPR Assessment

Although CBPR provides an opportunity for community voices to be heard, not all aspects of the community are represented in any given assessment. Specifically, community assessments primarily include community members who are willing and in a position to be able to work with us. This means individuals who complete assessments are slightly older, more likely to be employed, less likely to live in extreme poverty, and more educated than the average African American adult in Pemiscot County. As a result neither our findings nor our actions are representative of the entire community. Core partners are attempting to provide opportunities for new voices to influence our processes. Listening to multiple perspectives, new and existing, can help to ensure that data collection processes and procedures, and interventions, are inclusive and representative of the community-at-large.

Engaging New Partners Requires Orientation and Modification

Engaging new community and academic partners requires attention to orientation regarding the project history and principles, and often a modification of previous perspectives regarding research and community-academic partnerships. A core group of community and academic partners have been working on this project for nearly a decade. During this time, however, other partners have transitioned in and out. A challenge became how best to engage and integrate new academic and community partners and staff. Before inviting individuals to partner with us we review the aims of our project and our CBPR partnership principles with them. We found that initially some new partners are confused by our approach and the ways that community and academic partners are involved. We have learned the importance of reviewing and revisiting our CBPR principles and how these are operationalized with new partners, especially those working full-time on the project. However, it is important to recognize that some individuals have life and work experiences that challenge their ability to accept CBPR as a reasonable approach. Within the community, job opportunities that exist are mostly task oriented and hierarchical. These rarely provide opportunities for individuals to develop the power-sharing and process-oriented skills commonly used in a CBPR approach. Individuals who are able to acquire these skills in spite of the obstacles presented often leave the community (Barnidge, Baker, Motton, Rose, & Fitzgerald, 2011). For academics, many have been socialized to believe that the skills and perspectives they obtain during their training make them uniquely qualified to engage in the research process, analyze findings, and develop interventions. They may question the appropriateness of engaging community members as real partners in the research process. Academics must commit to developing the humility necessary to work within this context. Further, a commitment to mutual learning is necessary for community and academic partners alike to bridge the chasm of culture and knowledge.

Integrating Work into the Broader Community

When using a CBPR approach it is important to demonstrate not only how the data collected shapes project activities, but also to develop effective ways to integrate the work with that being done in other parts of the community. Partners, old and new, need to see that something is happening as a result of data collected. Although we were able to demonstrate how our assessments led to various project activities, we were often not as successful at integrating our work with that being done in other parts of the community (for example, economic development activities). It will continue to take time to overcome the history of exclusion.

SUMMARY

Our work started by focusing on individual and, to some extent, interpersonal determinants of CVD. This helped form a foundation to develop deeper relationships between academic and community partners. As these relationships developed we learned to use methods appropriate for the questions we wanted answered. In doing so, we have seen that the effectiveness of the methods used may be in part a function of partnership development. In our early stages (that is, the community forum), we heard discussions about the association between social determinants (for example, racism) and health, but it took increased trust and relationships within the community and between the community and academic partners to move from survey data (that is, community assessment) to methods that allow for deeper reflection (that is, photo-elicitation). Perhaps more importantly, it was through the use of these multiple methods and deep reflection with community and academic partners over time that we have been able to see why CVD is not seen by the community as strictly a function of health behaviors (for example, smoking, eating, physical activity). The use of multiple methods and actively engaging community and academic partners throughout the process has enabled us to outline the mechanisms through which individual, environmental, and social determinants influence health outcomes, and to develop interventions that address these multiple determinants.

KEY TERMS

African American

Cardiovascular disease

Partnership

Social determinants

DISCUSSION QUESTIONS

1. What are some specific ways that community and academic partners can work together to collect and analyze data? Do different methodologies lend themselves to different types of partner engagement?

2. What are unique strengths that each partner can bring to data collection, interpretation, and action planning? How might you structure engagement to build on the strengths of all partners?

3. What are some of the challenges that arise when community and academic partners work together in data collection, interpretation, and action planning?

4. What are some ways to structure data collection and analysis that engages all partners in the analysis of social determinants of health and the development of strategies to address these determinants?

REFERENCES

Baker, E. A., Metzler, M., & Galea, S. (2005). Addressing social determinants of health inequities: Learning from doing. *American Journal of Public Health, 95*(4), 553–555.

Baker, E. A., & Motton, F. (2005). Creating understanding and action through group dialogue. In B. Israel, E. Eng, A. Schulz, & E. A. Parker (Eds.), *Methods in community-based participatory research* (pp. 307–325). San Francisco: Jossey-Bass.

Barnidge, E., Baker, E. A., Motton, F., Rose, F., & Fitzgerald, T. (2010). A participatory method to identify root determinants of health: The heart of the matter. *Progress in Community Health Partnerships, 4,* 55–63.

Barnidge, E., Baker, E. A., Motton, F., Rose, F., & Fitzgerald, T. (2011). Exploring community health through the Sustainable Livelihoods Framework. *Health Education & Behavior, 38*(1), 80–90.

Braveman, P., & Gruskin, S. (2003). Defining equity in health. *Journal of Epidemiology & Community Health, 57,* 254–258.

Brownson, R. C., Baker, E. A., Boyd, R. L., Caito, N. M., Duggan, K., Housemann, R. A., et al. (2004). A community-based approach to promoting walking in rural areas. *American Journal of Prevention Medicine, 27*(1), 28–34.

Brownson, R. C., Housemann, R. A., Brown, D. R., Jackson-Thompson, J., King, A. C., Malone, B. R., et al. (2000). Promoting physical activity in rural communities: Walking trail access, use, and effects. *American Journal of Prevention Medicine, 18*, 235–241.

Brownson, R. C., Smith, C. A., Pratt, M., Mack, N. E., Jackson-Thompson, J., Dean, C. G., et al. (1996). Preventing cardiovascular disease through community-based risk reduction: The Bootheel Heart Health Project. *American Journal of Public Health, 86*, 206–213.

Commission on Social Determinants of Health. (2008). *Closing the gap in a generation: Health equity through action on the social determinants of health.* Geneva, Switzerland: World Health Organization.

Dahlgren, G., & Whitehead, M. (1992). *Policies and strategies to promote equity in health.* In World Health Organization (Ed.), (pp. 1–63). Copenhagen: World Health Organization.

Damaio, T., & Rothgeb, J. (1996). Cognitive interviewing techniques: In the lab and in the field. In N. Schwarz & S. Sudman (Eds.), *Answering questions: Methodology for cognitive and communicative processes in survey research* (pp. 177–196). San Francisco: Jossey-Bass.

Daniels, N., Kennedy, B., & Kawachi, I. (2003). *Is inequality bad for our health?* Boston: Beacon Press.

Department for International Development. (1999). Sustainable livelihoods guidance sheets. Retrieved March 31, 2011, from http://www.eldis.org/vfile/upload/1/document/0901/section1.pdf

Economos, C. D., Brownson, R. C., DeAngelis, M. A., Novelli, P., Foerster, S. B., Foreman, C. T., Pate, R. R. (2001). What lessons have been learned from other attempts to guide social change? *Nutrition Reviews, 59*(3 Pt 2), S40–S56; discussion S57–S65.

Frieden, T. R. (2010). A framework for public health action: The health impact pyramid. *American Journal of Public Health, 100*(4), 590–595.

Glanz, K., Lankenau, B., Foerster, S., Temple, S., Mullis, R., & Schmid, T. (1995) Environmental and policy approaches to cardiovascular disease prevention through nutrition: Opportunities for state and local action. *Health Education & Behavior, 22*(4), 512–527.

Goodman, R. M., Speers, M. A., McLeroy, K., Fawcett, S., Kegler, M., Parker, E., et al. (1998). Identifying and defining the dimensions of community capacity to provide a basis for measurement. *Health Education & Behavior, 25*(3), 258–278.

Graham, H. (2004). Social determinants and their unequal distribution: Clarifying policy understandings. *The Milbank Quarterly, 82*(1), 101–124.

Harper, S., Lynch, J., & Davey-Smith, G. D. (2011). Social determinants and the decline of cardiovascular diseases: Understanding the links. *Annual Review of Public Health, 32*, 39–69.

Israel, B., Schulz, A., Parker, E. A., & Becker, A. B. (1998). Review of community-based research: Assessing partnership approaches to improve public health. *Annual Review of Public Health, 19*, 173–202.

Kawachi, I., Kennedy, B., & Glass, R. (1999). Social capital and self-rated health: A contextual analysis. *American Journal of Public Health, 89*(8), 1187–1193.

Link, B., & Phelan, J. (2005). Fundamental sources of health inequalities. In D. Mechanic, L. Rogut, D. Colby, & J. Knickman (Eds.), *Policy challenges in modern health care* (pp. 71–84). New Brunswick, NJ: Rutgers University Press.

Link, B., Phelan, J., Meich, R., & Westin, L. (2008). The resources that matter: Fundamental social causes of health disparities and the challenge of intelligence. *Journal of Health and Social Behavior, 49*, 72–91.

Lloyd-Jones, D., Adams, R. J., Brown, T. M., Carnethon, M., Dai, S., Simone, G., et al. (2010). Heart disease and stroke statistics—2010 update. A Report from the American Heart Association Statistics Committee and Stroke Statistics Subcommittee. *Circulation, 121*, e1–e170.

McGinnis, J. M., Williams-Russo, P., & Knickman, J. (2002). The case for more active policy attention on health promotion. *Health Affairs, 21*(2), 78–93.

Mensah, G. A., Mokdad, A. H., Ford, E. S., Greenlund, K. J., & Croft, J. B. (2005). State of disparities in cardiovascular health in the United States. *Circulation, 111*(10), 1233–1241.

Minkler, M., & Wallerstein, N. (2008). Introduction to community-based participatory research. In M. Minkler & N. Wallerstein (Eds.), *Community-based participatory research for health: From process to outcomes* (2nd ed.). San Francisco: Jossey-Bass.

Missouri Department of Health and Senior Services (MDHSS). (2008). Leading cause of death profile for Pemiscot County residents by race. Retrieved December 10, 2008, from http://www.dhss.mo.gov/CommunityDataProfiles/index.html

National Center for Vital Statistics. (2006). Deaths: Final data for 2003. *National Vital Statistics Reports, 54*(13).

Patton, M. Q. (2002). *Qualitative research and evaluation methods* (3rd ed.). Thousand Oaks, CA: Sage.

Robert Wood Johnson Foundation. (2008). *Overcoming obstacles to health: Report from the Robert Wood Johnson Foundation to the Commission to Build a Healthier America.* Princeton, NJ: Robert Wood Johnson Foundation.

Schulz, A. J., Kannan, S., Dvonch, J. T., Israel, B. A., Allen, A., 3rd, James, S. A., et al. (2005). Social and physical environments and disparities in risk for cardiovascular disease: The healthy environments partnership conceptual model. *Environmental Health Perspectives, 113*, 1817–1825.

U.S. Census Bureau. (2011). *American factfinder.* Retrieved April 1, 2011, from http://factfinder.census.gov

Wang, C., & Pies, C. (2008). Using photovoice for participatory assessment and issue selection. In M. Minkler & N. Wallerstein (Eds.), *Community-based participatory research for health: From process to outcomes* (2nd ed., pp. 183–198). San Francisco: Jossey-Bass.

Warnecke, R. B., Oh, A., Breen, N., Gehlert, S., Paskett, E., Tucker, K. L., et al. (2008). Approaching health disparities from a population perspective: The National Institutes of Health Centers for Population Health and Health Disparities. *American Journal of Public Health, 98,* 1608–1615.

Wilkinson, R., & Marmot, M. (Eds.). (2003). *Social determinants of health: The solid facts* (2nd ed.). Copenhagen: World Health Organization.

Williams, D. (2005). Patterns and causes of disparities in health. In D. Mechanic, L. Rogut, D. Colby, & J. Knickman (Eds.), *Policy challenges in modern health care* (pp. 115–134). New Brunswick, NJ: Rutgers University Press.

Wong, M. D., Shapiro, M. F., Boscardin, W. J., & Ettner, S. L. (2002). Contribution of major diseases to disparities in mortality. *New England Journal of Medicine, 347*(20), 1585–1592.

Woodward, A., & Kawachi, I. (2000). Why reduce health inequalities? *Journal of Epidemiology and Community Health, 54*(12), 923–929.

Chapter 16

COLLABORATIVE MAPPING

FOR HEALTH EQUITY

MAKING PLACE VISIBLE

JASON CORBURN

ANNA YUN LEE

NEHANDA IMARA

SAMARA SWANSTON

This chapter highlights how map making is an essential aspect of community-based participatory research (CBPR) and offers two case studies about how community groups use map making to highlight health equity issues in their neighborhoods. We suggest that map making is as much a process as product, and that both help community members and researchers organize and prioritize information, make visible key data, challenge professional characterizations of whether or not a place is "healthy," and contribute to the important narratives of health equity that tend to influence decision makers as much as or more than abstracted data alone. In this chapter, we emphasize that map making for health equity, when driven by community member's local expertise, can challenge traditional health promotion research that often views residents as research subjects having a deficit of knowledge about the hazards and assets in their own neighborhoods and rarely is used to inform health-promoting action. Although map making can be used for multiple purposes, including the identification and definition of issues, for the purpose of this chapter we emphasize how mapping is used to inform action. Two specific cases of collaborative mapping processes—one from East Oakland, California and a second from Brooklyn, New York—provide concrete examples of the challenges and opportunities for community members, scientists, and decision makers interested in generating visual representations of community and professional knowledge.

Map making is a powerful analytic and data presentation tool that has a long history in social epidemiology and community health more generally. Throughout the modern history of epidemiology, **maps** of a range of community-level indicators have been used to highlight the spatial correlation between suspected social determinants of health and health inequities. Selected and now well-cited examples include Louis-René Villermé's maps of death rates and wealth by *arrondissement* or neighborhoods in 1840s Paris (Julia & Valleron, 2010); John Snow's maps of cholera by household and neighborhood water sources in 1858 London (Brody et al., 2000); and the maps of neighborhood conditions, family wealth, and health outcomes such as low birth weight by Alice Hamilton, Florence Kelley, Jane Addams, and the residents of Hull House in 1890 Chicago (Hull House Maps and Papers, 1895). The work of Hull House residents was especially important because it embodied many of the principles of CBPR, including an explicit *a priori* concern with equity, researchers partnering with residents, community members leading data gathering and mapping, and local people coauthoring and disseminating results. Over a century later, community-based epidemiology and mapping continue to use many of the same methods as the Hull House Progressive Era reformers, even as new spatial statistical methods, computer-based mapping, and Internet and hand-held communication devices have offered new techniques for **spatial data** analysis and presentation. As this chapter argues, community map making is essential for ensuring that the knowledge and benefits of CBPR reach everyone, as maps often take the percentages and abstract tabular data generated in research and connect it to a story about where people live, how they move through the world, and how to change features of their community that may be unhealthy and support characteristics that seem to promote well-being.

NEW TECHNOLOGY AND COMMUNITY MAPPING
FOR HEALTH

The last two decades have seen a rapid rise in the use of and access to Geographic Information Science, or research using geographic information systems (GIS), especially in the area of community health equity (Cromley & McLafferty, 2002; Gatrell & Elliot, 2009). In its most basic form, GIS allows users to create databases of quantitative information—such as census data, household surveys, addresses of polluting facilities, park size, number of vehicles traveling on a roadway, and a host of other community characteristics—and geo-reference this information, or place it on a map in relation to where people live. Spatial statistics can also be generated using GIS to explore correlations between, for instance, proximity to a hazardous exposure and a population health outcome. These quantitative analyses can then be used to generate visual representations of the data analysis in the form of maps. Yet, the use of GIS in CBPR, like other mapping tools, always raises questions of whether the **technology**—not community knowledge—might be driving representations of information, or whether community knowledge and organizing are being served by the use of technology and how information sharing and ownership is managed between GI scientists and community members? We aim to address these and other questions throughout this chapter.

Mapping technologies have also expanded beyond desktop GIS and now include such free and publicly accessible Web-based mapping tools such as Google Maps, MapServer, OpenStreetMap, and GRASS GIS, to name only a few (http://maps.google.com, http://Mapserver.org, http://www.openstreetmap.org, http://grass.fbk.eu). These Web-based tools have made sophisticated mapping available to community and nonprofit groups with limited resources, in part because they have centralized and made freely available very high-resolution background geographic data including satellite data, street photography, and building outlines. Importantly for CBPR, new social media, sometimes linked to mapping technologies, are reshaping definitions of community and how people see themselves in relationship with their surroundings, neighbors, and institutions—by mapping such things as access to food or the responsiveness of government agencies. For example, individuals and community-based organizations have mobilized citizens to send text messages and photos from mobile phones to track a range of community health "field" data that can be located on a map, many with additional geo-referenced data, such as incidents of violence, housing code complaints, dangerous streets and intersections, and pedestrian injuries (see, for example, http://www.crimemapping.com, http://www.everyblock.com, http://www.seeclickfix.com, http://www.infrastructurist.com/f-this/, http://www.appsfor democracy.org/stumble-safely, http://www.mybikelane.com, http://www.healthy city.org). In April 2010, days after the Deep Water Horizon Oil Spill in the Gulf of Mexico, a community-based organization called the Louisiana Bucket Brigade partnered with Tulane University's Disaster Resilience Academy to create a Web-based community map populated by local people sending text messages, e-mails, twitter feeds, or filling out a Web-based form that reported oil sightings, affected animals, odors, health effects, and other human impacts of the spill (http://oilspill .labucketbrigade.org/main). The project was enabled by new "crisis mapping" software that instantly places eyewitness reports into a publicly accessible map (developed by Ushahidi.org). Similar technologies are allowing community map makers to track identified community hazards and assets through time (that is, when during the day was the report sent) and space (that is, geographic location)— giving rise to sophisticated "time-space health biographies" that are enabling collaborative researchers to suggest that movement (and thus exposure) varies from person to person (for example, elderly versus adult versus young person) living in the same place (Kwan, 2009).

As we suggest throughout this chapter, map making using CBPR should be open to engaging with new technologies while also acknowledging its inherent limitations since low-cost mapping technology can help:

- Ensure community residents are valued coproducers of health knowledge;

- Offer a platform for community residents to express what matters to them and share this with a world of potentially new listeners and allies;

- Provide new forums for residents and researchers to collaboratively generate innovative solutions for persistent health inequities, and;

- Raise awareness among community members of the benefits and pitfalls of technology, such as the potential for overwhelming residents with too much information and creating a dependency on technology (Maantay, Maroko, Alicea, & Strelnick, 2009).

MAPPING AND MOVEMENT BUILDING

As we highlight throughout this chapter, no matter the technology used, map making can support CBPR and vice versa only when the process reflects norms of democratic science, including a commitment to transparency, an openness to critical scrutiny, a skepticism toward claims that too neatly support reigning values, a willingness to listen to countervailing opinions, a readiness to admit uncertainty and ignorance, and a respect for evidence gathered by local and professional experts (Corburn, 2005). Even when GIS-generated maps contribute to greater awareness of a community health equity issue, they may not contribute to community ownership over the issue, local power building, and a policy-advocacy coalition accountable to existing local organizations. For example, the highly-regarded maps of Chicago's neighborhood food deserts—communities lacking access to healthy food and their associated health disparities—developed by Mari Gallagher, used GIS to display community health inequities, but did not generate these maps through meaningful research partnership with community-based organizations (http://www.marigallagher.com). The maps did trigger a broader debate within Chicago over responsibility for these inequities, and community-based food justice organizations were involved later in these conversations, but the mapping project did not further core CBPR principles of equal collaboration, building on local assets, or community ownership. Because the assumptions underlying the computer map production are buried within the computer application itself, GIS may further hinder lay understanding of the mapping process. Yet, at the same time, the increased availability of mobile computing power might also lead to the democratization (or at least accountability) of map making, precisely because citizen groups may be able to offer their own computer-generated maps—as we will discuss in the case studies.

The "GIS revolution" in public health and planning has perpetuated an almost unfettered trust by both users and consumers of planning information in quantitative data as the most legitimate information for generating accurate spatial analyses, maps, and ultimately characterizing places. Another emerging implication is that the technology is beginning to frame social problems as only spatial research questions. Yet the most common errors, inaccuracies, and imprecision of GIS devolve from one of the technology's greatest strengths: the ability to collate and cross-reference many types of data and discrete datasets by location, called "geo-coding," in a single system. As new datasets are imported, the GIS can also inherit the errors of these new data and combine them with errors already in the system. Users of GIS often spend as much or more time "cleaning" disparate data sets to match up accurately with one another as they do devising strategies to visually analyze and display these same data.

Ensuring that map making is a democratic process owned and controlled by community members requires that local people, not outside researchers, define the geographic or other boundaries over what counts as part of the "community." The collaborative partnerships and knowledge generated through action research must be oriented toward existing **community organizing** and building goals, focus on mapping both assets and hazards, and aim to highlight issues that may be ignored or given scant attention by outsiders, particularly policymakers. In this process, mapping can facilitate learning about place and health equity relationships by both researchers and community members, particularly if the process is ongoing and dynamic, rather than a static, one-time effort. Finally, map making that extends CBPR must capture the broad, often cumulative, determinants of health in places and communicate this complexity easily and widely to residents and others beyond the community's boundaries. We summarize the key considerations for using spatial maps in CBPR in Table 16.1 below.

MAPPING FOR ENVIRONMENTAL JUSTICE IN EAST OAKLAND

In East Oakland, California, a community-based organization called Communities for a Better Environment (CBE) has worked to engage residents to document the hazards they are facing in an area called the "Hegenberger Corridor." The mission of Communities for a Better Environment (CBE) is to achieve environmental health and justice by building grassroots power in and with communities of color and working-class communities. Founded in 1978, CBE combines three major tools to support base building in order to impact social change: in-house community organizing, science-based advocacy, and legal intervention—the triad model. CBE's unique contribution is the integration of the three disciplines into a single organizational strategy to leverage facility-specific pollution prevention and regional policy progress that could not be achieved using organizing, science, or legal advocacy alone. The "Hegenberger Corridor" is a small area roughly 1.5 miles long by 0.8 miles wide, situated in the heart of the Elmhurst neighborhood

TABLE 16.1 Key Considerations For Using Spatial Maps in CBPR

CBPR Principles (Israel, B., Schulz, A. J., Parker, E. A., & Becker, A. 1998)	Examples of Mapping Considerations
Community as unit of identity	Different community organizations define geographic or other community boundaries
Build on strengths of community	Map assets, not just liabilities, hazards, etc.
Collaborative partnerships throughout Inquiry	Jointly defining, gathering, analyzing and presenting spatial data
Knowledge for action that benefits community	Maps that contribute to community organizing, awareness of ignored issues, and reframing problems can all highlight options for policy/ interventions
Colearning attends to inequities	Map making can help residents learn about their place as well as highlight features about their community ignored by outsiders
Cyclical and iterative processes	Maps not as static end points but constantly made and remade
Health as positive and ecological perspective	Capturing broad determinants of health in places and cumulative vulnerabilities
Broad dissemination of findings	Graphic and visualization of data can "translate" technical information for multiple audiences; results of Web-based mapping can be viewed by anyone with an Internet connection

in East Oakland, Alameda County, California, where residents are exposed to a series of industrial, transportation, and environmental hazards, such as the Oakland Coliseum, the 100-year old American Brass & Iron Foundry, the Interstate 880 Freeway and other transportation routes serving the Port of Oakland and the Oakland International Airport. The Interstate 880 highway alone brings over 200,000 vehicle trips per day through the Hegenberger Corridor, many of which are heavy diesel engine vehicles. The Port of Oakland is the fifth largest container seaport in the United States, handling 99% of containerized goods moving through Northern California, and is a major source of air pollution.

In the Hegenberger Corridor there are approximately 12,000 residents, over 95% of whom are people of color (49.1% Latinos, 42.6% African Americans, 3.5% Asian and Pacific Islanders, 2.7% whites), while East Oakland has a population of 116,509 residents (45% Latino, 39% African American, 24% White, and 7% Asian). According to the 2010 U.S. Census, the median household income of East Oakland is $37,166 compared to $40,055 for Oakland generally, and 58% of households are below twice the federal poverty level, compared to fewer than 18% in the City of Oakland. Rates of asthma hospitalizations among children under five years of age in East Oakland exceed the Alameda County average rate by two or more times (Alameda County Public Health Department, 2006). According to the 2008 Alameda County Public Health Department Report (ACPHD), *Life and Death from Unnatural Causes: Health & Social Inequity in Alameda County*, East Oakland residents have a life expectancy about ten years less on average than someone living only a mile away in the Oakland Hills (ACPHD, 2008). CBE brings its activism to a long legacy in East Oakland beginning with the rich grassroots organizing starting with the Black Panther Party in 1966. In its work in East Oakland, CBE aims to build on this legacy and partners with a number of local faith-based groups, housing advocacy coalitions such as Alliance of Californians for Community Empowerment (ACCE) and Causa Justa/Just Cause (CJJC), and community-based organizations such as At The Crossroads Homeowners Association (formerly Villa Bonita), Sobrante Park Neighborhood Collaborative, and Elmhurst and Brookfield Neighborhood Associations.

BUILDING LEADERSHIP THROUGH COMMUNITY MAPPING

In an effort to identify the key environmental hazards contributing to poor health in the community, to build a broader community health alliance, and to increase community knowledge of environmental justice issues, CBE partnered with researchers from the University of California, Berkeley, the University of Southern California, and Occidental College, who had a long history of conducting collaborative environmental health and justice research in California and other areas. In particular, CBE was interested in using a CBPR process to integrate mapping into their existing Leadership-Building Institute curriculum—a program that trains residents to be better organizers and advocates. The Leadership-Building Institute included a broad set of workshops and popular education activities that engaged community members to analyze East Oakland from their own perspectives.

CBE's organizing strategy in East Oakland aimed to explicitly build on the rich legacy of activism and social justice in the community, so local partners such as the Allen Temple Baptist Church—a faith-based institution organized in 1919—Tassafaronga Parks and Recreation Center, and several long-standing African-American neighborhood associations joined the Leadership-Building Institute. The idea was to start the mapping exercise with a discussion of the area's development and land use history by including local experts and to bring this historical knowledge into the contemporary mapping project.

The first activity for participants in the leadership academy was a community mapping exercise that located assets and challenges in East Oakland. Community residents developed their own hand-drawn maps and these were combined into a collective community vision. The hand-drawn maps were used as an icebreaker between participants and to identify characteristics of the physical environment for one of the Leadership Institute's first training sessions, "Environmental Justice: Communities Resisting Environmental Racism." Maps drawn by participants highlighted neighborhood problems, assets, and visions. The process was a way to share what residents already knew about the community with others from the same place. This allowed participants to discuss similarities and differences in their visions of their place and, as visions were combined into one map, made the hand-drawn map a rich representation of the community that everyone was deeply invested in since they could see "their own vision" in the map. This first exercise also enhanced community ownership over the process.

After the first exercise, the participants agreed to focus on identifying stationary and mobile air pollution sources and sensitive receptor sites in the Hegenberger Corridor. Subsequent leadership training sessions with community and academic partners included a review of the community redevelopment process and history in East Oakland, a primer on cumulative environmental impacts, and training in using Global Positioning System (GPS) for mapping. The academic partners worked with CBE lead organizer and research director to design the training for the mapping study only. All other aspects of the Leadership Institute's curriculum were designed by CBE and its community partners. The academic partners also conducted a "train the trainers" for CBE staff that included field mapping techniques and the use of GPS, and then CBE staff conducted the trainings for community members.

After agreeing to the geographic boundaries of the study, participants used iPaq handheld computers equipped with GPS and ArcPad GIS software. Paper worksheets were used to record observations, such as if trucks were idling, driving through residential streets, or carrying large containers of chemicals, and these were entered into a spreadsheet that would provide rich narrative descriptions of activities adjacent to environmental hazard and sensitive receptor sites. Community members walked every street in the defined study area to generate the maps and observation data over the course of two weeks; some areas were recorded twice for verification and duplicate data were omitted.

The community-gathered data were shared with the academic partners and, using GIS, maps were created by one of the academic partners. Maps were printed and shared with residents and also projected on the wall during meetings with CBE members, residents, community leaders and academic partners. Community generated maps were overlaid to allow for visual comparisons with hazard data obtained from publicly available data captured by the California Air Resources Board (CARB). The purpose of these meetings was to report back initial findings to the larger community and put the community-gathered data in the context of information used by regulatory agencies.

CBE staff and community leaders identified 216 hazards surrounded by 49 sensitive receptors, including day care and senior centers, only some of which are included in CARB's facility inventories. Diesel trucks were observed illegally driving through and idling for more than five minutes in residential areas, near schools, churches, and other sensitive receptors, causing traffic and pedestrian safety concerns and serving as magnets for crime and litter. This was an important observation to map because existing California regulation makes it illegal for diesel commercial vehicles weighing more than 10,000 pounds (such as delivery trucks, buses, big rigs), including sleeper berth trucks, to idle for more than five minutes. CBE staff and community leaders identified five "hot spots" of illegal diesel engine idling—some idling as long as five hours—and that many trucks were from the nearby Port of Oakland (Figure 16.1).

Community researchers also identified several gaps in the CARB inventory of polluters in the area. Community data revealed that there are 68 automobile-related businesses, as opposed to the nine listed on CARB's database (Figure 16.2). The mapping process also contributed to community members systematically documenting odors, oil spots on paved areas, and other potential environmental harms, as well as the lack of buffering between these businesses and residential areas. The connections between incompatible land uses and community health became apparent to community researchers and others as findings were shared.

FIGURE 16.1 Hegenberger Corridor Area, East Oakland, California and CBE-Mapped Sensitive Receptors, Hazards, and Diesel Truck Idling Locations

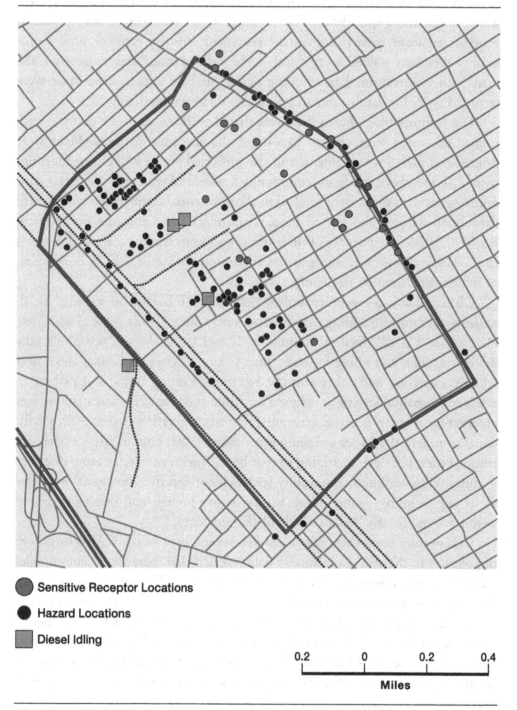

● Sensitive Receptor Locations

● Hazard Locations

■ Diesel Idling

0.2   0   0.2   0.4

Miles

From: Street Science: Community Knowledge and Environmental Health Justice. Jason Corburn, MIT Press, 2005, pg. 175. Reprinted by permission of the MIT Press.

FIGURE 16.2 Hegenberger Corridor, East Oakland, California, and Agency-Identified Hazards and Sensitive Receptors (Squares) & Community-Identified Hazards and Receptors (Circles)

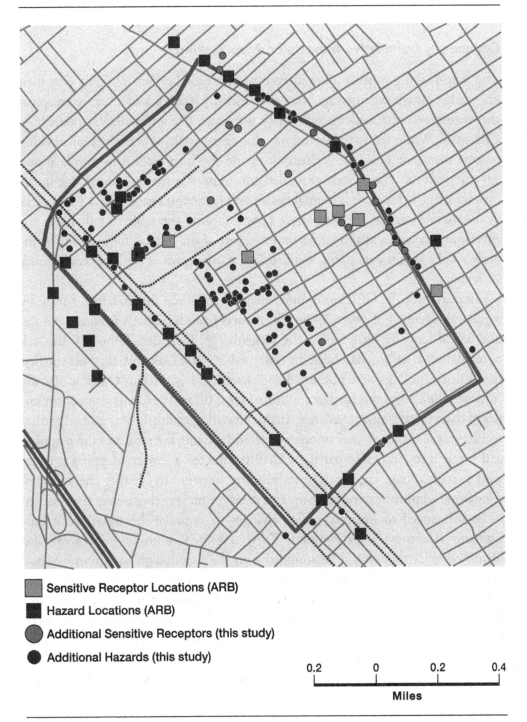

■ Sensitive Receptor Locations (ARB)

■ Hazard Locations (ARB)

● Additional Sensitive Receptors (this study)

● Additional Hazards (this study)

| 0.2 | 0 | 0.2 | 0.4 |

Miles

From: Street Science: Community Knowledge and Environmental Health Justice. Jason Corburn, MIT Press, 2005, pg. 175. Reprinted by permission of the MIT Press.

CBE used the maps and results to create a summary and peer-reviewed report in English and Spanish (www.cbecal.org/campaigns/oakland.html).

Community Cumulative Impacts on Map Making

The map-making process allowed community members to not only put their knowledge into data gathering, but also to identify hazards and sensitive receptors that regulators were missing and which were also not immediately apparent to CBE staff. While the maps were powerful visual tools, it was the map making process that gave CBE the legitimacy to use the information in outreach and advocacy efforts. The process grounded community voice and knowledge in the broader struggle for environmental health and justice and gave CBE a framework of *cumulative impacts*, to bring more people around the table to talk about the environmental and social justice solutions. Part of the process for building legitimacy was linking the mapping work to the broader goals of building community leadership.

Importantly, the CBE community maps highlighted the underestimation by regulatory agencies of potential health impacts from hazardous facilities and the number of sensitive receptors in the Hegenberger Corridor. Although this lack of regulatory attention had been documented in West Oakland, this was the first time similar findings were published and shared widely for East Oakland (Pacific Institute, 2002) and this further confirmed for CBE and residents that communities of color faced similar challenges in documenting multiple hazards and getting regulators to "see" their environment differently. Using the results of the mapping and input from academic partners, CBE conducted a Power Mapping exercise with participants in the Leadership-Building Institute to identify the agencies, regulators, administrative decisions, and decision makers themselves that needed to be influenced to institute policy changes to improve the situation in East Oakland (Democracy for America [DfA], 2009). Community members also identified allies that would be supportive in their campaign for environmental health and justice. One result of this exercise was that CBE demanded that CARB and EPA reevaluate their inventories and confirm or dispute the CBE findings—not the other way around, where community groups are often forced to defend what they know to regulators. The community-driven mapping process also allowed CBE to gain greater legitimacy from the broader East Oakland community, as members were acknowledged as cowriters of the study. A media event releasing the report celebrated the diversity and positive qualities of East Oakland—not just focusing on the hazards—and community members expressed the findings through hip-hop, songs, dance, and poetry. The report was distributed widely—from schools to the Web—and feedback was overwhelmingly positive and supportive.

Mapping follow-up included continuing to recruit members, developing a formal partnership with key East Oakland stakeholders, and building a series of CBPR projects that continue through today, including an air monitoring study for particulate matter (PM 2.5), a diesel truck survey, and a community health survey in 2009. Each research project laid a foundation that supported organizing. For example, the air monitoring study focused on areas where the first mapping study revealed that diesel trucks were idling illegally. In 2010, advocacy work with officials in the City of Oakland resulted in the city funding a comprehensive truck route study based on the initial findings of the community-based mapping and diesel truck survey. Some of CBE's current core campaign strategies, such as community-led Toxic Tours and The Freedom to Breathe initiative, which is focused on reducing pollution and promoting cleaner and healthier environment for East Oakland's workers and residents, continue to utilize the maps and knowledge generated in this CBPR process.

Community Mapping for Health Equity in Brooklyn, New York

In the Greenpoint/Williamsburg neighborhood of Brooklyn, New York, community groups and professionals have engaged in research partnerships and map making to address environmental health disparities. The Greenpoint/Williamsburg neighborhood is a low-income community in which several ethnic groups and polluting industries coexist. Latino, Hasidic Jewish, Polish immigrant, and African American families, along with young white families, live in a neighborhood where over 35% of residents live below the poverty line. In less than five square miles, the neighborhood houses over 30 waste transfer stations, the city's largest sewage treatment facility, and 17 toxic release inventory sites listed by the U.S. Environmental Protection Agency (EPA).

The community mapping project began after residents learned that the New York State Department of Environmental Conservation had scheduled a public hearing to review the operating permit of Radiac, a neighborhood low-level radioactive waste transfer and storage facility (see Corburn, 2005, for a more in-depth discussion of this case). In preparation for the hearing, students at El Puente Academy, a high school run by the community-based organization El Puente, organized a group called the Toxic Avengers to research and document existing environmental health burdens. After walking through the neighborhood with professionals and gathering existing environmental and health data, including information from the city's Department of Environmental Protection about facility location, students generated a map of their neighborhood (Corburn, 2005). The locations and type of facilities, data on facility pollution, and census demographic information were combined by the students to depict how they viewed their community (see Corburn, 2005, p. 175, for a copy of the map).

To create a sense of urgency that local pollution was compromising residents' health, the student map used skulls to mark local hazards and a background designed to look like an x-ray. Pictures of local facilities were included on the map to ensure that viewers recognized polluters by sight, not just by name, and each image was accompanied by brief text about the facility's environmental performance. Maps were placed around the community to alert residents about the upcoming hearing.

The Toxic Avengers' map helped organize over 200 residents to attend the Radiac hearing. The purpose was not necessarily to challenge existing data or how it was being interpreted for policymaking. Instead, El Puente, the community-based organization, used the map to argue that facilities should not be reviewed and permitted one at a time; rather, the hazardous exposures depicted on the map should be the focus of cumulative hazard assessment and the human health impacts from a number of polluters in the neighborhood (Ledogar, Garden Acosta, & Penchaszadeh, 1999). Of equal importance, the map helped organize the first multiethnic environmental health coalition in the neighborhood, the Community Alliance for the Environment (CAFE), whose members included three organizations—El Puente, the Polish-Slavic Center, and United Jewish Organizations—representing thousands of residents.

CONTESTED IMAGES: COMMUNITY AND PROFESSIONAL MAPS

Soon after the CAFE was formed, another community-based organization in the neighborhood was created to monitor environmental health from the community's vantage point, called the Watchperson Project. As part of their monitoring work, the Watchperson Project developed a community-based GIS accessible for all community members, and the organization partnered with Hunter College, City University of New York, to gather electronic data for their computer mapping and monitoring program. The academic partners provided some technical guidance in establishing the GIS, but research questions and priorities were set by community organizations.

Based on community mapping conducted by the CAFE and Hunter College, the U.S. EPA became interested in piloting its Cumulative Exposure Project (CEP) in the Greenpoint/Williamsburg neighborhood (Corburn, 2005). The CEP was initiated in 1994 by the EPA's Office of Policy, Planning and Evaluation to evaluate the cumulative exposures in communities from air, food, and drinking water with the aim of characterizing the multiple pollution burdens and associated health impacts from chronic and acute exposures. One aspect of the EPA's Cumulative Exposure study was to model the cancer and noncancer impacts from exposures to 148 hazardous air pollutants at the census-tract scale, a project later known as the National Air Toxic Assessment (NATA).

The EPA air toxics method and model was presented to community members in Brooklyn, and the Watchperson Project quickly realized that the model might be missing some significant sources of hazardous air pollutants. The EPA model used pollution data from the one New York State Department of Environmental Conservation air monitor in the Greenpoint neighborhood and the roughly fifty Toxic Release Inventory (TRI) sites registered with the EPA. Facilities are registered with the TRI only when they emit, store, or process at least 10,000 pounds of a toxic substance in a year. What the TRI database missed were small-source polluters—such as auto-body repair shops, printers, nail salons, and others—that did not meet the 10,000-pound threshold but were scattered throughout the neighborhood. According to community members commenting on the EPA analysis, the census tract aggregation of the NATA model was potentially going to "wash out" the block-to-block pollution differences that existed in the neighborhood.

The Watchperson Project partnered with Hunter College scientists, young people from a local high school, and community residents to walk the streets and, with the aid of maps, document the locations of polluting facilities and the type of operation. High school students were enrolled as part of a science class and Hunter College researchers partnered with the high school teacher to integrate pollution monitoring and community mapping into the curriculum. Watchperson Project staff trained other community members identified through their ongoing community environmental monitoring work. The Watchperson Project obtained a database of facilities from the New York City Department of Environmental Protection, Bureau of Air Resources Administration Management Information System (BARAMIS), that included permit data on over 3,000 facilities in the neighborhood that were required to file for an air emission permit, but were not regulated, such as apartment building boilers, auto-body paint shops, and printers. The community also launched field surveys to identify potential facilities not found in any agency database or incorrectly located through the wrong address. The community mapping effort aimed to capture whether the EPA model was going to miss important distinctions between city blocks and even within one block. The Watchperson Project and Hunter trained community mappers documented 15,167 distinct land parcels in the community and produced maps comparing the facilities used in the EPA model with facilities regulated by the DEP but which the dispersion model was not going to include (Figure 16. 3). This same group found over 1,000 potentially toxic air polluters that EPA was going to miss in its census-tract level assessment. These field survey data were entered into a geographic information system and joined with demographic and other land use data, such as school and day care facility locations. The community-generated maps were shared by the Watchperson Project leadership with the EPA and revealed the potential gaps in their exposure model.

The community-based mapping also highlighted that over fifty residential buildings had a printer, dry cleaner, or nail salon on the ground floor, presenting a potentially dangerous exposure for residents living upstairs and noting that there were no regulations or monitoring of these small-source emitters. Building on the findings from the community maps, a team of the Watchperson Project, Hunter College scientists and El Puente high school students and community researchers used funding from a Centers for Disease Control Asthma and Community Health grant to employ residents to do targeted air sampling in and around the buildings with polluting facilities on the ground floor. The samples revealed elevated concentrations of percholoroethylene, toluene, and xylene outside of homes and elevated concentrations of volatile organic compounds inside apartments located in buildings with one of the targeted facilities operating on the ground floor. The Watchperson Project estimated that as many as 183 apartments and approximately 550 residents were living above dry cleaning

FIGURE 16.3 Example of Block-by-Block Watchperson Project Map of Facilities EPA Modeling Was Missing

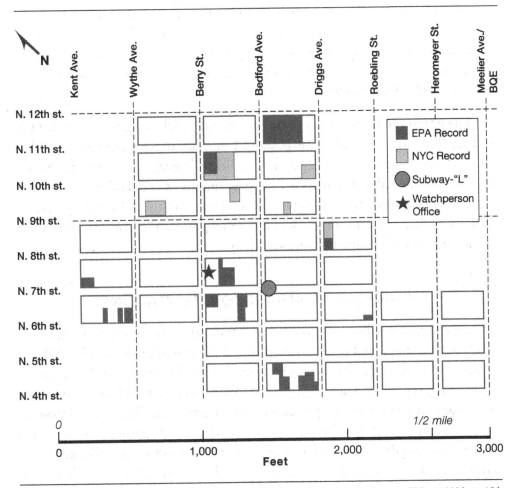

From: *Street Science: Community Knowledge and Environmental Health Justice.* Jason Corburn, MIT Press, 2005, pg. 194. Reprinted by permission of the MIT Press.

establishments and exposed to potentially dangerous concentrations of air toxics. Concentrations of "perc" inside apartments above dry cleaners were estimated to be close to 100 parts per million (PPM) while the EPA model had estimated *outdoor* concentration of perc in the community at less than 2 ppb (parts per billion), with a maximum-modeled census tract outdoor concentration of 39 ppb. According to Fred Talcott, project director of the CEP at EPA:

The average concentration found in apartments above dry cleaning establishments was on the order of 1,000 times higher than the outdoor concentration of "Perc" as predicted by our model in G/W. That to me is an illustration of a micro-level problem that would be completely obscured if you only looked at daily walking around concentration. Without the community group data set, we would have missed this. (Corburn, 2005, p. 195)

The group produced a map of their findings, which was used by the EPA in their final report on cumulative exposures. Community mapping helped validate what residents were already experiencing, helped bring this knowledge to the attention of the EPA, and helped raise new questions, validate new sources of data, new exposures, and new groups claiming access to the assessment process—all of which had a significant impact on the way professionals viewed community knowledge and environmental epidemiology.

CHALLENGES AND RECOMMENDATIONS

The cases presented here also raise some challenges for community members, activists, academics, and others attempting to use mapping to extend CBPR for health equity. First, organizing youth around scientific and health issues can be challenging, especially when engaged research projects demand long-term, multiyear commitments and young people may have limited available time. However, one recommendation from our experience is that the mapping process should *engage young people early and often*, especially as new technologies, Web and social media geared toward youth become commonplace as mapping tools. Partnering with youth can also ensure that map making is fun, tied to local culture and even a broader fundraising strategy, as CBE recognized in East Oakland. Engaging youth can also support mapping as a strategy to build new organizational capacity, leadership, and power, especially when community members drive the research questions, selection of appropriate data, and interpreting and presenting results.

A second challenge is that the rapid pace of technological change and sophistication may lead some groups to choose to leapfrog and start with the latest, most advanced tools. Our experience suggests that this rarely builds on local knowledge and may create an overdependency of community groups on technology and outside expert advisers. Hence, we suggest that mapping processes are most successful when they *build incrementally* from small to larger scale, from less to more complex, and from low to higher technology. This trajectory can be rather quick with skilled partnerships and collaborations, as Brooklyn activists moved from cartoons to GIS to sophisticated handheld environmental monitoring equipment in a relatively short time period. Ultimately, mapping can act as a key piece of an ongoing community-led research program.

A third challenge for mapping processes is to *focus on both bonding and bridging*, where bonding helps different CBOs and community members build trust and partnerships among themselves and bridging allows the mapping process and outputs to engage with unlikely allies and change agents, such as regulators and academic scientists. Often, the goal of a community mapping effort is to build community alliances and gather local knowledge or challenge an inaccurate characterization of a place done by outsiders, but not both. The cases presented here suggest that a both/and approach be explicit from the outset and designed into the mapping process.

Fourth, *linking concrete community health concerns with broader policy frames* and campaigns is another challenge of map making. An example of this was when CBE linked the neighborhood mapping of illegal truck idling and unregulated toxic sites to a policy campaign focused on preventing cumulative community environmental burdens. Characterizing one's community by selecting certain features to map always requires value judgments over what to leave out. Instead of viewing this as a weakness or limitation, we suggest that a community map-making process be explicit from the outset about the policy objectives and issue they are aiming to address, with place-based health inequities being one logical policy frame. Most cities, towns, and counties in the United States do not have detailed health determinant data that can be geocoded and mapped to show spatial distributions, making comparisons of community-gathered data to other administrative data sets a challenge. However, this also acts as an opportunity for community mapping efforts to fill a major gap in the field of population health and health disparities.

COMMUNITY MAPPING IN CBPR: OPPORTUNITIES AND LESSONS LEARNED

Community-mapping can act as a core method and process when using a CBPR approach and should be considered by all practitioners interested in building community knowledge and using that knowledge to inform action, leadership, organizing and ultimately improving the science of assessing health burdens in places. As these two cases have shown, when mapping processes embody the core principles of CBPR, they can contribute to the opportunities and lessons learned described below.

1. *Building a power/organizing base in communities of color.* In East Oakland the mapping process was embedded into a broader Leadership Institute, and in Brooklyn youth mapping helped galvanize a community to stop the siting of a potentially hazardous land use.

2. *Reframing community organizing priorities.* When Oakland and Brooklyn activists mapped their neighborhoods, they saw new assets and hazards and as a result reframed their organizing efforts around cumulative burdens.

3. *Highlighting local knowledge.* Mapping helped Oakland and Brooklyn community members document what they anecdotally suspected about environmental harms in their community, and that regulatory agencies charged with protecting communities were ignoring important local expertise of land uses.

4. *Linking work to health equity.* By mapping multiple toxic burdens in their community and engaging environmental health academics, both Oakland and Brooklyn activists used the mapping process to link their findings to larger policy debates about health equity and environmental justice.

5. *Demystifying research and environmental regulations.* The Oakland and Brooklyn community mapping acted as a "common language" that allowed a range of community members—young and old from different ethnic, language, and educational backgrounds—to understand and relate scientific processes to their lived experiences. The "democratization" of the research process and translation of science into policy helped to make public health science, which is often abstracted in percentages and numbers from people's daily lives, much more accessible to community members.

6. *Changing policy/improving lives.* In both the Oakland and Brooklyn cases, community-gathered information changed the way environmental regulators and other decision makers saw the hazards in these places and contributed to policy changes. More strict environmental and other policies were adopted as a result of community mapping that will reduce exposures to hazardous

pollutants in these neighborhoods and reduce health inequities. Just as important, regulatory agencies saw each community as legitimate experts in shaping new policies and made new efforts to include CBOs in future regulatory decisions. As both our cases highlighted, mapping health data can help improve living conditions in low-income, communities of color by offering compelling visual narratives of health disparities and concrete interventions to change these inequities. In our view, successful CBPR mapping processes are the means toward the end of greater health equity.

SUMMARY

Community mapping is one important tool to organize residents and extend the CBPR approach of ensuring that research contributes to action. In communities across the country, previously disempowered groups are partnering with academics and other groups to gather what they know, ask new research questions, visually share their findings, and hold decision makers accountable for persistent health inequities. As public health practitioners and social epidemiologists recognize that "place matters" for understanding why some populations in some places get sick more often and die prematurely, community mapping will be increasingly important for gathering information on the features and characteristics of places that influence well-being. Capturing both hazards and assets is crucial, and a CBPR approach is vital for ensuring that both residents and researchers engage in a collaborative process for deciding what information to capture, what role different technologies can play, what to display on maps, and how to share visual information within and outside the community. We have offered some reflections here on our own experiences, and acknowledge that similar processes may not be possible or necessary everywhere. What is crucial is that community members consider mapping as one part of an ongoing health equity advocacy and policy change strategy.

KEY TERMS

Community organizing

Maps

Spatial data

Technology

DISCUSSION QUESTIONS

1. What added value can maps that visualize complex environmental and health information bring to CBPR?

2. How can community members and researchers collaborate to map community information that isn't a static, one-time process?

3. How might maps help community members identify assets and hazards in their place and link these to inform concrete actions and policies?

4. How can mapping be an organizing tool in itself?

REFERENCES

Alameda County Public Health Department. (2006). *Alameda County health status report.* Retrieved November 11, 2010 from www.acphd.org/media/52956/achsr2006.pdf

Alameda County Public Health Department (ACPHD). (2008). *Life and death from unnatural causes: Health and social inequity in Alameda County.* Oakland, CA: ACPHD. http://www .acphd.org/user/services/AtoZ_PrgDtls.asp?PrgId=90, Accessed January 20, 2011.

Brody, H., Rip, M. R., Vinten-Johansen, P., Paneth, N., & Rachman, S. (2000). Map-making and myth-making in Broad Street: The London cholera epidemic, 1854. *The Lancet, 356*(9223), 64–68.

Corburn J. (2005). *Street science: Community knowledge and environmental health justice.* Cambridge, MA: MIT Press.

Cromley, E. K., & McLafferty, S. L. (2002). *GIS and public health.* New York: Guilford Press.

Democracy for America (DfA). 2009. *Power mapping: Step-by-step.* Campaign Academy Grassroots Campaign Training Manual. http://moveon.org/team/campaigns/GuideToPower Mapping.pdf, Accessed June 13, 2011.

Gatrell, A. C., & Elliot, S. J. (2009). *Geographies of health: An introduction* (2nd ed). West Sussex: Wiley-Blackwell.

Hull House Residents. (1895). *Hull House maps and papers.* New York: Thomas Y. Crowell.

Israel, B., Schulz, A. J., Parker, E. A., & Becker, A. B. (1998). Review of community-based research: Assessing partnership approaches to improve public health. *Annual Review of Public Health, 19*, 173–202.

Julia, C., & Valleron, A.-J. (2010). Louis-René Villermé (1782–1863), a pioneer in social epidemiology: Re-analysis of his data on comparative mortality in Paris in the early 19th century. *Journal of Epidemiology and Community Health.* doi:10.1136/jech.2009.087957

Kwan, M. (2009). From place-based to people-based exposure measures. *Social Science and Medicine, 69*(9): 1311–1313.

Ledogar, R. J., Garden Acosta, L., & Penchaszadeh, A. (1999). Building international public health vision through local community research: The El Puente-CIET partnership. *American Journal of Public Health, 89*, 1795–1797.

Maantay, J., Maroko, A. R., Alicea, C., & Strelnick, A. H. (2009). Geographic information systems, environmental justice, and health disparities. In N. Freudenberg, S. Klitzman, S. Saegert (Eds)., *Urban health and society: Interdisciplinary approaches to research and practice.* San Francisco: Jossey-Bass.

Pacific Institute. (2002). *Neighborhood knowledge for change.* Retrieved June 29, 2010 from http://www.pacinst.org/reports/environmental_indicators/

Chapter 17

PHOTOVOICE AS A

CBPR METHOD

A CASE STUDY WITH AFRICAN AMERICAN BREAST CANCER SURVIVORS IN RURAL EASTERN NORTH CAROLINA

ELLEN D. S. LÓPEZ

NAOMI ROBINSON

EUGENIA ENG

Photovoice is a participatory action research method that involves placing cameras in the hands of participants so that they may visually represent and communicate to others their lived experiences (Wang & Burris, 1994). During discussions about the meanings embedded within their photographs, participants are able to examine their worldviews and the events that shape them, and to communicate insights about their lives to others (Wang, Burris, & Xiang, 1996). The goals of photovoice are to enable people to:

1. Record and reflect their personal and community's strengths and concerns through taking photographs

2. Promote critical dialogue and knowledge about important issues through discussing their photographs

3. Reach policymakers and decision makers who can influence positive social change through hosting public forums and showings of their photographs.

When used in the context of a community-based participatory research (CBPR) approach, photovoice has the potential to enhance the quality and validity of research by drawing on local expertise to generate a new understanding about issues that participants deem important. Through sharing their knowledge with influential people to whom they might not normally have access, participants may forge relationships through which their insights can be used to catalyze individual and social change (Wang & Burris, 1997).

In this chapter we focus on the use of photovoice as an approach to research that is community-based and participatory. We first present a brief review of the origins, diverse applications, and theoretical underpinnings of photovoice. We then present a case example of a CBPR project we conducted using photovoice as the primary method of research. Finally, we share some of the challenges we encountered, and the lessons we learned from our experience and a review of the photovoice literature.

THE ORIGIN, USE, AND THEORETICAL
UNDERPINNINGS OF PHOTOVOICE

Photovoice **was** originally codified and applied by Caroline Wang, Mary Ann Burris, and colleagues while they were working in China's Yunnan province with rural village women. These women seldom had access to those who made decisions affecting their lives, both reflecting and reinforcing their social status (Wang & Burris, 1994). Photovoice afforded greater control to these village women over the ways their perspectives and life situations were depicted, discussed, and communicated to others. The women reached policymakers and decision makers through public showings and forums during which they presented and interpreted their photographs. The power of their photographs, coupled with text from their critical discussions, helped influence policymakers and decision makers to enact beneficial changes, such as constructing day-care facilities and water tanks in villages and establishing educational scholarships for rural girls (Wang & Burris, 1994).

Since its initial development, photovoice has been conducted with diverse populations around the world as a means to inform: needs and assets assessments (Wang, Cash, & Powers, 2000), program development (Zenkov & Harmon, 2009), program evaluation (Vaughn, Forbes, & Howell, 2009), and measurement development (Newman & Kanjanawong, 2005). Photovoice has also been applied with the goal of achieving enhanced levels of civic engagement, empowerment, and advocacy for typically underserved and marginalized populations such as women, youth, persons with disabilities, and people living with chronic diseases such as cancer, diabetes, and HIV/AIDS (Gant et al., 2009; Hergenrather, Rhodes, & Clark, 2006; Necheles et al., 2007; Wang, 2006). Over the years, photovoice has proven to be a flexible participatory method. Since its introduction, researchers and community partners have adapted the logistics of photovoice to meet their specific preferences, project aims, budgets, and other practical considerations (Wang, 2006).

Theoretical Underpinnings of Photovoice

Photovoice takes its theoretical and practical underpinnings from Freire's empowerment education for **critical consciousness** (Freire, 1970), feminist theory (Reinharz, 1992), and participatory documentary photography (Ewald, 1996; Wang & Burris, 1994). Each approach embodies a distinct set of underlying values which inherently acknowledges that the absence of research and information regarding underrepresented groups perpetuates powerlessness, and that political and power structures undermine the expertise individuals possess about their own lives and situations. Each approach strives to shift control over representation and knowledge generation from those in positions of power to those whose perspectives are seldom seen or heard. The idea is that knowledge gained from these perspectives can and should inform social change. All three approaches (critical consciousness, feminist theory, participatory documentary photography) identify the visual image as an important tool through which groups that have been ignored or marginalized by society can share knowledge and engage in illuminating discourse about the social and political forces that influence their daily lives (Ewald, 1996; Freire, 1970; Reinharz, 1992; Solomon, 1995; Weiler, 1994).

APPLICATION OF PHOTOVOICE: THE SURVIVING ANGELS— INSPIRATIONAL IMAGES PROJECT

Here we present the Surviving Angels—Inspirational Images Project as a case study of a CBPR collaboration that used photovoice as its principal method. Conducted over a three-year period between 1999 and 2002, our project represented a partnership comprising facilitators from a local self-help group for **African American breast cancer** survivors, 13 African American breast cancer survivors (self-named Surviving Angels) from three counties in rural eastern North Carolina, and academic researchers from the University of North Carolina at Chapel Hill (UNC-CH) School of Public Health. The Inspirational Images Project was the primary focus of first author Ellen López's doctoral dissertation. Through this collaboration, the Surviving Angels engaged in a photovoice project that entailed the following:

- Participating in a photovoice training session
- Documenting their experiences as rural African American breast cancer survivors by means of five photo assignments
- Participating in seven photo-discussion sessions
- Assessing the trustworthiness of findings that emerged during analysis of their discussions
- Planning and hosting an interactive forum to share findings and forge collaborations with influential people identified as being advocates for change

Preparing for the Photovoice Project Using a CBPR Process

Our project was guided by the testimonies from survivors and by a body of **cancer survivorship** and quality-of-life literature. A pilot study we conducted with two survivors helped to test the feasibility of using photovoice with African American cancer survivors, while we codeveloped the protocol used to conduct the Inspirational Images Project.

Background and Purpose

At the time of our study, for African American women in rural eastern North Carolina, cultural norms and beliefs promoted silence about breast cancer (Ashing-Giwa & Ganz, 1997). Work with rural African American communities in North Carolina found that older women remembered the long-standing social and historical conditions of inequality, such as a segregated health care system (Earp et al., 1997; Eng & Smith, 1995). These memories made it especially difficult for rural African American breast cancer survivors to express their quality-of-life (QOL) concerns. As perceptions of QOL are influenced by cultural and ethnic factors such as social norms, values, beliefs, and shared experiences (Hassey Dow, Ferrell, Leigh, Ly, & Gulasekaram, 1996), many of the concerns experienced by African American survivors were unique from those of other women.

At the time when the Inspirational Images Project was conducted, few studies had explored cancer survivorship for African American women (Northouse et al., 1999). Most QOL studies were based on white participants. Consequently, insufficient knowledge existed about the influence of ethnicity and culture on QOL (Leedham & Ganz, 1999). At that early stage of understanding African American breast cancer survivors' QOL concerns, our challenge was to clarify the role of race and ethnicity in shaping differential social and cultural contexts that led many African American survivors to live in silence with breast cancer.

The Need

The Inspirational Images Project was an offshoot of the North Carolina Breast Cancer Screening Program (NC-BCSP). NC-BCSP worked with African American communities in rural eastern North Carolina from 1991 through 2003 to successfully address barriers to cancer screening through establishing a network of lay health advisers (Earp et al., 2002; Earp, et al., 1997). NC-BCSP also sponsored a local self-help group for breast cancer survivors and their families. The We-Count program (pseudonyms are used for groups and individuals who participated in our project) was developed and facilitated by NC-BCSP community outreach specialist Helen Rock, who brought to the monthly meetings her own survivorship experiences.

The relationships developed by López and the other academic researchers who worked with NC-BCSP and We-Count, through which rapport and trust were established with several breast cancer survivors, formed the foundation of the Inspirational Images Project. As more was learned about survivors and their lives, it became apparent that many women obtained their survivorship support and information almost exclusively through We-Count. In fact, Ms. Rock often described the responsibility she felt as the primary resource to other survivors in her community. Our goal in forging a partnership with We-Count was to design and conduct a CBPR study that would enable breast cancer survivors to explore and voice their survivorship concerns so that a broader set of appropriate strategies could be developed to address them.

Our challenge was to use a research approach that would enable African American breast cancer survivors to communicate the social and cultural meaning of living in silence with breast cancer. López broached the idea of photovoice with Ms. Rock and Marian Sweet (another survivor who often cofacilitated We-Count meetings). Both agreed to participate in a pilot study to assess the feasibility of using photovoice with African American survivors in their community. Ms. Rock and Ms. Sweet represented variation in age, treatment regimen, time since diagnosis, and experience of recurrence. As such, they contributed different survivorship perspectives. As the women to whom other women turned for support and information, they also provided insight into how other survivors would react to the photovoice method and made suggestions, based on their own participation, for improving the study protocol.

Our pilot study was a small-scale photovoice project that included an introductory meeting and two sequences of photo assignments and audiotaped photo-discussion sessions. The photo assignments (developed with Ms. Rock and Ms. Sweet) included taking at least six pictures of the *"people, places and things that make your life enjoyable"* and *"the small, yet significant things that you have encountered as a breast cancer survivor and what you did to cope."* The pilot study also involved content analysis of taped discussions and a findings feedback session. During each photo-discussion session, Ms. Rock and Ms. Sweet shared and talked about their pictures. In addition, López used a structured process guide to elicit feedback about the extent to which the photovoice method was sensitive to participants' issues; feasible and enjoyable; and able to generate findings that accurately reflected participants' survivorship experiences.

During the findings feedback session, López reported back the themes that emerged through content analysis of the photo discussions. Ms. Rock and Ms. Sweet verified that the findings substantially captured their survivorship experiences, and were pleased at how effective the photos had been at triggering their critical discussions. They then agreed to collaborate in designing and conducting a larger photovoice project to benefit survivors and enhance the scope of We-Count. The subsequent Surviving Angels—Inspirational Images Project was tailored according to their feedback and guidance on issues ranging from the decision to use disposable cameras (because women might feel more comfortable carrying around an inexpensive throwaway camera than a more expensive digital camera) to the location and scheduling of photo-discussion sessions.

Research Methods to Achieve Objectives

The Inspirational Images Projects' specific aims were to achieve the following:

1. Engage breast cancer survivors in exploring how their QOL is perceived and addressed within their own social context.

2. Develop a conceptual framework of QOL and the impact of social and cultural factors.

3. Engage local policymakers and decision makers in reviewing findings to identify opportunities and initiate steps toward developing culturally appropriate interventions.

4. To achieve our aims, we used the photovoice method and data collection and analysis techniques of grounded theory. *Grounded theory* is a method of discovery where theory is generated from, or "grounded in," data that have been systematically collected through social research (Glaser & Strauss, 1967). Our photovoice and grounded theory data collection and analyses were guided by research questions posed to uncover rural African American breast cancer survivors' perceptions of their QOL needs; the physical, psychological, social, spiritual, and cultural factors that affect these perceptions; the strategies survivors develop to address their QOL needs; and the points in the survivorship process where interventions can be developed.

5. *Setting.* Ms. Rock recruited survivors from three rural counties located in the eastern coastal region of North Carolina. At the time of the project, all three counties ranked among the most economically deprived in North Carolina (U.S. Department of Agriculture, 2002), had populations less than 30,000, and were 45–60% African American (N.C. Office of State Budget and Management, 2011). Although each county had its own hospital, cancer patients and survivors often traveled 35–100 miles to larger towns for cancer care, support services, and stores that offered cancer-related products for African Americans (such as wigs, turbans, and prosthetics).

6. *Partners and Their Roles.* As coinvestigators and colearners, the Surviving Angels, community research advisers (CRAs), and researchers shared the

responsibility of decision-making power throughout the research process. Funding from Komen for the Cure enabled the project to hire Ms. Rock and Ms. Pleasant, two women who were well known and trusted in their communities as paid, part-time community research advisers (CRAs). As individuals who lived and worked in the project communities, the CRAs provided insights on local social and cultural norms that guided and shaped our research process (Goodman et al., 1998). Specifically, they participated in planning meetings, helped facilitate project-related activities, reviewed all protocols and materials, assisted survivors with the logistics of photovoice (such as providing transportation to meetings, picking up film for processing, and answering questions). They also used their community connections to secure a comfortable and convenient meeting house and provided access to survivors who would partner on the project.

The Surviving Angels contributed their expertise as women who had experienced cancer in their rural communities. They helped to guide the data collection and analysis through their participation in the photovoice process. The Angels clarified and interpreted preliminary themes that emerged from analysis of their photo discussions and assessed the trustworthiness of the findings and conceptual framework. They also took the lead in disseminating findings and forging relationships with influential people through a public forum and showing of their photographs, and they collaborated in sharing findings through other means, such as presentations at conferences and publications (López, Eng, Randall-David, & Robinson, 2005).

López and other academic partners contributed skills and experience as public health investigators and practitioners to develop a research protocol that would yield trustworthy findings. They also applied for funding, developed project-related materials, cofacilitated meetings, analyzed data, coauthored manuscripts and presentations, and worked with the CRAs to oversee the project's day-to-day activities.

Selecting and Recruiting Participants

Ms. Rock identified eligible participants from a database she maintained of the women who contacted her for breast health–related assistance, some of whom were members of We-Count. From her list, we used purposive sampling (Patton, 1990) to recruit survivors who met the following criteria: had completed their initial treatment; were willing to take photographs about their survivorship; were open to sharing their photos with a small group of survivors; and were able to commit to attending multiple meetings spanning several months.

Ms. Rock contacted potential participants and used information from our project factsheet and informed consent form (see Appendix K) to help describe the project, discuss what participation would entail, and answer questions. Survivors who showed interest in participating received an invitation to attend an informational training session. With permission, López called each invitee to introduce herself and answer questions. To reduce barriers to participation, we offered transportation and reimbursement for travel expenses.

Implementing the Photovoice Project Using a CBPR Process

Our photovoice process involved the following activities: a photovoice training, sequences of photo assignments and photo discussions, theoretical sampling, data management and grounded theory analysis, and data feedback and interpretation.

Training Photovoice Participants

The training session provided an initial encounter that promoted rapport and trust among CRAs, participants, and academic partners. Thirteen women attended the training, during which we discussed the project's goals, the photovoice process, and the concept of participatory research in which the survivors would be asked to take a role as active partners. The group also discussed power dynamics and ethical issues associated with using a camera, assessing personal safety when approaching a stranger to take their photograph, and the importance of expressing appreciation by offering to send individuals copies of their photographs (Wang, 1999). The women then received their disposable cameras, basic instructions on how to use them, and tips for taking successful photographs (for example, when in doubt, use your flash). The women tried out their cameras by taking pictures of each other, and role-played using the acknowledgment form (see Appendix L) that they would be using to obtain written permission prior to taking a person's photograph (Wang & Redwood-Jones, 2001).

During the training the women brainstormed ideas for photo assignments to identify specific aspects of their survivorship they wanted to explore, and to promote reflection on everyday experiences that might be important to their QOL, but too mundane to be regarded as noteworthy (Koch, 1970). They decided that their first photo assignment would be to *"take at least six pictures that represent information I wish I would have had as a survivor."*

Prior to ending the training session, the CRAs reminded the women that they would be contacting them to set a date and time to pick up their cameras for processing. The group then scheduled the first photo-discussion session. During the time between the training and photo-discussion session, López, CRAs, and Surviving Angels were often in contact to ensure that everyone was comfortable with the photovoice process.

Collecting Data: Photo-Discussion Sessions

The Angels took one month to complete each photo assignment, and after each assignment the group met for a three-hour discussion session. All sessions were audiotaped with permission. The sessions typically began by reviewing the project objectives and meeting agenda. López then presented the themes that emerged from analysis of previous sessions so that the Angels could discuss and clarify preliminary findings. This was followed by a "show and tell" activity during which each woman presented her photographs and explained how they related to the photo assignment. For example, for the photo assignment *"information I wish I would have had as a survivor,"* one Angel, Ms. Grace, presented her picture of trash bags filled with cans for recycling (Figure 17.1). She recounted that she did not know about financial aid programs that could help her pay for her cancer medications. She explained: *"Well, I had been saving cans before breast cancer, but after I got breast cancer it was more important that I save [them] financially. So that's the reason I saved the cans."*

The group then chose one or two photographs to discuss in-depth, guided by SHOWED, a six-step inductive questioning technique (Wallerstein & Bernstein, 1988). The SHOWED questions were:

1. What do you *See* in this photograph?

2. What is *Happening* in the photograph?

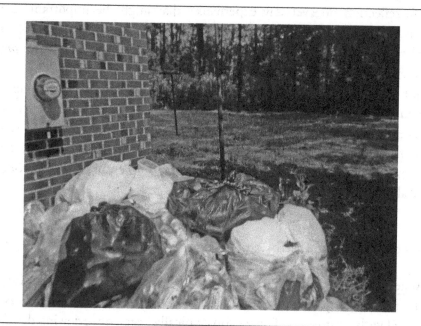

3.   How does this relate to *Our* lives?

4.   *Why* do these issues exist?

5.   How can we become *Empowered* by our new social understanding?

6.   What can we *Do* to address these issues?

This line of questioning helped move the Angels' discussions about their photographs from concrete to personal levels, then to a social analysis of the root causes of issues, and finally to identifying action steps for creating positive change (Wallerstein & Bernstein, 1988; Wang & Burris, 1997).

Sampling on Theoretical Grounds: Using Preliminary Findings to Guide Future Data Collection

At the end of each photo discussion the Angels summarized the themes they had heard. Using theoretical sampling (Glaser & Strauss, 1967), these new themes, as well as those that emerged during analysis of earlier sessions, helped to direct the avenues of inquiry that the women chose to explore during subsequent photo assignment and photo-discussion sequences. In addition, the Angels asked themselves, "Given what we have learned so far, what should we explore next? What should be our next photo assignment?" The answers to these questions helped the women develop their next photo assignment.

After five photo assignments and photo-discussion sequences (which occurred over a seven-month period because on two occasions participants opted to continue discussing the same assignment for two sessions), we began to hear the same information being repeated. At this point everyone agreed that no new information was being generated and that data saturation had been achieved (Glaser & Strauss, 1967; Strauss & Corbin, 1998).

Conducting Data Management and Grounded Theory Analysis

López took primary responsibility for data management and analysis with assistance from the CRAs. Immediately after each session, López listened to the audiotape to review the session and insert notes (about things such as body language and expressed emotions) (Sandelowski, 1995). She then had the tapes professionally transcribed, verbatim, and the transcripts became the raw data for grounded theory analysis using the qualitative management software Atlas.ti (version 4.2).

Grounded theory analysis involved reading through the transcripts multiple times and then breaking down the data analytically and assigning conceptual labels. For example, an Angel's recounting of praying to be cured was labeled "prayed for a cure." Data were then coded within and across the different transcripts and speakers, using the constant comparison method so that related concepts could be grouped into categories. For example, concepts such as "prayed for a cure" and "turning cancer over to G-d" were grouped into the category "relying on spiritual faith." Theory began to emerge as conceptual relationships among the categories became evident. For example, during analysis the category "relying on spiritual faith" emerged as an important strategy used by the Angels to address their QOL concerns. Analysis was complete when most of the categories could be unified around the central analytical ideas represented in the data (Strauss & Corbin, 1998).

Although the Angels chose not to be involved in reading and coding the transcripts, reviewing preliminary findings at each photo-discussion session provided them the opportunity to discuss, interpret, and clarify emerging concepts, themes, and conceptual linkages. For example, the group reported that some survivors receive the message from men that by having lost their breast, they had "lost their womanhood." Although the Angels verified that this theme was indeed grounded in the data, they clarified that it was not only men, but also women who contributed to the stigma of breast cancer and having undergone a mastectomy.

When the qualitative analysis was completed, we held a wrap-up findings meeting during which the Angels reviewed the final themes and conceptual model. While discussing each theme the Angels worked together to clarify any misconceptions and refined the findings until they credibly depicted what they wanted others to understand about their survivorship experiences (Kvale, 1995).

Developing a QOL Framework Grounded in Survivors' Experiences and Perspectives

From our analysis we developed a quality-of-life (QOL) framework (Figure 17.2) that brings to light how QOL is intricately tied to the socially ascribed status of being African American, a woman, and a cancer survivor. Through sharing their experiences, the Angels illustrated how the three social forces of racism, the stigma of cancer, and the cultural expectations of African American women (depicted in the center of the figure) drive four QOL concerns: seeking safe sources of support; adjusting to the role of "cancer survivor"; feeling comfortable about one's future; and serving as a role model to others (depicted in the four central ovals). The framework also suggests two specific individual-level strategies that survivors devise to achieve maximum QOL: relying on the spiritual faith (the inner ring) and maintaining social standing (the outer ring). (For an in-depth discussion of project results and the QOL framework, see López, 2002; López, et al., 2005.)

Addressing health issues from a strengths-based and ecological perspective is an established principle of the CBPR approach (Israel, Schulz, Parker, & Becker, 1998). The Angel's QOL framework shows how interventions might build on the personal strategies that survivors already employ to maximize QOL. It also illustrates how such interventions may address survivors' concerns by targeting

FIGURE 17.2 African American Breast Cancer Survivorship Quality-of-Life Framework Developed During Photovoice Study

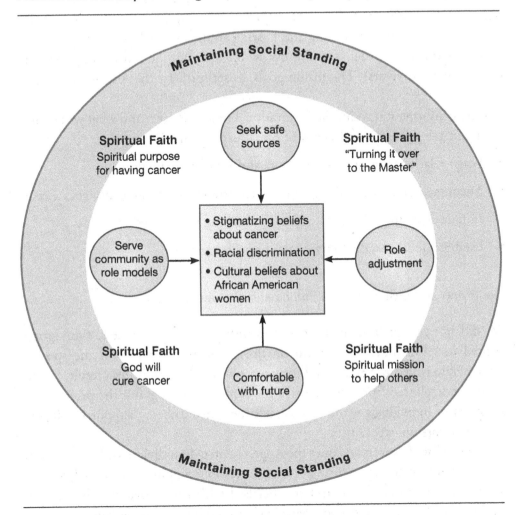

the social forces that operate as policies and practices of local organizations and institutions and as governing norms of their rural communities.

Sharing Findings with Local Policymakers and Decision Makers: Planning and Conducting a Forum

Congruent with the CBPR principle of disseminating findings to and by all partners (Israel, et al., 1998), a specific goal of photovoice is to enable participants to reach local policymakers and decision makers through public forums and showings of their photographs, with the aim of stimulating social action and change (Wang & Burris, 1994). Near the completion of our project the Angels took the lead in planning and hosting an interactive forum for influential advocates (people in their community whom they recognized as supporters of breast cancer survivors). The forum goals, as set forth by the Angels, were to:

- Share information about the Inspirational Images Project and what we learned about the strengths and needs of breast cancer survivors

- Forge relationships among survivors and influential advocates

- Encourage interest in taking action steps toward addressing survivors' needs

- Initiate steps toward taking action by forming task forces

- Establish local sustainability of the project

Identifying and Inviting Forum Participants: Influential Advocates

We did not recruit influential advocates until late in the process. Our group wanted to select individuals based on their influence in terms of the specific survivorship issues that emerged during our photo-discussions. As a result, forum guests were selected from an extensive list compiled throughout the project that consisted of individuals whom the Angels identified as being supportive during their survivorship experience.

From a list of over sixty names the Angels invited 43 individuals. Twenty-seven influential advocates representing diverse professions and interests participated in our forum; they were local elected officials, health care providers, clergy, legal service providers, cancer-support agency representatives, and academics.

Presenting Photographs and Engaging in Action-Oriented Discussion

The forum agenda featured photo displays, presentations about The Inspirational Images Project and what we learned, small-group work, issue prioritization, and future action planning steps. Upon arrival, forum participants walked around the venue (a local high school cafeteria) to view photo displays that featured 8-by-10-inch enlargements of the photographs taken and chosen by the Angels, along with explanatory statements quoted from the group's discussions. The displays also exhibited the photographs we took throughout the project to document our process and experiences. Several Angels then presented information about the Inspirational Images Project, including our rationale for conducting the project, the data collection and analysis methods, and the findings. Because the conceptual framework was not yet finalized, we decided to present a list of 10 themes (illustrated with quotations) that the Angels felt relayed important information about their survivorship experiences. For example, one of the themes exemplified the significance that both medical and spiritual intervention have in cancer treatment and survival: *"The survivor's comfort with her health care provider is strained when her provider does not respect her belief in prayer, and her belief that providers are created to do the Lord's work."*

To progress beyond merely presenting findings to the influential advocates to engaging them in discussion about QOL needs and strategies to address them, the forum participants divided into five small groups. Each group was lead by two Angels and focused on one of the 10 themes. The small-group objectives were to introduce a scenario (based on experiences shared by Angels during our photo discussions), use it to trigger discussion employing the SHOWED questioning technique, and then propose three strategies to address the theme discussed.

Prioritizing Needs and Initiating Plans for Taking Social Action

When the forum participants reconvened, representatives from each small group summarized their group's scenario and presented their three strategies. All of the strategies were written on newsprint, posted on a wall, and then grouped into categories. To prioritize future efforts, all participants came up to the wall to place stickers next to the three strategies they felt were most important to undertake to improve QOL for survivors (Figure 17.3). The strategies "educating clergy" and "educating male partners" about the needs of breast cancer survivors received the most votes.

Several Angels and influential advocates then volunteered to participate on task forces to develop each of the strategies, and scheduled a meeting to convene their groups. Prior to ending the forum, all the participants celebrated the Inspirational Images Project with a shared meal. To sustain the efforts and the newly forged relationships, one of the CRAs accepted responsibility for coordinating

FIGURE 17.3 Voting to Prioritize Future Efforts During Interactive Forum with Influential Advocates

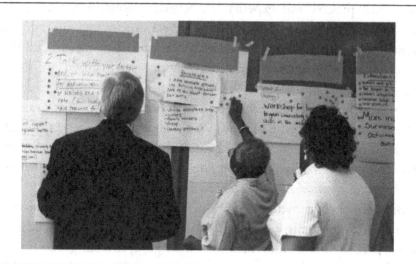

future project activities. Remaining project funds were budgeted to purchase a computer, printer, Internet access, and other supplies that would help facilitate project management.

Carrying Out Other Means of Disseminating Findings

In addition to sharing our findings with local Influential Advocates, our partnership (Angels, CRAs, and academic researchers) coauthored an academic article (López, et al., 2005) and copresented papers and posters at local and national meetings and conferences. (See Chapter Fourteen for a discussion of the development and implementation of dissemination procedures within a CBPR project.)

CHALLENGES

Here we share two specific challenges encountered while using photovoice within a CBPR approach, for which the principles of full participation and equitable decision-making power were paramount.

Achieving equitable decision-making power among all partners throughout the research process. At the beginning several women seemed to cede power and control to López (as the academic researcher), while they assumed the role of passive research subjects. For example, although survivors developed their own photo assignments, several were under the impression that the researchers had rigid ideas about specific photographs they should be taking. Because López and the CRAs did their best to convey otherwise and avoided making explicit suggestions about photographs, the CBPR approach was at first a source of confusion and distress to participants who wanted to make a good impression. This issue was epitomized during a photo discussion when one woman explained that she had taken a photograph of another survivor because she was "told" to do so.

Determining the optimal time for identifying and recruiting influential advocates so they could be involved and committed to improving survivorship QOL. Although Wang strongly suggests identifying influential advocates early in the photovoice process (Wang et al., 1996), we decided to recruit our advocates near the end of our project. Given the exploratory and inductive nature of the work, we felt that our influential advocates should be identified during our photo discussions so that their influence would be relevant to the specific themes that emerged. For example, if advocates had been identified at the outset of our project, one obvious choice would have been to recruit a representative for the local cancer support agency. Yet nobody from this agency was identified by the Surviving Angels as being an advocate. In fact, the Angels indicated that they rarely used the agency's resources because they perceived that it catered solely to white women.

Despite our rationale for recruiting advocates later in the project, there were drawbacks to this approach. Our partnership did not benefit from the advocates' involvement as partners, colearners, supporters, or advisers throughout the project, nor did we develop lasting and committed relationships with them. A recognized limitation of photovoice is that is does not shift to participants the power to decide policy (Wang, et al., 1996). During our forum, our goal was to set the stage for survivors and influential advocates to collaborate in developing and implementing culturally sensitive interventions. Yet, after forming the task forces it was a challenge to maintain commitment and involvement from advocates who had competing priorities.

LESSONS LEARNED—IMPLICATIONS FOR PRACTICE

Here we share several of the lessons we learned while conducting the Inspirational Images Project, and reviewing the photovoice literature.

Actively Solicit Local Expertise and Support to Develop and Conduct a Photovoice Project

From the very beginning of our planning process (conducting the pilot study with Ms. Rock and Ms. Sweet) and throughout the photovoice process (drawing from insights of CRAs, survivors, and researchers) to its completion (supporting CRAs to oversee future endeavors), our project benefited from local knowledge, contacts, and insights. As a result our partnership was able to conduct a project that was appropriate for working with African American survivors in rural communities.

Embrace the Flexibility of Photovoice by Adjusting Project Logistics Toward Specific Preferences, Cultural Context, Aims, Budget Constraints, and Other Practical Considerations

Our experiences and a review of the photovoice literature demonstrate flexibility in essentially all components of the photovoice process, including whether trainings are conducted with a group or individual participants, whether photo assignments are formulated by participants or predetermined by researchers, and how and to what extent photographs are discussed and interpreted. While the Surviving Angels project employed group photo-discussion sessions, other photovoice projects have used individual interviews during which each participant shares his or her photographs and their embedded meanings with only the researcher (Baker & Wang, 2006). Still, other projects have used a combination of individual interviews and group discussions (Brooks, Poudrier, & Thomas-MacLean, 2008). For example, in their study to explore the social context of cancer experiences from the perspectives of 12 Aboriginal women, Brooks and colleagues met individually with each woman to discuss her photographs. They then hosted a culturally responsive sharing circle workshop during which all of the women came together to meet each other and share their photos and stories (Brooks, et al., 2008).

Make Every Effort to Ensure a Safe and Open Environment During Photo Discussions

Feedback from the Angels suggests that they felt free to voice divergent opinions and comfortable sharing sensitive information about their survivorship experiences. This was facilitated by: having agreed-upon group norms to abide by throughout a photovoice project (for example, agree to disagree respectfully); integrating ample opportunities for group interaction and bonding (for example, icebreakers, shared meals, and celebrating cultural events and birthdays); and acknowledging up front the social, cultural, and economic factors that have historically resulted in difficulties achieving and maintaining authentic partnerships (Levy, Baldyga, & Jurkowski, 2003). For example, during our photo-discussion sessions, we tried to openly discuss racial tensions that might be due to López and other academics not being African American. This facilitated the Angels' feeling comfortable with broaching sensitive subjects pertaining to their perceptions of racial discrimination by white people.

Devote Time During Each Photo-Discussion Session to Reporting Back Preliminary Findings from Prior Sessions

Discussing emerging themes provided opportunities throughout our project for the Angels to be actively involved in theoretical sampling, data analysis, and interpretation, even if they chose to not be involved in reading and coding discussion transcripts.

Apply Flexibility and Creativity to Achieve the Final Goal of Reaching Policymakers and Decision Makers

For the Inspirational Images Project the Surviving Angels chose to plan and host an elaborate interactive forum to share findings and forge collaborations with influential people whom they identified as being advocates for change. Their decisions were based on their culture, preferences, and our project's aims and budget capacity. To achieve the goal of reaching policymakers and decision makers, other photovoice projects have used an array of strategies, including interactive forums, gallery showings, posters, and other displays (such as at art galleries, cafes, lunchrooms, public libraries, and other venues) (Castleden, Garvin, & Huu-ay-aht First

Nation, 2008), Internet galleries and postings (López et al., 2010), and presentations at organizational and community meetings, trainings, and conferences (Lorenz, 2010).

SUMMARY

Our experience demonstrates the utility of photovoice to explore the socially sensitive topic of cancer survivorship with African American breast cancer survivors from rural eastern North Carolina. Although the Surviving Angels were recruited to represent diversity on a range of sociodemographic characteristics, the photo discussions facilitated what one Angel described as "fellowship and togetherness." As a more equitable partnership evolved, this trusting bond was extended to all project partners, including academic researchers.

It has been asserted that partners in a participatory research endeavor should benefit from the new knowledge and skills they gain during the research process (Green et al., 1997). We found that by sharing control and ownership over the research process, colearning occurred and knowledge about important issues was brought to consciousness. As a result, the Angels, CRAs, and researchers were better able to see their own situations and the situations of others within a new light. Our partnership demonstrated increased critical awareness of how broad social and structural factors affect our own and other's lives. Partners recognized their ability to move beyond simply coping to taking action to influence their personal and social environment (Wallerstein & Bernstein, 1988; Wang et al., 2000).

The photovoice method provided the means for survivors to reach and forge relationships with influential people to whom they might not normally have access. The reactions from influential advocates who participated in the forum and their willingness to initiate collaborations with survivors suggested that the women's photographs, and what the women had to say about them, powerfully relayed the needs and strengths of rural African American breast cancer survivors. Although it was a challenge to sustain the task forces beyond the funding period, several survivors and a few committed influential advocates used the Inspirational Images Project as a foundation for collaboration, for example, by working with churches and civic organizations, and participating in city council meetings.

By sharing our process, we hope that those interested in conducting CBPR projects will better appreciate the flexibility inherent to the photovoice method. We are confident that with local insight, planning, and creativity, photovoice embodies the underlying principles of successful CBPR partnerships and endeavors. Our experience is but one of a multitude of projects that have demonstrated how photovoice can facilitate equitable collaboration and provide a mechanism through which new knowledge can be shared with others to promote taking action for positive social change.

KEY TERMS

African American

Breast cancer

Cancer survivorship

Critical consciousness

Photovoice

DISCUSSION QUESTIONS

1. Imagine that you are asked to complete the following photo assignment: Take 1–2 photographs that represent "A typical meal time for you."

    - What photographs would you take to complete this assignment? Why?

    - In what ways can/can't photographs provide a new or alternative way of exploring our everyday experiences?

    - Discuss some of the ethical implications associated with using the photovoice method. What strategies can be developed to reduce any risk of harm that might be incurred by researchers, photovoice participants, or the communities they represent?

    - When conducting a photovoice project, what are some of the factors that might impede equitable decision-making power among all partners? What strategies can partnerships develop to identify and address the dynamics that might relegate certain partners to play a more passive role throughout the research process?

REFERENCES

Ashing-Giwa, K., & Ganz, P. A. (1997). Understanding the breast cancer experience of African-American women. *Journal of Psychosocial Oncology*, *15*(2), 19–35. doi: 10.1300/ J077v15n02_02

Baker, T. A., & Wang, C. C. (2006). Photovoice: Use of a participatory action research method to explore the chronic pain experience in older adults. *Qualitative Health Research*, *16*(10), 1405–1413. doi: 10.1177/1049732306294118

Brooks, C., Poudrier, J., & Thomas-MacLean, R. (2008). Creating collaborative visions with aboriginal women: A photovoice project. In P. Liamputtong (Ed.), *Doing cross-cultural research: Ethical and methodological perspectives* (pp. 193–211). New York: Springer.

Castleden, H., Garvin, T., & Huu-ay-aht First Nation. (2008). Modifying photovoice for community-based participatory Indigenous research. *Social Science & Medicine*, *66*(6), 1393–1405. doi: 10.1016/socscimed.2007.11.030

Earp, J. A., Eng, E., O'Malley, M. S., Altpeter, M., Rauscher, G., Mayne, L., et al. (2002). Increasing use of mammography among older, rural African American women: Results from a community trial. *American Journal of Public Health*, *92*(4), 646–654.

Earp, J. A., Viadro, C. I., Vincus, A. A., Altpeter, M., Flax, V., Mayne, L., et al. (1997). Lay health advisors: A strategy for getting the word out about breast cancer. *Health Education & Behavior*, *24*, 432–451. doi: 10.1177/109019819702400404

Eng, E., & Smith, J. (1995). Natural helping functions of lay health advisors in breast cancer education. *Breast Cancer Research & Treatment*, *35*(1), 23–29. doi: 10.1007/BF00694741

Ewald, W. (1996). *I dreamed I had a girl in my pocket*. Durham: DoubleTake Books/Center for Documentary Studies.

Freire, P. (1970). *Pedagogy of the oppressed*. New York: Seabury Press.

Gant, L. M., Shimshock, K., Allen-Meares, P., Smith, L., Miller, P., Hollingsworth, L. A., et al. (2009). Effects of photovoice: Civic engagement among older youth in urban communities. *Journal of Community Practice*, *17*, 358–376. doi: 10.1080/10705420903300074

Glaser, B., & Strauss, A. (1967). *The discovery of grounded theory: Strategies for qualitative research*. New York: Aldine de Gruyter.

Goodman, R. M., Speers, M. A., McLeroy, K., Fawcett, S., Kegler, M., Parker, E., et al. (1998). Identifying and defining the dimensions of community capacity to provide a basis for measurement. *Health Education and Behavior*, *25*(3), 258–278. doi: 10.1177/ 109019819802500303

Green, L. W., George, M. A., Daniel, M., Frankish, C. J., Herbert, C. P., Bowie, W. R., et al. (1997). Background on participatory research. In D. Murphy, M. Scammell, & R. Sclove (Eds.), *Doing community-based research: A reader*. Amherst, MA: The Loka Institute.

Hassey Dow, K., Ferrell, B. R., Leigh, S., Ly, J., & Gulasekaram, P. (1996). An evaluation of the quality of life among long-term survivors of breast cancer. *Breast Cancer Research & Treatment*, *39*(3), 261–273. doi: 10.1007/BF01806154

Hergenrather, K. C., Rhodes, S. D., & Clark, G. (2006). Windows to work: Exploring employment-seeking behaviors of persons with HIV/AIDS through photovoice. *AIDS Education and Prevention, 18*(3), 243–258. doi: 10.1521/aeap.2006.18.3.243

Israel, B., Schulz, A., Parker, E., & Becker, A. (1998). Review of community-based research: Assessing partnership approaches to improve public health. *Annual Review of Public Health, 19*, 173–202.

Koch, K. (1970). *Wishes, lies, and dreams: Teaching children to write poetry.* New York: Harper & Row.

Kvale, S. (1995). The social construction of validity. *Qualitative Inquiry, 1*(1), 19–40.

Leedham, B., & Ganz, P. A. (1999). Psychosocial concerns and quality of life in breast cancer survivors. *Cancer Investigation, 17*(5), 342–348.

Levy, S. R., Baldyga, W., & Jurkowski, J. M. (2003). Developing community health promotion interventions: Selecting partners and fostering collaboration. *Health Promotion Practice, 4*(3), 314–322. doi: 10.1177/1524839903004003016

López, E. D. S. (2002). *Quality of life needs among rural African American breast cancer survivors from eastern North Carolina: Blending the methods of photovoice and grounded theory.* Unpublished dissertation, University of North Carolina at Chapel Hill.

López, E. D. S., Egensteiner, E., Andresen, E., Hannold, L., Lanzone, M., Vasudevan, V., et al. (2010). Evaluating photo-maps as tools for education, research, and empowerment. *Disability and Health Journal, 3*(2), e3.

López, E. D. S., Eng, E., Randall-David, E., & Robinson, N. (2005). Quality of life concerns of African American Breast Cancer Survivors within rural North Carolina: Blending the techniques of photovoice and grounded theory. *Qualitative Health Research, 15*(1), 99–115. doi: 10.1177/1049732304270766

Lorenz, L. (2010). Visual metaphors of living with brain injury: Exploring and communicating lived experience with an invisible injury. *Visual Studies, 25*(3), 210–223. doi: 10.1080/1472586X.2010.523273

Necheles, J. W., Chung, E. Q., Hawes-Dawson, J., Ryan, G. W., Williams, L. B., Holmes, H. N., et al. (2007). The Teen Photovoice Project: A pilot study to promote health through advocacy. *Progress in Community Health Partnerships, 1*(3), 221–229. doi: 10.1353/cpr.2007.0027

Newman, I. M., & Kanjanawong, S. (2005). Using photography to cross generational, linguistic, and cultural barriers to develop useful survey instruments. *Health Promotion Practice, 6*(1), 53–56. doi: 10.1177/1524839903259307

North Carolina Office of State Budget and Management. (2011). 2000 revised population estimates: http://www.osbm.state.nc.us/ncosbm/facts_and_Figures/socioeconomic_data/Population_estimates/demog/Countygrowth_2000.html

Northouse, L. L., Caffey, M., Deichelbohrer, L., Schmidt, L., Guziatek-Trojniak, L., West, S., et al. (1999). The quality of life of African American women with breast cancer. *Research in Nursing & Health, 22*(6), 449–460.

Patton, M. Q. (1990). Strategic themes in qualitative inquiry. In M. Q. Patton, *Qualitative evaluation and research* (2nd ed., pp. 37–72). Thousand Oaks, CA: Sage.

Reinharz, S. (1992). *Feminist action research: Feminist methods in social research.* New York: Oxford University Press.

Sandelowski, M. (1995). Focus on qualitative methods: Sample size in qualitative research. *Research in Nursing & Health, 18,* 179–183.

Solomon, J. (1995). Introduction. In J. Spence & J. Solomon (Eds.), *What can a woman do with a camera?* London: Scarlet Press.

Strauss, A., & Corbin, J. (1998). *Basics of qualitative research: Techniques and procedures for developing grounded theory* (2nd ed.). Thousand Oaks, CA: Sage.

U.S. Department of Agriculture: Economic Research Service. (2002). *1990 and 2000 Census poverty data: North Carolina Counties.* Retrieved June 25, 2012 http:www.ers.usda.gov/Data/Povertyrates/1989_1999/PovListpct.asp?st=NC&view=Percent

Vaughn, L. M., Forbes, J. R., & Howell, B. (2009). Enhancing home visitation programs: Input from a participatory evaluation using photovoice. *Infants & Young Children, 22*(2), 132–145. doi: 10.1097/01.IYC.0000348054.10551.66

Wallerstein, N., & Bernstein, E. (1988). Empowerment education: Freire's ideas adapted to health education. *Health Education Quarterly, 15*(4), 379–394.

Wang, C. C. (1999). Photovoice: A participatory action research strategy applied to women's health. *Journal of Women's Health, 8*(2), 185–192. doi: 10.1089/jwh.1999.8.185

Wang, C. C. (2006). Youth participation in photovoice as a strategy for community change. *Journal of Community Practice, 14*(1 & 2), 147–161. doi: 10.1300/J125v14n01_09

Wang, C. C., & Burris, M. A. (1994). Empowerment through photo novella: Portraits of participation. *Health Education Quarterly, 21*(2), 171–186. doi: 10.1177/109019819402100204

Wang, C. C., & Burris, M. A. (1997). Photovoice: Concept, methodology, and use for participatory needs assessment. *Health Education & Behavior, 24*(3), 369–387. doi: 10.1177/109019819702400309

Wang, C. C., Burris, M. A., & Xiang, Y. P. (1996). Chinese village women as visual anthropologists: a participatory approach to reaching policymakers. *Social Science & Medicine, 42,* 1391–1400.

Wang, C. C., Cash, J. L., & Powers, L. S. (2000). Who knows the streets as well as the homeless? Promoting personal and community action through photovoice. *Health Promotion Practice, 1*(1), 81–89. doi: 10.1177/152483990000100113

Wang, C. C., & Redwood-Jones, Y. A. (2001). Photovoice ethics: Perspectives from Flint Photovoice. *Health Education & Behavior, 28,* 560–572. doi: 10.1177/109019810102800504

Weiler, K. (1994). Freire and a feminist pedagogy of difference. In C. Lankshear & C. McLaren (Eds.) *Politics of liberation: Paths from Freire* (pp. 12–40). New York: Routledge.

Zenkov, K., & Harmon, J. (2009). Picturing a writing process: Photovoice and teaching writing to urban youth. *Journal of Adolescent & Adult Literacy, 52*(7), 575–584. doi: 10.1598/JAAL.52.7.3

Acknowledgments: We thank all of the Surviving Angels, Community Research Advisers, and researchers who participated on the Inspirational Images Project, and honor the memories of Surviving Angels and Advisers who are no longer with us. We further acknowledge Caroline Wang who created the photovoice method and coauthored the original version of this article. We also extend our gratitude to the North Carolina Breast Cancer Screening Program and the Lineberger Comprehensive Cancer Center for providing the foundation and support for our work. Our project was supported by the Susan G. Komen Breast Cancer Foundation through a dissertation research award (0100647), and the University of North Carolina at Chapel Hill (UNC-CH) through a University Research Council research grant, a graduate school dissertation fellowship, and a Center for Health Promotion and Disease Prevention traineeship. All project-related research protocol and materials were approved by the UNC-CH School of Public Health Institutional Review Board for Human Subjects.

Chapter 18

METHODS FOR COMMUNITY-BASED PARTICIPATORY POLICY WORK TO IMPROVE FOOD ENVIRONMENTS IN NEW YORK CITY

EMMA TSUI

MILYOUNG CHO

NICHOLAS FREUDENBERG

Many community health problems are caused or exacerbated by policies that make it difficult for individuals, neighborhoods, or organizations to create healthy environments. Increasingly, effective public health advocates must be able to identify, describe, and change health-damaging policies—processes that can be more meaningful and effective, yet also more complex, when they involve members of communities. In this chapter, we define **community-based participatory policy work** (CBPPW), an approach to policy activism that combines community-based participatory research and community-based policy advocacy. CBPPW thus incorporates research, outreach, communication, and mobilization activities.

Throughout the process of CBPPW, participants need to be able to collect and analyze information from a variety of sources and to use these analyses to guide their work, inform advocacy, target actions, and monitor implementation. In this chapter, our focus is on the methods that CBPPW practitioners use to collect, interpret, and apply the data that guide their activities. Readers who want more information on the political and advocacy strategies that CBPPW practitioners use to advance policy goals are referred to several recent discussions of this topic (Israel et al, 2010; Minkler, 2010; Minkler & Freudenberg, 2008; Themba-Nixon, Minkler & Freudenberg, 2010).

To illustrate the methods used in CBPPW, we draw from the experiences of three efforts to change food-related policies in New York City. These efforts have varying community roots and resource bases, and have worked toward the goals of representation and participation in different ways. However, all three define policy change as a priority, espouse social justice and reduction of health inequities, seek to bring new voices into the policymaking process, and are committed to improving the New York City **food environments** that shape health.

WHAT IS COMMUNITY-BASED PARTICIPATORY POLICY WORK?

Policy refers to an organization's planned activities to achieve a goal (Themba & Minkler, 2003). Policies can be public (for example, local, state or federal government) or private (for example, corporations or voluntary associations); short or long term; and a single action (such as a proclamation or law) or multiple actions across agencies (such as devolution of federal responsibilities to states). Although policies are intentional, a decision not to act or to ignore a problem is also a policy, even if not explicitly articulated. Public health professionals have long been involved in *policy analysis*, an assessment of the health impact of various approaches to solving a problem, and *policy advocacy*, efforts to change policies that harm health (Acosta, 2003; Brownson, Newschaffer, & Ali-Abarghoui, 1997; Christoffel, 2000; Israel et al., 2010; Minkler, 2010).

The literature on policy processes has typically been driven by stage models of policymaking (Kingdon, 2003; Longest, 2006; Steckler & Dawson, 1982). The early phases of a policymaking process are what Kingdon (2003) has called "agenda-setting," in which the agenda is "the list of subjects or problems to which governmental officials . . . are paying some serious attention at any given time" (p. 3), and what Longest has called "policy formulation" (2006). Steckler and Dawson (1982) divide these first steps into three phases, which include (1) problem awareness and identification, (2) problem refinement, and (3) setting policy objectives. We believe that these stage models provide useful overviews of the policymaking process. At the same time, we are struck by the complexity of the first stages of launching community-based policy change campaigns, especially while infusing them with meaningful and enduring participation on the part of diverse, often excluded groups. In our experience, some community groups find this first stage so frustrating or difficult that they abandon the effort before getting to later stages of the policymaking process. Thus, in this analysis, we place a special emphasis on the methods used in the earliest phases of CBPPW.

In this chapter, we discuss the **research methods** that the organizations we profile have used to collect, analyze, and present the evidence that will advance their policy goals. In the cases we discuss here, these methods contribute to and are complemented by several broader CBPPW strategies that include:

Using or creating processes to engage community members in shaping policy goals;

Cultivating and maintaining representativeness and participation;

Opening lines of communication with decision makers;

Strengthening community capacity to mobilize diverse constituencies in order to influence the policy process by building horizontal links with groups in other sectors and vertical links with groups working at other levels; and

Monitoring the implementation of policies.

The breadth of these strategies shows that, as in other participatory approaches, CBPPW differs from more traditional efforts at policy analysis and advocacy in several ways. First, it actively seeks the involvement of all relevant stakeholders, especially those traditionally excluded from the policy process (Themba & Minkler, 2003). Second, since it often starts with community perceptions of the problem, CBPPW may "frame" policy questions more broadly, frequently cutting across sectors (for example, health, education, criminal justice) and local, state and federal levels of government (Themba, 1999). Third, like other forms of participatory activity, CBPPW is rooted in the context in which it unfolds, requiring an analysis of the broader historical, social, cultural, and political dimensions of the problem and setting (Greenwood & Levin, 1998). Finally, CBPPW embraces both analysis and action, rather than stopping once analysis is complete (Israel et al., 2008). As these defining characteristics suggest, the principles of CBPR strongly inform the strategies and research methods of CBPPW.

FOOD-RELATED HEALTH CONDITIONS AND
FOOD POLICY IN NEW YORK CITY

Like other cities in the United States and around the world, New York City currently faces the linked problems of high rates of food-related health conditions, such as obesity and diabetes, and persistent hunger and food insecurity. These problems affect city residents who are poor and of color at much higher rates than those who are not. For instance, in New York City, 26.5% of people living under 200% of the federal poverty level (FPL) are obese, while 17.9% of people living over 400% of the FPL fit this category, a statistically significant difference (Raufman, Farley, Olson, & Kerker, 2007). Additionally, African American and Hispanic residents of New York City report having diabetes at almost twice the rate of white residents (Raufman et al., 2007). The many contributors to these disparities include a range of neighborhood characteristics, such as the reduced availability and higher prices of healthier foods (Jetter & Cassady, 2006), wide availability and active promotion of unhealthy food, especially in poor neighborhoods (Dinour, Fuentes, & Freudenberg, 2008), and lack of appropriate spaces for physical activity in low-income areas (Babey, Hastert, Yu, & Brown, 2008; Bennett et al., 2007).

In response to food insecurity and food-related health problems, many individuals and organizations have mobilized to advocate for healthier and more just food policies and systems at local and national levels, particularly in the last five years. This emerging food justice movement has already begun to have an effect in New York City, helping to create policies such as the requirement for calorie labeling in chain restaurants and the ban on trans fats, improving programs such as that which governs school food in New York City, and creating new programs such as the city's Green Cart initiative, which enables more mobile vendors to sell fruits and vegetables on the streets of low-income neighborhoods (Freudenberg, McDonough, & Tsui, 2011). This movement both creates new opportunities for the community-based initiatives described here and complicates the turf with a mix of allies and competitors.

By including city residents living in neighborhoods affected by food insecurity, obesity, and diabetes in policy and advocacy processes and making their perspectives a priority, the efforts we describe here have greater potential to meaningfully address problems in these places. To demonstrate how CBPPW unfolds on the ground, we describe as **case studies** three ongoing New York City food justice efforts that have collected, analyzed, and presented evidence in order to influence food policy. We have had varying levels of ongoing relationships with these efforts and base our report on our own observations and participation, interviews with leaders of the groups involved, and a review of relevant organizational documents, Web sites, and media reports. To set the stage for the second part of the chapter, Table 18.1 provides an overview of the methods that these groups have used to collect and analyze data to advance their CBPPW; we also introduce these organizations and describe the nature of their policy efforts.

Table 18.1 describes methods that each of our three case organizations have used to collect data on three different topics that are essential to the earliest phases of CBPPW: participant perceptions of the problem, the nature of the problem on the ground, and policy opportunities for addressing the problem. When formulated for studying urban food policy, these topics become: perceptions and experiences of food and food policy, the nature of food access and urban food environments, and policy opportunities and platforms. For each topic, we list examples of research tasks that the CBPPW teams completed to gather data on this topic, the specific methods that can be used for this task, and the types of research questions that might be posed for each task.

The Brooklyn Food Coalition

The Brooklyn Food Coalition (BFC) is a grassroots organization promoting food justice, food security, and a sustainable food system in Brooklyn. BFC was founded in the wake of a food justice conference, held in Brooklyn in March 2009 and attended by 3,000 people of all ages, and from a range of socioeconomic, racial/ethnic, and educational backgrounds. BFC has since grown to include members from many Brooklyn neighborhoods, and has created working groups on anti-racism, a 2012 conference, membership/governance, workers' rights newsletter, school food reform, research and mapping, and food policy.

TABLE 18.1 Research Methods for Community-Based Participatory Policy Work: Policy Formulation Phase

Task	Research Methods	Examples from Cases	Research Questions
Topic: Perceptions and experiences of food and food policy			
Eliciting various constituencies' definitions of priority problems	Surveys, focus groups, structured elicitation dialogues, conversations with community members	Everyday Democracy's Dialogue Circles process used by FLEJ	How do community members experience and define problems associated with food, the urban foodscape, and food systems?
Eliciting data on participant experiences with current policies	Surveys, focus groups, structured elicitation dialogues, conversations with community members	FLEJ Healthy Incentives Working Group survey of church members on SNAP and other policies; HEP School Food Campaign Survey	How do community members experience existing policies that shape access to food, the urban foodscape, and food systems?
Topic: The nature of food access and urban food environments			
Identifying, accessing, and understanding existing data sources to document problems associated with food and food environments	Review of public health, urban planning, food systems, and other relevant literatures	Development of HEP curriculum; BFC and FLEJ background research and grant proposals	What is known about how others have defined these problems?

(Continued)

TABLE 18.1 (*Continued*)

Task	Research Methods	Examples from Cases	Research Questions
Topic: The nature of food access and urban food environments			
Collecting and analyzing data on food environments	Surveys of consumers, structured observation/ assessment of food outlets, mapping community food resources	BFC Research and Mapping effort; HEP community food assessments	What challenges and resources currently exist in our local food environments?
Topic: Policy opportunities and platforms			
Policy scanning and analysis	Collaboration with policy experts to learn about possible policy solutions to the problems defined above, to analyze the degree to which existing/ possible legislation meets policy goals, and to assess relevance of policies existing elsewhere, literature review, document analysis	FLEJ Farm bill working group; BFC farm bill working group	How do existing and emerging legislative efforts address our policy goals? What policies implemented elsewhere address our policy goals?
Eliciting views on policy opportunities	Surveys, focus groups, structured elicitation dialogues, conversations with community members, email communications	BFC's cumulative policy platform developed through emailed critiques and additions	What policies in what formulations warrant our support and advocacy, given our organizational mission and policy goals?

Note: FLEJ = Faith Leaders for Environmental Justice. BFC = Brooklyn Food Coalition. HEP = Health Equity Project.

As in many community organizations, a central tension within BFC is around diversity and representativeness. Although BFC seeks to build "an inclusive, multi-racial, multi-cultural alliance" (Brooklyn Food Coalition, 2011) of Brooklyn residents, it operates with limited resources and must rely on the knowledge and skills of those members who have time and energy to give. So far, these have most often been white middle-class residents of Brooklyn, rather than poorer residents of color. To help address this, BFC has increased its outreach to more disadvantaged Brooklyn neighborhoods, and works to provide such supports as child care, dinner, and homework help for school-age children when it holds evening meetings. The issue of diversity has been a particular challenge for members of the food policy committee who, for the most part, joined because of a professional interest in food policy, and who tend to be more educated and affluent than the majority of Brooklyn residents.

In striving to do effective work on food policy that represents the interests of diverse Brooklynites, BFC has tried multiple approaches, often learning as much from its failures as its successes. Initially, a lawyer member of BFC with a strong interest in policy offered to lead the coalition's policy work. He produced detailed policy documents that connected ideas that he thought BFC members would support (for example, increased local sourcing of foods used by city agencies, increased support for composting) with specific legislative language. However, despite the fact that these ideas were perceived as well targeted and "at the center of our work," as one BFC leader said, they were not well received. A BFC leader explained the result: "What ended up happening was that people came in the room for these meetings, and there would be a stack of policy documents and they were like, huh? What is this? It didn't seem connected to what they were doing on the ground."

The solution seemed to be a more participatory approach, but the organization feared that it did not yet have the capacity to support that work. In a second and ongoing policy effort, BFC has worked to put this vision into action. Reflecting its commitment to participatory processes, BFC wanted to identify policies that warranted support and to develop procedures that engaged the broader membership. The organization began this process with an organization-wide policy summit that took place in fall 2010. Since then, a policy committee has formed and is working to establish structures and educational activities that will allow ongoing communication with and participation by other BFC members. As we will describe in the sections that follow, the topic of school food is one area where BFC has had particular success in learning about and organizing a diverse group of parents to influence policy. BFC's policy and research and mapping committees have also led the creation of what we view as CBPPW teams. These teams have used research to understand what is already known about food environments in Brooklyn, to collect primary data on retail food availability, and to understand the current policy landscape for the changes they would like to see. BFC's CBPPW teams are participatory in the sense that they are open to everyone and they actively recruit nonmember Brooklyn residents (particularly from communities of color).

Faith Leaders for Environmental Justice

Faith Leaders for Environmental Justice (FLEJ) was founded in 2007 by a group of individuals and organizations in New York City interested in mobilizing communities of faith around environmental justice issues. FLEJ is an interfaith collaborative program that includes more than 130 faith leaders and a network of seven faith and environmental organizations, several of which are umbrella or network organizations in their own right. Its work is centered on issues that affect the health of New York City residents with a focus on the neighborhoods of the South Bronx and Harlem.

One of the two key areas in which FLEJ is currently working is food justice. A primary initial goal of this work was to influence public policy through partnerships with nonprofit organizations and public officials and agencies. FLEJ focused its work on food access and sought to make healthy food more readily available by raising awareness and engaging churches and their members in initiatives like community-supported agriculture projects (CSAs), local food co-ops, community gardens, rooftop gardens, adopt-a-local-emergency-food-provider, food stamp outreach, advocacy for improvement in food and hunger policies, and support for supermarket creation in focal neighborhoods.

In the course of organizing these efforts, however, participants identified the need for a forum that would convene not only FLEJ's members, but also the faith community more broadly, food advocates, and public officials to develop a more representative community perspective in food justice advocacy efforts. The hope was that this forum would connect FLEJ staff and leaders more directly to existing faith-based and neighborhood grassroots organizations and would help to identify a limited number of policy goals that could focus and clarify existing grassroots efforts. In 2010, funding from the Centers for Disease Control provided the opportunity to create such a gathering.

FLEJ's one-day Food, Faith, and Health Disparities Summit in October 2010 utilized a data collection and discussion model developed by Everyday Democracy, a nonprofit organization that facilitates civic participation and community change (Everyday Democracy, 2011a). Specifically, Everyday Democracy uses a structured process to gather together "people of different backgrounds and views [to] talk and work together to solve problems and create communities that work for everyone" (Everyday Democracy, 2011b). This process is described in detail in the Methods section below, as are the efforts of the working groups that were created as a result of this process, which were still ongoing at the time this chapter was written. We consider FLEJ's CBPPW teams to include those who convened and participated in the one-day summit, and those who continue to participate in the working groups.

The Health Equity Project

The New York City Health Equity Project (HEP) was a partnership between the New York City Department of Health and Mental Hygiene (DOHMH), local youth organizations, and the City University of New York (CUNY) School of Public Health. Seeking to enhance its engagement with community organizations, DOHMH initiated HEP in order to increase its capacity for dialogue about health disparities with urban youth and to engage them in research and action to reduce food-related health disparities. DOHMH's structure, in which high-need neighborhoods were served by local District Public Health Offices (DPHOs), lent itself well to such a project. In 2008–2010, HEP was implemented in three DPHO neighborhoods: East Harlem, South Bronx, and North/Central Brooklyn, where the project was based. Responding to calls for productive academic-local health department collaboration (Livingood et al., 2007; Swain, Bennett, Etkind, & Ransom, 2006), DOHMH partnered with researchers at the CUNY School of Public Health who helped to conceptualize, design, and implement the project. HEP then sought partnerships with youth organizations that had prior experience in service learning, health programming, community mobilization around health or economic issues, and social justice education. HEP's focus on youth was based on the belief that young people have the time, energy, and passion to lead community movements and may constitute an untapped resource for public health (Checkoway & Gutiérrez, 2006) and for improving food environments (Kuo & Goodman, 2011).

With its workshop-based curriculum, the HEP ultimately trained more than 350 youth who undertook a range of research and action projects, some of which involved participatory policy research. The CBPPW teams in this case include the trainers and participating students at the various youth organizations. In the next section, we describe several of the approaches that students took in collecting data on their local food environments. An evaluation concluded that HEP was most successful in introducing youth to the social, economic, and political factors that shape food environments and to how health outcomes are influenced by food environments. In addition, the project was judged to have been somewhat successful in providing youth with community-based participatory policy research skills and engaging youth in documenting and then acting to change their neighborhood food environments (Tsui, Bylander, Cho, Maybank & Freudenberg, 2012).

METHODS FOR DATA COLLECTION, ANALYSIS AND PRESENTATION

BFC, FLEJ, and HEP's community-based participatory food policy efforts are structured in different ways and are at different stages of development. Additionally, their CBPPW teams were formed under different circumstances. For BFC and FLEJ, CBPPW work was initiated by those with more power and knowledge about the policy process who were already working and in many cases residing in these neighborhoods (for example, policy professionals who also happened to be BFC members and activist faith leaders working in the South Bronx and Harlem), and they sought to bring in those residents with less power and involvement. HEP was formed by those with more power and knowledge as well—and by groups based primarily outside of the neighborhoods in which they worked—but because of this, HEP sought even more proactively to let youth participants lead the team's research efforts. Because of their diversity, these efforts offer examples of the range of research methods that can be used in conducting CBPPW work, recognizing that not all methods were either appropriate or used by all three cases. In the following section, we elaborate on the research tasks and associated methods presented in Table 18.1.

Eliciting Various Constituencies' Definitions of Priority Problems

Participants in all three cases collected data early in the CBPPW process that articulated how and why constituents defined and experienced food systems as they do. CBPPW teams collected data on local experiences of food, the local food landscape, and perceptions of problems associated with the food system. The emphasis on the "local" and personal here should not be underestimated, as this seems especially critical in mobilizing people around policy. Thus, for example, it is not only information about levels of food access in neighborhoods that is needed to drive CBPPW; the organizations we feature as cases also elicited information about people's *experiences* of food. Experiences of food access may be part of this discussion, but in the cases we examine here, the dialogue needed to be framed more broadly to help residents and advocates better understand how food fits into the broader context of participants' lives.

Although surveys and focus groups might serve participants well for gathering these kinds of data during the early phases of CBPPW, our three cases used different data collection methods. FLEJ used the Everyday Democracy's "dialogue-to-change" process, which we consider to be a participatory form of eliciting residents' views on the impact of policy. Dialogue-to-change uses pedagogical processes developed by the Brazilian educator Paulo Freire (1970), which have previously been applied in public health to promote youth empowerment (Wallerstein & Bernstein, 1988; Wallerstein, 1994) and as an integral component of photovoice methodology (Wang & Burris, 1997). The dialogue-to-change method implemented at the FLEJ summit involved bringing together a wide cross section of community residents affected by a given problem to share their varied views and experiences through structured facilitated conversations in small groups. The full process, including the data elicitation, was governed by an issue guide developed by local food and health experts in conjunction with FLEJ and Everyday Democracy. In keeping with Everyday Democracy's principles, the more than 150 attendees at the summit itself were divided into "dialogue circles" that sought to maximize the diversity of race, ethnicity, gender, neighborhood, profession, and experience with food advocacy for each group. The groups then engaged in a series of four conversations led by trained facilitators: Making Connections, Food and Health Gaps, What Can We Do, and Moving to Action. Through this series of conversations, the dialogue circles moved from considering personal relationships and interests in food, food environments, and systems to thinking about these issues at the community and societal levels, and then developing a vision for a healthy food system in New York City. Participants also explored different perspectives on the roots of the problem and different approaches to addressing the problem, including what participants themselves could do. Each dialogue circle, which comprised 8–15 people, was responsible for proposing three action ideas. During dinner, the FLEJ leadership discussed the full set of ideas collected from all dialogue circles, conducted an informal thematic analysis, and distilled the most popular ideas into a list of possible working groups. Individuals from the groups then each chose a specific working group with which they would participate. The final working groups were: Business Outreach, Community Engagement, Farm Bill, Food and Voter Education, and Healthy Incentives.

At BFC, leaders believed their first policy efforts failed precisely because they did not adequately connect with members' perceptions of food-related problems on a personal level. As one leader explained, they are now working toward a way to "thread the needs and desires of the people in the neighborhoods through the core of [our] policy work." So far, BFC has typically used a data collection method that is oriented primarily around meeting-based conversations among members and nonmembers. In particular, BFC's outreach to parents at schools serving low-income students of color has created opportunities for learning directly from parents about how food policy work can become relevant to those most affected by health disparities, and social and economic dislocation. As one leader said, "In inventing an organization that embodies part of a people's movement, we had to be very flexible about how we function, so that we're reflecting the reality of what people seem to be telling us. We're not doing constant surveys and if we did . . . it wouldn't really reflect what people think anyway because we wouldn't be able to get to all of our people." This leader also noted that polling via online surveys may miss the many people who lack easy Internet access, an important portion of BFC's constituency. Data on perceptions of priority problems has thus been collected in the form of detailed neighborhood and committee meeting minutes, which are disseminated at meetings and via the Internet (for those who have access) to create a public archive and inform future BFC decisions and actions.

Eliciting Data on Participant Experiences with Current Policies

Just as the groups described in our cases found that collecting data on perceptions of priority problems was essential, they also put substantial energy toward collecting data on experiences and perceptions of current policies. The participatory nature of data collection on this topic allows such a process to provide insights into the shortcomings and unintended consequences of policies that a less participatory process might overlook. As suggested by the above cases, eliciting the local and personal side of policy perceptions is critical for at least two reasons. First, such a process ensures that policy recommendations emerge from the experiences of disenfranchised groups, rather than from outside experts, and thereby increases the likelihood that the proposed solutions will: (1) address the problems as experienced by the intended beneficiaries; and (2) be owned by participants in policy advocacy campaigns. Second, by eliciting the feelings connected to policy problems and solutions, advocates are better prepared to address the concerns of policymakers, who are often moved by emotional arguments ("My grandfather died of diabetes—I don't want the same for my children"). The following research methods that emerged from the cases point to the importance of recognizing that policy change is both an emotional and a rational process.

While the Dialogue Circles used by FLEJ provided a platform for collecting data related to policies as well as problems, one of the FLEJ working groups has moved toward developing a more targeted approach to collecting data on the manifestations of specific policies in constituents' everyday experiences. Specifically, when committee discussions identified a need for more data on experiences with the Supplemental Nutrition Assistance Program (SNAP, formerly called the Food Stamps program), the Healthy Incentives Working Group's coordinator facilitated a process for the working group's members to develop a church member survey that would generate data about how to improve healthy food consumption through incentives and public benefits, with a section specifically targeting people who receive SNAP benefits. The working group members were collectively involved in developing the survey questionnaire, suggesting questions that would investigate the topics of interest. The working group leader, who had training in survey research methods, then refined these questions and finalized the survey questionnaire. One of the key tensions that arose in these conversations was regarding the collection of demographic information. Although some of the group felt it was critical to gather this data in order to enhance understanding of local health disparities, others felt it was redundant with existing census data. Ultimately, there was consensus that it did make sense to collect demographic data. The group plans to tap into FLEJ's network of churches in the South Bronx, East Harlem, and Central Brooklyn to address congregations at the end of church services, describe the project, and ask members of the congregations to complete the survey. Included in the survey are questions about fresh produce consumption and availability in the neighborhood, the likelihood of using EBT for purchasing fruits and vegetables if the consumer received monthly discounts or reward points, the increased availability of produce at local bodegas, and questions assessing knowledge of how food stamps can be used (for example, at farmers' markets). The findings will inform the group's advocacy work for consumer-friendly improved incentives to encourage healthy food purchasing.

One of the major components of the HEP program was the development of a youth-led research project. These were generally designed as small-scale community food assessments (Pothukuchi, Joseph, Burton, & Fisher, 2002) focusing on documenting various aspects of local food environments, and are thus described in the next section. To investigate perceptions of one particular policy, however, HEP's CBPPW team designed and conducted a survey of more than 200 students at 17 high schools in Central Brooklyn and the South Bronx to develop a better understanding of students' perceptions of school food and the policies that shape what is served in their cafeterias. To collectively write the survey, students from participating youth organizations discussed their experiences of problems with school food, and developed questions that they wanted to ask other students about these and other problems. HEP trainers facilitated a brainstorming process to generate as many survey questions of different types as possible. The trainers then compiled questions and solicited comments from students on multiple drafts until a final survey questionnaire resulted. Students were then responsible for recruiting a convenience sample of students from their own schools and administering the survey over the course of approximately one month. The students involved in this research project later met with administrators of New York City's school food program to present their findings and recommendations, and to open lines of communication between students and school food administrators.

Identifying, Accessing, and Understanding Existing Data Sources to Document Problems Associated with Food and Food Environments

Across our three cases, efforts to synthesize and interpret existing data on the problems associated with food and food environments—primarily reviews of various literatures and reports—have typically been led by those members of CBPPW teams with more research and policy experience, and have taken place in all cases before full CBPPW teams were in place. Such data were critical, however, to helping to introduce CBPPW efforts to the larger community and to helping frame grant proposals to fund participatory work. For FLEJ, these reviews were undertaken by policy-savvy pastors and participating activist academics who reviewed public health, environmental health, and planning literatures to collect relevant data. Similarly, BFC's leadership and staff used their professional skills and networks to collect, critically review, and understand existing data on Brooklyn food environments, in order to complement and guide more participatory data collection as described in the next section. In HEP, the designers of the HEP curriculum—academics and public health practitioners, many of whom later functioned as trainers—were the ones who divided up literature review responsibilities and collaboratively evaluated the credibility of existing data on food in the HEP focal neighborhoods so that they could convey this to youth participants as a starting point for more personal and community-based explorations.

Collecting and Analyzing Primary Data on Food Environments

Although drawing from existing data sources to frame policy questions can be expedient and cost-effective, collecting primary data may be more compelling both to participants and to policymakers. Our cases provide two examples of methods used. First, the BFC CBPPW team is in the early stages of conducting a participatory mapping process, which will allow them to see how current policies are shaping food environments in their neighborhoods on the ground. As the BFC's Research and Mapping Committee leaders write, "We believe that a positive first step toward a healthy food environment is understanding the current terrain and that maps are one way to gain that understanding" (Brooklyn Food Coalition Research and Mapping Committee Community Food Survey, 2011). The food outlet mapping process was initiated by core members of BFC's Research and Mapping Committee and offers tools and a Web site through which participants can volunteer to map the location and offerings of food retail outlets in the borough (Brooklyn Food Coalition Research and Mapping Committee Community Food Survey, 2011), tools that are available as part of the downloadable supplement to this chapter. Anyone can participate in collecting data and all data are fully available to the public via the Internet. Typically, data collection days are organized by the BFC committee's leaders in conjunction with local community-based groups. For instance, youth employment programs might participate in the summer, and on Martin Luther King Day local service groups might spend several hours collecting data. Data collectors are oriented and trained by committee members, and a geographic area not already covered by the database is divided up among participants for data collection. A structured observation form is then filled out for each food outlet in the area and later entered into the public database.

HEP's community food assessments comprise another effort to document community food environments with primary data collection. In these projects, HEP students worked closely with trainers to define research questions about the availability of healthy and unhealthy foods, food pricing, and food advertising in their neighborhoods. The teams then jointly designed structured observation tools to help them collect data to answer these questions. Students collected the data, compiled it, and then used it to consider both local action projects and, in the case of school food, larger policy changes that could address the situation. (See Chapter Ten for another example of the development, evolution, and implementation of a food store audit.)

Policy Scanning and Analysis

The previous research tasks take up a charge well articulated by van Olphen and colleagues, who wrote, "Critical to making the case for policy change is 'doing your homework' and demonstrating that current approaches and programs are seriously inadequate" (2003, p. 375). However, a detailed understanding of the ways that existing and emerging legislative efforts address policy goals, and of relevant policies implemented elsewhere, is also necessary for effective CBPPW. In the cases described here, professional policy analysts have played a role in creating an organizational understanding of policies and policy opportunities. It is worth noting that policy professionals may be part of the convening organization, partners, or members of the "community."

Because BFC is a membership organization, the convening organization and the "community" are in many ways the same. The policy committee has several members who have extensive professional experience working in policy (including the head of a major hunger advocacy organization and a past employee of the mayor's office), and these members play a key role in policy scanning. By *policy scanning* we mean reviewing existing federal, state, and local policies for their relationship to the policy goals of BFC. Policy scanning typically involves a systematic review of legislative databases and advocacy reports, as well as interviews with key informants and policy experts. To maximize efficiency in the face of limited resources, at BFC, policy scanning is conducted by individuals in the group who have access to policy information through their social and professional networks. In practice, what this means is that when members of the committee come across information about policies that appear relevant, they share this information via e-mail with the full committee, usually starting with background information on a given policy, which is followed by discussion over e-mail or at meetings of a policy's promise and relevance to BFC's mission.

In a more focused policy analysis effort, BFC is working with a small group of university faculty and students who have expertise in the Farm Bill, the omnibus legislation that is the primary mechanism by which the federal government shapes agricultural and food policy, and a major priority for many advocates of healthy and affordable food. The academic team, with participation from policy committee members, has taken up the task of first reviewing other groups' Farm Bill platforms, as well as successes, failures, and advocacy alignments during past Farm Bill reauthorizations. These analyses will indicate specific policy opportunities, which then can be assessed for alignment with BFC's policy framework. The data collection and analysis processes involved are thus literature review, document collection and analysis, and conversations with advocates and policy-makers about opportunities to achieve BFC policy goals through changes to the Farm Bill.

Eliciting Views on Policy Opportunities

As BFC's work on scanning and analysis should make clear, discussions that take place during the analysis process often offer an opportunity to elicit constituent views on which policies in which formulations warrant a group's support and advocacy, given the group's specific organizational mission and policy goals. Other methods for gathering this kind of information—though not used in our cases—include surveys, focus groups, and structured elicitation dialogues, such as those used as part of Everyday Democracy's dialogue-to-change model. All of these are more formal methods than those used by BFC and would likely be more useful in a later stage of policy analysis.

LIMITATIONS AND CHALLENGES

Our analyses in this chapter suggest that each word in the label "community-based participatory policy work" presents challenges to the collection, analysis, and presentation of evidence to influence policy. How to navigate the notion of an effort that is "community-based" is the first hurdle. Some of the efforts we describe here started at the community level but most migrated between neighborhoods, cities, states, and the federal government, as the dictates of forming alliances and taking advantage of policy opportunities demanded. Both BFC and FLEJ, for example, were coalitions representing many different communities and with aspirations of citywide influence. Traditional conceptions of CBPR sometimes assume deep roots in a single specific geographic community, but for policy work this model may not always apply. In fact, given the limited abilities of a single community to change the higher-level policies that so powerfully shape communities, it may be beneficial to conceptualize a continuum of participatory policy work, from neighborhood to federal (or even global) levels, with the choice determined by the policy goals. Each level has its own political dynamics, data sources, and communications channels, requiring CBPPW researchers working across levels to master many systems.

"Participatory" is also a problematic concept. As our cases show, leaders struggle to engage many levels of participants, from disenfranchised and vulnerable populations to policymakers and elites. Usually, the strategies for bringing in different groups differ, adding to the complexity of the work. A core value of most CBPR proponents is that the process seeks to bring less powerful individuals and groups into policymaking. This may conflict with the role played by power analysis in most policymaking processes, which may encourage leaders to choose the most powerful allies in order to maximize the chance of policy success. On the other hand, an indiscriminate effort to engage as many groups as possible may obfuscate rather than clarify the central power dynamics of policy change.

"Policy" also has a complicating flexibility in our conceptualization of CBPPW work. We have defined this term broadly as "an organization's planned activities to achieve a goal" (Themba & Minkler, 2003), an approach that encompasses a wide variety of public and private, formal and informal, and policy- and practice-related organizational behaviors. This definition thus includes very different types of policy analysis and advocacy, making it difficult to define rules or principles that can guide action in all these arenas.

Another challenge is to define the types of evidence that CBPPW researchers collect and analyze. Traditionally, health policy researchers collect data on the incidence, prevalence, and costs of health conditions, the cost-effectiveness of various solutions, and public opinion on how problems should be prioritized and the acceptability of solutions. In our experience, CBPPW researchers also need to be able to elicit perceptions and emotional reactions to living conditions and policy options; conduct power analyses at the community, municipal, and national levels; analyze histories of previous relevant struggles; and assess qualitatively temporal changes and population differences in public attitudes through community forums and street outreach. This expanded notion of what constitutes research may challenge health researchers trained in more traditional approaches. Furthermore, the methods we describe in this chapter offer their own challenges. For example, as we have suggested, developing and maintaining participatory data collection and analysis processes requires striking a balance between rigor and feasibility, a balancing act that demands creativity and a commitment to neither oversell nor undersell what the data say.

In reflecting on the varied ideas included in the term *community-based participatory policy work*, we conclude that CBPPW work is not a single clearly defined entity but rather a porous and complex arena of activity. It is perhaps more helpful to consider a continuum of activities in each of four domains (community-based, participatory, policy, and research), ranging from more narrowly defined to more broadly defined. The multiple meanings of CBPPW work often make it difficult for groups to choose priorities—about policy goals, level of influence, sector of interest, or strategies to use. This may be especially true for food policy, which already has a dizzying array of options on the policy agenda. By having explicit discussions about where a group chooses to locate itself on the four domains, it may be possible to make more informed choices about policy goals and the methods that researchers can use to collect, analyze, and interpret evidence to advance these goals.

LESSONS LEARNED AND IMPLICATIONS FOR PRACTICE

Our experiences of participating in and studying these three cases suggest several lessons for CBPPW practitioners and their research partners.

Need for a Team with Diverse Skills

One key difference between traditional policy research and community-based participatory policy work relates to the question of who the initiator of a CBPPW project is and, more specifically, whether it is a group with existing policy expertise or not. Our cases provide different views of this. In the case of HEP, health department employees initiated collaboration with academics and youth organizations. In BFC's case, community members initiated the policy work, though for the most part, members of the policy committee leading this work had a preexisting interest in policy and, in some cases, significant policy expertise. In FLEJ, groups with policy expertise have been brought in to participate, and in several cases are leading working groups, but many other community members who have others kinds of expertise and skills are participating as well.

Though our cases do not show the full range of policy expertise, in CBPPW projects the initiator can come from any constituency, whether knowledgeable about policy or not. Over time, a CBPPW "team" is created, which includes those who are knowledgeable about policy and those who are knowledgeable about the manifestation of the policy problem on the ground. On the one hand, as BFC learned through their first effort at policy work, people with a professional interest or role in policy can be helpful in a CBPPW process, but their presence alone is not sufficient to comprise a CBPPW project. On the other hand, a diverse team that includes policy professionals may also be able to generate resources for doing this kind of work, as the inclusion of such professionals may confer pro bono access to expertise as well as an increased ability to write successful grants and secure funding.

Similarly, the breadth of research skills that a CBPPW team needs will vary by the effort's goals. Although epidemiologists and nutritionists can make important contributions to food policy work, a team may also need historians, policy analysts, or qualitative researchers skilled in focus groups and elicitation research. In the cases profiled here, CBPPW teams used their community, professional, and advocacy networks to find expertise they needed, allowing researchers with necessary skills to participate as team members or as occasional or one-time consultants.

Grant Funding Plays a Role in What Is Possible and When

Grant funding and resources can play an important role in how and when various CBPPW methods can be employed. For example, FLEJ funding from the Centers for Disease Control and Prevention allowed the group to host a diverse, large, and participatory summit meeting, setting the course for more participatory policy work. It also enabled them to hire Everyday Democracy, an organization skilled in eliciting community input into the policy process. Without this funding, their focus might have remained solely on food access, rather than encompassing the many working groups that are now a part of it. Conversely, the ability of youth groups to remain active participants in HEP greatly diminished after funding ended.

Tensions Around How Much Participation Is Needed at Various Decision Points

In the earliest phases of a CBPPW project, a wide range of decisions must be made: What are the most important aspects of the problem to this community? Who in this community needs to be represented? How can participation be increased? What kind of organizational or decision-making structures can support these efforts? Where are there policy opportunities? And importantly, what are our specific policy goals? Although the easiest and quickest path might be for those most interested in policy to answer these questions, this approach runs the risk of proposing solutions that are irrelevant or not supported by the communities they are meant to benefit.

Participants in our cases attempted to balance these tensions in different ways. After taking a top-down approach that was not broadly supported, the BFC took up new models, their current policy committee and school food network, which are highly attuned to the need for diverse participation from BFC's membership. HEP's experience was the reverse of this in many ways. The project's earliest cohort that conducted the school food research was mostly participatory and youth-led, but because of the lengthy nature of this process, fewer students received training or participated in research and action projects. In later cohorts, HEP attempted to reach a larger number of students, but found that the action projects became less policy oriented, and much more local and smaller scale in the transition. For FLEJ, increased participation through the Food, Faith, and Health Disparities Summit and the working groups that have followed have helped to expand the area of interest from food access (the initial focus after an assessment of church leaders' opinions) to the broad array of issues that the working groups are tackling.

CBPR researchers have long debated about how to find the right balance between the often time-consuming engagement of community residents in the research process and moving the research forward. In CBPPW work, we suggest two guidelines. First, policy work has to be sensitive to the external demands of the policy process: fixed dates for elections, votes on legislation, budgets, and so forth. If the consequence of fully engaging community members in the research process is missing policy deadlines, no one gains. With experience, groups can develop methods for getting quick and timely feedback from community constituents. A second suggestion is to specify in advance the areas of expertise that each team participant can contribute and to design processes for eliciting the specific expertise needed. For example, in the evaluation of an initiative to bring new supermarkets into a food desert, it is unlikely that community members will have opinions on which statistical tests to use to determine whether the observed change is statistically significant; however, community members are very likely to be able to contribute to an analysis of the human impact of bringing additional supermarkets to a neighborhood.

Coupling Education and Research Processes Can Help to Build Constituencies for Change

Combining the processes of education and gathering data from community members can help to increase and diversify participants, while at the same time doing so in ways that may be efficient in terms of time and resources. Training community residents to be researchers not only brings their perspectives into the data-gathering process but also develops their capacity to conduct policy research on other topics. Educating community-based researchers about how policymakers view evidence can increase the quality and utility of the data they gather and also prepare them to use this information effectively in later stages of advocacy. All three groups have used a variety of tactics to merge these two functions. This was a central premise on which HEP was based, and the reason for a structure that began with classroom instruction and ended with youth-led research and action. BFC is also making this approach central to their work. Specifically, in their work on the Farm Bill, policy committee members are seeking funding for community-based activities to educate Brooklyn residents about the Farm Bill, which they see as offering a unique opportunity for gathering community input on policy priorities. BFC has used this approach in their successful school food efforts as well. By creating parent and teacher committees within 16 schools in Brooklyn, BFC supports members of these school communities in researching and advocating for effective policy approaches in a range of school settings, while also continuing to learn about the needs and desires of these constituents.

Importance of Understanding How and Where Evidence Can Be Used Persuasively

Though not discussed extensively in this chapter, each of the cases required participants to operate at more than one level and branch of government and in more than one sector (for example, education, food, recreation, land use). For both advocates and researchers, this requires understanding the rules of the policy game within these levels and branches of government and the key players in the sector. It also requires an appreciation for the types of evidence that are most persuasive in these different settings. For example, city council members are often most moved by stories of problems that their constituents encounter, whereas executive agency leaders may find cost-benefit analyses of the proposed policy options more persuasive. Developing an understanding of the evidence preferences in both the political and policy worlds enhances a policy team's ability to achieve its goals.

SUMMARY

In this chapter, we explored the research methods used by those engaged in the early phases of community-based participatory policy work (CBPPW). To provide detailed examples of these methods, we drew from three collaborative efforts participating in the movement to increase food access and uphold food justice in New York City.

The methods we described can help CBPPW practitioners interested in food policy work to explore multiple topics, including: eliciting various constituencies' definitions of priority problems; eliciting data on experiences of current policies; understanding data that already exist to document problems associated with food and food environments; collecting and analyzing data on food environments; policy scanning and analysis; and eliciting views on policy opportunities. These explorations utilized specific methods ranging from literature reviews to surveys, elicitation dialogues, participatory mapping, and structured observation, among other methods.

Based on the efforts studied here, we noted several limitations and challenges, followed by several lessons learned about conducting research to support CBPPW. These included the need for a team with diverse skills, the degree to which the availability of funding can shape what is possible and when, the tensions that can emerge around participation at various decision points, the benefits of coupling education and research processes in building constituencies for change, and the importance of understanding how and where evidence can be used persuasively.

KEY TERMS

Case studies

Community-based participatory policy work

Food environments

Research methods

DISCUSSION QUESTIONS

1. What kinds of benefits and challenges can sustained community participation contribute to the early phases of a policy advocacy process?

2. Which research methods did the cases described use to collect, analyze, and interpret data to advance community-based participatory policy work? What other kinds of data collection methods might be used and how?

3. Which research methods described here are most relevant to other topics around which community-based participatory policy work might take place and why? For instance, which are most relevant to policy activism on HIV

prevention? Which are most relevant to policy activism to reduce rates of childhood asthma?

4. Why do CBPPW researchers need to understand policy and political processes at local, state, and national levels?

REFERENCES

Acosta, C. M. (2003). Improving public health through policy advocacy. *Community-Based Public Health Policy and Practice 8*, 1–8.

Babey, S. H., Hastert, T. A., Yu, H., & Brown, E. R. (2008). Physical activity among adolescents: When do parks matter? *American Journal of Preventive Medicine 34*(4), 345–348.

Bennett, G. G., McNeill, L. H., Wolin, K. Y., Duncan, D. T., Puleo, E., & Emmons, K. M. (2007). Safe to walk? Neighborhood safety and physical activity among public housing residents. *PLoS Medicine, 4*(10), e306, 1599–1607.

Brooklyn Food Coalition. (2011). Who we are. Retrieved June 26, 2011, from http://brooklynfoodcoalition.ning.com/page/who-we-are.

Brooklyn Food Coalition Research and Mapping Committee Community Food Survey. (2011). Food census. Retrieved June 26, 2011, from http://www.foodcensus.org/

Brownson, R. C., Newschaffer, C. J., & Ali-Abarghoui, F. (1997). Policy research for disease prevention: Challenges and practical recommendations. *American Journal of Public Health, 87*, 735–739.

Checkoway, B. N., & Gutiérrez, L. M. (2006). Youth participation and community change: An introduction. *Journal of Community Practice, 14*(1/2), 1–9.

Christoffel, K. K. (2000). Public health advocacy: Process and product. *American Journal of Public Health, 90*, 722–726.

Dinour, L., Fuentes, L., & Freudenberg, N. (2008). *Reversing obesity in New York City: An action plan for reducing the promotion and accessibility of unhealthy food.* CUNY Campaign Against Diabetes and Public Health Association of New York City. Retrieved June 26, 2011, from: http://www.phanyc.org/pdfs/2008unhealthyfoodreport.pdf

Everyday Democracy. (2011a). Homepage. Retrieved on June 26, 2011, from http://www.everyday-democracy.org/en/index.aspx

Everyday Democracy. (2011b). About us. Retrieved on June 26, 2011, from http://www.everyday-democracy.org/en/Page.AboutUs.aspx

Freire, P. (1970). *Pedagogy of the oppressed.* New York: Continuum.

Freudenberg, N., McDonough, J., & Tsui, E. (2011). Can a food justice movement improve nutrition and health? A case study of the emerging food movement in New York City. *Journal of Urban Health, 88*(4), 623–636.

Greenwood, D. A., & Levin, M. (1998). *Introduction to action research: Social research for social change*. Thousand Oaks, CA: Sage.

Israel, B. A., Schulz, A. J., Parker, E. A., Becker, A. B., Allen, A. J., & Guzman, J. R. (2008). Critical issues in developing and following CBPR principles. In M. Minkler, & N. Wallerstein (Eds.), *Community-based participatory research for health: From process to outcomes* (2nd ed., pp. 47–66). San Francisco: Jossey-Bass.

Israel, B. A., Coombe, C. M., Cheezum, R. R., Schulz, A. J., McGranaghan, R. J., Lichtenstein, R., Reyes, A .G., Clement, J., & Burris, A. (2010). Community-based participatory research: A capacity-building approach for policy advocacy aimed at eliminating health disparities. *American Journal of Public Health, 100*, 2094–2102.

Jetter, K. M., & Cassady, D. L. (2006). The availability and cost of healthier food alternatives. *American Journal of Preventive Medicine, 30*(1), 38–44.

Kingdon, J. W. (2003). *Agendas, alternatives, and public policies* (2nd ed.). New York: Longman Classics in Political Science, Addison-Wesley.

Kuo, B. D., & Goodman, E. (2011). The power and promise of youth's voices. *Childhood Obesity, 7*(1), 16–18.

Livingood, W. C., Goldhagen, J., Bryant, T., Wood, D., Winterbauer, N., & Woodhouse, L. D. (2007). A community-centered model of the academic health department and implications for assessment. *Journal of Public Health Management & Practice, 13*(6), 662–669.

Longest, B. B., Jr. (2006). *Health policymaking in the United States* (3rd ed.). Chicago: AUPH/ Health Administration Press.

Minkler, M. (2010). Linking science and policy through community-based participatory research to study and address health disparities. *American Journal of Public Health, 100*(Suppl 1), S81–S87.

Minkler M., & Freudenberg, N. (2010). From community-based participatory research to policy change. In H. E. Fitzgerald, C. Burack, & S. Seifer, (Eds.), *Handbook of engaged scholarship: The contemporary landscape (Vol. 2: Community-campus partnerships)* (pp. 275–294). East Lansing: Michigan State University Press.

Pothukuchi, K., Joseph, H., Burton, H., & Fisher, A. (2002). *What's cooking in your food system: A guide to community food assessment*. Community Food Security Coalition. Retrieved on June 26, 2011, from http://www.foodsecurity.org/CFAguide-whatscookin.pdf

Raufman, J., Farley, S. M., Olson, C., & Kerker, B. (2007). *Diabetes and obesity, summary of community health survey 2007*. New York City Department of Health and Mental Hygiene. Retrieved on June 26, 2011, from http://www.nyc.gov/html/doh/downloads/pdf/ community/CHS2007-Diabetes-Obesity.pdf

Steckler, A., & Dawson, L. (1982). The role of health education in public policy development. *Health Education Quarterly 9*(4), 275–292.

Swain, G. R., Bennett, N., Etkind, P., & Ransom, J. (2006). Local health department and academic partnerships: Education beyond the ivy walls. *Journal of Public Health Management & Practice 12*(1), 33–36.

Themba, M. N. (1999) *Making policy, making change: How communities are taking law into their own hands.* San Francisco: Jossey-Bass.

Themba, M. N., & Minkler, M. (2003). Influencing policy though community based participatory research. In M. Minkler & N. Wallerstein (Eds.), *Community-based participatory research for health* (pp. 349–370). San Francisco: Jossey-Bass.

Themba-Nixon, M., Minkler, M., & Freudenberg, N. (2008). The role of CBPR in policy advocacy. In M. Minkler & N. Wallerstein (Eds.), *Community-based participatory research for health: From process to outcomes* (2nd ed., pp. 307–322). San Francisco: Jossey-Bass.

Tsui, E., Bylander, K., Cho, M., Maybank, A., Freudenberg, N. (2012). *Engaging Youth in Food Activism in New York City: Lessons Learned from a Youth Organization*, Health Department, and University Partnership. Journal of Urban Health. Epub ahead of print. Retrieved on June 19, 2012 from, http://www.ncbi.nlm.nih.gov/pubmed/22696174

van Olphen, J., Freudenberg, N., Galea, S., Palermo, A. G., & Ritas, C. (2003). Advocating policies to promote community reintegration of drug users leaving jail. In M. Minkler & N. Wallerstein (Eds.), *Community-based participatory research for health* (pp. 371–389), San Francisco: Jossey Bass.

Wallerstein, N., & Bernstein, E. (1988). Empowerment education: Freire's ideas adapted to health education. *Health Education Quarterly, 15*(4), 379–394.

Wallerstein, N. (1994) Empowerment education applied to youth. In A. C. Matiella (Ed.), *Multicultural challenge in health education* (pp. 153–176). Santa Cruz, CA: ETR Associates.

Wang, C., & Burris, M. A. (1997). Photovoice: Concept, methodology, and use for participatory needs assessment. *Health Education & Behavior, 24*(3), 369–387.

Acknowledgments: The authors are deeply grateful to participants from the Brooklyn Food Coalition, Faith Leaders for Environmental Justice, and the Health Equity Project for their input into the development of this chapter and their admirable work to improve access to health via improving food environments throughout New York City. In particular, we thank Nancy Romer, Lisa Sharon Harper, Kim Bylander, Aletha Maybank, and the HEP staff members and youth organizations that participated as part of the Health Equity Project. Despite the contributions of many of these groups and individuals to this chapter, the interpretations and errors belong to the authors alone.

Chapter 19

CITIZENS, SCIENCE,

AND DATA JUDO

LEVERAGING SECONDARY DATA ANALYSIS TO BUILD A COMMUNITY-ACADEMIC COLLABORATIVE FOR ENVIRONMENTAL JUSTICE IN SOUTHERN CALIFORNIA

RACHEL MORELLO-FROSCH

MANUEL PASTOR

JAMES SADD

MICHELE PRICHARD

MARTHA MATSUOKA

Over the last three decades, California has distinguished itself as a hotbed of environmental justice (EJ) activism. The fuel behind this political momentum has been effective community organizing and advocacy by a variety of organizations seeking fundamental changes in **environmental health** policy and regulation at the regional and state levels. Within this context, it becomes clear that the recent focus of California policymakers on **environmental justice** is rooted in changing demographic realities of the state. Legislators representing crucial swing-vote communities have attained positions of political power that have enabled them to push forward environmental health and justice initiatives. Starting in 1999, the California legislature passed Senate Bill 115, a measure that directs the Governor's Office of Planning and Research to coordinate environmental justice initiatives across state agencies, including the California Environmental Protection Agency (Cal-EPA). Since then there have been several other regulatory initiatives to advance environmental justice in the state, guided in large measure by California's Environmental Justice Advisory Committee (Cal-EPA, 2003). In light of these political gains, state, regional, and local agencies have sought to engage environmental justice advocates in order to identify solutions to environmental health problems.

Although regulatory agencies have developed systems to ensure that decision making includes some form of community participation (such as access to information, public comment periods, and public meetings or hearings), these processes tend to be more focused on procedural justice and have not necessarily ensured equitable outcomes in regulatory, zoning, and siting decisions. Insuring that community participation in these policy and regulatory efforts is effective requires extensive preparatory work, including building capacity, and addressing language and scientific literacy needs. Moreover, if government agencies are to truly enhance effective public participation in the regulatory arena, they need to recall two key lessons from years of environmental justice organizing. First, diverse communities have important insights and localized knowledge about how environmental hazards may be affecting their health and well-being (Morello-Frosch et al., 2006). Second, although scientific analysis is critical to informed decision making, this expertise should not be the sole driver for whether and how agencies respond to environmental health and justice problems. Community organizations, which have traditionally had to muscle their way into the policymaking and regulatory process, should be viewed as a resource for broadening the range of voices and empowered to improve community environmental health in the most effective way possible. Community-based participatory research (CBPR) provides a means to address this issue, and there are multiple methods that community organizations and their academic partners have developed with the aim of enhancing community engagement in environmental justice issues in policymaking and regulation. The use of secondary data sources and community efforts to validate these information sources is one such method and will be the focus of this chapter.

This chapter discusses how the Los Angeles Collaborative for Environmental Health and Justice (the Collaborative) has applied a CBPR approach to conduct research using secondary data sources. We begin by describing how the Collaborative carries out its work. We then focus on the role that environmental health research plays in the Collaborative, including why we depend on secondary data analysis, and examples of how we collectively develop projects, interpret, and ground-truth data and disseminate study results. We also describe how the Collaborative has leveraged data to promote policy change. We briefly explore how our research model has sought to transform traditional scientific approaches to studying community environmental health. Finally, we conclude with a discussion of some of the challenges of our method and the lessons learned from our work.

LOS ANGELES COLLABORATIVE FOR ENVIRONMENTAL HEALTH AND JUSTICE: BACKGROUND AND THE PARTNERS INVOLVED

The Los Angeles Collaborative for Environmental Health and Justice (the Collaborative) was formed in 1996 when Communities for a Better Environment, a California-based environmental justice organization with strong organizing roots in Southern California, and the Liberty Hill Foundation, a Los Angeles–based community foundation specializing in grantmaking, technical assistance, and capacity building for community-based organizations, joined forces with academic researchers to study, fund, and support the burgeoning field of environmental justice.

At the intersection of environmentalism, social justice, and civil rights, the Collaborative emerged from a collective concern about the adverse health impacts of the urban environment on low-income communities of color. The Collaborative's work is driven by a shared perspective—based upon scientific evidence and residents' firsthand knowledge—that the elevated risk and incidence of asthma, cancer, and respiratory illnesses are linked to major pollution sources, such as factories, freeways, and goods movement corridors from the ports of Los Angeles and Long Beach. This work has been backed by over a decade of research demonstrating a regional pattern of clusters of polluting facilities, high concentrations of toxic **air pollution**, and high health risks in low-income communities of color

(Gauderman, 2004; Hricko, 2008; Morello-Frosch, Pastor, & Sadd, 2002; Pastor, Sadd, & Hipp, 2001; Sadd, Pastor, Boer, & Snyder 1999).

The Collaborative has grown significantly since its inception and now includes several community-based environmental health and justice organizations that have had significant success in cleaning up their communities and putting environmental health on the policy agenda. The Collaborative now includes a broad range of community-based organizations (CBOs) and research institutions that have contributed a growing sophistication and success in data analysis, community organizing, and policy advocacy. Collaborative members include:

- Coalition for a Safe Environment
- Communities for a Better Environment
- East Yard Communities for Environmental Justice
- Liberty Hill Foundation
- Occidental College
- Pacoima Beautiful
- University of California, Berkeley, School of Public Health and Department of Environmental Science, Policy and Management
- University of Southern California, Program for Environmental and Regional Equity
- Union de Vecinos

Despite its long history, the goals of the Collaborative have consistently remained twofold: (1) to improve environmental health in low-income communities of color in Southern California by conducting community-based participatory research on air quality and environmental justice; and (2) to build the capacity of community-based environmental justice organizations by linking research to policy advocacy and organizing at the local and statewide levels. Building on 15 years of work, the Collaborative continues to produce research on air pollution and its effects on the lives and health of residents living in the most affected and vulnerable areas of the Los Angeles region. Combining scientific data analysis with community knowledge and analysis, the Collaborative has provided funding and research to a cadre of community-based organizations that have been successful in reducing specific environmental health hazards such as: defeating a proposed Vernon Power Plant; legally challenging the South Coast Air Quality Management District's air pollution credit trading proposal; expanding public participation and health safeguards related to the expansion of the 710 freeway, a major goods movement corridor that stretches from the Ports of Los Angeles and Long Beach to the Inland Empire area of Southern California; and securing a community benefits agreement with the Port of Los Angeles for the TransPacific Container Corporation expansion project to pay container fees for off-port property air quality and community mitigation.

The Collaborative comprises the community-based organizations previously listed, the Liberty Hill Foundation, and a multidisciplinary research team with expertise from the fields of environmental health and epidemiology, biostatistics, economics and urban planning, and environmental science. All researchers came to the Collaborative with experience working with community partners and have focused much of their academic endeavors on supporting community economic development and improving environmental policymaking and regulation (Morello-Frosch, 2002; Morello-Frosch, Pastor, Porras, & Sadd, 2002; Pastor, Dreier, & Grigsby, 2000; Pastor, 2001; Sadd et al., 1999). Research team members have committed their academic careers to combining rigor, relevance, and reach— that is, conducting high-quality research that has relevance for policy and that simultaneously sustains training, outreach, and publications that engage diverse constituencies.

Recognizing that there was a range of simultaneous yet separate organizing, advocacy, and research approaches focused on advancing environmental justice in Southern California, Communities for a Better Environment and Liberty Hill initiated preliminary conversations with the researchers that culminated in the formation of the Collaborative. Residents in heavily affected neighborhoods had organized to challenge such environmental health problems, yet critical aspects of the EJ advocacy network in Southern California needed to be strengthened in several areas. First, environmental justice issues in the Southern California region had not been addressed in a holistic way that promoted an effective regional voice for community environmental health and social justice. Second, there was a paucity of scientific research documenting the regional character of environmental inequality in Southern California. Third, a regional focus on environmental justice research acknowledges that industrial clusters and land-use planning decisions are generally regionally rooted (Morello-Frosch, Pastor, Porras,

---

& Sadd, 2001; Morello-Frosch, Pastor, & Porras, 2001). Therefore, a coordinated strategy through a community-academic-foundation collaborative sought to build regional capacity and leadership by emphasizing community organizing to create public awareness, voice, and political pressure; legal and policy work to promote change; and scientific research on environmental health and demographics to help environmental justice groups more effectively engage in "data judo" with regulators and policymakers. Data judo is a process in which communities marshal scientific resources and expertise to conduct research and leverage the data necessary to support policy and regulatory change.

After a period of planning and some initial experience working together on small research projects, the Collaborative partners (that is, representatives from CBE, the Liberty Hill Foundation, and the research team) sought and successfully attained three years of funding support from The California Endowment, a statewide health foundation. The total grant was $1.7 million dollars, with 27% of the money supporting the organizing work of CBE, 55% going toward training, secondary grantmaking, and organizational capacity building to support EJ organizing and advocacy work throughout the area, and the balance (18%) supporting air pollution and environmental hazard studies on the South Coast Region). This grant was renewed to advance the work and grow the Collaborative and was also leveraged to secure funding from other foundations such as the California Wellness Foundation, the Ford Foundation, and the Kresge Foundation to support work on children's health, **cumulative impacts** analysis, and environmental justice.

Developing Approaches to CBPR on Environmental Justice

The experience of CBPR is well documented (Arcury, Quandt, & McCauley, 2000; Israel, Schulz, Parker, & Becker 1998; Minkler & Wallerstein, 2003; Shepard, 2000) and more recently, CBPR approaches in the area of environmental justice have gained wider recognition and funding support, largely through the many projects funded by the National Institute of Environmental Health Sciences, the U.S. EPA and private foundations (Brown et al., 2011). Despite the inherent challenges of bridging the academic and community organizing worlds to collect and interpret scientific data, one key asset of a CBPR approach is the involvement of residents who directly experience exposures and diseases of concern, provide firsthand knowledge, and encourage innovation in analytical techniques. Further, collaboration allows for substantive community involvement in several phases of the research process: formulating research questions; collecting and analyzing data; and disseminating results to diverse constituencies and the scientific community through peer-reviewed publications, popular reports, organizing, community presentations, and the media (Brown et al., 2011; Minkler & Wallerstein, 2003; Minkler, Vasquez, Tajik, & Petersen 2008; Morello-Frosch, Brown, Brody, Gasior, Rudgl, Zota, et al., 2011a).

The Collaborative has a unique decision-making structure to prioritize which research projects to undertake. Essentially any partner can bring a research idea to the table, but community partners largely shape decisions regarding research project priorities, timing, and design. Once these decisions are made, the research partners either independently or in close collaboration with community partners gather and validate the data; in the case of data collection that requires field work, community partners work closely with researchers to design study protocols and select study sites. In the case of secondary data analysis, the researchers conduct analysis independently, while ensuring that there are opportunities along the way for discussion and feedback from community partners regarding new ways to approach complex analytical questions and interpret findings. This decision-making and feedback structure for the research was developed shortly after the founding of the Collaborative through substantial discussion between CBE, Liberty Hill, and the research team. This structure was formalized in an early written document (see Appendix M), in order to balance the Collaborative's work load, ensuring that the researchers focus on initial commitments to fundamental research on environmental justice issues with regional relevance, and avoiding over-extending the Collaborative's resources by reactively responding to multiple requests to conduct specialized projects.

Operationally, the Collaborative has set up several processes to promote communication, continual internal feedback among partners, and evaluation of the work. Partners meet in person at least three times per year for an entire day to carry out the work, discuss issues or challenges that arise in projects, plan future endeavors, and assess whether and how the Collaborative achieves its project goals and objectives. These meetings are supplemented with periodic conference calls as necessary. The Collaborative also has retreats to plan new work and to strategize on the most effective way to integrate research and organizing efforts with political opportunities to promote policy and regulatory change that supports environmental justice. Within this context, community partners play a leading role in prioritizing and setting goals and objectives for the Collaborative's organizing, research, and advocacy work.

The Liberty Hill Foundation has assumed the primary role in managing the administrative work of the Collaborative, which includes: tracking budget and expenses, coordinating work on reports to funding agencies, and helping to facilitate strategic planning efforts to ensure that project goals and objectives are met. In addition to its grant-making, training, and capacity-building functions, Liberty Hill also supports the media advocacy and broader public communication efforts of the Collaborative.

When funding sources have allowed, the Collaborative has worked with an external evaluator who has evaluated the broader impact that the Collaborative has had in the policy arena by interviewing decision makers, regulatory officials, funding agencies, and members of Southern California's environmental justice community. The evaluator participates in all Collaborative meetings, providing ongoing feedback in addition to written process and outcome evaluations to Collaborative partners and funders. Finally, the Collaborative was also evaluated by an external research team as part of an outside project that sought to assess the policy influence of EJ CBPR projects nationwide (Minkler et al., 2008). (See Chapter Thirteen for an examination of the documentation and evaluation of a CBPR partnership using in-depth interviews and closed-ended questionnaires.)

Identification and Selection of Secondary Data

At the outset, Collaborative partners decided to rely primarily on secondary data analysis as the core of its research activities. (See Chapter Eighteen for an examination of the use of multiple methods for analyzing the impact of policies on public health.) However, more recently the Collaborative has sought to ground-truth the results of secondary data analysis as a way to systematically blend local knowledge of environmental hazards and sensitive land uses with official data sources (discussed below). Although primary data collection is generally viewed as the gold standard in research, it has some major drawbacks. First, primary data collection requires substantial financial resources and organizational capacity to carry out effectively. Second, primary data collection conducted in collaboration with community-based organizations with a clear stake in study outcomes is vulnerable to misguided criticism by the mainstream scientific community or skeptical policymakers who seek to marginalize CBPR research by arguing that methods suffer from systematic bias or lack objectivity (Anderton, 1996; Foreman, 1998). Given some of the high-stakes policy issues that community partners were grappling with, Collaborative members agreed that an effective way to address some of the persistent methodological challenges in the environmental justice research field would be to utilize secondary data collected by regulatory authorities such as the U.S. Environmental Protection Agency, the California Environmental Protection Agency, the California Air Resources Board, and others. In short, drawing from the experience of other mainstream environmental organizations, the Collaborative believed that analyzing the government's own data and supplementing this with community-engaged validation of study results would be a powerful way to draw regulatory attention to environmental justice issues.

Moreover, using secondary data sources allowed the Collaborative to take advantage of major advances in air emissions inventories, such as the Risk Screening Environmental Indicators, which provides toxicity-weighted hazard scores for air pollutant emissions from the Toxic Release Inventory, and EPA's National Air Toxics Assessment, which estimates exposure to outdoor air pollution on a national scale. Because of "Right-to-Know" laws that make this air pollution data publicly available, the research team was able to generate numerous studies that have built up the body of evidence on the significance of environmental inequality in Southern California. Secondary data analysis has allowed the Collaborative to economize and stretch out scarce resources for research, and to strengthen the power and legitimacy of its arguments in the policy arena by demonstrating that study results are based on data collected by federal and state agencies that in the eyes of skeptics may be viewed as more legitimate and scientifically "objective."

Analysis of Secondary Data

Part of what the Collaborative sought to do was document Southern California's environmental health "riskscape"—that is, demographic and geographic distributions of pollution burdens—in ways that are analytically rigorous and empirically compelling to residents, researchers, and policymakers. The analytical methods for this research involved the use of computer-based mapping, multivariate statistical analysis, environmental health risk assessment, and spatial statistics. To achieve this the research team developed indicators for assessing potential environmental inequalities, including: location of potentially hazardous industrial emission sources (Pastor et al., 2002); treatment storage and disposal facilities (TSDFs) (Pastor, Sadd, & Hipp, 2001; Sadd et al., 1999); and estimated health risks associated with outdoor air toxics exposures (Morello-Frosch, Pastor, & Porras, 2001; Morello-Frosch, Pastor, & Sadd, 2002; Pastor, Sadd, & Hipp, 2001; Pastor, Sadd, & Morello-Frosch, 2004; Sadd, Morello-Frosch, Scroggins, & Jesdale, 2011). Researchers used risk assessment tools to answer science-policy questions about the significance of ambient pollutant concentrations for distributions of cancer and respiratory risks among diverse communities (U.S. EPA, 1986a; 1986b); Cal-EPA, 1997a; 1997b; CAPCOA, 1993). This allowed researchers to address the question of whether there were patterns of environmental inequality and which communities bear the largest burdens of potential health impacts. Research results and conceptual issues were reported by the research team and regularly discussed at in-person Collaborative meetings and on conference calls involving the research team, community-based organizations, and Liberty Hill.

DISSEMINATION OF RESEARCH RESULTS TO ENHANCE COMMUNITY PARTICIPATION IN ENVIRONMENTAL POLICYMAKING AND REGULATION

Communication is critical to the Collaborative—in terms of engaging target audiences and helping them make a visceral connection to the issues of environmental justice. Whether it is through publishing study results or conducting "toxic tours" of communities affected by toxics, the interdisciplinary work of the research team, coupled with the organizing and advocacy experience of the CBO partners and Liberty Hill, enhances flexibility in how the Collaborative frames messages about community environmental health to diverse audiences including public health officials, regulators, urban planners, industry, the media, and policymakers.

In order to leverage research results and apply them toward promoting policy change, the Collaborative has developed various dissemination strategies. (Also see Chapter Fourteen for a discussion of the development of dissemination procedures within a CBPR partnership.) These include publication in peer-reviewed scientific and policy literature, media outreach, popular reports aimed at broad public audiences that are printed and posted online, and other public outreach materials. All decisions regarding dissemination activities are made collectively by the researchers, CBO partners, and Liberty Hill. Manuscripts are circulated and shared among Collaborative partners, and PowerPoint presentations developed by the researchers are posted on the Collaborative Web site to enable partners to utilize these materials in their work. The researchers take the lead on activities related to peer-reviewed publications, and CBOs and Liberty Hill take the lead in developing media strategies and community-based outreach. Since the beginning of the Collaborative, all partners agreed to prioritize publishing research in the peer-reviewed literature to ensure that results reach an academic audience as well as public health practitioners; this requires targeting journals in the fields of public health, sociology, urban planning, economics, political science, and public policy.

Media dissemination strategies have entailed interviews and the strategic publication of opinion page editorials in mainstream press outlets. Press coverage of the research and organizing work has appeared in the *Los Angeles Times, San Jose Mercury News, Sacramento Bee*, the *Wall Street Journal*, the *California Journal*, and smaller local media outlets, including Spanish-speaking outlets. Because of the bilingual capacity of members from the CBOs and the research team, the Collaborative has been able to do media outreach to Spanish-speaking press outlets.

A collectively defined popular and academic dissemination strategy has enabled the Collaborative to bring attention to the research and its implications for organizing and advocacy at the regional, citywide (Los Angeles), statewide, and national levels. Community partners play a central role in shaping media strategies related to dissemination of research results, often working to ensure that press coverage and op-ed pieces are timed to coincide with organizing campaigns to push policy change at either the local or statewide level. For example, media outreach and the placement of an op-ed piece in the *Los Angeles Times* discussing study results on the disparate impact of ambient air toxics exposures on residents of color was timed to coincide with major activities for a successful campaign to strengthen local air quality district rules governing facility emissions of carcinogenic compounds (Morello-Frosch, Pastor, & Porras, 2001; Pastor, Porras, & Morello-Frosch, 2000). Led by CBE, the Collaborative partners developed and implemented a similar media strategy to coincide with public hearings sponsored by the Cal-EPA regarding its proposed adoption of an environmental justice guidance document for the agency's programs and offices (Cal-EPA, 2003).

Collaborative partners collectively decide authorship for both media and academic publications. With one exception (Morello-Frosch, Pastor, & Sadd, 2002), community partners prefer to coauthor press articles (Morello-Frosch, Pastor, & Porras, 2001; Pastor, Porras, & Morello-Frosch, 2000), rather than coauthor research publications.

Collaborative partners have also developed other materials for dissemination, such as presentations, that can be tailored to diverse audiences. The researchers generally craft initial drafts of presentation materials and solicit feedback from community partners on their content and format. Both community partners and researchers use these materials to conduct presentations, and decisions about which partner is strategically best suited to make presentations on the Collaborative's work are decided collectively. Presentation materials are circulated electronically and posted on a password-protected Web site where they can be viewed, edited, downloaded, and shared among the Collaborative partners. Researchers have also published popular reports for broader public audiences. For example, in 2004 the Collaborative released a report, *Building a Regional Voice for Environmental Justice*, which summarized the Collaborative's research and documented the clear patterns of disproportionate health and environmental risks faced by low-income communities of color (Los Angeles Collaborative for Environmental Justice and Health, 2004). The report was among the first to address multiple sources of pollution, helping establish a research and policy framework that recognizes the cumulative impact of pollution and social stressors at the neighborhood level. In 2011, the Collaborative also released its report *Hidden Hazards*, which examines efforts to screen for, map, and characterize the cumulative impacts of environmental and nonenvironmental stressors in diverse neighborhoods within Southern California (Los Angeles Collaborative for Environmental Justice and Health, 2011). The methods and policy implications of this report are discussed in more detail below.

In the early years of the Collaborative, Liberty Hill administered an Environmental Justice Institute, which provided an important venue to conduct trainings for CBO staff on diverse topics such as GIS mapping and interpretation, media advocacy, reaching decision makers in the regulatory and policy arenas, and data collection techniques using air monitoring equipment such as DustTrak monitors for measuring fine particulate matter or through "bucket brigades" where organization staff are taught to build simple, low-cost air sampling devices using plastic buckets. Serving as the ultimate data judo tool, the use of these technologies has drawn regulatory attention to local air pollution problems in neighborhoods where fugitive emissions from nearby industries and transportation corridors have not been adequately addressed or monitored (Communities for a Better Environment, 2000; Pastor & Rosner, 2002).

LEVERAGING RESEARCH TO PROMOTE POLICY CHANGE

The Collaborative's strategy of linking research, organizing, and advocacy to promote regulatory reforms and policy change has contributed to some impressive victories at the regional and state levels. For example, early study results on the demographic distribution of air toxics and cancer risks in Southern California were leveraged by CBE and other environmental justice groups to compel the regional air quality authority in Southern California to adopt more stringent standards to significantly reduce cancer risks associated with air emissions from industrial facilities (Cone, 2000; Morello-Frosch, Pastor, Porras, et al., 2000). Each Collaborative partner played a central role in this policy victory. The researchers conducted data analysis demonstrating the disparate impact of carcinogenic air toxics on communities of color in the region, and Liberty Hill provided the financial and administrative support to back CBE's successful organizing campaign to tighten the standards. Collectively each partner implemented an effective media strategy: Liberty Hill leveraged its press contacts to ensure that the public hearings and community testimony were well covered by the media, CBE members conducted interviews with several reporters from mainstream and Latino press outlets, and the researchers worked closely with CBE to craft and place an op-ed piece in the *Los Angeles Times* that provided environmental health arguments supporting the proposed emission rule change.

Perhaps most significant in the policy change arena is the Collaborative's most recent effort to integrate secondary data analysis with local community knowledge to better guide decision making on air quality regulation and land use planning at the municipal and regional levels (Los Angeles Collaborative for Environmental Justice and Health, 2011). This work entailed the development of a quantitative Environmental Justice Screening Method (EJSM), which integrated a set of 23 health, environmental, and social vulnerability area-level measures in order to map and characterize cumulative impacts at the neighborhood level within the Southern California region (Sadd et al., 2011). The 23 metrics are organized and scored within three categories: (1) hazard proximity and land use; (2) estimated air pollution exposure and health risk; and (3) social and health vulnerability. The Collaborative sought to integrate the EJSM hazard location data which came from regulatory sources with the knowledge of community residents regarding the location and local effects of environmental stressors and sensitive land uses. Indeed, achieving a complete understanding of the cumulative impacts of environmental and social stressors requires input from community residents who observe the day-to-day activities of emission sources and find hidden hazards that are not recorded in government databases but which can be integrated into screening and mapping methods such as the EJSM.

In order to fill these data gaps, the Collaborative implemented a project called "**Ground Truthing**" to document community residents' observations of conditions "on the ground." Guided by the researchers, community partners gathered data about toxic emitters and their proximity to "sensitive receptors"— concentrations of people who are most vulnerable to pollution: the elderly, young children, and people with respiratory disease. More than sixty residents worked in teams to collect ground-truthing data in six neighborhoods. Community members were trained on the science of air pollution hazards, cumulative impacts, and social vulnerability. Training also covered databases maintained by state and federal regulatory agencies that contain the locations of facilities that require permits and report emissions. Community members learned to identify traditional air quality hazards, and also agreed to a list of land uses and facilities that they considered "sensitive" or "hazardous." Ground-truthing participants defined the geographic boundaries of the neighborhoods where data collection would occur, reviewed maps showing air quality hazards and sensitive land uses, and identified additional hazards and receptors of concern. Finally, after practicing on-the-ground data collection techniques, field teams were charged with:

- Verifying air quality hazard locations recorded in state regulatory agency databases;

- Verifying sensitive receptor locations (schools, child-care centers, playgrounds, urban parks, and health care facilities); and

- Mapping additional air quality hazards and sensitive receptors that were not included in the regulatory databases.

Using portable GPS receivers, residents recorded locations on Google Earth aerial photos with a street address, allowing for later verification using address geocoding. Teams also recorded observations such as trucks idling or passing through residential areas. Finally, residents conducted local air monitoring using DustTrak particulate monitors in specific areas of concern.

Ground-truthing revealed that hazardous facilities and land uses are more numerous than regulatory data suggest and that there are locational errors for many of these facilities. Sensitive land uses are also more numerous and many of these are located too close to hazards. The main findings were: (1) fine particulate levels in areas of concern often exceeded California ambient air quality standards; and (2) community residents found areas where diesel trucks congregate and idle for long periods, often near residential areas or other sensitive land uses. Figure 19.1 maps the Pacoima neighborhood ground-truthing results and Figure 19.2 illustrates the results of fine particulate monitoring for the Boyle Heights ground-truthing site. These figures demonstrate how ground-truthing data, when combined with standardized governmental information, provide an in-depth, picture of the multiple hazards that exist at the neighborhood level. These findings also verify community assertions that facility-by-facility regulation is piecemeal, uncoordinated, and inadequate in recognizing the cumulative impacts faced by residents.

Results from ground truthing have been used by the Collaborative to support improved scientific approaches for assessing the cumulative impacts of pollution from multiple emission sources on neighborhoods and vulnerable populations and the integration of the precautionary principle in environmental regulation and enforcement activities (Cal-EPA, 2003). The precautionary principle means that decision makers should be more proactive if scientific evidence strongly suggests, but does not yet fully prove, that a production facility or pollutant may be jeopardizing public health, particularly among communities that are overburdened by toxics and other health challenges. Similarly, the issue of cumulative impacts compels regulators to acknowledge that chemical-by-chemical approaches to regulation are not protective of public health due to the reality that communities are exposed to numerous pollutants from various sources and that it is important to assess exposures and health risks more holistically when setting standards to protect vulnerable populations.

Although pushing for these long-term, broad policy and regulatory reforms has been a mainstay of the Collaborative's work, these must be combined with

FIGURE 19.1 Results from Pacoima Ground-Truthing Area

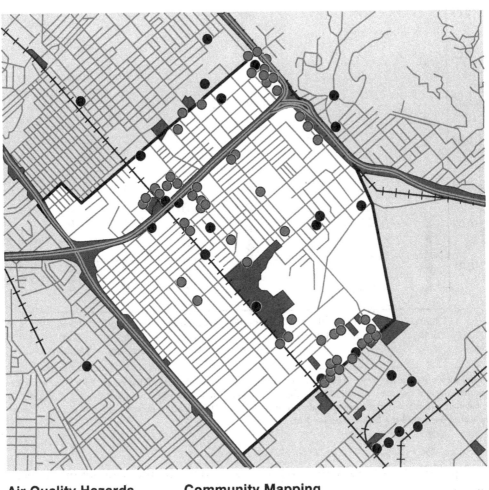

Air Quality Hazards
- ● Point Hazards
- +++ Railroads
- ■ Area Hazards

Community Mapping
- ● Air Quality Hazard

Pacoima is located in the San Fernando Valley, northwest of Los Angeles. In addition to air quality hazards recorded in state regulatory agency databases, community residents found numerous additional emissions facilities; these facilities are commonly clustered together, increasing the cumulative impact to the local neighborhood.

FIGURE 19.2 DustTrak Fine Particulate (PM2.5) Monitoring Results

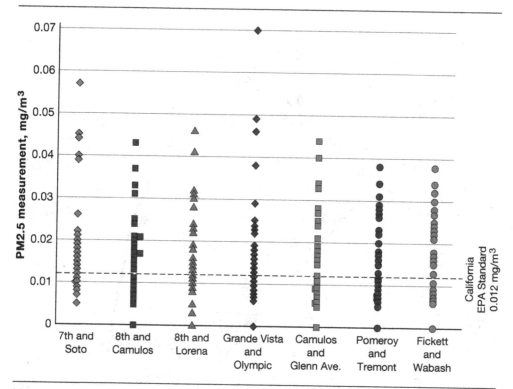

Measurements from each of seven test site locations are shown in vertical columns of data points. Each point represents one time-averaged measurement of PM2.5 at a given location, with a dashed horizontal line showing the California ambient air quality standard for fine particulate air pollution of 0.012 milligrams per cubic meter of air; points above the dashed line exceed this health-based standard.

local policy interventions that improve conditions in the short-term. Indeed, municipal government, with its broad authority over land use across a jurisdiction, can play a significant role in safeguarding communities from overconcentration of hazardous land uses and the development of so-called "hot spots." In fact, local planning and effective permitting and enforcement policies provide the most promising avenues for city and county governments to help overburdened communities deal with pervasive environmental problems over the short and long term. Therefore, as part of the Ground Truthing project, the Collaborative examined how municipal governments in California and elsewhere have adapted traditional planning and land use tools to address public health and safety problems associated with a concentration of industrial uses that persist despite regulation of individual establishments by state or federal agencies. A literature review and discussions with environmental health and justice organizations throughout the country enabled the Collaborative to learn from approaches that have been used by local and regional governments. This information was presented to an advisory group of environmental lawyers, land use experts, and environmental health advocates in Los Angeles for review and feedback. From this process, emerged a policy strategy, known as the *Clean Up, Green Up* campaign that identified specific steps for the City of Los Angeles to address cumulative impacts in vulnerable neighborhoods. This campaign has been guided by three principles:

- *Prevention:* Prevent further increase in the cumulative environmental impacts in overburdened communities.

- *Mitigation:* Clean up, reduce, and mitigate existing environmental hazards.

- *Revitalization:* Implement economic revitalization approaches and invest in green technologies to transform overburdened areas into healthy, sustainable, and vibrant communities with jobs for local residents.

This framework has helped the Collaborative develop strategies for addressing cumulative impacts, including adoption of a screening tool for planning and land use decision making to identify geographically defined areas that are most vulnerable and have a high concentration of hazardous land uses. This information can help the City establish supplemental use districts—a zoning designation which sets specific community standards and guidelines to prevent and reduce environmentally hazardous land uses, and to promote economic development and revitalization. Los Angeles has a precedent for using zoning designations to prevent new fast-food restaurants from opening in a number of South and Southeast Los Angeles neighborhoods. This designation gave city planners an opportunity to study the economic and environmental effects of the overconcentration of fast-food restaurants in these communities and to encourage more grocery stores, sit-down restaurants, and other amenities. Similarly, other zoning designations can require certain businesses to meet specific conditions to harmonize the establishment with its surroundings, even though the service or product is regulated by another agency. Cities can impose sanctions against operators who do not comply with required operating conditions for permits and conduct public hearings, thus providing a mechanism for residents to have a voice in the decision-making process that shapes their community environment.

As part of the *Clean Up, Green Up* campaign, the Collaborative has pushed the City to increase the use of health impact assessments (HIA) as an interdisciplinary approach to assess the health impacts of proposed policies, plans and projects with an explicit concern for socially excluded or vulnerable populations using a combination of quantitative, qualitative, and participatory techniques (Cole, Wilhelm, Long, Fielding, & Kominski, 2004; Corburn & Bhatia, 2007). HIAs could be more effectively folded into the more traditional environmental impact assessment (EIA) process that has been a mainstay of decision making in city planning. Finally, the Collaborative has sought the creation of a mitigation fund through a structure of regulatory fees and fines or penalties for violations in order to enable associated permitting, inspection, and compliance functions in affected neighborhoods, and to also provide a source of revenue to reduce environmental hazards through improvements to existing uses. Cities often apply mitigation funds to reduce localized impacts for intensive commercial or industrial activities. In many jurisdictions, fees or fines collected as part of the inspection and enforcement process are put into trust funds for specific kinds of mitigation with a nexus to project impacts, such as parks or environmental improvement projects.

Through the *Clean Up, Green Up* campaign, Collaborative partners have been pressuring city officials, including officials in the Los Angeles mayor's office, city council members, as well as other decision makers and agency officials to take action to address the findings from the *Hidden Hazards* report and adopt health protective approaches in land use planning and decision making. One of the primary targets of these advocacy efforts has been to encourage the City's Planning Department to adopt many of these strategies, particularly the zoning designations, and application of mitigation funds to address the cumulative impacts of environmental and social stressors in L.A. neighborhoods. This strategic decision to focus on the Planning Department (and Planning Commission) is because of the precedent of applying zoning designations and mitigation funds which can be expanded to address community environmental health issues. For example, the City has applied GIS approaches to map medical marijuana outlets in relation to schools and other sensitive uses; established special districts for historic preservation; and required new liquor stores to go through a rigorous permitting process. Through its research and advocacy strategy, the Collaborative has shown that these same planning and policy tools can be creatively applied to address the overconcentration of industrial land uses that pose significant environmental hazards to human health, not just in overburdened communities, but the region as a whole.

Transforming Traditional Approaches for Researching Community Environmental Health

The Collaborative strategy for conducting research and interpreting and disseminating study results has sought to transform traditional approaches to research on community environmental health. There are three primary ways the Los Angeles Southern California EJ Collaborative has promoted new approaches to community-based participatory research on environmental justice by emphasizing secondary data analysis.

1. *Moving "upstream":* This upstream/downstream analogy takes its title from an oft-used metaphor about preventive health: Villagers notice helpless people floating downstream and develop increasingly sophisticated ways to rescue them, yet no one ventures upstream to find out why people are falling into the river in the first place (Steingraber, 1997). Causally linking pollution with potentially adverse health effects is a tough challenge in the field of environmental health, particularly when populations are chronically exposed to complex chemical mixtures (Institute of Medicine, 1999). Improving epidemiological and exposure methods is one route to addressing this issue. Nevertheless, environmental justice advocates have argued that in the never-ending quest for better data and unequivocal proof of cause and effect, researchers can lose sight of a basic public health principle—namely, the importance of disease prevention (Morello-Frosch, Pastor, & Sadd, 2002). As a result, the Collaborative has supported a multipronged approach to environmental health research. The first approach seeks to improve methods, such as exposure assessment, to better understand the relationship between pollution exposures and environmentally mediated disease. (See Chapter Twelve to learn more about using CBPR in exposure assessment.) The other method uses environmental risk assessment and secondary data analysis when there is a paucity of human epidemiological data to show cause and effect between pollution exposures and disease. The third approach entails ground truthing to verify the accuracy of regulatory data. This

mixed-methods approach circumvents the regulatory paralysis that can occur when definitive human data are lacking, and provides crucial tools to keep policymaking and regulation moving forward. Moreover, this work accounts for the cumulative impacts of environmental and social stressors (Morello-Frosch, Zuk, Jerrett, Shamasunder, & Kyle, 2011; NAS, 2008).

2. *Promoting an "eco-social" outlook:* By connecting social inequality with environmental degradation and community health, the Collaborative's research provides a framework for understanding the impact of discrimination on the environmental health of diverse communities. This framework also raises the challenge of whether disparities in exposures to environmental hazards play an important role in health disparities (Morello-Frosch et al., 2011b). The Collaborative's research focus looks beyond individual or lifestyle factors, such as smoking and diet, and toward the environmental and socioeconomic factors that shape distributions of people and pollution. For this reason researchers draw extensively from the field of social epidemiology to inform research on environmental health and social justice (Krieger, 2001). This framework enables the examination of issues such as segregation, inequality, and community empowerment as possible drivers of environmental inequality (Adler & Rehkopf, 2008; Morello-Frosch & Lopez, 2006; Morello-Frosch, Jesdale, Sadd, & Pastor, 2010; Morello-Frosch et al., 2011b).

3. *Ensuring active community involvement:* Community partners are the final arbiters of how the Collaborative prioritizes research projects, based on advocacy work and organizing needs. This ensures that the research the Collaborative pursues is relevant to the residents and the neighborhoods where they live. Nevertheless, implementing CBPR strategies to address environmental health issues facing communities of color invites open skepticism from critics seeking to challenge the premise of environmental justice and the role of communities in the research process (Foreman, 1998). As a result, the research team and the community partners have been vigilant about methodology and statistical strategies in their approach to secondary data analysis and interpretation of results; indeed, the Collaborative's research faces scrutiny from diverse reviewers, including academic peers, policymakers, and regulators and, ultimately, the test of community wisdom. Despite its challenges, this approach to connecting community and academic partners to secondary data analysis enhances the rigor,

methodological integrity, and most important, the relevance of research for environmental policymaking.

Challenges and Limitations of Emphasizing Secondary Data Analysis

The Collaborative has had to address certain challenges inherent in using secondary data analysis in the context of a CBPR approach to support organizing and policy advocacy. In contrast to other methods that engage communities directly in developing study designs and collecting data, by its very nature secondary data analysis limits the depth of community engagement in the research process. Moreover, reliance on secondary data sources can also narrow the scope of research questions that a community partner may be able to pursue. Overcoming this limitation requires that the Collaborative devote extra time for community partners to review and give feedback on data analysis as it evolves, and ultimately to actively engage in framing the interpretation of study results. For example, community partners have been interested in examining environmental justice questions related to asthma severity and incidence in the South Coast region, but comprehensive, individual-level data on the communities of interest are not readily available. However, the research team was able to address this issue indirectly by conducting an ecological study using noncancer risk assessment to estimate respiratory hazards associated with ambient air toxics exposures among Los Angeles schoolchildren (Morello-Frosch, Pastor, & Sadd, 2002; Pastor, Sadd, & Morello-Frosch, 2002; Pastor, Sadd, & Morello-Frosch, 2004). Ground-truthing efforts can also effectively facilitate the integration of local knowledge and data gathering into secondary data analysis.

Other challenges include managing the research needs and expectations of other environmental justice organizations. Given the proliferation of neighborhood-level organizations that are addressing myriad environmental health concerns, there is an ever-increasing demand for localized research projects which could easily drain the resources of the research team and the Collaborative as a whole. In any situation of scarce resources, the challenge for the Collaborative has been to effectively prioritize the deployment of time and money. After much discussion, the Collaborative collectively decided that a CBPR research strategy based on secondary data analysis would be an effective and efficient approach to promote policy change in a way that would not overwhelm the capacities of the academic partners or unduly burden the organizational resources of community partners. Upon its formation, the Collaborative developed a decision-making structure in which its original community partner, CBE, had the ultimate say on prioritizing research projects and shaping strategies for the dissemination of study results. Although the number of community partners involved with the Collaborative has since increased, this decision-making structure continues as it compels the academic partners to share control over the research agenda, while still preserving the scientific integrity of the analytical work.

Therefore, the Collaborative has prioritized secondary data analysis on regional and statewide environmental justice questions in order to build a body of evidence to inform specific actions such as tightening air quality rules, adopting cumulative exposure strategies for regulation, and pushing for cleaner, safer schools.

LESSONS LEARNED AND LOOKING TOWARD THE FUTURE

The history of the Collaborative offers lessons that transcend CBPR approaches to promoting policy change and that can inform productive alliances between funders, community-based organizations, and the academy. The first lesson is to *build the base to move policy*. Often when community-based organizations engage with academic partners in scientific research and succeed in gaining entry as a valid stakeholder in the policy arena, there is the danger of abandoning the work of organizing. Yet the primary reason community groups are invited to the policy table is the political pressure rooted in an organized community base. Strategically, Collaborative partners believed that a CBPR approach emphasizing secondary data analysis rather than primary data collection would allow community partners to engage effectively in research without pulling organizational and staff resources away from core organizing functions. The ongoing role of the Liberty Hill Foundation enabled the Collaborative to nurture new community voices by expanding the number of CBO partners directly involved in the work, providing critical training and capacity-building opportunities, and providing resources to mobilize communities to participate in public policy debates and decision making.

The second lesson is to *build organic relationships between partners*. This Collaborative was not convened in response to a Request for Proposals, but rather early partners (the research team and CBE) had already formed deep relationships based on prior environmental justice work in the South Coast region. This is not something that can be easily replicated, but it suggests the importance of proactively forming academic-community collaboratives and the need to scale up those partnerships that are authentic and sustainable. The success of the Collaborative model and the strength of the partner relationships have sustained the work during periods when funding was abundant and even when funding had temporarily run dry. The ability of the Collaborative to sustain its research, grow the number of CBOs involved, and expand its organizing and advocacy work within the Southern California region over the last fifteen years is firmly rooted in the partners' collective commitment to the goals of the Collaborative's work and the unique CBPR method of leveraging secondary data analysis to promote policy change. Utilizing secondary data analysis as the core of the Collaborative's CBPR research strategy has also enabled the academic partners to keep the research portion of the Collaborative active during temporary lulls in the funding stream over the years.

The third lesson flows from the second: *make long-term investment in change* through multiyear campaigns and funding streams. There is a tendency among many foundations to think in terms of short-term progress, particularly given the pressures to show accountability, demonstrate measurable outcomes, and make a smooth transition to long-term sustainability. These expectations can have the unintended effect of promoting opportunistic partnerships that have difficulty completing projects or those that focus primarily on grantsmanship. Active leadership by the Liberty Hill Foundation has resulted in multiyear investments by several foundations. This has allowed the Collaborative to think beyond short-term outcomes and work to build a regional framework for social and policy change. Ultimately, building community capacity to promote changes in environmental policy and regulation requires a regional approach. Indeed, shutting down a chromium plating facility operating near an elementary school requires a well-organized neighborhood or parent-teacher organization, but advocating for tighter rules on facility siting and emissions to protect *all* schoolchildren region-wide requires empowering organizations across neighborhoods, racial divides, and economic strata as well as ensuring that the organizations have the technical and organizational capacity to effectively engage in the planning and rule-making process. Achieving this goal requires building in flexibility that allows partners to nimbly respond to opportunities and challenges, shifting directions and resources as necessary.

More important, however, is the Collaborative's desire to support the replication of the collaborative model, with its pillars of research, organizing, advocacy, and community capacity-building, to other regions. This long-term goal of replication and ensuring its sustainability requires resources. Although start-up monies have been critical for supporting single-issue campaigns and coalitions, developing a framework to achieve sustainable social and political change for environmental justice requires a significant long-term investment. Some large foundations and government agencies like the National Institute of Environmental Health Sciences have taken on this challenge by investing in academic-community collaboratives that are inclusive and participatory (Brown et al., 2011; NIEHS, 2011; O'Fallon & Dearry, 2002). Yet, much of this work is still conducted on the margins as few agencies and foundations invest significant resources to support long-term work that *integrates* research and advocacy.

SUMMARY

The achievements of the Collaborative show that the marginal has slowly evolved to become mainstream: from its origins in typically unfunded "participatory action research" and 1960s federal programs' requirements for public involvement, community-based participatory research (CBPR) has grown significantly over the last two decades, largely through federal and private foundation funding in the 1990s. The results of CBPR projects are now well represented at conferences and published in major journals, and methods are now taught in college and graduate schools (Brown et al., 2010). The work of the Los Angeles Collaborative for Environmental Health and Justice demonstrates that CBPR projects that emphasize secondary data analysis in their approach to promoting environmental justice can be powerful agents for policy change without compromising scientific rigor. These partnerships not only promote good science, but science that is focused on important problems that have an impact on the lives of real people while enhancing community capacity and participation in research and advocacy—all of which can ultimately improve the regulatory and policy-making process. In light of this, government agencies and foundations need to proactively support this CBPR work. Increased long-term investment in this work would also encourage more academic researchers to engage with community organizations in pursuit of scientific research that addresses the real-world environmental health challenges faced by communities of color and the poor. Ultimately, promoting the development of new community-academic collaboratives in other regions nationwide will be critical to broadening constituencies and deepening public understanding of the connections between social justice, racial equality, public health, and environmental sustainability.

KEY TERMS

Air pollution

Cumulative impacts

Environmental health

Environmental justice

Ground truthing

DISCUSSION QUESTIONS

1. How can community-based participatory research on environmental health and justice issues improve the rigor, relevance, and reach of science?

2. How can different forms of expertise, including local community knowledge and scientific analysis, be effectively integrated and disseminated to diverse stakeholders to improve policy and regulation in ways that better protect community environmental health?

3. How does community engagement in the scientific enterprise affect theories of disease causation in the field of environmental health and, conversely, how does it affect community perceptions and strategies for addressing local environmental health problems?

REFERENCES

Adler, N. E., & Rehkopf, D. (2008). U.S. disparities in health: Descriptions, causes, and mechanisms. *Annual Review of Public Health, 29,* 235–252.

Anderton, D. L. (1996). Methodological issues in the spatiotemporal analysis of environmental equity. *Social Science Quarterly, 77,* 508–515.

Arcury, T., Quandt, S. A., & McCauley, L. (2000). Farmers and pesticides: Community-based research. *Environmental Health Perspectives, 108,* 787–792.

Brown, P., Brody, J., Morello-Frosch, R., Tovar, J., Zota, A., & Rudel, R. A. (2011). Measuring the success of community science: The Northern California Household Exposure Study. *Environmental Health Perspectives*. doi:10.1289/ehp.1103734

Brown, P., Morello-Frosch, R., Brody, J., Altman, R. G., Rudel, R. A., Senier, L. et al. (2010). Institutional review board challenges related to community-based participatory research on human exposure to environmental toxins: A case study. *Environmental Health, 9*, 39. doi: 10.1186/1476–069X-9–39

Cal-EPA. (1997a). *Technical support document for the determination of noncancer chronic reference exposure levels.* Berkeley: California Environmental Protection Agency, Office of Environmental Health Hazard Assessment, Air Toxicology and Epidemiology Section.

Cal-EPA. (1997b). *Toxic air contaminant identification list summaries.* Sacramento: California Environmental Protection Agency, Air Resources Board.

Cal-EPA. (2003). *Recommendations of the California Environmental Protection Agency (Cal/EPA) Advisory Committee on Environmental Justice to the Cal/EPA Interagency Working Group on Environmental Justice.* Sacramento: Cal-EPA Advisory Committee on Environmental Justice.

CAPCOA. (1993). *Air toxics "Hot Spots" program: Risk assessment guidelines.* Sacramento: California Air Pollution Control Officers' Association.

Cole, B., Wilhelm, M., Long., P., Fielding, J., & Kominski, G. (2004). Prospects for health impact assessment in the United States: New and improved environmental impact assessment or something different? *Journal of Health Politics Policy and the Law, 29*, 1153–1186.

Communities for a Better Environment. (2000). *The bucket brigade manual.* Oakland, CA: CBE.

Cone, M. (2000, March 18). AQMD Tightens cancer rule; pollution: Regulation will force large industries to cut risk posed by emissions in residential areas. Both businesses and environmentalists find fault with the new standard. The *Los Angeles Times*, p. 5.

Corburn, J., &. Bhatia, R. (2007). Health impact assessment in San Francisco: Incorporating the social determinants of health into environmental planning. *Journal of Environmental Planning and Management, 50*, 323–341.

Foreman, C. (1998). *The promise and peril of environmental justice.* Washington, DC: Brookings Institution.

Gauderman, W. (2004). The effect of air pollution on lung development from 10 to 18 years of age. *New England Journal of Medicine, 9*, 1057–1067.

Hricko, A. (2008). Global trade comes home: Community impacts of goods movement. *Environmental Health Perspectives, 116*(2), A80.

Institute of Medicine. (1999). *Toward environmental justice: Research, education, and health policy needs.* Washington, DC: Committee on Environmental Justice, Health Sciences Policy Program, Health Sciences Section, Institute of Medicine: 14–21.

Israel, B. A., Schulz, A. J., Parker, E. A., & Becker, A. B. (1998). Review of community-based research: Assessing partnership approaches to improve public health. *Annual Review of Public Health, 19*, 173–202.

Krieger, N. (2001). Theories for social epidemiology in the 21st century: An ecosocial perspective. *International Journal of Epidemiology, 30*, 668–677.

Los Angeles Collaborative for Environmental Justice and Health. (2004). *Building a regional voice for environmental justice.* Los Angeles: Liberty Hill Foundation.

Los Angeles Collaborative for Environmental Justice and Health. (2011). *Hidden hazards: A call to action for healthy, livable communities.* Los Angeles: Liberty Hill Foundation.

Minkler, M., Vasquez, V. B., Tajik, M., & Petersen, D. (2008). Promoting environmental justice through community-based participatory research: The role of community and partnership capacity. *Health Education & Behavior, 35*(1), 119–137.

Minkler, M., & Wallerstein, N. (2003). *Community-based participatory research for health.* San Francisco: Jossey-Bass.

Morello-Frosch, R. (2002). The political economy of environmental discrimination. *Environment and Planning C, 20*, 477–496.

Morello-Frosch, R., Pastor, M., & Porras, C. (2001, June 3). Who's minding the air at your child's school? *Los Angeles Times*, M3.

Morello-Frosch, R., Pastor, M., Porras, C., & Sadd, J. (2001). Environmental justice and Southern California's "riskscape": The distribution of air toxics exposures and health risks among diverse communities. *Urban Affairs Review, 36*(4), 551–578.

Morello-Frosch, R., Pastor, M., Porras, C., & Sadd, J. (2002). Environmental justice and regional inequality in Southern California: Implications for future research. *Environmental Health Perspectives, 110*(Suppl 2), 149–154.

Morello-Frosch, R., Pastor, M., & Sadd, J. (2002). Integrating environmental justice and the precautionary principle in research and policy-making: The case of ambient air toxics exposures and health risks among school children in Los Angeles. *Annals of the American Academy of Political and Social Science, 584*, 47–68.

Morello-Frosch, R., & Lopez, R. (2006). The riskscape and the color line: Examining the role of segregation in environmental health disparities. *Environmental Research, 102*(2), 181–196.

Morello-Frosch, R., Zavestoski, S., Brown, P., McCormick, S., Mayer, B., & Gasior, R. (2006). Embodied health movements: Responses to a "scientized" world. In K. Moore & S. Frickel (Eds.), *The new political sociology of science: Institutions, networks, and power* (pp. 244–271). Madison: University of Wisconsin Press.

Morello-Frosch, R., Jesdale, B., Sadd, J., & Pastor, M. (2010). Ambient air pollution exposure and full-term birth weight in California. *Environmental Health, 9*, 44. doi:10.1186/1476-069X-9-44

Morello-Frosch, R., Brown, P., Brody, J., Gasior, R., Rudel, R. A., Zota, A., et al. (2011a). Experts, ethics, and environmental justice: Communicating and contesting results from personal exposure science. In G. Ottinger (Ed.) *Environmental justice and the transformation of science and engineering*. Boston: MIT Press.

Morello-Frosch, R., Zuk, M., Jerrett, M., Shamasunder, B., & Kyle, A. D. (2011b). Understanding the cumulative impacts of inequalities in environmental health: Implications for policy. *Health Affairs, 30*(5), 879–887.

NAS. (2008). *Science and decisions: Advancing risk assessment.* Washington, DC: National Research Council Committee on Improving Risk Analysis Approaches Used by the U.S. EPA.

NIEHS. (2011). *Partnerships in environmental and public health.* Available at: http://www.niehs.nih.gov/research/supported/programs/peph/index.cfm

O'Fallon, L. & Dearry, A. (2002). Community-based participatory research as a tool to advance environmental health sciences. *Environmental Health Perspectives, 110*(Suppl 2), 155–159.

Pastor, M. (2001). Common ground at ground zero? The new economy and the new organizing in Los Angeles. *Antipode, 33*(2), 260–289.

Pastor, M., Dreier, P., & Grigsby, J. E. (2000). *Regions that work: How cities and suburbs can grow together.* Minneapolis: University of Minnesota Press.

Pastor, M., Porras, C., & Morello-Frosch, R. (2000, March 16). The region's minorities face major health risks from pollution: Justice demands that the AQMD cut emissions. *Los Angeles Times.*

Pastor, M., & Rosner, R. (2002). Communities armed with bucket take charge of air quality. *Sustainable solutions: Building assets for empowerment and sustainable development.* New York: The Ford Foundation.

Pastor, M., Sadd, J., & Hipp, J. (2001). Which came first? Toxic facilities, minority move-in, and environmental justice. *Journal of Urban Affairs, 23*(1), 1–21.

Pastor, M., Sadd, J., et al. (2002). Who's minding the kids? Pollution, public schools, and environmental justice in Los Angeles. *Social Science Quarterly, 83*(1), 263–280.

Pastor, M., Sadd, J., & Morello-Frosch, R. (2004). Reading, writing and toxics: Children's health, academic performance, and environmental justice in Los Angeles. *Environment and Planning C 2*, 271–290.

Sadd, J., Pastor, M., Boer, J. T., & Snyder, L. D. (1999). "Every breath you take ...": The demographics of toxic air releases in Southern California. *Economic Development Quarterly, 13*(2): 107–123.

Sadd, J., Pastor, M., Morello-Frosch, R., Scroggins, J., & Jesdale, B. (2011). Playing it safe: Assessing cumulative impact and social vulnerability through an environmental justice screening method in the South Coast Air Basin, California. *International Journal of Environmental Research and Public Health, 8*, 1441–1459.

Shepard, P. (2000). Achieving environmental justice objectives and reducing health disparities through community-based participatory research and interventions. *Successful models of community-based participatory research.* Research Triangle Park, NC: National Institute of

Environmental Health Sciences, pp. 30–35. Available at: http://portal.hud.gov/hudportal/documents/huddoc?id=DOC_12485.pdf

Steingraber, S. (1997). *Living downstream: An ecologist looks at cancer and the environment.* Reading, MA: Perseus Books.

U.S. EPA. (1986a). Guidelines for carcinogenic risk assessment. Washington, DC: U.S. Environmental Protection Agency: 33992–34003, *Federal Register, 51*(185).

U.S. EPA. (1986b). Guidelines for the health risk assessment of chemical mixtures. Washington, DC: U.S. Environmental Protection Agency: 34014–34025, *Federal Register, 51*(185).

Chapter 14

DEVELOPING AND
IMPLEMENTING GUIDELINES
FOR DISSEMINATION

THE EXPERIENCE OF THE COMMUNITY ACTION AGAINST ASTHMA PARTNERSHIP

EDITH A. PARKER

THOMAS G. ROBINS

BARBARA A. ISRAEL

WILMA BRAKEFIELD-CALDWELL

KATHERINE K. EDGREN

ASHLEY O'TOOLE

DONELE WILKINS

STUART BATTERMAN

TOBY LEWIS

Ensuring that findings are disseminated to the communities studied is an important aspect of all public health research endeavors. This is especially true in community-based participatory research (CBPR), because a fundamental tenet of CBPR is to use the knowledge generated to inform action with the community involved in the research (Chen, Diaz, Lucas, & Rosenthal, 2010; Gagnon, 2011; Green et al., 1995; Israel, Schulz, Parker, & Becker, 1998; Montaya & Kent, 2011). For this to happen, the research design and methods must include a plan for the translation and **dissemination of research results** so that these findings can inform and be incorporated into community efforts for change at the individual, organizational, community, and policy levels (Ahmed & Palermo, 2010; deKoning & Martin, 1996; Farquhar & Wing, 2003; Green et al., 1995; Israel et al., 1998). Despite the potential usefulness of creating a dissemination plan, there are few examples in the literature of how to engage all partners in determining the structure and products of the dissemination process. In this chapter, we discuss the experience of the Community Action Against Asthma partnership in involving community and academic partners in establishing and then implementing a process to disseminate findings in a timely and understandable fashion to participants, community members, health practitioners, government officials, academics, and policymakers.

OVERVIEW OF THE COMMUNITY ACTION AGAINST ASTHMA PARTNERSHIP

Community Action Against Asthma began as a research project of the Michigan Center for the Environment and Children's Health (MCECH) and is affiliated with an already existing community-academic partnership, the Detroit Community-Academic Urban Research Center (Detroit URC) (see Chapter Thirteen for a more detailed description of the Detroit URC). The Detroit URC had identified childhood illnesses related to the environment as a priority area for research. In 1998, the Detroit URC board successfully competed for funding from the Children's Environmental Health Research Initiative, awarded by the National Institute of Environmental Health Sciences (NIEHS) and the U.S. Environmental Protection Agency. This five-year award enabled the Detroit URC to establish MCECH as a coordinating structure for the following three studies of childhood asthma: a laboratory-based, mouse model study to determine if the mechanism of chronic pulmonary inflammation due to children's repeated exposure to allergens is mediated by excessive local production of chemokines (the *chemokines* project); a household intervention study to reduce environmental triggers for childhood asthma (Parker et al., 2008); and an epidemiological study of the relationship between ambient and indoor air quality exposures (for example, ozone and particulate matter) and children's lung function and other asthma-related health indicators.

The epidemiological and intervention studies were conducted with the same participant population and guided by the same steering committee (described later) and therefore were combined into one larger project, named Community Action Against Asthma (CAAA). In year two, CAAA applied for and received an additional grant to focus on reduction of environmental triggers at the neighborhood level. This project, referred to as Community Organizing Network for Environmental Health (CONEH) (Parker et al., 2010), was incorporated into the CAAA activities and administered by the steering committee. The initial funding period for the three MCECH studies (the mouse model project, the household intervention, and the epidemiological study) ended in October 2004 when funding for MCECH was not renewed. The CONEH study ended in June 2005.

With the end of MCECH and then CONEH, the CAAA partnership went without funding until May 2007. During this period, the CAAA SC continued to apply for research grants and write publications, and continued to meet quarterly to discuss grant progress as well as dissemination activities. In May 2007, CAAA received two NIEHS-funded R01 projects, the "Air Filter Intervention study" (Batterman et al., 2012; Du et al., 2011); and the "Diesel Exposure study." These two projects did not share the same participants but were both guided by the CAAA steering committee (SC). Subsequent to the implementation of these two projects, the CAAA partnership has received an EPA-funded grant, the "Near-Roadway Exposure to Urban Air Pollutants" (NEXUS) study and another NIEHS-funded R01, "The Asthma, Infections, Roadways and Youth Study" (AIRWAYS). (See Table 14.1 for description of CAAA projects and types of dissemination activities.) All CAAA research projects have followed the dissemination guidelines described in this chapter, though the focus will be on the initial process of developing and implementing the guidelines in the context of the initial household intervention, exposure assessment, and CONEH research studies.

CAAA follows the set of CBPR principles originally adopted by the Detroit URC to guide the research process (Israel et al., 1998). The work of CAAA is guided by a steering committee (SC) that includes representatives from community-based organizations, health services institutions, and academia (see Acknowledgments for a list of the partner organizations). The CAAA SC meets monthly and is actively involved in all major phases of the research and intervention, for example, defining the research questions, designing survey instruments, hiring key staff, and designing research and intervention activities such as educational materials and incentives for participants (Edgren et al., 2005; Parker et al., 2003). In 1998, to ensure that CAAA project results would be disseminated according to the CBPR principles, the SC established a dissemination committee to develop guidelines and operating procedures for project dissemination, which are the focus of this chapter.

The geographical focus area for the initial CAAA projects was eastside and southwest Detroit. Eastside Detroit is predominantly African American and southwest Detroit is the area of the city where the largest percentage of Latinos resides. With subsequent projects, CAAA has expanded to the Northwest of Detroit (predominantly African American) and into Dearborn (30% of the population of Middle Eastern descent).

TABLE 14.1 CAAA Projects and Dissemination Activities

Project	Purpose	Dates	Types of Dissemination Activities
MCECH-affiliated Household Intervention	Reduce household asthma triggers	1999–2004	Comm. forums; academic conferences and publications; fact sheets, presentations to community groups; classroom teachings; newsletters; media interviews
MCECH-affiliated Epidemiological Study	To study combined effects of indoor and outdoor air quality on children with asthma	1999–2004	Comm. forums; academic conferences and publications; fact sheets, presentations to community groups; classroom teachings; feedback to project participants; newsletters; media interviews
Community Organizing for Environmental Health (CONEH)	Neighborhood and policy organizing to reduce environmental triggers for asthma	2000–2005	Comm. forums; academic conferences and publications; fact sheets, presentations to community groups; classroom teachings; presentations to elected/govt. officials; policy briefings; newsletters; media interviews
Air Filter Intervention Study	Test effects of air filters in reducing PM and improving children's asthma-related health	2007–2012	Academic conferences and publications; fact sheets, presentations to community groups; classroom teachings; feedback to project participants
Diesel Exposure Study	Characterize relationship between exposure to vehicle exhaust (particularly diesel) and aggravation of childhood asthma	2007–2012	Academic conferences and publications; fact sheets, presentations to community groups; classroom teachings; feedback to project participants

(Continued)

TABLE 14.1 *(Continued)*

Project	Purpose	Dates	Types of Dissemination Activities
Near Roadway Exposure to Urban air Pollutants (NEXUS)	Further examines the impact of vehicle emissions on near-road air quality and relationship of respiratory viral infections and exposure to vehicular exhaust in children with asthma	2010–2012	Academic conferences and publications thus far (additional dissemination activities forthcoming)
Asthma, Infections, Roadways and Youth Study (AIRWAYS)	Further explores the relationship of respiratory viral infections and exposure to vehicular exhaust in children with asthma	2011–2016	Study initiated 2011.

FORMATION AND FUNCTIONS OF THE CAAA DISSEMINATION COMMITTEE

In 1998, during the first year that CAAA was established, SC members identified three issues regarding dissemination. First, they wanted to ensure that the dissemination of research findings reached both academic and community audiences and in a timely fashion. Second, the SC wanted to build and guide the capacity of all CAAA partners, including but not limited to the academic partners, to communicate results through a range of channels as soon as the results would become available. Especially in view of the potentially significant policy ramifications of project results, the SC agreed that project findings presented by different partners in different venues needed to be highly consistent. The SC was concerned that without a standardized summary of the findings, information might be presented differently by various SC partners and these differences might be used to discredit the findings. Finally, the SC wanted to ensure that both academic and community representatives would always **copresent at conferences** and coauthor publications on CAAA methods and findings.

Hence, in the fall of 1999, the SC decided to form the dissemination committee (DC) to develop guidelines for dissemination activities and oversee decisions around dissemination. The SC asked one of the academic principal investigators to serve as chair of the DC and to write a first draft of a set of guidelines to direct the work of the DC for review and input by the full SC. This draft outlined the potential role of the dissemination committee (for example, outlining core articles, reviewing and approving requests for use of data and access to data, and determining and prioritizing methods of dissemination of findings), suggested criteria for determining coauthorship on academic manuscripts, and proposed that committee membership be composed of five academic and two community partners (representing the different cores and projects of MCECH). Upon reviewing this draft, the SC's community members noted that community representation on the DC needed to be equal to that of academic representation. Thus representation on the DC was set at six academic partners and six community partners.

Recruiting and Selecting Members

The selection processes for the academic and the community members of the DC differed slightly. Through discussion by the SC, academic members asked the leaders of the various MCECH components to serve on the DC. These leaders included the MCECH principal investigator; the intervention, epidemiological, and chemokines project leaders; and the leaders of MCECH's Biostatistics and Exposure Assessment Facilities Cores. The rationale was that these persons would be knowledgeable about the types of data and results that would be generated from their projects and also because of a desire to protect the time of those faculty members who were more junior in their careers. For the DC community member positions, volunteers from the SC were solicited, with an emphasis on ensuring that there were an equal number of members from both eastside and southwest organizations. Community members who volunteered became members of the DC. Once membership was decided, the DC met monthly from January through June 2000. As will be described later, the activities of the DC were assumed by the SC in July 2000.

The DC agreed to make decisions through a consensus process used previously by the Detroit URC (Israel et al., 2001). When considering a particular issue, all members were asked if they could agree to a proposed decision with at least 70% of their support (as opposed to having to support the decision by100%). Using this rule, proposed decisions were discussed and modified, if necessary, until all DC members could support the decision by at least 70%. The proposed decisions were then added to the next SC meeting agenda for discussion and final approval.

Developing Dissemination Guidelines and Related Issues

During DC meetings, members discussed, developed, and revised the draft dissemination guidelines and related issues and agreed on recommendations to make to the SC (discussed later) for decisions about: developing a process for selecting partners to copresent at professional conferences; revising and finalizing the dissemination guidelines; establishing ground rules for coauthorship; and drafting a proposed list of core articles and presentations to be developed from the partnership's projects. (See Chapter Four for a discussion of another partnership's development of dissemination guidelines.)

Selecting Partners to Copresent at Conferences

At the first meeting of the DC, members discussed at length the procedure for selecting CAAA partners to copresent at conferences. Committee members recognized the importance of presentations at national and local venues as a vehicle for disseminating research results as well as for emphasizing the CBPR partnership between CAAA researchers and community members. DC members' discussion of including, whenever possible, a community copresenter with an academic copresenter addressed the following issues and suggestions:

- The CAAA dissemination policy should articulate procedures that would avoid resentment among SC members and staff who might like to copresent but were not chosen to do so.

- The selection criteria for copresenters should include level of participation in the project and attendance at the monthly SC meetings, ability to present a quality and informed presentation, and comfort in presenting in a public venue. Acknowledging that not all persons participating in CAAA would have public-speaking skills and experience, the DC discussed the possibility of offering training in public speaking.

- Requests to copresent at a conference should be brought to the SC for approval. If this were not possible, owing, for example, to time constraints imposed by due dates for abstracts, the person(s) requesting permission to copresent at a conference would contact all SC members via phone, e-mail, or fax for approval.

- Because CAAA's academic partners often receive information about conferences that community partners do not receive, they have an extra responsibility to notify community partners in a timely fashion to allow adequate opportunities for the DC to follow the dissemination policy.

- Two guiding principles for CAAA's dissemination process have been to ensure that all presentations are made with the knowledge and approval of the SC and that the authority of community partners is equal to that of academic partners in deciding who speaks for the whole group.

To ensure equitable copresentation at conferences, one academic partner suggested the adoption of the Rose Bowl Principle. This refers to the policy followed at that time by the Big Ten athletic conference (which includes the University of Michigan) for determining which team will participate in the Rose Bowl football game when two teams have identical records. The policy states that the team that has participated less recently in the Rose Bowl will be selected. Hence, the SC should select copresenters who either have not presented before or have not presented as recently as other potential presenters.

Establishing Ground Rules for Coauthorship

The DC wanted to follow standard guidelines for authorship, such as those of the International Committee of Medical Journal Editors, which states that all authors must have made substantial contributions to each of three activities (in either oral or written form): (1) conception and design, or analysis and interpretation; (2) drafting the article or revising it critically for important intellectual content; and (3) review and approval of the final version to be published (International Committee of Medical Journal Editors, 2004). The DC also wanted to make explicit what was meant by a "substantial contribution" in a way that ensured recognition of **community coauthorship** as well as academic partners as authors. The definition of coauthorship, as agreed to and written into the dissemination guidelines, was "active participation in the conception and design or analysis and interpretation, measured directly by number of hours of input on collecting, processing, and interpreting data; indirectly by time and energy spent supervising a junior researcher in the acquisition, processing, and interpretation of data; or both." Though not stated in the guidelines (perhaps because it was recognized from the start as an implicit requirement of all dissemination activities), all manuscripts must include both community and academic partners as coauthors. As described later, the DC then developed a process for proposing manuscripts for publication and presentations, determining their priority, and identifying the lead and coauthors for each.

Further Revising and Finalizing Dissemination Guidelines

The DC took approximately three months to develop and further revise the dissemination guidelines, carrying out such tasks as adding a section on procedures for selecting participants to copresent at conferences, as just described. An ad hoc committee of the DC was formed for the purpose of further revising the guidelines. Members of this ad hoc committee drafted a statement of rationale and operating philosophy, and after approval by the DC, this statement was merged with the already existing description of dissemination procedures. This final document was adopted by the SC and titled the "Philosophy and Guiding Principles for Dissemination of Findings of the Michigan Center for the Environment and Children's Health (MCECH) Including Authorship of Publications and Presentations, Policies and Procedures, Access to Data, and Related Matters" (see Appendix J).

Drafting a Proposed List of Core Publications and Presentations to Be Developed from the Project

As part of its duties around dissemination, the DC asked its academic members to draft a proposed list of core articles for publications and presentations on findings from the initial CAAA studies. Core articles were defined as those central to the main hypotheses described in the initial proposal. The SC agreed that once those core articles were determined by the DC, other members of the broader CAAA team could propose additional topics for publication and presentation. Over the course of four months, the academic members drafted a list that went beyond the initially proposed core articles and included 35 possible topics in seven broad areas (such as methodology, exposure assessment, and intervention-related). Later, when the teams began writing, they realized that many of these topics were not sufficient for stand-alone articles and they combined topics into a smaller number of manuscripts.

The DC approved the list and expected that the lead author for data-driven articles would come from the academic members of the research team, because they would be the best versed in the details of study design and analysis. The DC also suggested adding articles on findings that were not data-driven, such as lessons learned about different participant incentive options, noting that the lead author for these articles would come from the community members of the research team. The DC acknowledged that even in the CBPR literature, community partners rarely served as the lead author, perhaps, as noted by a community member of the DC, because community partners tend to be "the doers, not the writers." Hence, CAAA's contribution to furthering the influence of CBPR could be to build the capacity of community partners to take the lead in disseminating findings to an academic audience. A category of articles entitled "other qualitative methodological," with seven possible topics, was added to the list to cover these possible manuscripts. As will be discussed later, to date there have been no articles in which the lead author was a community partner in either the initial CAAA studies for which this list was applicable or the subsequent CAAA studies. The DC prioritized the overall list of possible articles and identified seven manuscripts that were to be completed first. These manuscripts were mostly descriptive and were chosen because they did not require data results (which were not yet available) and they would describe the various aspects of the study so that future manuscripts would not have to include such details on the study methodology and could instead refer to these earlier articles.

Establishing Procedures for Feedback to the Community

The DC also discussed and established initial procedures for disseminating information to the community. For example, the DC established a process for which any inquiries from the media would be directed to the project manager, who would determine which academic and community members would be best to involve, depending on their expertise and availability. The DC also decided to have a fact sheet about the project and key findings, which would be updated quarterly, as well as a newsletter to disseminate information and to serve as a retention tool for participants. (This generation of project fact sheets has continued with the newer CAAA studies.) Processes for some community-wide dissemination activities (such as **community forums** and meetings with policymakers) were not specified by the DC but were later handled by the SC, as described in the next section.

Transition of DC Responsibilities to the SC

After six months, questions arose during a DC meeting about the continuing need for a separate DC or whether its ongoing functions should be part of the SC's responsibilities. Attendance at DC meetings was becoming a problem; sometimes not enough members were present to establish a quorum. Consequently, DC members decided that after the dissemination procedures were in place, they would meet less frequently and much of the DC business would be carried out by fax, e-mail, and mail.

With the SC's adoption of the "Philosophy and Guiding Principles for Dissemination," the DC ceased to meet. Although there was never an explicit discussion and decision about disbanding the DC, the SC began handling dissemination issues at its monthly meetings. This occurred due to a combination of factors, including: with the adoption of the dissemination procedures, the SC had a roadmap to use in making dissemination-related decisions; all but two members of the SC were members of the DC; and the time required placed an excessive burden on community partners who participated in both the DC and the SC.

IMPLEMENTATION OF THE GUIDELINES: EXAMPLES OF DISSEMINATION DECISIONS AND ACTIVITIES

The dissemination activities of CAAA are varied and have included presentations and materials tailored to academic audiences, the SC itself, the broader community, and participants in the CAAA research projects. The following section focuses primarily on how the dissemination guidelines were initially implemented in the first CAAA studies, with some examples from subsequent CAAA studies.

Selecting Representatives for Conferences and Meetings

For the most part, the selection of copresenters for conferences and meetings have followed criteria and procedures as described earlier and outlined in the dissemination guidelines (see Appendix J). The selection of academic partners has often been the most clear-cut process, depending as it has on the nature of the meeting and the subject to be presented (for example, results of the intervention, results of the epidemiological study, air quality monitoring). Whenever possible, academic partners, who are more junior in experience, have been selected to help them gain further experience and recognition.

The DC had worried about potential disagreements over which community partners would copresent, but this has not occurred. For example, during the third meeting of the DC, one of the academic researchers notified the members that a community member was needed to copresent with an academic partner at a national conference on CBPR, sponsored by NIEHS. After discussion of the focus of the conference and the presentation that had been requested, one community partner nominated another community partner to present based on her involvement and knowledge of CAAA and the relevance of her previous work to the presentation. The rest of the committee supported this nomination and the "nominee" agreed to copresent. This has continued to be the case with subsequent project presentations.

In general, selection of attendees for conferences became a more informal process than originally proposed by the DC. For example, for each conference presentation or meeting invitation, the dissemination guidelines spelled out that the SC would develop a list of the people who were eligible, based on their level of participation, their knowledge and experience, and the SC's desire to ensure that a variety of members were offered this opportunity. In actuality, academic members who were either submitting conference abstracts or had been invited to present would ask for volunteers or would suggest a person (based on the presentation topic) and request SC approval.

Approving Abstracts and Abstract Authorship for Conference Presentations

The DC also discussed the need for a process for submitting abstracts for SC approval before they were officially submitted for review by conference organizers. Noting that abstracts were sometimes "last-minute" submissions, the DC discussed ways to ensure that the abstracts would be reviewed by the SC without jeopardizing their timely submission. The DC suggested that SC members create a list of the conferences and meetings (and their abstract submission deadlines) that the SC would like partners to attend, so that to the extent possible, last-minute approvals and submissions could be avoided. However, this list was never formally developed in the initial CAAA projects nor in subsequent projects, perhaps reflecting the fluid nature of conference opportunities.

The DC also adopted and implemented the following procedure for abstract submission. The interested person (if other than the lead researcher) would first submit the abstract to the lead researcher of the project that was the subject of the abstract, for his or her approval. The lead researcher would then send the abstract to the SC. If time permitted, this process happened before an SC meeting so that the abstract could be discussed at the meeting. If this were not possible, SC members were asked to respond by telephone or e-mail to say whether they had any questions or concerns with the abstract and whether or not they approved the abstract. This approval process was one of passive consent, that is, if SC members did not respond about the abstract, it was agreed that they approved its content and coauthorship. This process has been followed in subsequent CAAA projects.

Selecting Lead Authors and Coauthors for Manuscripts

As noted earlier, in the initial project, the DC drafted and prioritized a list of core articles for publications and presentations. This process has been followed by subsequent CAAA projects, with some adjustments. Initially, the SC selected lead authors for core articles, from the principal investigators or coinvestigators of the project. In subsequent projects, the principal investigators or coinvestigators proposed articles with coauthorship to the SC for their approval. Writing teams were then determined, based on the topic and the involvement of SC members in that particular aspect of the project. Once a writing team was named, the lead author brought the writing team together, either in person or by telephone conference call, at which time he or she either presents a draft outline for discussion by the group or spends this time working with the group to create an outline. The lead author would be responsible for writing the first draft, basing it on this outline and discussion and consulting with the coauthors as needed. This first draft would then be shared with the coauthors for their review and feedback, and the lead author would make revisions in light of the coauthors' comments, repeating this process until the article is ready to be submitted. The early stages of this process could involve several meetings of the writing team, with the subsequent review and revisions handled via e-mail and regular mail and telephone conversations.

Handling Requests for Use of Data

The DC also developed a procedure for requesting permission to use data from the CAAA project. As part of this procedure, anyone interested in using the data for a purpose other than writing a core article needed to complete the "Request for Use of Community Action Against Asthma Data" form. The form required the applicant to answer the following questions.

1. Are you requesting this data for personal or for organizational use? Please explain.

2. Please describe in detail what data you are requesting from CAAA, both with respect to scope and desired format.

3. Please describe in detail for what purposes you wish to obtain this data and how the data will be used. Include in your description how this use of the data will benefit the Detroit community, as appropriate to the intended purpose, and how this use otherwise will follow community-based participatory research principles (a copy of these principles is attached to the form).

If necessary, the requester is asked to come to an SC meeting to further explain the request and answer questions. In addition, all requesters who are allowed to use data are required to come to an SC meeting to present the findings of any analysis performed with CAAA data. To date, four doctoral degree students, one master's degree student and another affiliated Detroit-URC project, the Healthy Environments Partnership (HEP), have requested and used CAAA data. For the students, the use was for their theses. For HEP, they used CAAA exposure assessment data from the epidemiological study for two of their three monitoring sites in their initial research study (see Chapter Seven for description of HEP).

Discussing How to Handle Dissemination Requirements for Affiliated Projects

Within months of development of the dissemination policies and procedures, an investigator from another university approached the CAAA SC about collaborating on an additional exposure assessment project. This new project, which was to take place during one of CAAA's seasonal assessments, would require parking a mobile laboratory (contained in a specially modified tractor-trailer) beside one of the primary schools where CAAA was conducting ongoing air quality monitoring using equipment placed on the school roof. The investigator wished to use data from the CAAA epidemiological project to augment data collected by the mobile laboratory (which would conduct animal experiments assessing the effects of exposures to concentrated pollutants in the air on the animals' lung function). The DC was concerned about how data from the two projects would be shared and wanted to ensure that all results from this new project would be shared with community members in a way that complied with CAAA's dissemination guidelines. The DC recognized that the investigator of the proposed new project did not use a CBPR approach, but felt that he might be open to learning more about and following the principles of CBPR, especially in this project. After much discussion the DC suggested that CAAA draft a letter of agreement that stipulated the requirements for dissemination, and the SC agreed with this suggestion. The letter of agreement included the following requirements: any manuscripts that originated from this new project must include coauthors from CAAA, the CAAA data manager and biostatistician must be informed of any additional analysis undertaken by others, and CAAA must be kept abreast about the work and progress of this new project (through such means as formal presentations of results to the CAAA steering committee). The CBPR principles and the dissemination policies and procedures were attached to the letter of agreement. The new investigator agreed to the requests in the letter of agreement and subsequently presented project results to the SC on several occasions.

Feeding Back to Participants and the Wider Community

The DC initially, and later the SC have been active in developing and implementing mechanisms for feedback to study participants and the larger community for all CAAA studies. Methods of feedback have included fact sheets about the project and general project findings, individualized feedback sheets for project participants (including, in some cases, individualized meetings to explain the results), and a series of forums for project participants and the broader community.

Fact Sheet Development and Distribution

One of the initial decisions of the DC was to create a fact sheet about the project. The DC proposed that the fact sheet be developed in layperson's language, updated quarterly, and distributed within the community. The DC felt these fact sheets could serve as the main source of information for informal presentations by SC members and staff in the Detroit community and could also be distributed directly to interested community members, legislators, and government officials. The intent of the fact sheets was to give an overview of the CAAA intervention and epidemiological projects, share data findings as they emerged, and also include relevant findings from other research projects on similar topics. The SC has been instrumental in the development of the fact sheets for all CAAA projects. SC members provide input on focus and content and ensure that the sheets are understandable and culturally and linguistically appropriate for the intended audiences. (See the downloadable supplement for this chapter for examples of fact sheets from the CAAA projects.)

Individualized Feedback to Project Participants

As part of CAAA's first epidemiological study, lung function assessments were performed twice daily over two weeks in each season, with a handheld, digitized peak flow device. Two academic physician members of the SC worked closely with SC community partners to develop a clear and useful format for sharing this inherently complex data with project participants. Results were also mailed to all physicians of the participating children, if the caregivers had requested CAAA to do so. In the subsequent Diesel Exposure and Air Filter Intervention studies, lung function results were also fed back to participating families. CAAA staff members presented the lung function feedback forms during a visit to the participant's home. Staff reviewed the forms with the child and their caregiver, and encouraged them to share the results with their physician. (See the downloadable supplement for this chapter for examples of Lung Function Feedback Reports.)

Individualized feedback on indoor air quality was also presented to the 15 families who participated in the intensive air sampling component of the first epidemiological study. The academic partners involved in this component worked with project staff to develop individualized feedback sheets. These sheets showed the levels of particulate matter (PM) 2.5 and ozone in each individual home compared to the aggregate levels of all 15 homes and to the overall EPA National Ambient Air Quality Standards for outdoor levels of PM 2.5 and ozone. These sheets were shared with the families during a meeting in which the academic partners gave an overview presentation of what they had found, explained the results, and then were available to meet with the families to answer their questions. In the Air Filter Intervention study, more extensive air monitoring data were made available, so the individualized feedback to the 126 participating households was more detailed and also included information about how to reduce the levels of the particular exposure. These data were also presented to participants during an in-home visit by trained project staff. (See the downloadable supplement for this chapter for examples of individualized feedback on air quality provided to participants in the intensive air sampling component of the initial CAAA, and a feedback sheet on in-home exposures provided to participants in the Air Filter Intervention study.)

Community Forums

In the fourth year of the initial CAAA projects, as preliminary results became available, the SC conducted a series of forums to feed back the results to the broader community and project participants. A subgroup of the SC, consisting of project field staff, two academic partners, and two community partners, developed a proposed plan for the forum and shared it with the SC for input and modification. Initially, the SC planned to have a single forum for both project participants and other interested community groups, but on further discussion the SC chose to hold separate forums. Some of the academic partners suggested that the results should first be presented to the participating families for their information and reactions before being presented to the wider community. Following this suggestion, the SC decided to have two separate family forums for participants (one in eastside and one in southwest Detroit) before staging a community forum for the wider community. The SC also felt that having two separate family forums would make it easier for participants from these separate intervention areas to attend a forum. These two forums were held on successive Saturdays and lasted two hours each.

The format of the family forums consisted of a welcome by project staff, presentation of intervention and air quality research results by the academic partners, questions and discussion, and a small-group exercise in which the family participants were asked to respond to a set of questions developed by the planning committee and aimed at increasing understanding of the findings. CAAA served refreshments, distributed door prizes, and provided transportation and child care to ensure that participants could attend. The southwest and eastside family forums were attended by 25 and 19 adults, respectively. Forum participants also included adult caregivers from CAAA participant families and guests of the immediate families (friends and additional family), numerous children who either went to the child-care room or participated in forum activities, and several CAAA staff, researchers, and SC members.

The community-wide forum was held a few weeks after these two initial family forums and focused more on the results of the air quality and health effects investigations. This emphasis was proposed by the planning committee and approved by the SC, both of whom felt that community members would be more interested in this aspect of the study than in the results of the intervention. Members of community-based organizations, governmental agencies and officials, families who had participated in the study, and individual community residents who had attended previous CAAA events or had worked for CAAA in data collection activities were invited to attend the community-wide forum. This larger forum was attended by 41 individuals, including CAAA family participants, staff members of locally elected officials (a state representative and a county commissioner), agency representatives, advocacy workers, and community members. Many of these individuals and groups were identified through an assessment performed by the staff of the community organizing component of CAAA with the active involvement of the SC. (For more information on these forums, see Lopez et al., 2005; Edgren et al., 2005.)

CHALLENGES

The CAAA SC has experienced a number of challenges in creating and implementing guidelines for disseminating research findings in a community-based participatory fashion. We describe these challenges in this section, and in the next section we present the lessons we have learned for handling these challenges and implications for practice.

Adhering consistently to the dissemination guidelines. One of the challenges CAAA has faced involved situations in which academic members of CAAA were invited to speak about the project at national meetings or conferences. When this occurred, the invited person would let the conference organizers know that due to the participatory process of the CAAA partnership, presentations were normally copresented by an academic and a community partner. Often the organization or conference planner would agree to pay for two persons to copresent, but sometimes the organization did not have enough funds to sponsor more than the academic person originally invited. If project funds were not available to pay for the community partner's expenses, the situation was discussed openly at SC meetings. In general, community partners understood the constraints and the academic partner would present alone.

Another challenge involved meeting deadlines for submitting abstracts and responding to invitations to present at conferences when these occurred in between the monthly meetings of the DC (and subsequently the SC). A combination of e-mail, phone, and fax messages was used to communicate between the abstract submitter or the invitee and the rest of the SC. Though not as ideal as a face-to-face discussion at a SC meeting, this system seemed to work fairly well.

A third challenge in adhering to the dissemination guidelines was that of balancing dissemination activities with other project demands. All research projects face this tension between ongoing project implementation and data collection and dissemination activities. Yet the additional dissemination-related activities needed in a CBPR approach can increase the difficulty of achieving a balance between ongoing implementation and dissemination of findings. During the initial CAAA project period, not all of the activities outlined in the dissemination guidelines happened as originally planned. For example, although the original intention of the DC was to have all fact sheets updated quarterly, SC members' and project staffs' occupation with project implementation activities left little time for further data analysis or even recognition that updating of the fact sheets had fallen behind schedule. Another example is that feedback to the participants about their lung function results happened much later than was intended in the first CAAA epidemiological project. Much of this delay was due to the ongoing project implementation duties of the members of the research team. The community partners and field staff were understandably frustrated by the delay in presenting these results to participants, and the academic members were frustrated at the lack of resources to make this happen sooner. The process for feedback went much more smoothly and the feedback was more timely in the Air Filter Intervention and Diesel Exposure studies, perhaps due to lessons learned in the first project period.

Ensuring up-to-date involvement of community partners in the data analysis process. CAAA also has faced challenges related to involving community partners in data analysis and informing them of the data analysis steps. For all CAAA projects, as agreed upon by the SC, data preparation and analysis have been conducted at the partner university. Community partners involved in writing articles and papers usually viewed the data in table form, after preliminary data analyses had been conducted. In the initial CAAA intervention and epidemiological projects, perhaps due to the large amount of data collected, data cleaning and analysis took what seemed to community partners to be a very long time. Although the academic members of the SC gave semi-annual reports about preliminary findings, community members of the SC were rarely kept up to date about the progress of data cleaning and analysis. In addition, it became clear toward the end of the project that community members had not been well informed about the complexity of data cleaning and analysis and the time it typically took. This resulted in frustration about the delay in feeding back results to the community and in completing and submitting manuscripts about project results. In the subsequent CAAA projects, more attention was paid at SC meetings to data feedback and updates on data cleaning and analysis.

Achieving a balance between dissemination and feedback to community and academic audiences. CAAA also has faced the challenge of achieving a balance between dissemination to community audiences, through such means as fact sheets and forums, and dissemination to academic audiences, through such means as journal articles. Israel and colleagues (1998) have identified the considerable time it takes to develop and maintain relationships and to involve all partners in the research process as a challenge for academics participating in CBPR. Although some aspects of preparing for disseminating results to community members (for example, data analysis and the preparation of visual displays) can also be useful in manuscript development, the time spent disseminating results to community members can be time that is taken away from writing manuscripts for publication. In the fifth year of the initial CAAA projects, concerns related to productivity (defined by the funder as manuscript submission and publication) were discussed. SC members considered ways to ensure that academics had the time needed to produce manuscripts while also ensuring that dissemination to the community continued. They discussed having community members of the SC take the lead on presenting at community venues. This strategy had been discussed by the DC (and was the impetus for the development of the fact sheets), but such presentations did not occur. SC members decided that community members serving on the SC would need to receive training on data interpretation and presentation and would need to have additional resources (such as stipends) because these activities would be over and beyond their everyday duties. Despite intentions to pursue this approach in the future, CAAA has not done so, primarily due to time demands on the community and academic partners and lack of resources to direct to this endeavor.

Ensuring that dissemination is culturally sensitive. Another challenge faced by CAAA was that of ensuring that dissemination took place in a culturally sensitive manner in keeping with the tenets of cultural humility (Tervalon & Murray-García, 1998). This is a challenge faced by many CBPR partnerships (Boyer, Mohatt, Pasker, Drew, & McGlone, 2007; Pufall et al., 2011). Given that CAAA now works with four different geographical communities, involving white, African American, Arab American, and Latino participants, issues of culture are important in designing community feedback activities. All project materials, including fact sheets about project results, have been produced in English and Spanish (those specific to the Diesel Exposure study, are also produced in Arabic). In addition, at the forum for the initial CAAA projects in southwest Detroit (which is the area with the largest percentage of Latinos in Detroit) and at the community-wide forum, a Spanish interpreter was present to provide simultaneous interpretation. CAAA also hired an interpreter for the one deaf project participant. To ensure that project materials were appropriate to the African American and Latino cultures with which CAAA was working, SC members and project staff of these ethnicities reviewed all dissemination materials (including presentations at the forum) and offered suggestions to improve them.

Involving partners with differing experience and expertise. As the DC had recognized at the beginning of the project, not all partners had the same level of experience and expertise in preparing manuscripts or presenting at conferences. Seeking to ensure that persons with less experience and expertise were not excluded, the DC suggested processes for capacity building (for example, conducting mock presentations before the scheduled meeting so persons would gain experience and feedback). In addition, academic partners realized that being a coauthor might be a new experience for some of the partners and have considered multiple ways of obtaining comments and ideas on each article from all partners. For example, some partners preferred to suggest changes and edits through direct conversation rather than in writing.

LESSONS LEARNED AND IMPLICATIONS FOR PRACTICE

The Value of and Need for Joint Academic-Community Participation in All Dissemination Activities

The SC has found that involvement of academic and community members in all dissemination activities has greatly enhanced the efforts of the CAAA partnership. As expected, community partners bring expertise on venues for community dissemination as well as advice on "breaking it down," as they refer to the process of helping the academic members deliver research results in language that is accessible to community members. Similarly, academic partners bring their experience in writing presentations and publications for academic audiences. Partners also contribute to each other's traditional area of expertise in dissemination-related activities. For example, our community members, who coauthor manuscripts and copresent at conferences, raise issues about interpretation of results and offer valuable input on content and writing style, which serve to make these presentations and manuscripts much stronger. And as noted before, academic members in the initial CAAA projects were the ones to raise concerns about presenting results at a community forum before first presenting the results to project participants.

As described in this chapter, the presence of structures (for example, a steering committee and its subcommittees) and processes (for example, frequent meetings, written dissemination guidelines) that foster relationship building and trust facilitate the joint participation of academics and community members in dissemination activities. We would suggest that all research partnerships develop initial structures and processes as a first step toward joint participation in disseminating research results. (See the chapters in Part Two in this volume for further discussion of ways to ensure joint collaborative participation, and Chapter Four for a specific description of another partnership's experience with dissemination guidelines.)

The Need to Recognize That Dissemination Is Time-Consuming and May Not Be Part of the "Job Description" of All Partners and That Projects Should Address How to Compensate Partners for Their Time and Contributions and How to Acknowledge What They Do

Stoecker (2003) noted that in a CBPR project, community members may be asked to "participate in ways they aren't interested in or don't have time for" (p. 102). This may be especially true for some aspects of dissemination, such as involvement in coauthoring manuscripts or copresenting papers at national conferences and meetings, because these tasks are not part of the usual duties of most community partners. For example, as described earlier, despite much discussion and actual identification of potential manuscript topics for which community members can take the lead, to date no community member has served as lead author for a manuscript. Thus, resources that enable community members to involve themselves in this type of dissemination need to be identified and provided.

Stoecker's observation (2003) may also apply to academic partners. Traditionally, academics are rewarded for their participation in certain scientific dissemination activities, such as peer-reviewed publications and, to a lesser extent, presentations. Other forms of dissemination, such as community presentations, authoring fact sheets about research findings, and individual presentations to project participants, however, are not recognized and rewarded by most tenure and promotion systems or by funding agencies (such as the National Institutes of Health). In addition, many academic researchers are not familiar with and have not been trained in how to involve nonacademic researchers as coauthors and copresenters, and may not have the skills or orientation to do so effectively.

To address these issues, research partnerships need to consider dissemination when they are developing the initial proposal. For example, providing stipends for community members that more accurately reflect their desired involvement in dissemination activities may allow them to participate more intensively. In addition, continued efforts are needed on the national level, first, to educate academic institutions on the importance of dissemination activities in the community as a form of translation of research findings and the importance of recognizing this type of dissemination in the tenure and promotion process and, second, to educate funding agencies about the need to acknowledge these types of dissemination activities in evaluating the "productivity" of CBPR projects. Examples of progress in this regard are the University of North Carolina at Chapel Hill, Gillings School of Global Public Health's Faculty Promotion and Tenure policies (2012), which specifically includes this type of dissemination activities and products as criteria for demonstrating excellence in public health practice, as well as the peer-reviewed Community Campus Partnership for Health Community Engaged Scholarship for Health, which is an online mechanism for peer-reviewing, publishing, and disseminating products of health-related community engaged scholarship that are in forms other than journal articles (www.ccph.info).

The Need to Develop an Appropriate Mechanism for Identifying and Deciding on Dissemination Issues and Guidelines

When the SC formed the dissemination committee, it was with the understanding that the DC would continue to function throughout the life of the project. As noted earlier, however, the DC ceased to meet after the guidelines were developed and the SC took on the duties of the DC. In retrospect it was unrealistic to add another layer of meetings and responsibilities to the work of SC members. We recommend a process that involves forming a short-term, ad hoc committee to focus on developing dissemination guidelines, with the understanding that once the guidelines are developed the partnership's governing body would implement them. We further suggest the incorporation of a standing "update" agenda item on dissemination for each meeting of the partnership, even if no dissemination-related events have taken place. This would encourage ongoing discussion on the progress made in data analysis and foster more open discussion and the education of all partners about what is involved in the data preparation and analysis process.

The Need to Budget Adequate Resources for Dissemination Activities

As suggested earlier, resources to compensate community partners for their participation in dissemination-related activities need to be included in grant proposals. In addition, funds for dissemination activities (for example, for materials and refreshments for community forums, translation of materials into appropriate languages, and interpretation services for forums and meetings) should be included in project budgets. Finally, resources are needed to cover staff time required to carry out dissemination related activities.

SUMMARY

Dissemination of research findings in ways that are understandable and helpful to community members is a crucial component of CBPR. In this chapter we have shared our experience in establishing and implementing a process for dissemination of research results using a CBPR approach. Although we have had successes in our dissemination activities, we also acknowledge the challenges we have faced and the need to continually improve upon our efforts. We have been energized by the positive and enthusiastic reaction to our efforts to share the results of our research with the project participants and community members who have made efforts possible and to do so in a way that acknowledges the contributions of both community and academic partnership members. This positive reaction has strengthened our belief in the importance of community-academic participation in the dissemination of research findings to the project participants and community members who will most benefit from knowing and applying these results to foster community change.

KEY TERMS

Dissemination of research results

Community coauthorship

Copresent at conferences

Community forums

DISCUSSION QUESTIONS

1. What are some of the key issues and components that need to be considered in developing dissemination guidelines for a CBPR partnership?

2. What are some of the challenges of ensuring equal participation of community and academic partners in dissemination activities?

3. What might a CBPR partnership do to ensure that community members have the opportunity for equal participation in dissemination activities?

REFERENCES

Ahmed, S. M., & Palermo, A. G. (2010). Community engagement in research: Frameworks for education and peer review. *American Journal of Public Health, 100,* 1380–1385.

Batterman, S., Du, L., Mentz, G., Muhkerjee, B., Parker, E., Godwin, C., et al. (2012). Particulate matter concentrations in residences: An intervention study evaluating stand-alone filters and air conditioners. *Indoor Air, 22*(3), 235–252.

Boyer, B. B., Mohatt, G. V., Pasker, R. L., Drew, E. M., & McGlone, K. K. (2007). Sharing results from complex disease genetics studies: A community-based participatory research approach. *International Journal of Circumpolar Health, 66,* 19–30.

Chen, P. G., Diaz, N., Lucas, G., & Rosenthal, M. S. (2010). Dissemination of results in community-based participatory research. *American Journal of Preventive Medicine, 39,* 372–378.

Du, L., Batterman, S., Parker, E., Godwin, C., Chin, J. Y., O'Toole, A., et al. (2011). Particle concentrations and effectiveness of free-standing air filters in bedrooms of children with asthma in Detroit, Michigan. *Building and Environment, 46,* 2303–2313. http://dc.doi.org/10.1016/j.buildenv.2011.05.012

deKoning, K., & Martin, M. (Eds.). (1996). *Participatory research in health: Issues and experiences.* London: Zed Books.

Edgren, K. K., Parker, E. A., Israel, B. A., Lewis, T. C., Salinas, M. A., Robins, T. G., & Hill, Y. R. (2005). Community involvement in the conduct of a health education intervention and research project: The Community Action Against Asthma Project. *Health Promotion Practice, 6,* 263–269.

Farquhar, S., & Wing, S. (2003). Methodological and ethical considerations in community-driven environmental justice research: Two case studies from rural North Carolina. In M. Minkler & N. Wallerstein (Eds.), *Community-based participatory research for health* (pp. 221–241). San Francisco: Jossey-Bass.

Gagnon, M. L. (2011). Moving knowledge to action through dissemination and exchange. *Journal of Clinical Epidemiology 64,* 25–31.

Green, L. W., George, M. A., Daniel, M., Frankish, C. J., Herbert, C. J., Bowie, W. R., et al. (1995). *Study of participatory research in health promotion.* Ottawa: Royal Society of Canada.

International Committee of Medical Journal Editors. (2004). *Uniform requirements for manuscripts submitted to biomedical journals.* Retrieved July 7, 2004, from http://www.icmje.org

Israel, B. A., Lichtenstein, R., Lantz, P., McGranaghan, R., Allen, A., Guzman, J. R., et al. (2001). The Detroit Community-Academic Urban Research Center: Development, implementation and evaluation. *Journal of Public Health Management and Practice, 7*(5), 1–19.

Israel, B. A., Schulz, A. J., Parker, E. A., & Becker, A. B. (1998). Review of community-based research: Assessing partnership approaches to improve public health. *Annual Review of Public Health, 19*, 173–202.

Lopez, E. D. S., Parker, E. A., Edgren, K. K., & Brakefield-Caldwell, W. (2005). Lessons learned while using a CBPR approach to plan and conduct forums to disseminate research findings back to partnering communities: A case study from Community Action Against Asthma, Detroit, Michigan. *Metropolitan Universities Journal, 16*(1), 57–76.

Montaya, M. J., & Kent, E. E. (2011). Dialogical action: Moving from community-based to community-driven participatory research. *Qualitative Health Research, 21*, 1000–1011.

Parker, E. A., Israel, B. A., Brakefield-Caldwell, W., Keeler, G. J., Lewis, T. C., Ramirez, E., et al. (2003). Community Action Against Asthma: Examining the partnership process of a community-based participatory research project. *Journal of General Internal Medicine, 18*, 558–567.

Parker, E. A., Israel, B. A., Robins, T. G., Mentz, G., Xihong, L., Brakefield-Caldwell, W., et al. (2008). Evaluation of Community Action Against Asthma: A community health worker intervention to improve children's asthma-related health by reducing household environmental triggers for asthma. *Health Education & Behavior, 35*, 376–395.

Parker, E. A., Chung, L., Israel, B. A., Reyes, A., & Wilkins, D. W. (2010). Community organizing network for environmental health: Using a community health development approach to increase community capacity around reduction of environmental triggers. *Journal of Primary Prevention, 31*(1–2), 41–58.

Pufall, E. L., Jones, A. Q., McEwen, S. A., Lyall, C., Peregrine, A. S., & Edge, V. L. (2011). Community-derived research dissemination strategies in an Inuit community. *International Journal of Circumpolar Health, 70*, 532–541.

Stoecker, R. (2003). Are academics irrelevant? Approaches and roles for scholars in community-based participatory research. In M. Minkler & N. Wallerstein (eds.), *Community-based participatory research for health* (pp. 98–112). San Francisco: Jossey-Bass.

Tervalon, M., & Murray-García, J. (1998). Cultural humility vs. cultural competence: A critical distinction in defining physician training outcomes in medical education. *Journal of Health Care for the Poor and Underserved, 9*(2), 117–125.

University of North Carolina at Chapel Hill. (2012). *Gillings School of Global Public Health's faculty promotion and tenure policies.* Retrieved from: (http://www.sph.unc.edu/images/stories/faculty_staff/acad_affairs/documents/aptmanualrevision_2010–04–07.pdf)

Acknowledgments: Community Action Against Asthma is a community-based participatory research initiative investigating the influence of environmental factors on childhood asthma, and is a partnership of the Detroit Community-Academic Urban Research Center (www.detroiturc .org). CAAA has involved collaboration among the Detroit Department of Health and Wellness Promotion, the University of Michigan Schools of Public Health and Medicine, the Henry Ford Health System, the Michigan Department of Agriculture Office of Pesticides and Plant Management, and the following community-based organizations: Community Health and Social Services Center, Friends of Parkside, Warren-Conner Development Coalition, Kettering/Butzel Health Initiative, Butzel Family Center, Latino Family Services, United Community Housing Coalition, Detroiters Working for Environmental Justice, and Detroit Hispanic Development Corporation. We thank these partners for their contributions. CAAA has been and currently is funded by the National Institute of Environmental Health Sciences (grants PO 1-ES09 5 89, RO 1 ES10688, R01-ES014566, R01-ES014677, R01-ES016769;) and the U.S. Environmental Protection Agency (grant R826710–01, RD-83411701).

APPENDIXES

Appendix A

INSTRUCTIONS FOR

CONDUCTING A FORCE

FIELD ANALYSIS

ADAM B. BECKER

BARBARA A. ISRAEL

ALEX J. ALLEN III

Force field analysis is a group process activity that enables a group to identify and document the forces for and against reaching a specific desired state of affairs or achieving a specific goal (Johnson & Johnson, 2008; Lewin, 1944). This process is not one in which solutions per se are identified but one in which the facilitating factors for achieving a goal or objective and barriers to doing so are enumerated as part of a process of identifying and prioritizing potential action steps. Facilitating a thorough force field analysis can take one to two hours to complete and can be carried out over more than one group meeting.

PROCEDURE

1. Introduce the basic process (described in steps 3–6). If possible, practice on a sample proposed change or goal. State both the proposed change and the issue or problem situation to which it relates.

2. Draw this diagram on newsprint, chalkboard, or whiteboard:

Issue or problem: _____

_____

Proposed change (ideal state/goal): _____

_____

_____

Forces for ──────────▶	◀────────── Forces Against
(the proposed change, ideal state, or goal)	(the proposed change, ideal state, or goal)
(list of forces)	(list of forces)

NOTE: For discussion of the use of this force field analysis activity, see Chapters Three and Five.

3. Following a discussion within the group, write the issue or problem statement identified by the group in clear and precise language next to the "Issue or problem" heading in the diagram. Write the group's proposed change or the ideal state or goal (that is, how things would be if the problem did not exist) next to the "Proposed change" heading. Explain the diagram stating that "forces for" are those that would facilitate the proposed change and "forces against" are those that would be barriers to the proposed change. (Such forces can relate to, for example, individuals, organizations, policies, community history and context, and need to be forces that actually exist already in the community.) Ask the group to list the forces that go in these two columns. Discussion of the lists should be withheld until all anticipated forces for and against are listed. The facilitator should write down the forces identified verbatim in the appropriate columns.

4. Ask the group to identify which "forces for" can be strengthened or harnessed and which "forces against" can be decreased. Circle those forces that seem to be the most important for achieving the ideal state or goal and mark with an "x" those that the group thinks need to be researched and discussed in more depth.

5. As needed, identify group members who will research each force marked with an "x" and ask them to bring their findings back to the next group meeting to share with the group.

6. For each important "force for" ask the group to list as many responses or action steps as possible that would increase its effect. For each important "force against" ask the group to list possible responses or action steps that might reduce its effect or eliminate it completely. The group should then select the most appropriate action steps and make plans for implementing them.

REFERENCES

Johnson, D. W., & Johnson, F. P. (2008). *Joining together: Group theory and group skills* (10th ed.). Boston: Allyn & Bacon.

Lewin, K. (1944). Dynamics of group action. *Educational Leadership, 1*, 195–200.

FULL VALUE CONTRACT

MICHAEL YONAS

ROBERT ARONSON

NETTIE COAD

EUGENIA ENG

REGINA PETTEWAY

JENNIFER SCHAAL

LUCILLE WEBB

Our beliefs and values must be alive in our team and in our work. We must have an agreement among the group members to work together to achieve the goals that have been developed during our time together. Shared goals and expectations are essential to team or group alignment and commitment.

Inherent in this process is the belief that every group member has value and by virtue of that value has the right and responsibility to give and receive open and honest feedback. Such feedback is a positive affirmation of individual value and respect. Below is a list of what we as a team have said that we value about working together to achieve our goals:

As a team, we will value:

- Mutual respect

- A willingness to stay at the table

- Speaking from our own experience

- Perseverance

- Teamwork

- Humor

- Critical listening

- Accountability to team members and to the team

- Fun

- Honesty

- Conflict

- Humility

- A willingness to be uncomfortable

- Confidentiality

- Acknowledgment of people's strengths

See Chapter Four for a discussion of the development and application of this Full Value Contract.

By agreeing to the terms of this "contract" and our stated values, we are investing our time, experiences, and commitment in the success of the team and community-building process. We are acknowledging the value of the process, as well as the value of all the people that it involves. With this agreement, we can move ahead with a more realistic understanding of what cooperative work and community requires.

Finally, we agree that any products, research or otherwise, are the property of the group and cannot be reproduced or published without consent of the group.

Signature:_____ Date: _____

COLLABORATIVE

REVISED BYLAWS

ADOPTED/AMENDED:
(MONTH, DAY, YEAR)

MICHAEL YONAS

ROBERT ARONSON

NETTIE COAD

EUGENIA ENG

REGINA PETTEWAY

JENNIFER SCHAAL

LUCILLE WEBB

ARTICLE I: NAME

The name of the organization is **Greensboro Health Disparities Collaborative**, hereinafter known as the Collaborative. It is a nonprofit coalition operating under the umbrella organization, the Partnership Project (EIN 421594926).

ARTICLE II: MISSION, GOAL, AND STRATEGY

Section 1—Mission

The mission of the Collaborative is to establish structures and processes that respond to and build the capacity of communities and institutions in defining and resolving issues related to racial and ethnic disparities in health. Thus, the results of the work of the Collaborative will be used to reduce racial and ethnic disparities in health and health care.

We function as an anti-racist coalition that values: mutual respect, a willingness to stay at the table, speaking from our own experience, perseverance, teamwork, humor, critical listening, accountability to individual team members and to the team as a whole, fun, honesty, conflict, humility, a willingness to be uncomfortable, confidentiality, and acknowledgment of people's strengths.

Section 2—Goal

The overall goal of the Collaborative is to improve health in communities by addressing systemic discrepancies related to disparities in health and health care.

Section 3—Strategy

The overall strategy of the Collaborative is to examine and explore the systemic causes for the racial disparities in health that exist in specific communities and to do so in the context of community-based participatory projects integrated with anti-racist community organizing designed to increase institutional awareness of structural racism and strengthen the capacity of communities to assess and to address their own unique health-related problems.

See Chapter Four for a discussion of the development and application of these Bylaws using a CBPR approach.

- To decrease ethnic and race-based health and health care disparities.

- To build an improved interdisciplinary methodology and knowledge of measuring racial disparities in health and health care delivery, access, and quality

- Following the community-based participatory research approach and principles, to design and conduct studies on the effect of institutional racism on health and health care that can be used in other areas of North Carolina and nationwide.

To focus on Undoing Racism™ and develop systems of accountability to the community in the areas of health and health care.

ARTICLE III: MEMBERSHIP

Section 1—Eligibility

Voting membership must include a simple majority of membership coming from the community, community-based organizations, or both.

Recruitment for voting membership shall be extended by invitation to anyone in the Greater Greensboro community or a member of the affiliated institutions involved in the work of the Collaborative.

Voting membership is granted after:

a) Approval by Membership Committee;

b) Approval by majority vote of voting members;

c) Completion of the People's Institute Undoing Racism™ training and acceptance and signing of the Full Value Contract (which includes the Collaborative's values of: mutual respect, a willingness to stay at the table, speaking from our own experience, perseverance, teamwork, humor, critical listening, accountability to individual team members and to the team as a whole, fun, honesty, conflict, humility, a willingness to be uncomfortable, confidentiality, and acknowledgment of people's strengths); and

d) Completion of other training requirements, as specified by the Collaborative.

Section 2—Representative Membership Make-Up

Membership shall include representatives from at least one community-based organization, at least one health organization, and at least one academic institution.

> A community-based organization is nongovernmental, benefits a constituency in the community with which it works, is governed by people who are served by it, and can demonstrate accountability to the community.

> A health department or organization protects the public's health and benefits a specific constituency.

> An academic institution can be public or private.

Section 3—Annual Dues

The amount required for annual dues shall be $25 each year for voting members, unless changed by a majority vote of the members at the Collaborative's annual meeting or any special meeting called by the Collaborative. Active members reconfirm their commitment to the Collaborative through paying their annual dues and signing the Full Value Contract on an annual basis.

Section 4—Membership

Active membership is contingent upon being up to date on membership dues, and any other Collaborative requirements such as continuing education sessions. Membership dues may be waived for persons experiencing financial hardship; the treasurer will report such instances to the Executive Committee while maintaining the confidentiality of the member experiencing hardship. Active members will be those members whose dues are paid or who have had their dues waived. All active members are eligible to partake in voting for Executive Committee members or any other matters requiring a vote. "Friends of the Collaborative" will be individuals who are interested in maintaining a relationship with the Collaborative and who serve as a valuable resource to the Collaborative. **All Friends of the Collaborative must have undergone the Undoing Racism™ training to maintain membership status**. Friends of the Collaborative will be dues-paying members and stay on the Collaborative e-mail list, but are not active members and do not have voting rights. A Friend of the Collaborative can change to active status contingent upon meeting the requirements of membership as specified in Article III, Section 1.

Section 5—Rights of Members

Each voting member shall be eligible to cast one vote for all matters requiring a vote.

Section 6—Change in Membership Status, Resignation, and Termination

Any member may resign through consultation with a member of the Executive Committee. All resignations will be reported to the Membership Committee. Resignation shall not relieve a member of unpaid dues, or other charges previously accrued. A member shall be terminated from the Collaborative, through action of the Executive Committee, for demonstrated unethical conduct, or for any conduct that violates the Full Value Contract.

ARTICLE IV: MEETINGS OF MEMBERS

Section 1—Regular Meetings

Regular meetings of the members shall be held periodically at a time and place agreed upon by the Collaborative members.

Section 2—Special Meetings

Special meetings may be called by the chair, a simple majority of the Executive Committee, or a simple majority of the Collaborative members.

Section 3—Notice of Meetings

Printed or electronic notice and agenda for each meeting shall be given to each voting member not less than 14 days prior to the meeting.

Section 4—Distribution of Meeting Minutes

Meeting minutes shall be sent out by the Secretary or a designated member of the Collaborative within 14 days following the meeting.

Section 5—Quorum

In order to transact business, a simple majority of voting membership shall constitute a quorum.

Section 6—Voting

All issues to be voted on shall be decided by a simple majority of those voting members present at the meeting in which the vote takes place.

ARTICLE V: EXECUTIVE COMMITTEE

Section 1—Officers and Duties

The officers of the Collaborative shall be a chairperson, a vice-chair person, a secretary, an assistant secretary, and a treasurer (chair and vice-chair may have cochairs or assistants at the discretion and vote of the Collaborative membership), all of whom shall be members of the Executive Committee. The Executive Committee shall also include chairs of the standing committees of the Collaborative.

The chair shall convene regularly scheduled Collaborative meetings and shall preside or arrange for other members of the Executive Committee to preside at each meeting in the following order: vice-chair, secretary, assistant secretary, treasurer. The chair shall call to order all meetings of the Collaborative, establish for all such meetings an agenda, appoint members to all standing and special committees, report the transactions of the office. In addition, the chair shall perform all such duties as custom and parliamentary usage requires. The chair of the Collaborative shall report to the Board of the Partnership Project.

The vice-chair shall chair committees on special subjects as designated by the Executive Committee. The vice-chair shall assist the chair in the administration of the affairs of the Collaborative, and during the absence of or at the request of the chair, shall officiate meetings.

The secretary shall be responsible for keeping records of the Collaborative's actions, including overseeing the taking of minutes at all Collaborative meetings, sending out meeting notices, distributing copies of minutes and the agenda to each Collaborative member, and assuring that records are maintained. The secretary shall make a report at each Collaborative meeting. The secretary must inform the assistant secretary when he or she will be absent from a meeting.

The assistant secretary shall be responsible for taking minutes at Collaborative meetings and sending out meeting notices when the secretary is unable to attend a meeting. The assistant secretary will turn in minutes to the secretary for the secretary to distribute at the next meeting.

The treasurer shall collect yearly dues, keep track of memberships, and report the expenses and balances of the Collaborative. She or he sends out a letter in September to the membership requesting payment of the $25 yearly dues and signing the Full Value Contract, both to be returned by mail or at a meeting of the Collaborative no later than November 15. Because the Collaborative is under the aegis of the Partnership Project and does not maintain a separate money account, all financial business is carried out in conjunction with the Partnership Project. The Partnership Project treasurer provides an ongoing report of the balance, expenses and income to the Collaborative, which is in turn reported to the Collaborative membership by the Collaborative's treasurer at each Collaborative meeting.

The chair of the Membership Committee shall be responsible for membership lists, voting eligibility, and other duties as outlined in Article VI, Section 2, and will report relevant information at each Collaborative's regular meeting, as deemed necessary.

The chairs of other standing committees, as identified and outlined in Article VI, Section 2, shall be responsible for reporting relevant business matters for the respective Committees at each of the Collaborative's regular meetings, as deemed necessary.

Section 2—Terms

All Officers shall serve one-year terms at the beginning of the Collaborative's fiscal year (January 1st), and are eligible for reelection.

Section 3—Vacancies

When a vacancy on the Executive Committee exists midterm, the secretary will solicit and receive nominations from Collaborative members. These nominations shall be sent out to Collaborative members with the regular meeting announcement, to be voted upon at the next Collaborative meeting. These vacancies will be filled only to the end of the particular Executive Committee member's term.

Section 4—Resignation, Termination, and Absences

Resignation from an Executive Committee must be in writing and received by the Secretary. An Executive Committee member may be removed for other reasons by a 2/3 vote of the Executive Committee or majority vote of the Collaborative.

Section 5—Special Meetings

Special meetings of the Executive Committee shall be called upon the request of the chair, or a simple majority of the Executive Committee. Notices of special meetings shall be sent out by the secretary to each Executive Committee member at least 14 days in advance.

ARTICLE VI: COMMITTEES

Section 1—Appointments

Members of all standing and special committees are appointed by the chair of the Collaborative. Except where otherwise specified in the bylaws, all committee chairs are appointed by the chair of the Collaborative.

All committee members are appointed to serve for the duration of the term of the chair who appointed them. The appointment may not exceed one year in length, but members may be reappointed by the next chair.

Section 2—Standing Committees

a. Executive Committee

The Executive Committee shall be composed of the chair, vice-chair, secretary, assistant secretary, treasurer, and chairs of the standing committees. It shall operate by majority rule. The Committee has responsibility for supervision of the structure and operational framework of the Collaborative. The Executive Committee must approve and monitor the budget, and all expenditures must be within budget. Any major change in the budget must be approved by the Executive Committee. The fiscal year shall be the calendar year (January to December). Annual reports are required to be submitted to the Collaborative showing income, expenditures, and pending income. The financial records of the organization are public information and shall be made available to the membership.

In addition, it shall adopt interim policies which shall be in effect until the next meeting of the Collaborative and develop an annual report for the Collaborative which will be distributed to the membership on an annual basis.

b. Membership and Bylaws Committee

The Membership and Bylaws Committee shall consist of at least three members. It shall be responsible for determining whether members continue to meet the standards for active membership and for contacting members regarding attendance requirements. It shall be responsible for keeping an accurate record of the membership.

The committee shall also review proposed amendments to the bylaws and properly formulate proposed amendments for vote; it also may propose amendments for vote as it deems necessary. The chairperson shall report proposed amendments to the Executive Committee, clarify intent, and act as a resource person as needed.

c. Nominating Committee

The Nominating Committee shall consist of at least three members, one of whom shall be the immediate past chair who will serve as chair of the committee. The committee shall be responsible for nominating at least one candidate for the office of chair, one candidate for the office of vice-chair, one candidate for secretary, one candidate for assistant secretary, and one candidate for treasurer. It shall announce its nominees to Collaborative members and allow input from Collaborative members at least one month prior to the scheduled annual meeting.

The election results shall be determined by a simple majority of votes at the Annual Meeting of the Collaborative. Those elected shall begin their term at the beginning of the Collaborative's fiscal year.

d. Publications and Dissemination Committee

The Publications and Dissemination Committee shall establish criteria and guidelines for publications that might arise out of Collaborative activities. For specific details related to the operations of the Publications and Dissemination Committee, refer to the Collaborative's Guidelines on the Publication and Dissemination Committee, which was approved in July 2006.

e. Planning and Outreach Committee

The Planning and Outreach Committee shall be responsible for developing the public relations plan for the Collaborative including, but not limited to, issues of official names, press releases, printed materials describing the Collaborative, and individuals authorized to speak for the Collaborative. The committee will offer guidance and support to the coalitions in developing press reports and other information publicizing the Collaborative's activities. Publicity materials for the Collaborative should be reviewed by the Publications and Dissemination Committee so as to assure that standard terminology is being used for the Collaborative and its projects. This committee is also responsible for education and community awareness around the work of the Collaborative. It shall be responsible for dissemination of information to the general public and for hosting health awareness forums. It is responsible for promotion of community awareness and in engaging community partners in outreach efforts.

f. Budget and Finance Committee

The Budget and Finance Committee shall be responsible for proposing an annual budget of the Collaborative. It shall also be responsible for planning and monitoring any grant-related budgets in cooperation with the Collaborative's respective research partners.

Section 3—Special Committees

Special committees or ad hoc committees may be appointed by the chair or by a simple majority of the Executive Committee as the need arises.

ARTICLE VII: AMENDMENTS

Section 1—Amendments

These bylaws may be amended when necessary by a simple majority of the Collaborative members. Proposed amendments must be submitted to the Membership and Bylaws Committee for review and recommendation before being submitted to the Executive Committee before Collaborative membership voting.

ARTICLE VIII: GIFTS, BEQUESTS, AND GRANTS

The Collaborative, through the Executive Committee, is hereby authorized to receive contributions, gifts, bequests, and grants for the advancement of the purpose of the Collaborative.

Certification

These bylaws were approved at a meeting of Collaborative by a unanimous vote of the Collaborative on MONTH, DAY, YEAR.

COMMUNITY MEMBER

KEY INFORMANT

INTERVIEW GUIDE

EUGENIA ENG

KAREN STRAZZA

SCOTT D. RHODES

DEREK M. GRIFFITH

KATE SHIRAH

ELVIRA MEBANE

ntroduction: Hello, my name is _____ I'm going to be leading our interview today. This is _____, who will be taking notes and helping me during our discussion. We will be here about sixty minutes to talk to you about living in your community and your opinions concerning the strengths of your community and the challenges it faces. Your insights and opinions on these subjects are important, so please say what's on your mind and what you think. There is no right or wrong answer.

General Information About the Community

1. Please describe your role in the community. (Probe: How long have you lived here?)

2. Describe the community.

3. What do people in the community do for a living? (What is their source of income?)

4. How do people from the community get around?

5. What do people do for fun?

6. How are people involved in politics (for example, voting, talking with community leaders, elections)?

7. How do people of different races (ethnicities/backgrounds) interact within the community?

8. How involved are churches in the lives of people in the community (for example, attend church, participate in church groups)?

Assets and Needs of the Community

9. What are some of the best things about the community (for example, resources, agencies, social gatherings and support, physical environment)?

NOTE: See Chapter Five for a discussion of the development and implementation of this key informant interview guide within a CBPR project. We acknowledge Leo Allison for his contributions to this appendix as it appeared in the first edition of the book.

10. What do you think are the major issues and needs community members face (for example, children, income, elderly, safety, housing, disability, health, sanitation, pests)?

11. Which needs do you feel are the most important for the community to address?

12. What do you wish could happen for the community in the next 5–10 years?

Problem Solving and Decision Making

13. What kinds of community projects have been started during your time here? How would you explain their success or lack of it?

14. If you were going to try to solve a community problem, who would you try to involve to make it a success?

Services and Businesses

15. What services or programs do community members use? (Do those services come here or do residents go to them?)

16. What services or programs do community members need?

17. Where do people go to buy things like food, clothing, medicine, household items, and so on?

Recommended Individuals to Interview

18. Is there anyone else with whom we should speak about the community (for example, service providers, residents)? Are you willing to get permission for us to contact them?

    - Describe the specific person or organization.

    - Why do you think their opinions and views would be helpful for us to hear?

Recommendations for Community Forum

19. We plan to conduct a forum this spring to share the information we have gathered with the community. Would you be interested in helping us plan this event?

20. Do you have any ideas regarding how to get people to attend (for example, time, place, publicity)?

21. Who else do you think should help us coordinate this forum?

Additional Information

22. Is there anything else you would like to share about the community?

23. Thank you again for your participation.

Appendix E

SELECTED HEALTHY

ENVIRONMENTS PARTNERSHIP

MEASURES BY SURVEY

CATEGORIES, INDICATING

SOURCE OF IDENTIFICATION

FOR INCLUSION AND

SCALE ITEMS

AMY J. SCHULZ

SHANNON ZENK

SRIMATHI KANNAN

BARBARA A. ISRAEL

CARMEN STOKES

Measure	Identified by	Source
Neighborhood Context		
Municipal services	Steering committee, focus groups	Developed for this study
Recreational resources	Steering committee, focus group, existing literature	Adapted from East Side Village Health Worker Partnership; Schulz et al., 1998, http://www.sph.umich.edu/urc, and REACH Detroit Partnership, http://www.sph.umich.edu/reach/
Food resources	Steering committee, focus groups, existing literature	Adapted from the East Side Village Health Worker Partnership survey, http://www.sph.umich.edu/urc, and from Michigan BRFSS http://michigan.gov/mdch/0,1607,7-132-2945_5104_5279_39424—,00.html; Frazier, Franks, and Sanderson 1992; Gentry et al., 1985.
Sense of community	Steering committee, focus groups, existing literature	Adapted from East Side Village Health Worker Partnership; Parker et al., 2001.
Neighborhood participation	Steering committee, focus groups, existing literature	Items adapted from Goodman et al., 1998; some new items written for this study.
Stressors		
Duke life events inventory	Existing literature, focus groups	Blazer, Hughes, and George, 1987; George et al., 1989; Hughes et al., 1988.
General perceived stress	Existing literature, focus groups	Cohen and Williamson, 1988.
Work stress	Existing literature, focus groups	Karasek, Gardell, and Lindell, 1987.
Financial vulnerability	Existing literature, focus groups	James, Keenan, Strogatz, Browning, and Garrett, 1992.
Discrimination	Existing literature, focus groups	Adapted from Williams, Yu, Jackson, and Anderson, 1997; new response categories added based on focus groups.
Safety stress	Existing literature, focus groups	Schulz, Parker, Israel, and Fisher, 2001; Schulz et al., 2004.
Police stress	Existing literature, focus groups, pilot testing	Items adapted from East Side Village Health Worker Partnership, some new items written for this study.

Family stress	Existing literature, focus groups	Adapted from Schulz et al., 2001, 2004; some items created for this study.
Immigration stress	Focus groups, existing literature	Adapted items and created items based on focus group; Marin, G., Sabogal, Marin, B., Otero-Sabogal, and Perez-Stable, 1987.
Neighborhood social environment	Focus groups, steering committee, existing literature, pilot testing	Some items created based on focus groups; Adapted some items from Sampson, Raudebush, and Earls, 1997.
Neighborhood physical environment	Focus groups, steering committee, existing literature, pilot testing	Some items created based on focus groups; Adapted some items from East Side Village Health Worker Partnership.
Health-Related Behaviors		
Alcohol intake	Existing literature, focus groups	Block, Coyle, Hartman, and Scoppa 1994.
Tobacco use	Existing literature, focus groups	Adapted from BRFSS, http://www.cdc.gov/brfss/questionnaires.htm; Frazier, Franks, & Sanderson 1992; Gentry et al. 1985.
Physical activity	Existing literature, focus groups	Adapted from BRFSS, http://www.cdc.gov/brfss/questionnaires.htm; Frazier et al. 1992.
Nutrient intake	Existing literature, focus groups	Adapted from Block et al., 1994, 1986.
Health screening	Existing literature, focus groups, steering committee	NHANES, http://www.cdc.gov/nceh/dls/nhanes.htm
Social Integration and Social Support		
Social support	Focus groups, existing literature	Strogatz, et al., 1997; James et al., 1987.
Spiritual support	Focus groups, existing literature	Pargament, Koenig, and Perez, 2000.
Organizational membership	Focus groups, existing literature	Adapted from East Side Village Health Worker Partnership survey.

(Continued)

Measure	Identified by	Source
Psychosocial Indicators		
John Henryism Scale for Active Coping	Existing literature	James, Strogatz, Wing, and Ramsey, 1987.
Beck hopelessness scale	Existing literature, focus groups	Beck, Weissman, Lester, and Trexler, 1974.
Anger or hostility	Existing literature, focus groups	Spielberger et al., 1985.
Symptoms of depression (CES-D)	Existing literature, focus groups	Radloff, 1977.
Composite International Diagnostic Interview (CIDI)	Existing literature, focus groups	Wittchen, 1994; WHO, 1991.
Health Outcome Indicators		
Self report diagnosis (blood pressure, diabetes, etc.)	Existing literature, focus groups	Adapted from NHANES, http://www.cdc.gov/nceh/dls/nhanes.htm
Physical activity limitations	Existing literature	Roscow and Breslau, 1966.
General self-rated health status	Existing literature, focus groups	Idler and Benyamini, 1997.
Blood pressure	Existing literature, focus groups	Guidelines adapted from James et al., 1992.
Overweight/obesity (Height, weight, hip, waist)	Existing literature, focus groups	Guidelines adapted from James et al., 1992.

NOTE: See Chapter Seven for a discussion of the development and administration of this survey questionnaire using a CBPR approach. We acknowledge Mary Koch for her contributions to this appendix as it appeared in the first edition of the book.

REFERENCES

Beck, A. T., Weissman, A., Lester, D., & Trexler, L. (1974). The measurement of pessimism: The hopelessness scale. *Journal of Consulting and Clinical Psychology, 42*(6), 861–865.

Blazer, D., Hughes, D., & George, L. K. (1987). Stressful life events and the onset of a generalized anxiety syndrome. *American Journal of Psychiatry, 144*(9), 1178–1183.

Block, G., Hartman, A. M., Dresser, C. M., Caroll, M. D., Gannon, J., & Gardner, L. (1986). A data-based approach to dietary questionnaire design and testing. *American Journal of Epidemiology, 124*, 453–469.

Block, G., Coyle, L. M., Hartman, A. M., & Scoppa, S. M. (1994). Revision of dietary analysis software for the Health Habits and History Questionnaire. *American Journal of Epidemiology, 139*, 1190–1196.

Centers for Disease Control and Prevention, Division of Adult and Community Health, & National Center for Chronic Disease Prevention and Health Promotion. *Behavioral Risk Factor Surveillance System Online Prevention Data, 1995–2002* (BRFSS.). Retrieved 2004, from http://www.cdc.gov/brfss/

Centers for Disease Control and Prevention, National Center for Environmental Health, & Division of Laboratory Science. (2004). *The National Health and Nutrition Examination Surveys (NHANES).* Retrieved June 8, 2004, from http://www.cdc.gov/nceh/dls/nhanes .htm

Cohen, S., & Williamson, G. (1988). Perceived stress in a probability sample of the United States. In S. Spacapan, & S. Oscamp (Eds.), *The Social Psychology of Health.* Newbury Park, CA: Sage.

Eastside Village Health Worker Partnership, www.sph.umich.edu/urc/projects/esvhwp.html

Frazier, E. L., Franks, A. L., & Sanderson, L. M. (1992). Using behavioral risk factor surveillance data. In National Center for Chronic Disease Prevention and Health Promotion (U.S.). Office of Surveillance and Analysis (Ed.), *Using Chronic Disease Data: A Handbook for Public Health Practitioners.* Atlanta: Centers for Disease Control and Prevention.

Gentry, E. M., Kalsbeek, W. D., Hogelin, G. C., Jones, J. T., Gaines, K. L., Forman, M. R., et al. (1985). The behavioral risk factor surveys: II. Design, methods, and estimates from combined state data. *American Journal of Preventive Medicine, 1*(6), 9–14.

George, L. K., Blazer, D. G., Hughes, D. C., & Fowler, N. (1989). Social support and the outcome of major depression. *British Journal of Psychiatry, 154*, 478–485.

Goodman, R. M., Speers, M. A., McLeroy, K., Fawcett, S., Kegler, M., Parker, E. A., et al. (1998). Identifying and defining the dimensions of community capacity to provide a basis for measurement. *Health Education & Behavior, 25*(3), 258–278.

Hughes, D. C., Blazer, D. G., & George, L. K. (1988). Age differences in life events: A multivariate controlled analysis. *International Journal of Aging and Human Development, 27*(3), 207–220.

Idler, E. L., & Benyamini, Y. (1997). Self-rated health and mortality: A review of twenty-seven community studies. *Journal of Health and Social Behavior*, *38*(1), 21–37.

James, S. A., Strogatz, D. S., Wing, S. B., & Ramsey, D. L. (1987). Socioeconomic status, John Henryism, and hypertension in blacks and whites. *American Journal of Epidemiology*, *126*(4), 664–673.

James, S. A., Keenan, N. L., Strogatz, D. S., Browning, S. R., & Garrett, J. M. (1992). Socio-economic status, John Henryism, and blood pressure in black adults: The Pitt County Study. *American Journal of Epidemiology*, *135*(1), 59–67.

Karasek, R. T., Gardell, B., & Lindell, J. (1987). Work and non-work correlates of illness and behavior in male and female Swedish white collar workers. *Journal of Occupational Behavior*, *8*, 187–207.

Marín, G., Sabogal, F., Marín, B., Otero-Sabogal, R., & Perez-Stable, E. J. (1987).Development of a short acculturation scale for Hispanics. *Hispanic Journal of Behavioral Sciences*, *9*, 183–205.

Pargament, K. I., Koenig, H. G., & Perez, L. (2000). The many methods or Religious coping: Development and initial validation of the RCOPE. *Journal of Clinical Psychology*, *56*, 519–543.

Parker, E. A., Lichtenstein, R. L., Schulz, A. J., Israel, B. A., Schork, M. A., Steinman, K. J., et al. (2001). Disentangling measures of individual perceptions of community social dynamics: Results of a community survey. *Health Education & Behavior*, *28*(4), 462–486.

Radloff, L. S. (1977). The CES-D: A self-report depression scale for research on the general population. *Applied Psychological Measurement*, *1*, 385–401.

REACH Detroit Partnership, www.sph.umich.edu/reach/

Roscow, I., & Breslau, N. (1966). A Guttman health scale for the aged. *Journal of Gerontology*, *21*(4), 556–559.

Sampson, R., Raudebush, S., Earls, F. 1997. Neighborhoods and violent crime: A multilevel study of collective efficacy. *Science*, *277*, 918–924.

Schulz, A. J., Parker, E. A., Israel, B. A., Becker, A. B., Maciak, B. J., & Hollis, R. (1998). Conducting a participatory community-based survey: Collecting and interpreting data for a community health intervention on Detroit's east side. *Journal of Public Health Management and Practice*, *4*(2), 10–24.

Schulz, A. J., Parker, E. A., Israel, B. A., & Fisher, T. (2001). Social context, stressors and disparities in women's health. *Journal of the American Medical Women's Association*, *56*(4), 143–149.

Schulz, A. J., Israel, B. A., Estrada, L., Zenk, S. N., Viruell-Fuentes, E. A., Villarruel, A., et al. (2004). Engaging community residents in assessing their social and physical environments and their implications for health. Presented at the American Public Health Association Annual Meeting, Washington, DC, November 6–10, 2004.

Spielberger, C. D., Johnson, E. H., Russell, S. F., Crane, R. J., Jacobs, G. A., & Worden, T. J. (1985). The experience and expression of anger: Construction and validation of an anger expression scale. In M. A. Chesney & R. H. Rosenman (Eds.), *Anger and Hostility in Cardiovascular and Behavioral Disorders* (pp. 5–30). Washington, DC: Hemisphere.

Strogatz, D. S., Croft, J. B., James, S. A., Keenan, N. L., Browning, S. R., Garrett, J. M., et al. (1997). Social support, stress, and blood pressure in black adults. *Epidemiology*, *8*(5), 482–487.

Williams, D. R., Yu, Y., Jackson, J., & Anderson, N. B. (1997). Racial differences in physical and mental health: Socioeconomic status, stress and discrimination. *Journal of Health Psychology*, *2*(3), 335–351.

Wittchen, H. U. (1994). Reliability and validity studies of the WHO composite international diagnostic interview (CIDI): A critical review. *Journal of Psychiatric Research*, *28*, 57–84.

World Health Organization. (1991). *International Classification of Diseases (ICD-10)*. Geneva: WHO.

PROMOTING HEALTHY

LIFESTYLES AMONG WOMEN

FOCUS GROUP SUMMARY ANALYSIS FORM: EASTSIDE AND SOUTHWEST DETROIT— PROCEDURES AND EXAMPLE QUESTIONS

EDITH C. KIEFFER

YAMIR SALABARRÍA-PEÑA

ANGELA M. ODOMS-YOUNG

SHARLA K. WILLIS

GLORIA PALMISANO

J. RICARDO GUZMÁN

Focus Group Summary Analysis Form: Eastside Detroit Focus Group

Group: _X_ Pregnant _____ Postpartum

Place: Butzel Family Center

Date: 08/18/01

Date that this summary was filled out:

_____

Moderator's Name: _____

Assistants' Names: _____

_____

General notes about focus group and participants:

(Include information such as what was the atmosphere of the group. Did the people participate actively or was there much silence? Was there any question(s) that caused more participation? Was there any question(s) that caused less participation? Please do not include information on this sheet that identifies the participants.

How should you use these pages?

Please give a summary of the responses of the focus group for the following questions. Write the general feelings of the participants (for example, "the majority of the participants said that . . .") and also the variety of responses (for example, "the people mentioned the following barriers for a healthy diet . . ."). Do not forget to include the opinions of the people that said things outside of the general opinion of the group (for example, "the majority of people said . . . , but a participant [or a few] said . . ."). Include specific quotes. If you need more space to write please write on the other side of the page. If you use another page please number the question that you are summarizing. Thank you for your help.

NOTE: See Chapter Nine for a discussion of the development and administration of this focus group protocol.

Examples of Questions and Summary (in italics):

WEIGHT/BODY IMAGE-GENERAL

What influences the way you think about your ideal size, shape and weight?

Women discussed influences on their ideas about ideal body weight, size, and shape. Some women talked about wanting to be the same size they were when they were younger. For others, getting heavier was something they accepted as going along with getting older and having children. Women also talked about comparing their own weight and shape with that of other women.

Probe: before, during, after pregnancy

Have your ideas about your ideal weight changed since you were younger?

Probe: What caused these ideas to change?

PROGRAM IDEAS

If you had the power to create a program to help women and their families, including helping them to eat a healthy diet and to exercise during and after pregnancy, what would it be like?

Probe:

What activities would it include?

Who would plan and lead the activities? (including characteristics, skills)

Where would it be?

Who should participate? (including characteristics of women, participation of

husband/partner, child, etc.?)

How would you inform and motivate potential participants?

What other services would be needed to help women to participate?

What would definitely have to be included in order for you to participate?

PROMOVIENDO ESTILOS DE VIDA SALUDABLES ENTRE MUJERES

Spanish Language Version Used in Southwest Detroit

RESUMEN DEL ANALISIS DE GRUPO FOCAL

Grupo: __X__ Embarazadas _____ Después del parto

Lugar: Latino Family Services

Fecha: 06/29/01

Fecha en la que se llenó este resumen:

_____

Nombre de la Moderadora: _____

Nombre de la Asistente: _____

Notas generales sobre el grupo y participantes:

(Incluya información, como cuál fue la atmósfera del grupo. ¿La gente participó activamente o había mucho silencio? ¿Hubo alguna pregunta que creó mucha participación? ¿Alguna pregunta creó poca discusión? Por favor no incluya información en esta hoja que pueda identificar a las participantes.

¿Cómo se usa esta hoja?

Favor de dar un resumen sobre las respuestas del grupo focal de los siguientes temas. Escriba el sentimiento general de las participantes (por ejemplo, "la mayoría de los participantes dijeron que . . .") y también la variedad de respuestas (por ejemplo, "las personas mencionaron las siguientes barreras para una alimentación saludable . . ."). No olvide incluir las opiniones de la gente que han dicho cosas fuera de la opinión general del grupo (por ejemplo, "la mayoría de la gente dijeron . . . , pero una participante [o unos cuantos] dijo . . ."). Incluya citas específicas. Si necesita más espacio para escribir por favor escriba detrás de la página. Si usa otra página por favor enumere la pregunta que está resumiendo. Gracias por su ayuda.

616 ● APPENDIX F

Ejemplos de Preguntas, y Resumen (en cursiva)

PESO/APARIENCIA FÍSICA

¿Cómo ustedes se han sentido con los cambios en peso, talla o figura durante su embarazo ?

Las mujeres hablaron de varias experiencias relacionadas con a subir o bajar de peso durante sus embarazos. Aunque algunas mujeres se sentían cómodas con los cambios en su peso, talla, y figura durante sus embarazos, a otras no les gustaban tales cambios.

Indagar: ¿Por qué esto es importante?

¿Qué piensan las personas que son importantes en su vida de estos cambios? (pareja/esposo, mamá, papá, etc.)

¿Cuán importante es para las mujeres volver al peso, talla, o figura que tenían antes del embarazo?

Indagar: ¿Cuáles son las razones?

IDEAS PARA PROGRAMAS

Si ustedes tuvieran el poder de crear un programa para ayudar a mujeres y a sus familias a que tengan una dieta saludable y a hacer ejercicio durante y después del embarazo, ¿En qué consistiría este programa?

Indagar:

¿Qué actividades debe incluir?

¿Quién planearía y dirijiría tales actividades? (incluyendo las características y las abilidades de esas personas?

¿En donde se llevaría a cabo?

¿Quiénes deben participar? (¿Qué tipo de mujeres? ¿Qué tal la participación de esposos/parejas, novios, hijos(as), etc.)?

¿Cómo informarían y motivarían a la gente a participar?

¿Qué otros servicios se necesitarían para ayudar a las mujeres a participar?

FIELD NOTES GUIDE

NICOLE S. BERRY

CHRIS McQUISTON

EMILIO A. PARRADO

JULIO CÉSAR OLMOS-MUÑIZ

Informant code: _____

Interviewer name: _____

Date: _____

Location of interview: _____

Time of interview: _____

Observational notes: What you observe about the informant, the place or environment in which the interview takes place, anything that is not recorded by the tape recorder.

Examples:

- Description of the location where the interview takes place

- If there are other people present during the interview

- Observations about the informant:

    Is he or she nervous? Shy? Calm?

    Does the informant seems to easily understand the questions that you ask?

Methodological notes: Comments on the process of the actual interview.

Examples:

- Comments about the interview guide

    Changes in the order of questions

    Difficulties with certain questions or themes

- Length of the interview

- Interruptions

Theoretical notes: Refer to the objectives of the interview. Here is where you, the interviewer, start to analyze the information that the informant is giving you. You want to start to answer your basic research questions:

NOTE: See Chapter Eleven for a discussion of the use of these guidelines for taking field notes of ethnographic interviews within the context of a CBPR project.

- How have gender roles changed as a result of the process of migration to the United States and what do those changes mean for men and for women who experience them?

- How has decision making changed since the individual or couple came to the United States?

- What impact does gender role change have on the sexual behavior of the individual or couple?

- What are the different gender roles and their corresponding attributes as described by the informant?

- How does social or familial support influence a couple's relationship?

- What does the informant know or think about HIV and HIV-related risks?

Here you can also write about new themes that come up from the interview—if the informant talks about themes that are relevant to the study, but are not included in the guide. Try to identify reoccurring themes—a subject or experience that the informant talks about repeatedly.

Personal notes: How you felt doing the interview.

Examples:
- "I felt uncomfortable asking her about her sex life because this informant is a very religious person."

- "I felt like he answered the questions honestly and openly. He was very open with me, but I did notice that he became hesitant and timid when I asked him questions about his migration history."

- "I felt tired today and started to lose my concentration about halfway through the interview. I asked her if we could take a break for a couple of minutes to have a glass of water so that I could wake up."

IN-DEPTH, SEMI-STRUCTURED
INTERVIEW PROTOCOL

DETROIT COMMUNITY-ACADEMIC URBAN RESEARCH CENTER, DETROIT URC BOARD EVALUATION 1996–2002

BARBARA A. ISRAEL

PAULA M. LANTZ

ROBERT McGRANAGHAN

J. RICARDO GUZMÁN

INTERVIEW QUESTIONS ASKED IN 1996

1. The Urban Research Center (URC) has been in existence for about a year. Last October was when the first introductory meetings for the URC took place. Can you tell me what you had hoped the URC would accomplish during its first year? What were your expectations for the initial year of the URC?

   Probe: Would you say you had high or low expectations for the first year?

2. Has the URC met your expectations for the first year? Has it exceeded these expectations?

   Probes: If fallen short of expectations, why do you think this happened? Were your expectations too high to begin with? If exceeded expectations, why do you think this happened? Were your expectations too low to begin with?

3. What have been the URC's major accomplishments thus far? Name two or more.

4. What have been the major barriers or challenges facing the URC thus far? Name two or more.

5. I would like to know what you hope the URC will accomplish during the next year and then beyond. First, what do you want the URC to tackle and accomplish over the next year? Second, what do you want the URC to have accomplished by the end of the first five years, which will be the fall of the year 2000?

6. What sort of challenges or barriers do you foresee for the URC over the next few years? Do you have any recommendations for how the URC can meet these challenges or reduce these barriers?

7. What have you personally learned from your association with the URC? Has it expanded your knowledge at all, or helped you to develop or refine any skills? Has it helped you professionally in any way?

NOTE: See Chapter Thirteen and Lantz et al., 2001 for an examination of the development and use of this instrument. We acknowledge Diana Kerr for her contributions to this appendix as it appeared in the first edition of the book.

8. Has your organization's affiliation with the URC provided any tangible benefits yet? What does your organization hope to accomplish by its affiliation with the URC?

9. Could you please give me some examples of exchanges of information, assistance, or support between your organization and other organizations in the URC? Do you think that these exchanges would have happened without the establishment of the URC?

   Probe for examples that don't involve URC staff or university faculty/staff.

10. What sort of gap or need does the URC have the potential to fill? What would be the consequences of not having a Community-Academic Urban Research Center in Detroit?

11. Evaluation question 1: What would you like to learn from an evaluation of the URC? One way to think about that difficult question is to think about what questions you would like us to be able to answer about the URC four years from now.

    Probe: What do you think an evaluation should try to show?

12. Evaluation question 2: There are six goals of the URC (show them). Do you have any other goals for the URC that are not on this list?

    Probe: What are indicators of success for the URC? What are some indicators of problems or lack of success?

ADDITIONAL INTERVIEW QUESTIONS ASKED IN 1999

1. What factors have facilitated the accomplishments of the URC? What structures and processes instituted by the URC have been important in establishing and maintaining collaborative relationships among the different partners?

2. To what extent has the URC created new relationships among the organizations or partners participating?

3. Do you think that community interests have been represented and assured in the research projects that have been developed and implemented by the URC? Please explain why or why not.

4. To what extent and how has the URC helped communities recognize and work with their assets and local resources in its projects?

5. The last few questions refer to the role of the Centers for Disease Control and Prevention (CDC) in the development of the Detroit URC. In general, how have CDC priorities and policies influenced the direction of the URC? In what capacities has the CDC helped the URC foster and develop community-based participatory research? What recommendations would you give to CDC regarding how to improve their Urban Research Centers program?

6. Thinking about other communities who may want to establish their own partnerships for community-based participatory research, what would you say worked well about the process by which the URC developed its partnership? What would you recommend they do differently?

ADDITIONAL INTERVIEW QUESTIONS ASKED IN 2002

1. In what ways is the work of the URC benefiting the community? How could the URC improve its benefits to or value for the community?

2. Has your organization's affiliation with the URC resulted in any *costs or problems* for your organization? How about for you personally?

3. During the recent past, the URC has attempted to open up lines of communication with policymakers and policy experts at the local, state, and federal level. What do you think of the URC's policy activities to date? What do you recommend for future activities in this area?

4. Future funding from the CDC for URC infrastructure and research projects is uncertain. How do you think the loss of CDC funding would affect the URC? How would it affect your organization's participation in URC activities? How should the URC best explore options for future funding?

REFERENCE

Lantz, P., Viruell-Fuentes, E., Israel, B. A., Softley, D., & Guzman, J. R. (2001). Can communities and academia work together on public health research? Evaluation results from a community-based participatory research partnership in Detroit. *Journal of Urban Health,* 78(3), 495–507.

Appendix I

CLOSED-ENDED SURVEY

QUESTIONNAIRE

DETROIT COMMUNITY-ACADEMIC URBAN RESEARCH CENTER, DETROIT URC BOARD EVALUATION 1997–2007[1]

BARBARA A. ISRAEL

PAULA M. LANTZ

ROBERT J. McGRANAGHAN

J. RICARDO GUZMÁN

RICHARD LICHTENSTEIN

ZACHARY ROWE

Organization and Structure of Meetings	1997	1999	2001	2002	2007
1. I find URC board meetings useful.	—	X	X	X	X
2. The URC board meetings are well organized.	X	X	X	X	X
3. Background materials (agendas, minutes, etc.) needed for meetings are prepared and distributed well enough in advance of meetings.	—	—	—	—	X
4. We discuss important issues at URC meetings.	—	—	—	X	X
5. I wish we spent more time at board meetings hearing about and discussing URC projects.	—	—	X	X	X
6. The board meetings are held too frequently.	X	X	X	X	X
7. We do not accomplish very much at URC board meetings.	—	—	—	X	—
8. I believe that we adequately address all of the agenda items at the URC meetings.	X	X	X	X	X
9. When I want to place something on the meeting agenda, I am comfortable with the process.	X	X	X	X	X
10. I would like more of a voice in determining agenda items for the URC board meetings.	X	X	X	X	—
11. When the URC board makes decisions, appropriate follow-up action is taken by staff.	X	X	X	X	X
12. When the URC board makes decisions, appropriate follow-up action is taken by URC board members.	—	X	X	X	X
13. The opinions of some individuals on the URC board get weighted more heavily than they should.[2]	X	X	X	X	X
14. One person or group dominates at URC board meetings.	X	X	X	X	X
15. New members receive adequate orientation to allow them to become effective members of the board.	—	—	—	—	X

Trust	1997	1999	2001	2002	2007
16. Relationships among URC board members go beyond the individuals at the table, to include member organizations.	—	X	X	X	—
17. I am comfortable requesting assistance from other board members (when I feel that their input could be of value).	—	X	X	X	X
18. I can talk openly and honestly at the URC Board meetings.	X	X	X	X	X
19. I am comfortable expressing my point of view at URC board meetings.	X	X	X	X	X
20. I am comfortable bringing up new ideas at the URC board meetings.	X	X	X	X	X
21. URC board members respect each other's points of view even if they might disagree.	X	X	X	X	X
22. My opinion is listened to and considered by other Board members.	X	X	X	X	X
23. In the past year, my willingness to speak and express my opinions at board meetings has: increased, stayed same, decreased, don't know.	X	X	X	X	—
24. Over the past year, the amount of trust between URC board members has: increased, stayed same, decreased, don't know.[3]	—	X	X	X	X
25. In the past year, the URC board members' capacity to work well together has: increased, stayed same, decreased, don't know.	X	X	X	X	—
26. How much trust is there between partners now? A lot, moderate amount, not much, don't know.[4]	—	X	X	X	X
27. In the next year, how much trust do you expect to see between partners? A lot, moderate amount, not much, don't know.	—	X	X	X	—

Board Decisions	1997	1999	2001	2002	2007
28. I am satisfied with the overall way in which the URC board makes decisions.	—	—	X	X	X
29. All board members have a voice in decisions made by the group.	—	—	X	X	X
30. It often takes the URC board too long to reach a decision.	—	—	X	X	X
31. Decisions about URC resources are made in a fair manner.	—	—	X	X	X
32. URC board members work well together to solve problems.	—	—	X	X	X

Impact	1997	1999	2001	2002	2007
33. The board of the URC has been effective in achieving its goals.	X	X	X	X	X
34. The work of the URC has brought benefits to my community.[5]	X	X	X	X	X
35. Participation in the URC has increased my knowledge and understanding of the other organizations represented.	—	X	X	X	—
36. Participation in the URC has increased my knowledge of family and community health issues during the past year.	X	X	X	X	X
37. Participation in the URC has increased my knowledge of health disparities and social determinants of health.	—	—	—	—	X
38. Participation in the URC has increased my organization's capacity to conduct community based research.	—	X	X	X	X
39. My organization uses knowledge generated by the URC.	—	X	X	X	X
40. I believe that other, nonmember health and human service agencies in the Detroit area *know about* the URC and its initiatives.	—	X	X	X	X
41. I believe that other, nonmember health and human service agencies in the Detroit area *use knowledge* generated by the URC.	—	X	X	X	X
42. URC-affiliated projects are improving health outcomes for people in Detroit.	—	—	—	—	X

General Satisfaction	1997	1999	2001	2002	2007
43. I am generally satisfied with the activities and progress of the URC during the past year.	X	X	X	X	X
44. I have a sense of ownership in what the URC does and accomplishes.	X	X	X	X	X
45. I am satisfied with the types of proposals that the URC has submitted.	—	X	X	X	X
46. I am satisfied with the types of projects that the URC has implemented.	—	X	X	X	X
47. I frequently think of having my organization sever its affiliation with the URC.	X	X	X	X	X
48. I have adequate knowledge of the URC budget, URC resources, and how resources are allocated.	—	X	X	X	X
49. Thus far, the URC has distributed available resources in a fair and equitable manner.	X	X	X	X	X
50. I would like to have more input regarding the allocation of URC resources.	—	X	X	X	X
51. I am satisfied with the visibility of the URC within Detroit.	—	—	—	—	X
52. I am satisfied with the URC's efforts to translate research and evaluation results into information and programs that can improve health in Detroit.	—	—	—	—	X
53. I am satisfied with the URC board's attention to the *financial sustainability* of the Center.	—	—	—	—	X
54. I am satisfied with the URC board's attention to the *ongoing sustainability of relationships* within the partnership.	—	—	—	—	X
55. I am satisfied with the URC board's attention to *building the capacity of all partners* to participate actively in the work of the board.	—	—	—	—	X

Strategic Planning	1997	1999	2001	2002	2007
56. Our strategic planning process resulted in the development of concrete goals and objectives.	—	—	—	—	X
57. Our strategic planning process resulted in the development of appropriate strategies to accomplish our goals and objectives.	—	—	—	—	X
58. Our strategic planning process has helped to sustain the URC.	—	—	—	—	X

URC Policy Impact	1997	1999	2001	2002	2007
59. The URC has been effective in informing policymakers and key government officials about the URC and its initiatives.	—	X	X	X	X
60. Partners have increased their policy-related activities as a result of their involvement with the URC.	—	—	—	—	X
61. Involvement with the URC has provided support for policy issues my organization feels strongly about.	—	—	—	—	X
62. The URC has been effective at translating research findings into policy-relevant documents and educational materials.	—	—	—	—	X
63. The URC has been effective at translating research findings into policy change.	—	—	—	—	X

Community-Based Participatory Research and Centers for Disease Control and Prevention (CDC)	1997	1999	2001	2002	2007
64. It is important that policymakers and key government officials are informed about the URC and its initiatives	—	X	X	X	X
65. The URC is following its own community-based research principles in its projects.	—	X	X	X	—
66. Community interests are well represented in URC activities.	—	X	X	X	—
67. CDC staff in Atlanta play an important role in helping the URC foster and develop community-based participatory research.	—	X	X	X	—

Community-Based Participatory Research and Centers for Disease Control and Prevention (CDC)	1997	1999	2001	2002	2007
68. The CDC is supportive of what we are trying to do in our URC.	—	X	X	X	—
69. Length of membership on board, since 1995: between four and eight years, less than four years.	—	—	—	—	X
70. Served as a member of a URC subcommittee	—	—	—	—	X
71. Served on a Steering Committee of one of the URC's affiliated projects/partnerships.	—	—	—	—	X
72. Served as a copresenter or presenter representing the URC or one of its affiliated projects at a conference, training, or workshop/seminar.	—	—	—	—	X

Participation in Board Meetings	1997	1999	2001	2002	2007
73. Please indicate approximately how many times over the last year you have attended URC board meetings: never, 1–3, 4–6, 7–9, 10–11 times.	—	—	—	—	X

Assessment of Participation	1997	1999	2001	2002	2007
74. I am satisfied with my level of participation in the URC board.	—	—	—	—	X
75. I have taken advantage of opportunities to influence the work of the URC board.	—	—	—	—	X
76. I devote time outside of board meetings to URC activities or projects.	—	—	—	—	X
77. My participation in the URC board is limited by the capacity of my organization.	—	—	—	—	X

Board Operations and Capacity	1997	1999	2001	2002	2007
78. The URC has a clear vision of what it aspires to achieve.	—	—	—	—	X
79. The URC vision has been translated into concrete, measurable goals that we aim to achieve.	—	—	—	—	X

Board Operations and Capacity	1997	1999	2001	2002	2007
80. There is a general agreement about the mission of the board.	—	—	—	—	X
81. There is general agreement about the goals and objectives of the board.	—	—	—	—	X
82. Board members agree on the strategies the URC uses in pursuing its priorities.	—	—	—	—	X

Board Operations and Capacity	1997	1999	2001	2002	2007
83. The URC board effectively represents the diversity of our communities.	—	—	—	—	X
84. Community interests are well represented in URC activities.	—	—	—	—	X
85. The URC board thinks strategically.	—	—	—	—	X
86. The URC board is well managed.	—	—	—	—	X
87. The URC is following its own community-based participatory research principles.	—	—	—	—	X
88. Board members take responsibility for getting work done.	—	—	—	—	X
89. In the past year, URC board members' capacity to work well together has increased.	—	—	—	—	X

Communication	1997	1999	2001	2002	2007
90. Board members communicate effectively with each other during meetings.	—	—	—	—	X
91. Communication between URC staff and board members is effective.	—	—	—	—	X
92. Information communicated within the URC partnership is relevant.	—	—	—	—	X
93. Board members communicate effectively with each other outside of meetings.	—	—	—	—	X

Benefits of URC Involvement	1997	1999	2001	2002	2007
94. Increasing recognition and respect for my organization in Detroit.	—	—	—	—	X
95. Increasing my knowledge and understanding of the other organizations and projects represented on the board.	—	—	—	—	X
96. Increasing my professional knowledge and skills to address health-related issues being studied by URC-affiliated projects.	—	—	—	—	X

Benefits of URC Involvement	1997	1999	2001	2002	2007
97. Developing new collaborative relationships between my organization and other URC partner organizations.	—	—	—	—	X
98. Working with communities with whom my organization has previously had little contact.	—	—	—	—	X
99. Getting funding for my organization.	—	—	—	—	X

Challenges/Limitations Associated with URC Involvement	1997	1999	2001	2002	2007
100. URC activities do not address my organization's goals and interests.	—	—	—	—	X
101. Membership in the URC requires a considerable time commitment.	—	—	—	—	X
102. My (or my organization's) opinion is not valued within the URC.	—	—	—	—	X
103. There is too little funding for my organization's participation in the URC.	—	—	—	—	X
104. The requirement to include funds for URC infrastructure support in new affiliated-project grant proposals is satisfactory.	—	—	—	—	X
105. The partner organizations on the board do not adequately represent the interests of our community.	—	—	—	—	X
106. The board's process for approving new URC projects is satisfactory.	—	—	—	—	X

Challenges/Limitations Associated with URC Involvement	1997	1999	2001	2002	2007
107. The board's process for identifying/ inviting new board members is satisfactory.	—	—	—	—	X
108. The board's process for deciding who becomes the lead fiduciary organization for a new project is satisfactory.	—	—	—	—	X

Benefits Compared to Challenges Associated with URC Involvement	1997	1999	2001	2002	2007
109. From your organization's perspective, do the benefits of participation in the URC appear to outweigh the costs at this point? (Yes/No)	—	—	—	—	X
110. From your personal perspective, do the benefits of participation in the URC appear to outweigh the costs at this point? (Yes/No)	—	—	—	—	X

NOTES

[1] All questions used five point Likert scale response categories ranging from strongly agree to strongly disagree unless otherwise noted.

See Chapter 14, Lantz et al. 2001 and Schulz et al. 2003 for an examination of the development and use of this instrument. With acknowledgment to Shawn Kimmel for his role in the partnership evaluation conducted in 2007.

[2] Versions prior to 2007 read: Certain individuals' opinions get weighed more than they should.

[3] 2007 version reads: The amount of trust between URC Board members has increased over time. Response categories changed to Likert-type scale (strongly agree to strongly disagree).

[4] 2007 version reads: There is a high level of trust between URC Board members. Response categories changed to Likert-type scale (strongly agree to strongly disagree).

[5] Versions prior to 2007 read: The URC can have a positive effect on the community.

REFERENCES/SOURCES

Granner, M. L., & Sharpe, P. A. (2004). Evaluating community coalition characteristics and functioning: A summary of measurement tools. *Health Education Research, 19*(5), 514–532.

Lantz, P. M., Viruell-Fuentes, E., Israel, B. A., Softley, D., & Guzman, J. R. (2001). Can communities and academia work together on public health research? Evaluation results from a community-based participatory research partnership in Detroit. *Journal of Urban Health, 78*(3), 495–507.

Schulz, A. J., Israel, B. A., & Lantz, P. M. (2003). Instrument for evaluating dimensions of group dynamics within community-based participatory research partnerships. *Evaluation and Program Planning, 26,* 249–262.

Some questions used in 2007 were adapted from the Prevention Research Center of Michigan, *Community Board Process Evaluation Survey,* 2005.

Some questions used in 2007 were adapted from Allies Against Asthma, "Coalition Self-Assessment Survey," 2002; originally developed by Erin Kenney, PhD, and Shoshanna Sofaer, DrPH, School of Public Affairs, Baruch College, City University of New York, 2000.

PHILOSOPHY AND GUIDING PRINCIPLES FOR DISSEMINATION OF FINDINGS OF COMMUNITY ACTION AGAINST ASTHMA INCLUDING AUTHORSHIP OF PUBLICATIONS AND PRESENTATIONS, POLICIES AND PROCEDURES, ACCESS TO DATA, AND RELATED MATTERS

EDITH A. PARKER

THOMAS G. ROBINS

BARBARA A. ISRAEL

WILMA BRAKEFIELD-CALDWELL

KATHERINE K. EDGREN

DONELE J. WILKINS

The DC develops policies and procedures for decision making about dissemination as it applies to MCECH activities and findings. Dissemination activities might be in the form of papers, presentations, news releases, newsletters, or through other resources. Presentations might be to academics, to funding agencies or potential funding agencies, or to community members. We are eager to use these opportunities in a spirit of partnership that lessens the gap between academics and nonacademics. Our goal is to have a process that ensures high quality and is fair, inclusive, and allows people to grow in their skills, knowledge, and experiences. It is the university's responsibility to ensure that community partners are involved in decision making. We also recognize this will be a challenge, particularly when decisions need to be made quickly. Having a process where we keep everyone informed means that we have to do things a bit differently. We are committed to maintaining feelings of mutual respect and trust and are hopeful that the policies and procedures developed will foster that. If policies are not followed, the person who did not follow the policy must attend the next Steering Committee meeting and make a clear presentation to the group.

The duties, rights, and responsibilities of the DC include:

- Outlining core articles and presentations based on the original grant and potential conferences and journals for submission, and proposing writing teams including designation of first authorship for these core articles and presentations.

- Reviewing and approving new proposals (which shall include motivation, research questions, variables to be used, members of the writing team, and first authorship) from interested members of the research team for "non-core" articles and presentations.

   Policy: The decision as to whether an abstract should be submitted, and under whose names, should come to the Steering Committee. Preferably, a presentation should be made first to them.

- Developing, in consultation with the MCECH Steering Committee, guidelines, and procedures to ensure that information about the project and its

NOTE: See Chapter Fourteen for an examination of the development and application of these dissemination guidelines.

findings are presented to the media and at public meetings in a consistent and accurate fashion.

Policy: When trying to decide about which representatives of the project should attend a conference, the criteria of quality and fairness will be used. To ensure a high-quality presentation, the following items regarding possible presenters will be considered by the Steering Committee:

- Involvement in project-related activities.

- Length of time of involvement with the project.

- Meeting attendance.

- Supervisor's evaluation (in the case of project staff).

- Attendance at mini-workshops/in-services about the project.

- To ensure fairness, we adopt the "Rose Bowl Principle," which states that if several people are able to make a high-quality presentation, someone who has not been before would be chosen.

Procedure: The Steering Committee or its designees will develop a list of the people who are eligible to attend a conference because of their participation, knowledge, and fairness issues.

Policy: Regarding Conference Attendance, the preference for the decision is to go to the Steering Committee for approval. If time does not permit, Steering Committee members will be either called or faxed and approval sought in this way. Once notified, it is the Steering Committee member's responsibility to reply within the time frame set by the person requesting the decision.

- Reviewing any and all requests for use of data and access to data by members of the research team and outside agencies or persons (for example, for dissertations, presentations, publications, FOIA, and so on).

- Determining and prioritizing methods of dissemination of findings to the CAAA steering committee and Detroit communities.

- Developing and implementing strategies to enhance the national and international visibility and prominence of CAAA by means such as generating lists of anticipated conferences and meetings, presentation topics, and speakers at which CAAA should present.

Authorship and presentation guidelines:

- Only those actively participating in the academic work of the project will be eligible for authorship. Active participation means substantial intellectual contribution to the publication in question, and may be measured directly by physical hours of input on acquisition, processing, and interpreting of data; or indirectly by time and energy spent supervising a junior researcher in the acquisition, processing, and interpretation of data; or a combination of both. Those making such contributions will be recognized in the authorship of manuscripts. Nonacademic assistance in the form of funding grants, administrative work, and secretarial work will not be the basis of authorship but will be expressly acknowledged in presentations and publications.

- Criteria for first authorship are expected to include responsibility for coordinating and facilitating the work of the writing team—for example, scheduling and facilitating meetings, overseeing data analysis, writing all or most of the first draft of a manuscript, handling communication with journals—together with significant other relevant activity on the CAAA project itself.

- Taking the lead on presentations will not necessarily result in lead authorship for resulting manuscripts; this will be decided by the Steering Committee in consultation with the writing/presentation team.

- Any person who gains permission to use any portion of the data set and conducts statistical analyses independent of the work of the data manager must provide written documentation (including statistical programs used, creation of new variables, data output, and so on) to the data manager within a few weeks of the activities conducted using the data.

- In its deliberations, the SC will especially strive for sensitivity to the needs of junior members of Research Team (for example, research scientists, doctoral students) with respect to areas such as authorship and meeting presentations.

- Opportunities will be organized for members of the research team to deliver practice presentations to other research team members before their scheduled conference presentations.

- A centralized, accessible, numbered filing system for every manuscript and abstract that is published or produced by CAAA will be established.

INSPIRATIONAL

IMAGES PROJECT

FACT SHEET AND INFORMED CONSENT FORM FOR STUDY PARTICIPANTS

ELLEN D. S. LÓPEZ

NAOMI ROBINSON

EUGENIA ENG

WOULD YOU LIKE TO PARTICIPATE IN THIS RESEARCH PROJECT EXPLORING BREAST CANCER SURVIVORSHIP?

Why am I being asked to participate in this project?

- This project is being done to learn about how African American women in your community who have experienced breast cancer feel about their lives as survivors. The project will give you the opportunity to discuss the challenges you have encountered, what you have done to make your life better, and what more can be done in the future to make sure that you and other women who experience breast cancer have an easier time.

- The purpose of this project is to provide the means for you and a small group of other survivors to voice your needs to influential people (local decision makers and product/service providers).

- The goal of the project is that by sharing your survivorship experiences and concerns with influential people, programs and support services will be developed to better meet your needs and improve the quality of life of African American breast cancer survivors in rural eastern North Carolina.

What will I be asked to do?

- If you choose to participate in the project, you and a group of at least 10 other survivors will be given disposable cameras so that you can take pictures that "trigger" discussions about your experiences and concerns as breast cancer survivors. At the completion of the project there will be a public forum where you and the other project participants will have the opportunity to present your photographs, the information learned from discussing your photographs, and your suggestions on how to address your survivorship needs and concerns to influential people in your community.

How long will this project take? How often will we meet for the project?

- This project should take about 10–14 months to complete and will involve you, the other project participants, and university researchers coming together

NOTE: See Chapter Seventeen for a discussion of how this form was used to recruit participants into a breast cancer survivorship CBPR project. We acknowledge Caroline Wang for her contributions to this appendix as it appeared in the first edition of the book.

about once per month. If you choose to participate you will be invited to attend the following sessions:

- *Project Training Session* (3 hours): During this session we will all come together to discuss details about the project and what participation involves. If you decide to participate you will be asked to sign the agreement statement on the last page of this form. This will show that you fully understand what being a part of this project entails. You will then receive a disposable camera and tips on how to use it. Then you will have the opportunity to practice using your camera. At the end of the training you and the other project participants will decide on the topic you would like to explore with your cameras. This is called a "photo assignment." You will also decide on a date and time when you will all come back together to discuss the photographs you have taken.

- *Photo-Discussion Sessions* (about 5–7 monthly sessions at 3 hours each): This is where the fun really begins! You, the other project participants, and the researcher will all come together to share and discuss your photos. After several of the photos have been discussed you and the other participants will decide what your next photo assignment will be.

- *Findings Session* (2 hours): After you and the other participants feel that you have learned enough about your survivorship experiences and concerns you will all come together to discuss the main themes and topics that came from your photos and discussions. As a group, you will then decide how well the themes relay what you want others to understand about your survivorship experiences.

- *Forum* (4 hours): The forum is the chance for everyone in the project to *celebrate* all that has been accomplished! Most important, you will also have the option to present what has been learned during the project to influential people in your community and discuss with them how programs and services can be developed to improve the lives of breast cancer survivors. As a group, everyone who participates in the project will decide *how* to present what has been learned during this project to these influential people. *You do not have to be a part of this presentation if you do not want.*

- *Other public displays of your photos:* You will also have the opportunity to publicly display your photos and the words you used to describe them so that even more people in your community can learn about how women experience breast cancer. If you *do* choose to display your photographs and words, you will decide which photographs to display, how they should be displayed, and where they should be displayed (for example, public library, town hall). *You do not have to participate in any public displays to be a part of this project.*

Will you be taping our photo-discussion sessions?

- Yes. What you have to say during the photo discussions is important. Therefore the sessions will be audiotaped. If you ever want to have the tape recorder turned off for a while during the discussion sessions, say so, and it will be turned off immediately.

Are there any risks involved with taking part in the project? Will I feel uncomfortable?

- Taking part in the project *should not* put you at risk for physical harm. You *may* feel uncomfortable going out to take pictures, but any concerns you may have will be discussed during project meetings. Also, you may feel uncomfortable discussing your breast cancer. *You will never be required to discuss any issues that make you feel uncomfortable.*

What will I get out of taking part in the project? Will I get paid?

- You will *not* be paid to be in the project. You *will* be offered light refreshments at each discussion session. You will also receive copies of every photograph you take for the study. Further, any film left over in your camera can be used to take pictures of anything or anyone you would like for free.

Do I have to pay for anything to take part in the project?

- You will *not* have to pay for anything to take part in the project. You can use the cameras at no cost to you. You will also be reimbursed for any travel expenses involved with getting to and from the meetings. The only cost for being in the project is the time you allow for taking the photographs and coming to project-related meetings.

Will people know that I took part in the project?

- To ensure *confidentiality*, if you wish, you can pick a made-up name to use during the project so that nobody will see your real name associated with the project. Further, what people say during the discussions is confidential, so it will be required that you never tell any specific things that are said by other group members during these discussions.

Do I have to participate? Can I stop being in the project whenever I want?

- You *do not* have to participate in this study. Further, you are free to stop being in the project at any time, for any reason.

Has this study been approved by the University of North Carolina at Chapel Hill?

- Yes. This study has been approved by the University of North Carolina at Chapel Hill (UNC-CH) School of Public Health Institutional Review Board on Research Involving Human Subjects.

What if I have any questions about the project or my participation?

- If you ever have any questions about this study, please feel free to contact [contact person's name, phone number, e-mail address].

Do you have any questions about the project?	[ ] Yes (write questions below or ask contact person) [ ] No

If you are interested in participating in this project, *please read the following agreement statement very carefully*. Then, if you would still like to participate, please sign and date this form and return it to [contact person's name]. You will be given a copy of this form to keep in case you have any questions or concerns at a later date.

Agreement statement:

By signing this consent form, I agree to participate in the project. I also understand and agree that unless otherwise notified in writing, the University of North Carolina at Chapel Hill assumes that permission is granted to use my photograph(s) and text from project-related sessions for project-related presentations, publications, exhibits, or other educational purposes.

Participant Signature _____ Date _____
Staff Signature _____ Date _____

Appendix L

INSPIRATIONAL

IMAGES PROJECT

INFORMED CONSENT FORM FOR ADULTS WHO MAY APPEAR IN PHOTOGRAPHS

ELLEN D. S. LÓPEZ

NAOMI ROBINSON

MAY I TAKE YOUR PICTURE?

What am I being asked to do?

- You are being asked to give me your permission to take your picture.

- Why are you taking these pictures?

- I am part of a group of breast cancer survivors and university researchers that is exploring breast cancer survivorship. We are taking pictures that we can bring back and share with our group. We hope the pictures will help us to discuss topics about survivorship that might normally be difficult to bring up.

How will you use the pictures?

- After I have taken my pictures, I will share them with the group, and we will discuss why I took them, and how they relate to survivorship issues. There is also the possibility that some of the photographs I take will be included in public exhibits or presentations.

Will people know that I had my picture taken for your project?

- Your name will never be revealed during any of the discussions, presentations or exhibits. Still, there is the chance that somebody may recognize you.

What will I get out of having my picture taken for your project?

- All pictures will be kept in a secure place by one of the researchers and me. If you wish, I will send you a copy of the picture(s) I take. *If you would like a copy, please write your name and address at the end of this form.*

Do I have to allow you to take my picture?

- No. You do not have to allow me to take your picture.

NOTE: See Chapter Seventeen for discussion of how this form was used to obtain permission to take a photograph as part of a breast cancer survivorship CBPR project. We acknowledge Caroline Wang for her contributions to this appendix as it appeared in the first edition of the book.

Has this project been approved?

- Yes. This project has been approved by the University of North Carolina at Chapel Hill School of Public Health Institutional Review Board on Research Involving Human Subjects.

Who can I contact if I have any questions about the project?

- If you ever have any questions or concerns please call [contact person's name, number].

If you are willing to have your picture taken, please read the following agreement statement very carefully. Then, please sign and date this form and return it to me. I will give you a copy of the form for your records.

Agreement statement:

By signing this consent form, I agree to have my pictures taken. I also understand and agree that unless otherwise notified in writing, the University of North Carolina at Chapel Hill assumes that permission is granted to use my pictures(s) for *project-related* discussions, exhibits, and presentations.

Your Signature_____ Date:_____

Photographer's Signature_____ Date:_____

If you would like a copy of your picture(s) please print your name, street number, street name, city, and zip code.

_____

_____

_____

_____

Thank you!

Appendix M

SOUTHERN CALIFORNIA

ENVIRONMENTAL JUSTICE

COLLABORATIVE

PARTNERSHIP AGREED-UPON MECHANISM FOR DECIDING ON RESEARCH ACTIVITIES

COMMUNITIES FOR A BETTER ENVIRONMENT,

LIBERTY HILL FOUNDATION,

AND THE RESEARCH TEAM

While all the partners want to protect the time allocated for fundamental research, we have agreed that the contours or subjects of action research should be largely determined by Communities for a Better Environment (CBE). Although the research team could decline a particular task for various reasons, and should research load issues emerge, as noted below, from joint conversations, it is our collective sense that CBE has the best notion of the overall organizing agenda and therefore can indicate what action research would be most useful. Of course, trade-offs will need to be acknowledged: more work on a particular research project will lead to less on another. It is probably the responsibility of the research team to raise these trade-offs and it is our collective responsibility to take them seriously and make hard choices.

Criteria for deciding to take on research tasks:

Primary responsibility of the researchers would be to CBE.

1. Partners must bring action research ideas to the whole Collaborative.

2. Research must be affiliated with environmental justice (EJ) campaign work in Los Angeles.

3. Research must be relevant to the goals of the Collaborative.

4. Research should be influenced and prioritized by its relevance to projected EJ policy outcomes defined by the Collaborative.

5. At least one conference call and one face-to-face meeting by the whole Collaborative are needed to decide to take on an action research task.

6. CBE should lead in tying action research tasks to organizing agenda.

7. Trade-offs in the action research arena should be discussed and acknowledged.

8. The research team should continue making progress on the fundamental research front, sharing both results and research designs for discussion and agenda setting on this front as well.

NOTE: See Chapter Nineteen for a discussion of how this document was developed and used to guide the work of the Collaborative.

9. The Collaborative must build in a process to popularize and disseminate research results (multilingual fact sheets, posters, maps, newsletters).

10. Research should include an analysis of cumulative exposure.

In this process the Collaborative must:

Fully integrate, cross-train, and dialogue among partners to achieve the following:

1. Create a plan to share web and other technology with activists and community members to improve their ability to access needed information.

2. Coordinate the community-focused research projects and the state policy research and an action plan with CBE.

3. CBE should frequently engage in interval analysis (including Power analysis) to reflect on whether policy goals are being reached.

4. CBE should plan their participation as facilitators for the EJ Institute.

INDEX

A

Academic-community research partnerships, developing, 48–49

Accessibility, 109

Action-Oriented Community Diagnosis (AOCD), 136, *See also* United Voices of Efland-Cheeks, Inc.; benefits of, 154; case study research design, 141–142; and colearning, 152; community forum planning committee, 153; competencies necessary for conducting, 139–140; conducting, 141–142; constructivist research paradigm, 140–141; as critical first step in program planning/ evaluation, 138–139; data collection and analysis, 142–143, 153; data interpretation, sustaining movement from, 153; dissemination, 143; duration/time required to complete, 143; forum planning committee, 143; gaining entry, 146, 151, 153–154; key to, 154–155; origins of, 137–140; participant observation, 146; partnership approach, 154; positivist research paradigm, 141; postpositivist research paradigm, 141; purpose of, 154; range of concepts/skills required by, 152–153; research design and methods, 140–143

Advocacy: goals, setting, 82; housing advocacy coalitions, 471; organized efforts, 164; and photovoice, 491; policy, 280, 519–521; services, 253; skills, 180

African Americans, *See also* Rural African-American community: and Detroit community, 253, 255; diabetes in, 521; economic/political marginalization, 14; rate of heart disease among, 521; and research, 14; and United Voices of Efland-Cheeks, Inc., 144–145

Agency for Healthcare Research and Quality, 7

Agreeing to disagree, and conflict, 86

Air Filter Intervention Study, 408, 409

Air pollution, 14; and containerized goods, 470; effects of, 551; fugitive emissions from nearby industries and transportation corridors, 560; National Air Toxics Assessment, 556;

Citizen power, gradation of, 98

Closed-ended survey questionnaires, 371, 375, 382–386; challenges, 386–389; data analysis, 384; data collection, 384; data feedback/interpretation/discussion, 384–385; lessons learned, 389–393; limitations, 386–389; practice implications, 389–393; program changes based on results, 385–386; survey questionnaire, development of, 383–384

Coad, N., 97

Coauthorship: defined, 414; rules, establishing, 413–414

Colearning: and Action-Oriented Community Diagnosis (AOCD), 152; and CBPR, 10; focus groups, 252, 297

Collaboration, community ethnographers, 312

Collaborative map making, 463–488

Collaborative model, ethnography, 308

Collaborative research, 5

Collaborative survey development, 198

Columbia University Children's Environmental Health Center, and West Harlem Environmental Action (WE ACT), 61–62

Communities for a Better Environment (CBE): mission of, 469–471; Toxic Tours/The Freedom to Breath initiative, 477

Community-academic partnerships, 269

Community Action Against Asthma (CAAA), *See also* Dissemination committee, CAAA: Air Filter Intervention Study, 408, 409; Asthma, Infections, Roadways and Youth Study (AIRWAYS), 408, 410; CBPR

principles, 408; challenges, 424; Community Organizing Network for Environmental Health (CONEH), 407, 409; culturally sensitive dissemination, ensuring, 426; data analysis process, 425; Diesel Exposure Study, 408, 409; dissemination activities, budgeting adequate resources for, 430; dissemination committee, 410–416; dissemination decisions/activities, examples of, 416–423; dissemination issues/guidelines, need to develop a mechanism for identifying and deciding on, 429; dissemination to community audiences/academic audiences, achieving a balance between, 425–426; EPA-funded grant, 408; experience/expertise, 427; geographical focus area for CAAA projects, 408; joint academic-community participation in dissemination activities, 427–428; lessons learned, 427–430; MCECH-affiliated Epidemiological Study, 409; MCECH-affiliated Household Intervention, 409; Near-Roadway Exposure to Urban Air Pollutants (NEXUS) Study, 408, 410; NIEHS-funded R01 projects, 408; partnership, 405–433; "Philosophy and Guiding Principles for Dissemination," 414, 416; practice implications, 427–430; projects/dissemination activities, 409–410; steering committee, 407–408; time-consuming nature of dissemination, 428–429

Community Action Against Asthma (CAAA) partnership, 26–27, 200

Community Action Agencies, 98

Community Alliance for the Environment (CAFE), 478–479

Community assessment, 135, 162; and CBPR, 163–166

Community assets, 48

Community-based ethnographic participatory research (CBEPR), 307

Community-based organizations (CBOs), 47; activities, encouraging active participation in, 56; and food environments, 297; perspective, 54–55

Community-based participatory policy work (CBPPW), See also Food environments, in NYC: Brooklyn Food Coalition (BFC), 522–526; challenges, 536–537; compared to traditional efforts at policy analysis/advocacy, 520–521; data collection, 528–536; defined, 518; diverse skills, need for, 538–539; education and research processes, coupling, 540–541; evidence, how/where to use persuasively, 541; evidence researchers collect/analyze, 537; Faith Leaders for Environmental Justice (FLEJ), 526–527; food justice case studies, 522; grant funding/resources, 539; Health Equity Project (HEP), 527; to improve food environments in NYC, 517–545; lessons learned, 538–541; limitations, 536–537; participant experiences with current policies, eliciting data on, 530–532; participant tensions, 539–540; policy formulation phase, research methods for, 523–524; policy opportunities, eliciting views on, 535–536; policy questions, framing of, 520; policy scanning/analysis, 534–535; practice implications, 538–541; primary data on food environments, collecting/analyzing, 533–534; priority problems, eliciting constituencies' definitions of, 529; synthesis/interpretation of existing data on food/food environment problems, 532–533

Community-based participatory research (CBPR), 4, 5, 198, 226, 306–307; achieving an effective collaborative process, evaluating progress toward, 25; acknowledgment of community as unit of identity, 8–9; Action-Oriented Community Diagnosis (AOCD), 21; balance between knowledge generation and intervention for mutual benefit of all partners, 10; CBPR process used to modify interviewer training protocols, 23; colearning/capacity building among partners, 10; as collaborative approach to research, 16; collaborative map making, 463–488; and community assessment, 163–166; community assessment and diagnosis, 20–21; community-based ethnographic participatory research (CBEPR), 24; conceptual model, 63; core components, 11–13; cultural competence, 15–16; cultural humility, 15–16; cultural safety, 14–15; defining the issue or health problem, 22; dissemination of results to partners, 11; effective group process in, 69–96; ethnographic methods, 21–22; exposure assessments, 24–25; facilitation of collaborative, equitable partnership in all phases of research, 9;

feedback and interpretation of findings, 26; Food Environment Audit for Diverse Neighborhoods, 24; funding opportunities supporting partnership approaches to research, 5; group process methods and facilitation strategies, 20; and health inequities, 13–18; Healthy Environments Partnership, 22–23; infrastructure for equitable participation in decision making, 20; Inspirational Images Project, 28; interviewer training manual, development with members of Apsáalooke Nation, 225–248; knowledge/skills, demand for, 7–8; Los Angeles Collaborative for Environmental Health and Justice, 28–29; map making, 27; NYC food environments, policy work to improve, 517–545; partnership formation and maintenance, 19; partnership success, 60; permutations/reformulations of processes, 46; phases in conducting, 11–13; photovoice, 27–28; pregnancy, strategies to maintain healthy diets and physical activity levels in, 23; principles of, 8–13; process methods tools/procedural documents/data collection instruments, 29; in public health, 6; relevance of, for professionals, 6–7; and strengths/ resources within community, 9; sustainability, long-term process and commitment to, 11; systems development using a cyclical and iterative process, 10–11; university-community research partnerships, 19–20; utilizing principles of, 60; workshops, 6–7

Community-Based Participatory Research for Health (Minkler/Wallersein), 17

Community-Campus Partnerships for Health, 121

Community-centered research, 5

Community coauthorship, 414

Community ethnographers, 310–312; administration of the survey, 316; CBEPR partnership, 311–312; CBEPR process, stages of, 312–313; collaboration, 312; developing the grant proposal (stage 1), 313; ethnographers, checking in with, 316–317; ethnographic training, 315–316; ethnosexual survey, 314–315; findings, analyzing, 317–321; major causes of HIV, identification of, 313–314; moving from concept to process (stage 2), 314–317; study background, 310; study setting, 310–311; team members, 312; team size, 312

Community forum planning committee, AOCD, 153

Community, getting to know, 48

Community Health and Social Services Center, Inc. (CHASS), 254

Community Health Centers, 98

Community involved research, 5

Community maps, *See also* Community mapping; Map making: ArcPad GiS software, 472; bonding/bridging, focusing on, 483; building a power/ organizing base in communities of color, 484; building knowledge incrementally, 483; building leadership through, 471–478; and CBPR, 483–485; challenges, 482–483; characterizing one's community by selecting features to map, 483; as common language, 484; community cumulative impacts on, 476–477; community-gathered data, sharing of, 473; community organizing priorities, reframing, 484; concrete community health with broader policy frames, 483; contested images, 478–482; exercise, 472; gaps in the CARB inventory of polluters, 473–476; global positioning system (GPS), 472; hazards/sensitive receptors, 473–474; for health equity in Brooklyn, New York, 477–478; health equity, linking work to, 484; improving lives using, 484–485; local knowledge, highlighting, 484; mapping follow-up, 477; paper worksheets to record observations, 472–473; policies, changing, 484–485; recommendations, 482–483; young people, engaging, 482

Community Organizing Network for Environmental Health (CONEH), 407–408, 409

Community participation, 98

Community partnerships: CBPR processes, permutations and reformulations of, 46; common identities, 45; community-based organizations (CBOs), 47; criteria for academic partners, 56; developing and maintaining, 43–68; guidelines for clarifying involvement with, 62–63;

insider-outsiders, 45; partnership development and maintenance, 47; working to deepen participation of, 57

Community-wide assessment, Men on the Move CBPR project, 443; findings/action steps taken based on, 446–447; partner engagement in, 446

Conceptual framework for assessing, partnerships, 372–374

Confidentiality, respecting, 79

Conflict, 11, 15, 19–20; addressing, 71, 77, 86–87; agreeing to disagree, 86; building in structures to deal with, 62; conflict management procedures (CMPs), 114–116; within ethnography, 180; interpersonal, 86; management, 86–87, 101, 111, 114, 139, 443, 448; negotiation, 114; resolution, 372, 373, 377; resolution committee, 115–116

Consensus decision making, 89

Continuum of Community Involvement, Impact, Trust, and Communication Flow, 98–101, 121

Corburn, J., 463

Crisis mapping software, 467

Critical consciousness, 492

Cross-sectional food audits, 293

Cultural competence, 15–16, 57

Cultural humility, 15–16, 57; areas of focus, 16

Cultural interpretation, 307

Cultural safety, 14–15; achieving within a CBPR partnership, 15; influence of cultural factors on relationships between professionals and communities, 15

Culturally supported interventions (CSIs), 58

Culture Box, 89

Culture-centered interventions, 51–52

Cumulative Exposure Project (CEP), and EPA, 479

Cumulative impacts, 476

D

Data analysis: closed-ended survey questionnaires, 384; Community Action Against Asthma (CAAA), 425; focus groups, 262–264; Healthy Environments Partnership (HEP), 283–284; in-depth, semistructured interviews, 381

Data collection: Action-Oriented Community Diagnosis (AOCD), 142–143, 153; closed-ended survey questionnaires, 384; community-based participatory policy work (CBPPW), 528–536; ethnography, 175–178; focus groups, 258–259; Food Environment Audit for Diverse Neighborhoods (FEAD-N), 291–292; Healthy Environments Partnership (HEP), 200; Healthy Homes, 346–348; Inspirational Images project, 496, 500–501; Men on the Move CBPR project, 455–456; methods, 374–375; partnerships, 374–375; photovoice, 499–500; Seattle-King County Asthma Program (SKC-AP), 350

Data feedback: closed-ended survey questionnaires, 384–385; focus groups, 264–266

Decision making, 87–89; consensus, 89; decentralized, 85–86; equitable, 101–102, 109, 110, 120; influence, 199

Deep Water Horizon Oil Spill (Gulf of Mexico), 467

Detroit Community-Academic Urban Research Center (URC), 26, 200, 253, 371; board, 376–377; evaluation subcommittee, role of, 377–379; formative evaluation, 377; funding, 376; and Michigan Center for the Environment and Children's Health (MCECH), 407–409; overall goal of, 376; participatory evaluation, 377; partnership background, 376–377

Detroit URC Board, 84

Diabetes: in African Americans, 521; and East Side Village Health Worker Partnership (ESVHWP), 281

Diesel Exposure Study, 408, 409

Direct observation, food audits, 279

Disaster Resilience Academy (Tulane University), 467

Disrespect, and ethnography, 180

Dissemination: AOCD, 143; Community Action Against Asthma (CAAA), 416–423, 429

Dissemination committee, CAAA, 410–416; coauthorship, defined, 414; coauthorship rules, establishing, 413–414; community coauthorship, 414; community forums, 416; core articles for publications and presentations, proposal list of, 414–415; developing, 412–415; dissemination guidelines, developing, 412–415; feedback procedures, 415–416; formation of, 411; International Committee of Medical

Journal Editors, 413–414; partner selection to copresent at conferences, 412–413; recruiting/selecting members, 411–412; representation on, 411; revising/finalizing, 414; transition of responsibilities to the steering committee, 416

Dissemination guidelines, 26–27, 102, 116–119, 405–433; abstracts/abstract authorship, approving for conference presentations, 418; adhering to, 424; balancing dissemination and chickadees with other project demands, 424–425; community forums, 422–423; deadlines, meeting, 424; dissemination decisions/activities, examples of, 416–423; dissemination requirements for affiliated projects, discussing how to handle, 420; fact sheet development/distribution, 421; feedback to study participants and the larger community, 421; implementation of, 416–423; individualized feedback to project participants, 421–422; lead author, identification of, 118–119; lead authors/co-authors for manuscripts, selecting, 418–419; Publications and Dissemination Committee, 118; representatives for conferences/ meetings, selecting, 417; Request for Use of Community Action Against Asthma Data form, 419–420; use of data, handling requests for, 419–420

Diverse partnerships, strategies for working, 89–90

Duran, B., 43

Dust samples, 337

E

East Oakland, Alameda County, California, Hegenberger Corridor, 469–471, 476

East Side Village Health Worker Partnership (ESVHWP), 281–282, 297–298; Detroit food stores, early observations of, 282–283; and diabetes, 281; Healthy Eating and Exercising to reduce Diabetes (HEED) project, 282; informal food store observations, 283

Ecological modeling, 169

Economic assessment, Men on the Move CBPR project, 447–448; findings/ action steps taken based on, 448; partner engagement in, 447–44

Economic Opportunity Act (1964), 98

Edgren, K. K., 405

El Centro Hispano (ECH), 310–312

.emic, 134

Eng, E., 3, 133, 489

Environmental exposure assessment methods, asthma, 337–340

Environmental Protection Agency (EPA), 336, 407, 477; and Cumulative Exposure Project (CEP), 479

Epidemiological and intervention studies, of children's lung function/ asthma-related health indicators, 407

Equitable decision making: accessibility, 109; achieving consensus on developing infrastructure for, 120–121; format, 109; literacy, 109; policies for, 120; with regard to investigators/ research process, 120; structures for,

Green Cart Initiative (NYC), 521

Greensboro Health Disparities Collaborative, 102; conflict management procedures (CMPs), 114–115; dissemination guidelines in, 118; establishment of, 103; Full Value Contract (FVC), 104–106; human subjects training, 107–108; membership in, 113–114; mission, 103; nontraditional investigators, 108; planning grant, 103; role of process in development of bylaws, 112–113; Undoing Racism™ training, 104–106; vision and leadership, 103

Griffith, D., 133

Grounded theory, 496

Group dynamics in CBPR research, 69–96; appropriate group size, establishing, 73–74; elements of, 71–72; equitable participation, 73–77; group membership, 72–73; open communication, 73

Group structure, ethnography, 322

Gustat, J., 69

Guzmán, J. R., 249, 369

H

Harmful environmental exposures, assessment of, 336–337

Head Start program, 98

Health disparities, 254

Health Education & Behavior, 7

Health Equity Project (HEP), 527–528; CBPPW efforts, 528; City University of New York (CUNY) School of Public Health, 527; food survey, 532; formation of, 528; New York City Department of Health and Mental Hygiene (DOHMH), 527; participant tensions, 539–540; workshop-based curriculum, 528; youth-led research project, 532; youth trained in research/action projects, 528

Health inequities, and community-based participatory research (CBPR), 13–18

Healthy Eating and Exercising to Reduce Diabetes (HEED) project, 282

Healthy Environments Partnership (HEP), 22–23, 80, 200, *See also* Food Environment Audit for Diverse neighborhoods (FEAD-N); Food environments, in NYC; HEP focus groups; administrative sources of data, 200; agendas, 214; air quality data collection, 200; application of survey results, 210–211; bidirectional communication across multiple dimensions, 218; biomarker data collection, 200; contributions, demonstrating value of, 216–217; contributions of CBPR work in Chicago, 284–285; data analysis, 283–284; data collection methods, 200; decision-making issues, 215; defined, 199; dissemination of survey results, 210–211; field period, oversight of, 205–208; focus groups, 200–203, 213, 219; food audit, 279, *See also* Food Environment Audit for Diverse Neighborhoods (FEAD-N); food environment audit, 287–288; food frequency questionnaire, 200; geographic distance and difference, addressing, 213; history, 199–201; implications for practice from, 211–218; initiation of, 199–200;

photo-elicitation group interviews, 451–452; readiness, importance in determining utility of various methods, 454–455; soft skills class evaluation, 443, 449–450; walking trails, 439

Mentorship, 266; inclusive models, 59; multidimensional and nonhierarchical process, 59; up, down, and peer mentoring, 50, 58–60

Messengers for Health on the Apsáalooke Reservation, 226–227, 229, 238

Michigan Center for the Environment and Children's Health (MCECH), 407–409

Michigan Department of Community Health, 264

Minkler, M., 43

Model Cities Program, 98

Moderators, focus groups, 268; background, 268; recruitment, 260; training, 256–257, 260; training workshops for, 257

Morello-Frosch, R., 547

Mothers Moving to a Healthy Future (*Madres/Moviendose a un Futuro Saludable*), 265

Motton, F., 435

N

Nair, S., 161

National Air Toxic Assessment (NATA), 479

National Cancer Institute's Center to Reduce Cancer Health Disparities Community Networks Program (NCI), 5

National Center on Minority Health and Health Disparities, 445

National Congress of American Indians Policy Research Center, 121

National Institute of Environmental Health Sciences (NIEHS), 407

National Institute of Nursing Research (NINR), 310

National Institute on Minority Health and Health Disparities' Community-Based Participatory Research Initiative (NIMHD), 5

National Institutes of Health (NIH), Clinical and Translational Science Awards Program, Community Engagement Core, 5

Native American Cancer Research Corporation (NACR), 230

Native Americans, and research, 14

Native Research Network (NRN), 51–52

Navajo Nation, Institutional Review Board, 60

Near-Roadway Exposure to Urban Air Pollutants (NEXUS) Study, 408, 410

New social movements, key innovation of, 51

NIEHS-funded R01 projects, Community Action Against Asthma (CAAA), 408

Nominal group technique (NGT), employing, 75

Nontraditional investigators, 108

Norms, establishing, 77–78

North Carolina Breast Cancer Screening Program (NC-BCSP), 494

North Carolina Community-Based Public Health Initiative Consortium, 102; conflict management procedures (CMPs), 114–116; dissemination guidelines in, 117; human subjects